AF352367

Ulcer Disease

CLINICAL PHARMACOLOGY

Series Editor

MURRAY WEINER

Division of Clinical Pharmacology and Toxicology
University of Cincinnati
College of Medicine
Cincinnati, Ohio

Additional Volumes in Preparation

Ulcer Disease

Investigation and Basis for Therapy

edited by

Edward A. Swabb

G.D. Searle & Co.
Skokie, Illinois

Sandor Szabo

Harvard Medical School
and
Brigham and Women's Hospital
Boston, Massachusetts

Marcel Dekker, Inc.   **New York • Basel • Hong Kong**

RC
821
.U44
1991

Library of Congress Cataloging-in-Publication Data

Ulcer disease : investigation and basis for therapy / edited by Edward
   A. Swabb, Sandor Szabo.
        p.   cm. -- (Clinical pharmacology; v. 17)
      Includes bibliographical references and index.
      ISBN 0-8247-8226-7
      1. Peptic ulcer--Treatment.   I. Swabb, Edward A.
   II. Szabo, Sandor. III. Series.
      [DNLM: 1. Anti-Ulcer Agents--therapeutic use. 2. Clinical Trials.
   3. Peptic Ulcer--physiopathology. 4. Peptic Ulcer--therapy. W1
   CL764H v. 17 / WI 350 U362]
   RC821.U44   1991
   616.3'43--dc20
   DNLM/DLC
   for Library of Congress   91-13085
                                                                  CIP

COPYRIGHT © 1991 MARCEL DEKKER, INC. ALL RIGHTS RESERVED

Neither this book nor any part may be reproduced or transmitted in any form or by
any means, electronic or mechanical, including photocopying, microfilming, and
recording, or by any information storage and retrieval system, without permission in
writing from the publisher.

MARCEL DEKKER, INC.
270 Madison Avenue, New York, New York 10016

Current printing (last digit):
10 9 8 7 6 5 4 3 2 1

PRINTED IN THE UNITED STATES OF AMERICA

Preface

This book gives medical researchers and practicing clinicians a review of the origins, presentations, therapies, and human investigation of ulcer disease.

Ulcer disease has a multifactorial etiology and ultimately results in an unfavorable imbalance between aggressive and defensive factors. Epidemiological invesigations have revealed significant morbidity and mortality associated with ulcer disease. This disorder can have various presentations, such as the nonspecific ulcer syndrome in general practice, gastropathy associated with nonsteroidal anti-inflammatory agents, and gastrointestinal bleeding.

Antacids, surgery, and histamine H_2-receptor antagonists continue to be established therapies of ulcer disease. However, interest is also focused on new pharmacological modalities, such as sucralfate, bismuth subcitrate, prostaglandin analogs, and sulfhydryl and nonsulfhydryl antioxidants. Endoscopic examination of ulcer disease has, with advances in medical instrumentation technology, led to endoscopic methods of treatment of ulcers, although controversy remains regarding optimal techniques.

Underlying the therapy of ulcer disease is the conduct of human investigation. Academic investigators, independent clinical research organizations, the pharmaceutical industry, and governmental regulatory agencies have all played major roles in developing methods for human investigation of anti-ulcer agents. Statistical considerations play a major role in the design of clinical trials of anti-ulcer agents. The proliferation of clinical trials has provided opportunities for meta-analysis of similar studies. The current practice of developing an anti-ulcer drug in countries such as the

United States and Japan is a focus of interest and is continuing to evolve. Cost-effectiveness of treatment of ulcer disease is being investigated more frequently, due to escalating overall costs of medical care in many countries.

We hope that the reader will find useful the diversity of topics included in this book, in view of the multidisciplinary nature of investigating and delivering to patients effective and safe therapies for ulcer disease.

Edward A. Swabb
Sandor Szabo

Contents

THERAPIES

HUMAN INVESTIGATION

Contents   **vii**

Contributors

Pietro Andreone, M.D.   Senior Research Fellow, University of Bologna, S. Orsola Hospital, Bologna, Italy

Mario Baraldini, M.D.   Senior Research Fellow, University of Bologna, S. Orsola Hospital, Bologna, Italy

Ralph E. Bennett, M.D.   Rheumatologist, Arthritis Center, Phoenix, Arizona

G. Bianchi Porro, M.D., Ph.D.   Chairman, Gastrointestinal Unit, L. Sacco Hospital, Milan, Italy

Joe A. Bollert, Ph.D.   Executive Vice-President, Institute for Biological Research and Development, Inc., Irvine, California

Fiorenza Bonvicini, M.D.   Senior Research Fellow, University of Bologna, S. Orsola Hospital, Bologna, Italy

Frank P. Brooks, M.D., Sc.D.   Emeritus Professor of Medicine and Physiology, School of Medicine, University of Pennsylvania, Philadelphia, Pennsylvania

T. Edward Bynum, M.D.   Associate Professor, Harvard Medical School, Boston, Massachusetts

Esam Z. Dajani, Ph.D., F.A.C.G.   Director of Clinical Research, G. D. Searle & Co., and Professor of Pharmacology, Chicago Medical School, Chicago, Illinois; and Professor of Medicine, University of California, Los Angeles, California

Janet D. Elashoff, Ph.D.   Department of Biomathematics, University of California, Los Angeles, and Director, Cedars-Sinai Medical Center, Los Angeles, California

Hugo E. Gallo-Torres, M.D., Ph.D., F.A.C.G.   Medical Officer, Division of Gastrointestinal/Coagulation Drug Products, Food and Drug Administration, Rockville, Maryland

Giovanni Gasbarrini, M.D.   Professor of Medicine, Department Head, University of Bologna, S. Orsola Hospital, Bologna, Italy

Fred Halter, M.D.   Professor of Medicine, Gastrointestinal Unit, University Hospital, Inselspital, Bern, Switzerland

Michael P. Hocking, M.D.   Associate Professor, Department of Surgery, University of Florida College of Medicine and the Gainesville Veterans Administration Medical Center, Gainesville, Florida

Colin W. Howden, M.D., M.R.C.P.   Senior Registrar, Department of Medicine and Therapeutics, University of Glasgow, Western Infirmary, Glasgow, Scotland

Richard Hunt, M.D., F.R.C.P. (Edinburgh), F.R.C.P.C., F.A.C.G.   Professor of Medicine, Head of the Division of Gastroenterology, McMaster University Medical Centre, Hamilton, Ontario, Canada

Tibor Jávor, M.D., Sc.D.   Professor of Medicine, Medical University of Pécs, Pécs, Hungary

Gary G. Koch, Ph.D.   Professor, Department of Biostatistics, School of Public Health, University of North Carolina, Chapel Hill, North Carolina

Guenter J. Krejs, M.D.   Professor and Chairman, Department of Internal Medicine, Karl Franzens University, Graz, Austria

John H. Kurata, Ph.D., M.P.H.   Director of Research, Department of Family Medicine, San Bernardino County Medical Center, San Bernardino, and Associate Adjunct Professor, Division of Family Medicine, University of California, Los Angeles, School of Medicine, Los Angeles, California

Shiu-Kum Lam, M.D., F.R.C.P. (Edinburgh), F.R.C.P. (London), F.R.C.P. (Glasgow), F.R.A.C.P.   Professor of Medicine and Chief of the Division of Gastroenterology and Hepatology, University of Hong Kong Queen Mary Hospital, Hong Kong

M. Lazzaroni, M.D.   Senior Assistant, Gastrointestinal Unit, L. Sacco Hospital, Milan, Italy

Richard B. Lynn, M.D.   Instructor of Medicine, Division of Gastroenterology, Jefferson Medical College, Thomas Jefferson University, Philadelphia, Pennsylvania

I. N. Marks, M.B.Ch.B., F.R.C.P., F.A.C.G.   Professor of Gastroenterology, Gastrointestinal Clinic, Groote Schuur Hospital, and Department of Medicine, University of Cape Town, Cape Town, South Africa

Takeshi Miwa, M.D.   Professor, Tokai University School of Medicine, Isehara, Japan

John G. Moore, M.D.   Chief, Gastroenterology Section, Department of Medicine, Salt Lake Veterans Affairs Medical Center, Salt Lake City, Utah

Gyula Mózsik, M.D., Ph.D., Sc.D.(Med.)   Professor of Medicine, Medical University of Pécs, Pécs, Hungary

Karl E. Peace, Ph.D., F.A.S.A.   President, Biopharmaceutical Research Consultants, Inc., Ann Arbor, Michigan

Stefano Pretolani, M.D.   Senior Research Fellow, University of Bologna, S. Orsola Hospital, Bologna, Italy

Jeffrey B. Raskin, M.D.   Professor of Medicine, Division of Gastroenterology, Department of Medicine, University of Miami School of Medicine, Miami, Florida

André Robert, M.D., Ph.D.   Senior Scientist, Safety Pharmacology, The Upjohn Company, Kalamazoo, Michigan

Sanford H. Roth, M.D.   Medical Director, Orthopaedic Center for Excellence, Humana Hospital and Arthritis Center, Phoenix, Arizona

Roland A. Sauer, M.S.*   Institute for Biological Research and Development, Inc., Irvine, California

Michael H. Smolensky, Ph.D.   Professor of Environmental Sciences and Pulmonary Medicine, University of Texas, School of Public Health and School of Medicine and Center for Medical and Public Health Chronobiology, Health Science Center—Houston, Houston, Texas

Anders Walan, S.E., M.D., Ph.D.   Associate Professor, Senior Director of Clinical Research, AB Hässle, Mölndal, Sweden

Donald E. Wilson, M.D.   Professor and Chairman, Department of Medicine, State University of New York Health Science Center, Brooklyn, New York

E. R. Woodward, M.D.   Professor of Surgery, University of Florida College of Medicine and the Gainesville Veterans Administration Medical Center, Gainesville, Florida

Harvey E. Zimmerman, M.A.   President, Spectrum Research Services, Inc., Warwick, Rhode Island

---

*Present affiliation: Pacific Research Network, San Diego, California

Ulcer Disease

ORIGINS

1

The Pathophysiology of Peptic Ulcer: An Overview

RICHARD B. LYNN

Jefferson Medical College, Thomas Jefferson University,
Philadelphia, Pennsylvania

FRANK P. BROOKS

School of Medicine, University of Pennsylvania,
Philadelphia, Pennsylvania

I. INTRODUCTION

Pathophysiology is the knowledge of how normal physiological processes are altered in disease. It is not a substitute for etiology [1]. However, in diseases where a cause has not been found, the features of the pathophysiology may provide clues leading to the identification of causes and may offer guidance in the development of new methods of treatment.

The gastric mucosa is normally exposed to powerful aggressive factors such as hydrochloric acid and pepsin and is protected by a variety of defensive factors such as mucus and bicarbonate secretion, mucosal blood flow, and cellular regeneration. Peptic ulcers are believed to develop when there is an imbalance of these opposing forces, either because of increased secretion of acid or pepsin or because of impairment of mucosal resistance, or a combination of these factors. In the first part of this review we will examine each of these factors separately.

One of the most important recent trends is the recognition that not all peptic ulcers share the same pathophysiology. Acute ulcers, for example, arise under different clinical circumstances, follow a different clinical course, and respond differently to treatment than chronic ulcers. There are conflicting opinions as to the significance of differences in the abnormalities between gastric and duodenal ulcers [2–4]. In this chapter we provide an overview of the pathophysiology of the three main categories of peptic ulcer: acute ulcers and erosions, chronic and recurrent gastric ulcer, and chronic and recurrent duodenal ulcer. Within these three main groups are important subcategories.

Peptic ulcers are classified in Table 1 [5]. The morphological distinctions between erosions, acute ulcers, and chronic ulcers are shown in Figure 1 [6]. It is clear that there are major differences in the pathophysiology within the three major categories of peptic ulcers. Among this heterogeneous group, we will try to identify subgroups of patients in whom an aggressive factor or impairment of a specific resistance factor might play a predominant role in ulcerogenesis.

Table 1 Peptic Ulcers

Acute ulcers[a]
    Acute ulcers in patients with extensive burns: Curling's ulcer
    Acute ulcers in patients with lesions in the central nervous system: Cushing's ulcer
    Acute ulcers in patients exposed to aspirin and other drugs, acute alcoholic binges, or bile
        reflux
    Acute ulcers in patients subjected to nonspecific stress
    Acute ulcers in patients at the extremes of age: neonates, children, and the elderly
    Acute ulcers in patients who eventually follow the clinical course of chronic or recurrent ulcer
Chronic and recurrent ulcers
    Gastric ulcers
        corpus or fundus ulcer
        antral or prepyloric ulcers
        pyloric channel ulcers
        combination of gastric and duodenal ulcers
        ulcers resistant to healing under treatment
    Duodenal ulcers
        uncomplicated duodenal ulcers
        bleeding duodenal ulcers
        perforated duodenal ulcers
        gastric outlet obstruction due to duodenal ulcer
        ulcers resistant to healing under treatment
    Recurrent ulcers after surgery
        anastomotic ulcers
        recurrent duodenal ulcer
    Hormonally induced ulcers
        Zollinger-Ellison syndrome—gastrinoma
        retained antrum
        G-cell hyperplasia
    Esophageal ulcers
        Ulcers adjacent to Meckel's diverticulum

---

[a]Often superficial and characterized clinically by bleeding; recurrence rate is low once the ulcer heals.

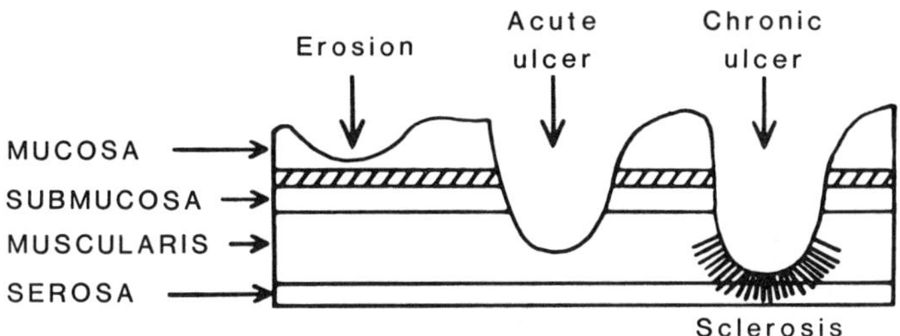

FIGURE 1 Diagrammatic illustrations of acute and chronic gastric mucosal lesions. (Modified from Sava G. Ulcerations et ulcere aigus de l'estomac. Fr Med 1967; 30:274.)

II. AGGRESSIVE FACTORS

A. Hydrochloric Acid

The role of acid secretion in the pathophysiology of acute peptic erosions and ulcers varies widely in the different categories of lesions and will be discussed with the other features of the subclassified groups. A unifying feature is that all peptic ulcers occur in mucosa exposed to acid or pepsin secretions. Ulcers in all three categories heal more rapidly when acid secretion is neutralized or inhibited. Healing rates in duodenal ulcer are significantly correlated with acid suppression, but in gastric ulcer there is no clear relationship between acid suppression and ulcer healing [7]. Only in patients with chronic duodenal ulcer has it been convincingly shown that basal and maximal acid output are higher than in normal subjects. However, there is considerable overlap, with many duodenal ulcer patients having acid secretory rates that are in the normal range. Chronic gastric ulcer, especially in the corpus, is associated with low acid secretion, but again there is a large overlap, with many patients falling within the normal range. In patients with acute peptic ulcers the role of acid secretion remains controversial. These findings suggest that whereas acid plays an essential role in ulcerogenesis and may be the predominant factor in chronic duodenal ulcers, in gastric ulcers and acute peptic ulcers other factors must also be involved.

The gastric mucosa is normally impermeable to hydrogen and sodium ions, despite the presence of major concentration gradients across the mucosa. If this mucosal barrier becomes leaky because of either overwhelming acid concentrations in the lumen or some impairment of resistant forces, then hydrogen ions can enter the mucosa and sodium ions can flow into the gastric contents. According to Davenport's concept illustrated in Figure 2 [8], hydrogen ions release histamine and stimulate cholinergic nerves, resulting in stimulation of acid and pepsinogen secretion, an increase in mucosal blood flow, and an increase in capillary permeability. The net effect is a loss of protein and blood into the contents of the stomach. Davenport [9] provided experimental evidence that aspirin, under conditions such that it could cross

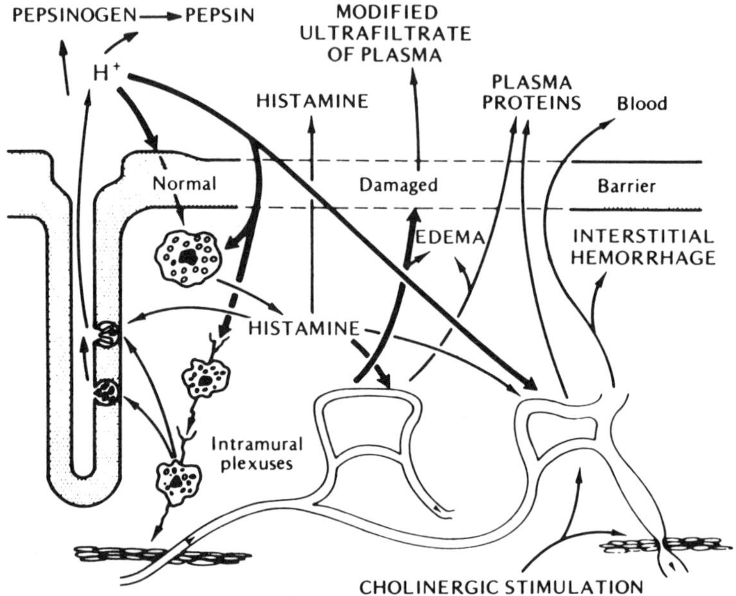

FIGURE 2 Pathophysiological consequences of the back-diffusion of acid through the broken gastric barrier. (From Davenport HW. Salicylate damage to the gastric mucosal barrier. N Engl J Med 1967; 276:1312, with permission.)

the lipid cell membrane, injures the mucosal barrier of vagally denervated fundic pouches in dogs, so that the events just listed can occur. He subsequently demonstrated that ethanol and bile salts have similar effects.

B. Pepsin

Pepsins are proteolytic enzymes that are secreted as inactive precursors, pepsinogens, which on exposure to the acidic environment of the stomach are converted to the active enzyme pepsin. Pepsins have maximal activity at pH 2–3.3, lose their activity above pH 5, and are irreversibly denatured at alkaline pH. Because gastric juice contains both pepsin and hydrochloric acid and their levels of secretion vary in parallel, it is difficult to determine the relative importance of each in ulcerogenesis. There is a considerable amount of evidence from experimental models of peptic ulcer disease that pepsin is a major contributor to the disease process [10]. Infusing acid into rat stomachs induces experimental ulcers. These ulcers can be prevented by adding a pepsin inhibitor [11] or by using an anticholinergic agent to inhibit both acid and pepsin secretion while continuing to infuse acid [12]. However, there are many important differences between rat and human gastric function. For example, pepsinogen can be classified into two immunochemically distinct types, pepsinogen I (PG I) and pepsinogen II (PG II). In humans, PG I and PG II are both present in the fundic gland mucosa of the stomach, but PG II alone is present in the antrum and proximal duodenum. In rats the gastric mucosa of the fundus and antrum contain proteases that share antigenic determinants with human PG II but not with PG I [13]. Thus, results using experimental models of ulcer formation must be interpreted with caution.

In patients with duodenal ulcer the duodenal pH is lower than in control subjects and clearly low enough to support peptic activity but not low enough for direct "caustic" damage to the duodenal mucosa [14–16]. Rather, the reported values are well within the range needed to support peptic activity. Thus, although both acid and pepsin are necessary for ulcer formation, it may be that pepsin is the agent that damages the mucosa. The role of hydrochloric acid may be mostly supportive of the pepsin activity.

C.   The *Helicobacter* (*Campylobacter*) *pylori* Story

Helicobacter pylori (formerly known as *Campylobacter pylori*) is a bacterium found only in association with gastric mucosa, and *H. pylori* infection is frequently associated with antral gastritis. *Helicobacter pylori* infections have been found in the antrum of approximately two-thirds of patients with gastric or duodenal ulcers [17]. In one endoscopist's experience, 95.5% of patients with active duodenal ulcer had *H. pylori* gastritis in foci of gastric metaplasia within the duodenal bulb [18]. *Helicobacter pylori* is an acid-sensitive organism that inhabits the surface of the gastric epithelium and the overlying mucus in the neutral pH environment. The bacterium secretes urease, which splits urea into alkaline ammonia, thus further buffering its environment. It has been suggested that *H. pylori* causes mucus depletion and thus renders the mucosa more vulnerable to injury. Obviously the *H. pylori* story is very incomplete, and much needs to be learned about the relationship between *H. pylori* and ulcers of the stomach and duodenum and about the mechanisms that might mediate the injury.

Persistent infection with *H. pylori* might explain the high recurrence rate in peptic ulcer disease. In a recent prospective study of 63 patients with either duodenal or gastric ulcers, all but one were found to have gastritis and *H. pylori* infection. After 4 weeks of therapy with either cimetidine or colloidal bismuth subcitrate, all but two patients had healing of their ulcers. In all patients treated with cimetidine there was persistence of *H. pylori* infection. In contrast, 45% of patients treated with colloidal bismuth subcitrate cleared their *H. pylori* infection at 1 month, and many of these remained uninfected at 12 months after treatment [19]. It remains to be shown whether clearing the *H. pylori* infection will reduce the incidence of recurrent ulcers in these patients.

III.   RESISTANCE FACTORS

A.   The Mucus–Bicarbonate Barrier

Acid or peptic secretions found under physiological conditions are generally accepted to be noxious and potentially damaging to the gastric or duodenal mucosa. Usually under these conditions the gastric and duodenal mucosa are able to defend themselves. Recently, the mechanisms of this defense have received much attention and several important factors have been identified. Which factors play critical roles and which factors are defective in ulcer patients has not yet been worked out.

In the stomach, mucus and bicarbonate secretion work together to maintain a layer of near neutral pH on the surface of the epithelial mucosa as demonstrated in Figure 3 [20]. The barrier that protects this nonacidic layer and the underlying mucosa has the task of slowing the diffusion of hydrogen ions down the very steep gradient from the acidic lumen and of neutralizing the acid that does get through. We will consider the many components of this barrier individually.

Gastric mucus is secreted by epithelial cells and mucus cells in glands. It is 95% water and 5% glycoprotein. Mucus forms a viscous gel, one role of which is to keep the thin neutral layer "unstirred" and prevent it from immediately mixing with the acidic lumenal contents. Williams and Turnberg [21] used in vitro methods to demonstrate that although it is mostly water, acid diffuses three to four times more

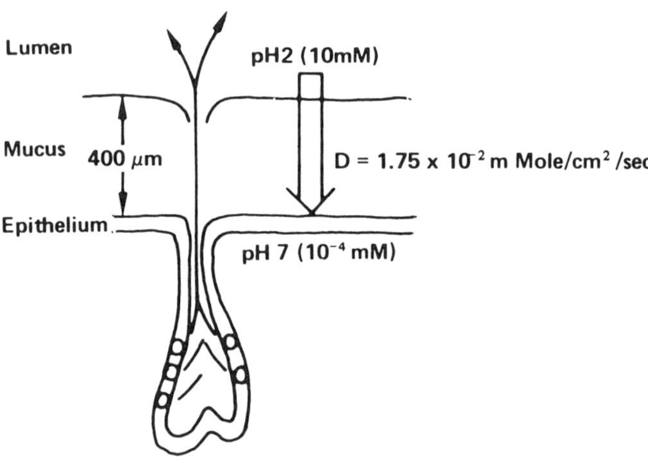

FIGURE 3   Calculated values for characteristics of the mucus layer. The low diffusion coefficient (D) would be insufficient alone to account for a neutral pH at the epithelium, when luminal pH = 2, unless mucus was being secreted at an unlikely high rate from the epithelium. (From Turnberg LA. Resistance factors I: "mucus-bicarbonate" barrier. In Brooks FB, Cohen S, Soloway RD, eds. Peptic ulcer disease. New York: Churchill Livingstone, 1985:218.)

slowly through a thin layer of mucus than through an equally thin layer of water. The mechanism of this effect is unclear, but its advantage is obvious. Additionally, the mucus is constantly turning over, with the mucus nearest the lumen sloughing off and new mucus being secreted on the epithelial side of the barrier. This "current" of mucus against the acid gradient might contribute a little to slowing the rate of acid diffusion. It has been observed that exposure of the gastric mucosa to an irritant such as 1 M NaCl increases the resistance to a subsequent exposure to a strong irritant. One of the responses of the gastric mucosa to the superficial damage of the mild irritant is rapid exfoliation of surface epithelial cells and the release of mucus and fibrin to form a "mucoid cap" over the damaged site [22]. In a recent experiment, Wallace found that this mucoid cap did not appear to be responsible for the increased resistance after mild irritation [23]. It is difficult to assess the role of mucus in the pathogenesis of peptic ulcers or to define abnormalities of mucus in ulcer patients, because there is no useful way to measure mucus or its function. Kurito et al. [24] developed a method of measuring the viscosity of gastric juice, which correlates with the macromolecular glycoprotein concentration. They found that the gastric juice viscosity in active and healing gastric ulcer patients was significantly lower than that in the scarring stage or in hospitalized control patients. Whether this correlation between gastric juice viscosity and the pathophysiologic state of gastric ulcers implies a role in pathogenesis is unclear.

Bicarbonate is secreted by the oxyntic, antral, and duodenal mucosa. Bicarbonate is actively transported across the luminal membrane of surface epithelial cells. In the antrum, bicarbonate is also passively secreted, accounting for about one-third of antral alkali secretion [25]. The total magnitude of this gastric alkalinization is only about 5–10% of maximal acid output. Thus this alkali secretion does not serve to neutralize the overwhelming acidity in the lumen, but it does manage to maintain a neutral environment over the mucosa. Using pH microelectrodes, Turnberg and his associates [26,27] have demonstrated that when the luminal bulk phase was pH 2, the epithelial surface within the mucus layer was maintained at pH $\sim$ 7.

In addition to mucosal bicarbonate secretion, other processes may play important roles in supplying bicarbonate to the gastric mucosal barrier or in helping to neutralize invading hydrogen ions when the barrier is impaired. "Alkaline tide" occurs when for each hydrogen ion secreted into the lumen of the stomach by a parietal cell, a bicarbonate ion is released into the bloodstream on the basal side of the epithelium. The vascular organization in the oxyntic mucosa as described by Gannon et al. [28] allows the bicarbonate released into the capillary effluent of the gastric pits to then continue on to flow in the capillaries of the bicarbonate–secreting mucosa. Thus at times of active acid secretion, the gastric mucosa most vulnerable to acid damage is bathed in an especially alkaline capillary blood flow. The supply of bicarbonate is aided by the increase in blood flow to the gastric mucosa that occurs with meals and in response to mucosal injury.

The ability of the above mechanisms to maintain the pH gradient across the mucus–bicarbonate barrier is limited. Increasing the acidity of the luminal fluid to pH 1.4 overwhelmed the barrier, resulting in a drop in pH adjacent to the epithelium within a few minutes [29]. Aspirin in combination with an acidic lumen will rapidly cause a decrease in the pH gradients across the barrier. Whether this effect of aspirin is mediated by prostaglandins or is a direct effect of the epithelial cell and diminishes its ability to secrete bicarbonate is not clear. Of course, whatever the cause of injury— whether peptic, toxic, or ischemic—the result is acidification of the gastric epithelium. The extent of mucosal injury, erosion, and ulceration will depend upon the severity of the acidification and the body's ability to clear this infiltration of hydrogen ions by increased blood flow, repair of the mucus–bicarbonate barrier, and repair of the epithelial cell layer.

Injury to the gastric mucosa due to thermal, mechanical, or hyperosmolar agents or after ingestion of various foods may result in superficial damage to the epithelium, with subsequent cell death and sloughing. The exfoliated epithelial cells can be rapidly replaced by epithelial cells that migrate from adjacent areas or from cells in the crypts beneath the injured area. This process, known as reconstitution or restitution, can cover the denuded area in minutes and does not require mitotic proliferation or inflammation. This method of reestablishing the epithelial cell layer and thus restoring the integrity of the mucus–bicarbonate barrier may be a major mechanism of defense of the gastric mucosa. If the injury is deep enough that it disturbs the basal lamina, healing will take substantially longer and require inflammation and mitotic proliferation [30].

The mucus–bicarbonate barrier in the duodenum is less well understood. The duodenum has the capacity to secrete bicarbonate independent of Brunner's glands and secretion from the pancreas or liver. Studies in rats have suggested that acid in the duodenal lumen stimulates alkalinization initially by an increase in mucosal permeability, allowing a passive influx of bicarbonate, followed by a cellular, prostaglandin-dependent active secretion of bicarbonate [31].

While duodenal ulcers are generally associated with acid hypersecretion, some of these patients do not hypersecrete, and in this population possible defects in defensive factors must be considered. There is some evidence that the proximal duodenum has impaired bicarbonate secretion in duodenal ulcer patients [32]. The best experimental model of duodenal ulcer is the cysteamine-induced duodenal ulcer in rats. Cysteamine-induced ulcers, like duodenal ulcers in humans, are associated with acid hypersecretion and hypergastrinemia. In this model, it has recently been reported that there is decreased bicarbonate secretion by the mucosal epithelium of the proximal duodenum [33]. Clearly, further study in humans will be needed to determine the significance of these findings.

B. Mucosal Blood Flow

The patterns of blood flow can be divided into mucosal, submucosal, and muscular and are illustrated in Figure 4. The mucosa is the metabolically most active tissue and

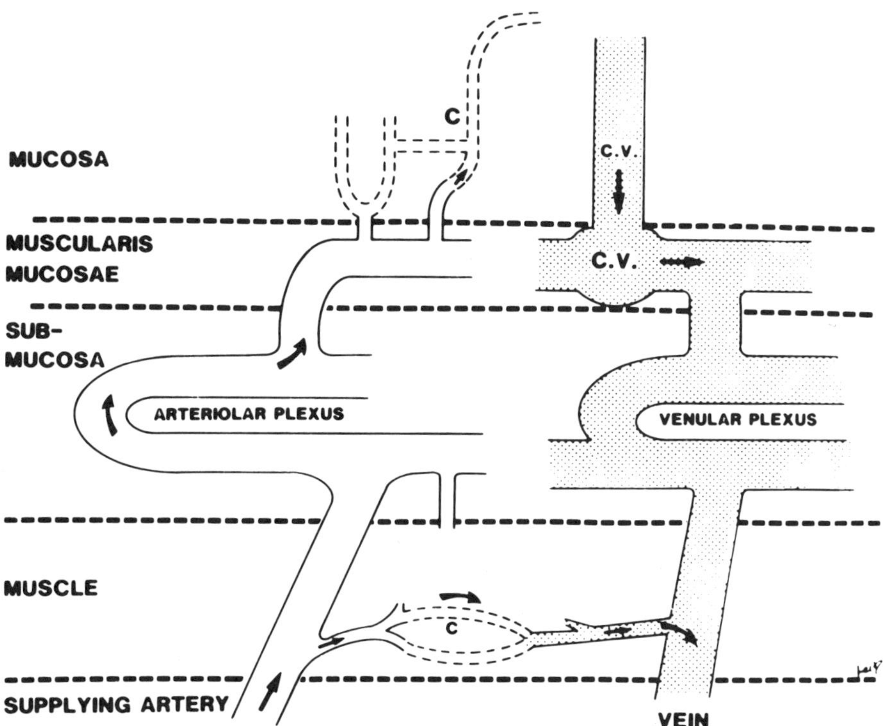

FIGURE 4 Diagram of the microcirculation of the stomach. Diversion of blood from muscle to mucosa or vice versa can occur by varying resistance in the arteries supplying muscle or mucosa, since the arteries are arranged in parallel, without the need for invoking mucosal shunts. (From Guth PH. Fed Proc 1984; 43:13.)

receives the largest share of blood. The submucosa has an extensive plexus of vessels containing arteriovenous shunts as well as branches to the mucosa. Blood can flow through the shunts, thus bypassing the mucosa, or the shunts can close, directing more blood to the mucosa. Beginning with the cephalic phase, a meal is a major stimulus, causing an increase in both the total and mucosal gastric blood flow [34].

The increase in mucosal blood flow is not necessary for acid secretion but probably plays a supportive role [35]. The increase in mucosal blood flow is controlled by the autonomic nervous system, hormones, and paracrine substances as summarized in Figure 5 [36]. Vagal cholinergic inputs are important for vasodilation. Sympathetic stimulation causes potent vasoconstriction. However, with continued sympathetic stimulation, there is an "autoregulatory escape," with blood flow recovering within minutes. In addition to these external controls, there is "autoregulation" that maintains a relatively constant mucosal blood flow in the face of fluctuating arterial blood

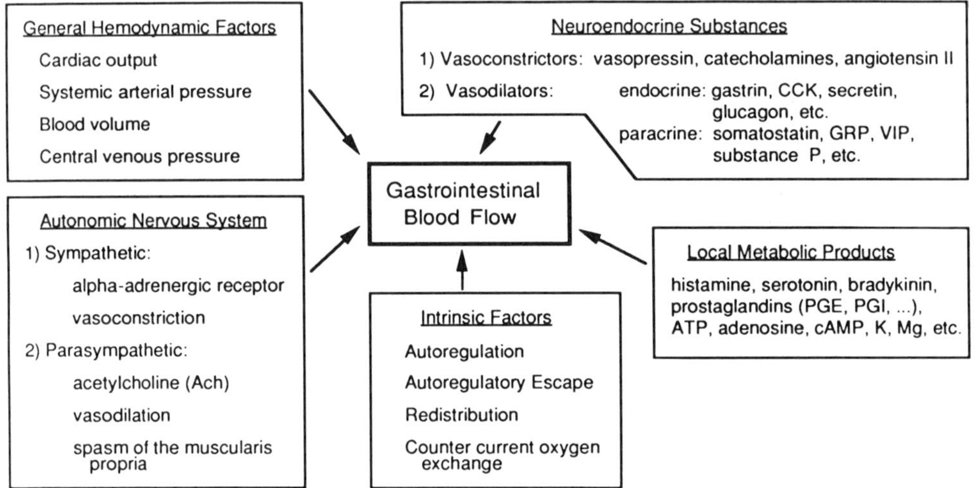

FIGURE 5 Factors regulating physiological microcirculation in the gastrointestinal tract. (From Yabana T. Stress induced vascular damage and ulcer. Dig Dis Sci 1988; 33:753.)

pressure. Finally, there are local metabolic mechanisms that maintain a stable uptake over a wide range of blood flows.

Gastric mucosal ischemia is frequently postulated as a cause of gastric ulcers. Many studies using experimental models of stress ulcers such as hemorrhagic shock in the rat have suggested that decreased mucosal blood flow is an important mechanism of stress ulceration. However, the overall evidence is not conclusive, and the role of ischemia is poorly defined. The important role of mucosal ischemia may not be due to direct injury but rather to decreased oxidative phosphorylation and cellular metabolism of epithelial cells, which result in decreased ability to secrete bicarbonate to buffer the influx of acid [29].

C.   The Role of Prostaglandins

Prostaglandins are a central component in our understanding of the pathophysiology of peptic ulcer disease. Exogenous prostaglandins can protect the gastric mucosa from an incredible variety of insults. They have effects on most of the other aggressive and defensive factors we have discussed so far. Parenteral prostaglandins potently inhibit basal acid secretion and acid secretion stimulated by histamine, pentagastrin, and cholinergic drugs. The mechanism of this antisecretory effect is unclear but seems to be a direct effect on the parietal cell at a site after the gastrin, histamine, and cholinergic receptors.

Importantly, prostaglandins exhibit strong protective effects at much lower doses than are needed for their antisecretory effects. This ability to confer mucosal protection without decreasing acid secretion is called *cytoprotection*. The mechanism of this cytoprotection is unclear, but there are many candidates. One observation is that prostaglandins given systematically stabilize the potential difference across the mucosa. Whether this is due to some specific effect on the epithelial cells of the mucosa or is rather the cumulative result of the other effects of prostaglandins is not known.

Exogenous prostaglandins stimulate bicarbonate secretion by the gastric mucosa. Prostaglandins stimulate the secretion of mucus in experimental animals, in humans, and in preparations of isolated mucosal cells [37]. Both of these effects enhance the mucus–bicarbonate barrier, but how essential they are for maintaining this barrier is not certain. Prostaglandins exert a vasodilator effect to maintain gastric mucosal blood flow. This may be important in supporting normal function and in response to injury, enhancing the ability to remove acid that has penetrated into the mucosa. The ability of prostaglandins to ameliorate those ulcers where ischemia is thought to play an important role, such as stress ulcers, and in animal models of stress ulcers, may be due to this property of increasing mucosal blood flow. Interestingly, prostaglandin E_2 (PGE_2) blocked ethanol-induced vascular injury [38], and this may be the mechanism of preventing mucosal injury. As discussed later, this may be due to decreased responsiveness to vasoactive mediators of injury.

Another approach to the issue of cytoprotection is to study the effects of prostaglandins on repair. Lacy and Ito [39] use the experimental model of ethanol-induced hemorrhagic lesions in the stomach in rats. Review of rat stomachs microscopically revealed two grades of injury, the grossly visible hemorrhage lesions and superficial mucosal injury that was not grossly apparent. Pretreatment of the rats protected against the hemorrhagic lesions but did not prevent the superficial type of injury. Because reconstitution of the epithelial layer by migrating cells rapidly replaces the sloughed cells, this brief superficial injury is easily missed. Robert [40] concludes that cytoprotection does not apply to the surface epithelium but rather to the gastric mucosal tissue underneath the epithelium, protecting it from becoming necrotic and hemorrhagic. Although prostaglandins may not accelerate migration of epithelial cells, by protecting the underlying tissue including the basal lamina they can facilitate reconstitution of the epithelium if blood flow is maintained for the energy-dependent epithelial restitution.

Prostaglandins are a complex group of chemicals with a multiplicity of derivatives, precursors, and metabolites. Malagelada [41] reviews the many problems with prostaglandin research and makes the point that "investigations employing exogenous prostaglandins may be somewhat misleading in that they do not reflect the physiological endogenous prostaglandin mix." To address the question of the effect of endogenous prostaglandins, Schepp et al. [42] studied the effects in rats of varying the dietary content of linoleic acid, a precursor in the synthesis of many prostaglandins. Diets supplemented with excess linoleic acid (10%) resulted in increased gastric lumen release of PGE_2, decreased basal and pentagastrin-stimulated acid output, and decreased the area of cold-restraint gastric mucosal lesions. Pretreatment with indomethacin abolished the effects of the supplemental diet. These results suggest that increased chronic dietary intake of linoleic acid caused the above-described events because of augmented synthesis of endogenous prostaglandins in the gastric mucosa.

Where prostaglandins fit into the pathophysiology of peptic ulcer disease is unclear. Furthermore, in no subgroup of patients has a defect in prostaglandins been found. The only subgroup of patients in which prostaglandins can be convincingly implicated are the erosions and ulcers secondary to nonsteroidal anti-inflammatory drugs.

Although the mechanism of prostaglandin activity is still controversial, there is little doubt that prostaglandins accelerate the healing of acute and chronic ulcers of the stomach and duodenum at rates comparable to those of other standard therapies. However, successful healing with prostaglandins does not protect against recurrence [43].

IV. ACUTE PEPTIC ULCERS

The diagnosis of acute gastric ulcers or erosions can be made with considerable accuracy now by early fiberoptic upper gastrointestinal endoscopy. A common clinical feature is bleeding, which presents as hematemesis or melena. Perforation is a particularly serious but infrequent (15%) presenting finding. Pain is a very uncommon symptom. Acute lesions in some cases appear to have specific etiologies, for example, aspirin and nonsteroidal anti-inflammatory agents. Other acute lesions are associated with certain clinical situations such as burns, brain injury, or the so-called stress ulcers occurring after major surgery, trauma, or life-threatening medical illness. Although the hallmark of acute lesions in the stomach and duodenum is that they heal and do not recur, there remain a few patients who present initially with clinical, endoscopic, and radiological evidence of acute ulcers and subsequently follow a course typical of chronic recurrent gastric or duodenal ulcer. We will consider each subgroup of acute ulcers and erosions separately and emphasize findings of pathophysiology that are unique to each.

A. Acute Erosions and Ulcers in Patients with Severe Burns (Curling's Ulcer)

Burns involving more than a third of the body surface area are associated with an increased risk of acute erosions or ulcerations of the upper gastrointestinal tract. Often, there is a single ulcer (the classical Curling's ulcer) located in the duodenum. The most striking observation is the relationship between the percentage of the body surface area burned and the incidence of ulcers. Figure 6 shows the correlation based upon patients seen at the Army Burn Center during the period 1967–1969 [44]. Note that about 40% of the patients with burns covering more than 70% of the body surface developed ulcers. Another interesting correlation, based on 20 patients, was

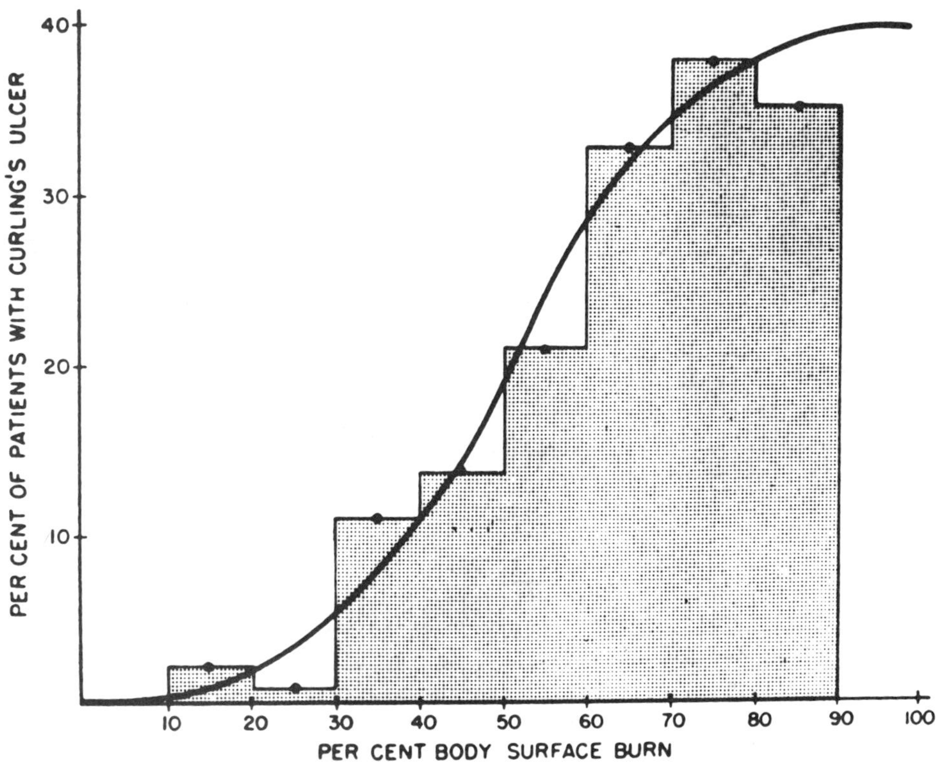

FIGURE 6 Incidence of Curling's ulcer as related to burn size in patients at the Army Burn Center 1967–1969. (From Pruitt BA, Foley FD, Moncrief JA. Curling's ulcer: a clinical pathology study of 323 cases. Ann Surg 1970; 172:529.)

the inverse relationship between 12-hr acid output and the extent of the burn [45] (Fig. 7). In the Army Burn Center study there was no evidence of hypergastrinemia [46].

Since the early 1970s a remarkable change has occurred. At the Army Burn Center during 1968–1969, gastrointestinal bleeding was present in 69% of patients examined. This incidence fell to 1% in 1978 and 1979 [47]. Improved control of dehydration and sepsis as well as prophylactic use of antacids and H_2 blockers might explain this improvement. To further study the role of acid, a small group of patients received antacids to maintain a gastric pH of 7.0. This group had a marked decrease in bleeding compared to a control group who did not receive antacids [48]. These results suggest that acid plays at least a permissive role in the development of erosions and ulcers in burned patients.

The only evidence for a decrease in local defense mechanisms comes from rather

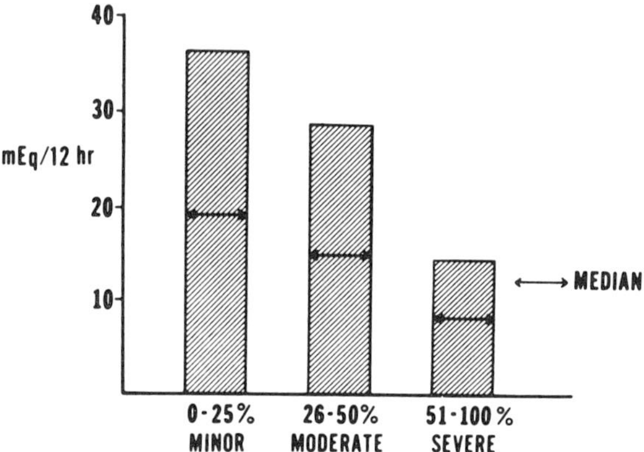

FIGURE 7 Relation of 12-hr acid output to extent of burn. (From Harrison AM, Gaisford JC, Wechsler RL. Gastric secretion in the burned patient. J Trauma 1972; 12:1042.)

imprecise measurements showing a decrease in the secretion of gastric mucus [49,50]. The endoscopic evidence of local ischemia as the first indication of the formation of an erosion points out the need for quantitative methods for measuring gastric mucosal blood flow in regional areas [5].

B. Acute Erosions and Ulcers in Patients with Injuries to the Central Nervous System (Cushing's Ulcer)

In a large series of patients with head injury, bleeding into the gastrointestinal tract was noted in 17% of patients [51]. In general, the incidence of bleeding correlated with the severity of the injury. These lesions may occur anywhere from the proximal esophagus to the distal duodenum. In Vietnam, Stremple et al. [52,53] compared acid outputs prospectively in soldiers with head, spinal cord, or abdominal injuries. Figure 8 illustrates that hypersecretion of patients with head injuries lasted only 4–5 days. Overall, some investigators have reported a high incidence of gastric acid hypersecretion and basal hypergastrinemia in patients with CNS injury, whereas others have not. This lesion too has become much less common, coincident with prophylactic treatment with antacids and H_2 antagonists. As in burn patients, localized ischemia has been demonstrated early in the evolution of ulcers.

C. Drug-Induced Erosions and Ulcers

Almost all healthy subjects develop stomach erosions or subepithelial hemorrhages after taking ordinary aspirin by mouth for a week. In 82 patients with rheumatoid arthritis receiving chronic treatment with aspirin, endoscopy revealed that 14 had gastric ulcers and 33 had erosions [54]. This suggests that there is mucosal adaptation

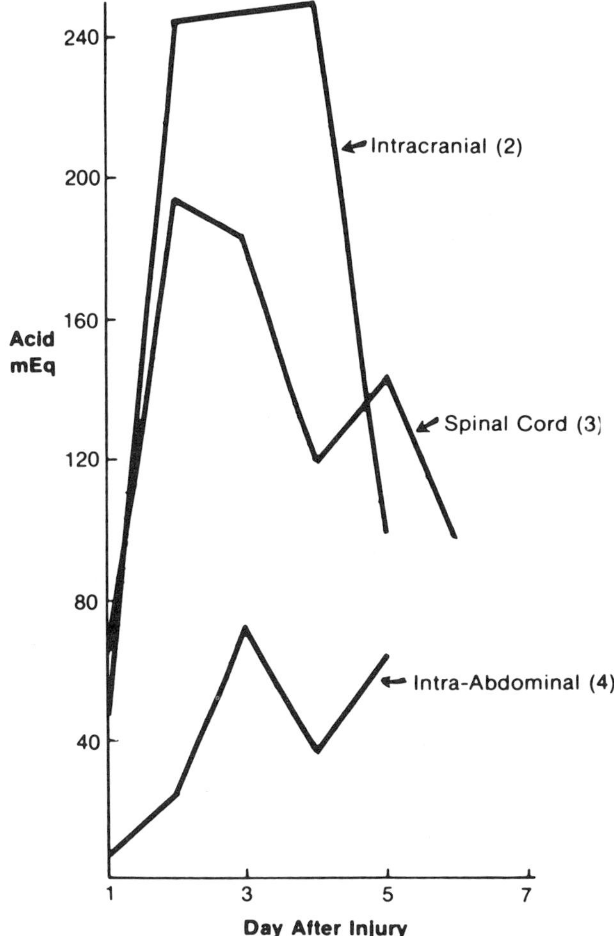

FIGURE 8 Daily changes in mean acid output of nine bleeding patients according to site of injury (normal is 84 ± 36 mEq/24 hr). (From Stremple JF, Malot MD, MacNamara J, et al. Posttraumatic gastric bleeding: prospective gastric secretion composition. Arch Surg 1972; 105:179.)

to continued administration of aspirin. In both cases enteric-coated aspirin produced fewer lesions. Salicylates given intravenously to healthy subjects did not affect the gastric mucosal barrier or produce morphological changes, despite salicylate blood levels comparable with those of oral administration associated with gastric lesions [55,56]. These results favor a local topical site of action of aspirin on the mucosa. Symptoms of abdominal distress were common, but lesions were seen frequently in asymptomatic patients and normal subjects. Other nonsteroidal anti-inflammatory agents also cause symptoms and erosions but usually less frequently than aspirin [57,58].

Absorption of salicylate depends upon the pH of the gastric contents. With no buffering, 12% of aspirin is absorbed in 10 min, whereas less than 1% is absorbed when gastric contents are buffered at pH 7 [59]. Hunt et al. [60] proposed that mucosal damage is related to the amount of aspirin absorbed and for this reason the mucosal damage correlates with the acidity of the gastric contents. Aspirin enters the cells of the gastric mucosa and inhibits mitochondrial oxidative phosphorylation with a resulting increase in cell permeability and a decrease in the secretion of mucus and bicarbonate. In spite of damage to cell organelles, the tight junctions remain relatively intact. The formation of prostaglandins is reduced, and the transmucosal potential difference falls. These events disrupt the defensive barrier of the gastric mucosa enough to allow back-diffusion of hydrogen ions and ensuing injury to the mucosa as Davenport described. The surface cells slough, exposing erosions that may enlarge and rupture superficial blood vessels. Deeper areas of hemorrhage occur in gastric glands. The rate of cell shedding is proportional to the dose of aspirin.

Alcohol ingested in large amounts over short periods of time readily causes gastric mucosal injury and is a common cause of upper gastrointestinal bleeding. The patterns of injury include hyperemia, edema, mucosal and submucosal hemorrhage, and mucosal necrosis. As for aspirin, investigations into the pathophysiology have reported a variety of disturbances that result in impairment of the mucosal defensive barrier. The effect of alcohol on the stomach of rats has been investigated extensively. A recent study combined gross morphological, videomicroscopic, histochemical, and pharmacological approaches [61]. Diffuse mucosal hyperemia was present within 1 min of ethanol contact. The onset of venoconstriction (9 sec post-ethanol) preceded arteriolar dilatation (16 sec). This study found that the ethanol-induced hyperemia was reduced by a lipoxygenase-selective inhibitor and H_1-antihistamine but not by indomethacin or cimetidine. The authors postulated that within seconds of topical contact, ethanol causes mast cells to release the vasoactive substances histamine and leukotriene C_4 (LTC_4), resulting in venoconstriction and subsequent hyperemia. Prostaglandin E_2 blocks ethanol-induced hyperemia [62], perhaps by decreasing responsiveness to these vasoactive mediators.

Bile salts are believed to cause "bile reflux gastritis," characterized by multiple erosions and diffuse bleeding. This problem typically occurs in patients who have undergone a partial gastrectomy and a gastrojejunostomy of the Billroth II type. Bile salts are further implicated by the observation that healing often occurs following a Roux-en-Y diversion of bile flow into the jejunum distal to the gastrojejunostomy. However, the association between bile salts and gastric mucosal injury is less convincing than for aspirin or alcohol. There is a lack of correlation between bile reflux and gastric injury, and it is uncertain whether bile salts or some other component of duodenal contents is the primary injuring agent [63]. Furthermore, Roux-en-Y diversion does not always heal the gastritis.

Bile acids, when applied above their critical micellar concentrations, can cause solubilization of membrane lipid [64]. However, Duane and associates [65] reported that the severity of the resultant injury is unrelated to the critical micellar concentration of taurine-conjugated bile acids but is directly proportional to their absorption by the mucosa.

D. Stress Ulcers

Stress ulcers include those acute erosions or ulcers associated with trauma, sepsis, or life-threatening disease, excluding burns, intracranial injuries, and mucosa-damaging drugs. Other risk factors for stress ulcers include major operative procedures, respiratory failure, peritonitis, jaundice, renal failure, and hypotension.

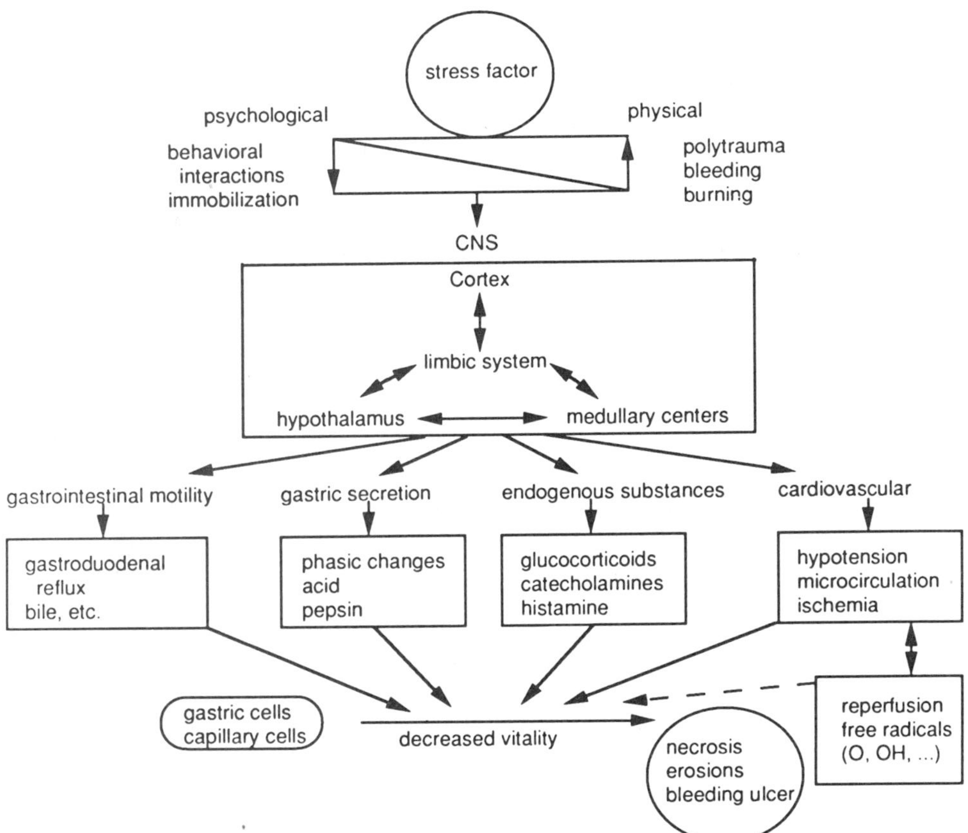

FIGURE 9 Various pathogenetic factors that may be associated with stress ulcer formation. (From Ref. 33 of paper by Yabana [34].)

These lesions are typically found in the proximal stomach within the boundaries of the acid-secreting mucosa. However, lesions can be found as distally as the second or third portion of the duodenum [66].

Studies of gastric acid secretion have produced conflicting results. Gastric intramural pH, calculated from the pH of gastric juice and the arterial P_{CO_2}, was decreased in patients at the greatest risk of major stress ulcer bleeding [67]. Stress ulcer formation probably involves multiple pathogenetic factors. One such model, shown in Figure 9, has been proposed by Jennewein and Hammer [68]. This model emphasizes the role of the central nervous system in mediating the effects of both physical and psychological stresses. These stresses affect the limbic system, most notably the hypothalamus, which is the regulatory center of both the autonomic nervous system and the neuroendocrine system. There is much experimental evidence for the role of various central nervous system centers. For example, electrical stimulation of the amygdala in cats induced ulcers within 4 hr. The effect is blocked by vagotomy [69]. Recent evidence suggests that thyrotropin-releasing hormone (TRH) might play an important role as the central mediator of stress resulting in ulceration. TRH injected intracisternally induced gastric ulcerations in rats [70].

Endoscopic studies report that lesions begin as focal areas of ischemia [71]. There are a variety of experimental models of physical and psychological stress ulceration in the rat. Although many findings have been reported, they are generally inconclusive. Ischemia of the gastric mucosa as the primary pathophysiological event has received some support from experimental evidence, as reviewed earlier in Section III.B. The recent decrease in incidence is due in large part to the use of prophylactic alkalinization of gastric contents in intensive care unit patients but also to improve care in general, avoidance of hypotension, better diagnosis and treatment of sepsis, and so on.

V.   CHRONIC PEPTIC ULCERS

Without a better understanding of their etiology, the classification of chronic peptic ulcers remains arbitrary. Features that are associated with gastric ulcer over duodenal ulcer are older age, increased frequency of other medical illnesses, reduced gastric acid secretion with ulcers in the corpus or fundus, and atrophic gastritis. Significant genetic influences seem to divide patients along these lines as well. Relatives of patients with gastric ulcers tend to have gastric ulcers but not duodenal ulcers. Duodenal ulcers occur three times as often in siblings of patients with duodenal ulcer as in the general population [72]. Crean and Spiegelhalter [73] compared symptoms and clinical aspects of gastric and duodenal ulcers. They found that pain on a daily basis, age greater than 56, and female gender were more likely to be associated with gastric ulcer than with duodenal ulcer. Although patients with both types of ulcers reported that their pain lessened with food, pain that worsened with food favored gastric ulcers.

Another, innovative classification of ulcer patients is according to their birth-cohort. The recent decline in the incidence of duodenal ulcer and the fluctuations of incidence and other variables over time have provoked this type of evaluation. The lives of patients born in certain years or generations are greatly influenced by the sociological trends such as smoking or urbanization, economic trends such as industrialization and automation, and other factors such as wars, migrations, or substantial changes in standard of living. Sonnenberg and Sonnenberg [74] report that changes of peptic ulcer mortality did correlate with changes in birth-cohort risks. Using birth-cohort analysis they report a number of findings and suggest the interesting hypothesis that increased physical work perhaps linked with increased food consumption makes one more susceptible to duodenal ulcer.

A. Chronic Gastric Ulcers

Within this group as well there probably exists considerable heterogeneity. Chronic gastric ulcers can be categorized by location into three groups: ulcers proximal to the incisura (corpus), those between the incisura and the pylorus (antral or prepyloric ulcers), and those occurring either concomitantly with duodenal ulcers or in patients who have had both gastric and duodenal ulcers at different times. Table 2 lists the functional abnormalities in patients with gastric ulcers of the corpus [5]. Obviously, reflecting the heterogeneity of gastric ulcer patients, not all patients will show a given abnormality.

Patients with gastric ulcers above the incisura exhibit hyposecretion of hydrochloric acid compared with normal subjects or patients with duodenal ulcer. Patients with antral or prepyloric ulcers or gastric ulcers in combination with duodenal ulcers

Table 2 Abnormalities in Patients with Gastric Ulcer in the Corpus

Hyposecretion of gastric HCl and pepsin
    Basal acid output
    12-hr night secretion
    Maximal or peak acid output (decreased parietal cell mass)
    Response to a meal
Fasting and postprandial hypergastrinemia (G-34)
Decreased gastric antral gastrin content
Decreased release of pancreatic polypeptide in response to a meal
Decreased mucosal prostaglandin content
Increased bile reflux
Incompetent pylorus
Reduced amplitude of gastric antral contractions
Delayed gastric emptying
Decreased gastric mucosal blood flow

have acid-secretory patterns similar to those of duodenal ulcer patients. In both situations, healing is improved with H_2 blockers, suggesting that acid plays an important, perhaps permissive, role in ulcerogenesis. In patients with corpus ulcers, serum gastrin levels are increased and antral gastrin content is decreased, which is believed to reflect increased release.

Abnormal gastric motor function results in delayed emptying and bile reflux. Decreased mucosal blood flow has been reported. The high incidence of ulcers at the junction of the corpus and antrum might be related to the presence of a large sling muscle at that location. Smoking and the ingestion of caffeinated beverages and salicylates are risk factors. An important feature of chronic gastric ulcers is their tendency to heal and recur. Recurrences, which reach 50% in one year, may be asymptomatic. A variety of available agents accelerate healing and decrease the recurrence rate. Perhaps a better understanding of the aggressive factors and the inadequacies of defensive barriers will allow for more effective prevention of recurrence.

B.   Chronic Duodenal Ulcers

Like acute ulcers and chronic gastric ulcers, chronic duodenal ulcers are probably a heterogeneous group of disorders [75]. The lesion is usually in the duodenal bulb, and the natural course is one of healing and recurrence. The clinical impression is that after a period of 10–15 years of recurrent ulcers the disorder becomes less severe [5]. Genetic findings of an increased prevalence of HLA-B12 and blood group O might identify subgroups of patients at increased risk [76].

Table 3 lists the functional abnormalities found in patients with duodenal ulcer [5]. Duodenal ulcer patients as a group have hypersecretion of gastric acid, but a considerable number of individuals overlap with matched controls [77]. There is increased basal acid output, 12-hr night secretion, and maximal acid output. The latter correlates with an increased parietal cell mass in hypersecretors. The response to a variety of stimuli is increased, including sham feeding and insulin hypoglycemia, which are the most purely vagally mediated responses and are abolished by vagotomy. Whether vagal tone or responsiveness is abnormal in duodenal ulcer patients has not been proved. The ratio of basal acid output to peak acid output reflects resting vagal tone. In duodenal ulcer patients with elevated ratios, sham feeding failed to increase acid output. These results identify a subgroup of duodenal ulcer patients with high resting vagal tone, which is not further increased by sham feeding [78]. Duodenal ulcer patients have an increased response to balloon distention of the antrum that is thought to be mediated by a pyloro-oxyntic reflex independent of gastrin [79]. Perfusion of the duodenum with a 10% peptone solution produced an acid output twice as large as duodenal ulcer patients as in normal subjects [80]. The mechanism of this abnormal response is not known. In one study the abnormal response of duodenal ulcer patients to a meal was due to a prolonged period of gastric acid secretion and an

Table 3   Abnormalities in Patients with Duodenal Ulcer

Hypersecretion of gastric HCl
    Basal acid output
    12-hour night secretion
    Maximal or peak acid output to histamine or pentagastrin (increased parietal cell mass)
    Increased response to stimulation
        sham feeding
        insulin hypoglycemia
        gastric distention
        intestinal phase of secretion
        response to a meal
Other secretory abnormalities
    Excessive vagal stimulation
    Excessive duodenal acid load
    Qualitatively abnormal mucus
    Hypersecretion (exocrine and endocrine) of pepsinogens
    Failure of inhibition of gastric acid secretion
Increased sensitivity of secretory processes: response to gastrin and calcium
Abnormal histamine metabolism
Endocrine abnormalities and disorders of regulation
    Inappropriate release of gastrin
    Impaired negative feedback: effect of gastric HCl or inhibition of gastric release
    Impaired control of somatostatin release
Abnormalities in mucosal defense mechanisms
    Decreased mucin secretion
    Decreased availability of prostaglandins
    Decreased salivary secretion
Abnormalities in blood flow
Abnormalities in gastric motor function
    Increased phasic antral contractility
    Accelerated gastric emptying
Abnormal psychodynamics
Genetic factors: HLA-B12 antigens, blood group O, and nonsecretor status present in excessive
    numbers compared to general population

abnormally rapid delivery of acid to the duodenum [81]. In this study the acid load delivered to the duodenum after a meal was four to five times that in normal subjects (Fig. 10) [81]. One possible explanation for the increased acid output is failure of normal acid inhibitory mechanisms. Despite many reported observations, there are no firm answers.

The role of gastrin in duodenal ulcer has received much attention. Antral G-cell mass, antral content of gastrin, and fasting serum gastrin levels have compared

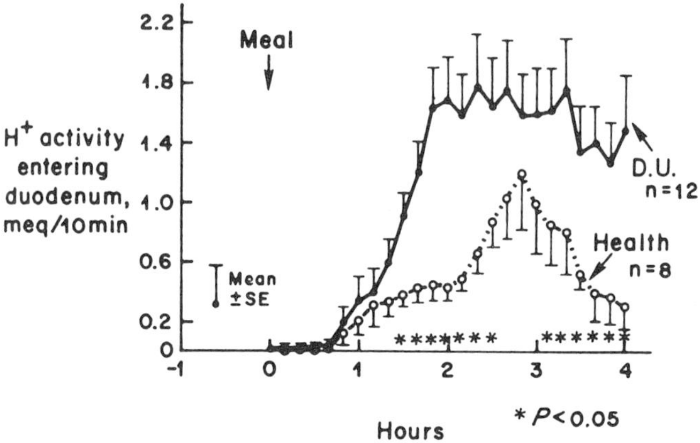

FIGURE 10 Duodenal hydrogen load after meals in patients with duodenal ulcer (DU) and healthy volunteers (Health). *Significant differences ($P < 0.05$) at each 10-min interval. (From Malegelada JR, Longstreth GF, Deering TB, et al. Gastric secretion and emptying after ordinary meals in duodenal ulcer. Gastroenterology 1977; 73:992.)

variably between duodenal ulcer patients and normal subjects. There seems to be a group of duodenal ulcer patients with increased gastrin release in response to a protein meal. Decreased inhibition of gastrin release in response to somatostatin has been suggested. To further study the relationship of these two hormones, Harty et al. [82] used cultured antral mucosa obtained by endoscopic biopsy of duodenal ulcer patients and controls. Antral mucosal explants from duodenal ulcer patients contained less somatostatin and in response to stimulation with cAMP released more gastrin and less somatostatin than did those from normal controls. This is further evidence for an alteration of the local (paracrine) inhibitory effects of somatostatin in duodenal ulcer patients. An important observation is that the fasting serum gastrin concentrations, although normal in patients with duodenal ulcer, are actually inappropriately high considering the acidic pH of antral contents [83].

In the experimental model of duodenal ulcer in rat produced by cysteamine, it was found that serum gastrin levels were elevated and there was a decrease in gastric and duodenal mucosal somatostatin levels [84,85]. The pH must be lowered to ≤ 2.5 to inhibit gastrin release in duodenal ulcer patients, whereas in normal controls pH 3.5 is sufficient. Hypersecretion of pepsinogen I occurs in about two-thirds of patients with duodenal ulcer. Basal secretion of pepsinogens was increased in patients with active duodenal ulcer and fell as the ulcer healed [86].

Gastric-duodenal motility may play a role in duodenal ulcers. In the rat model of cysteamine-induced duodenal ulcer, cysteamine inhibited gastric motility and markedly increased the force of duodenal contractions [87] and decreased the movement of pancreatic bicarbonate from the distal to the proximal duodenum [88]. Duodenal mucosal defense mechanisms and blood flow are areas of active investigation, but because the duodenum is more difficult to study than the stomach, our understanding of these processes lags behind that of the stomach. Psychodynamics in duodenal ulcer patients has been extensively studied, but no clear answers have emerged.

The ability of acid-reducing agents to accelerate healing of duodenal ulcers so successfully attests to the importance of the gastric acid/pepsin aggressive factors in ulcerogenesis. However, the high healing rate on placebo, ulcer resistance to therapy, and the tendency of ulcers to recur even on maintenance therapy suggests that much of the pathophysiology of duodenal ulcer remains to be explained.

VI. CONCLUSION

Peptic ulcer disease continues to be a major clinical problem. Advances have been made in our understanding of its epidemiology, physiology, clinical characteristics, and pathophysiology. These advances have helped us classify the heterogeneous group of ulcer patients into distinct subgroups that might have specific etiologies. With this reductionist approach, perhaps we will gain the understanding of the pathophysiological mechanisms we will need to better treat these patients.

REFERENCES

1. Wormsley GK. Duodenal ulcer: does pathophysiology equal aetiology? Gut 1983; 24: 775–80.
2. Ginsberg AL. The ulcer controversy. Dig Dis Sci 1981; 26:149.
3. Kirk RM. Are gastric and duodenal ulcers separate diseases or do they form a continuum? Dig Dis Sci 1981; 26:149–153.
4. Rotter JJ. Gastric and duodenal ulcers are many different diseases. Dig Dis Sci 1981; 26:154–160.
5. Brooks FP. The pathophysiology of peptic ulcer: an overview. In Brooks FP, Cohen S, Soloway RD, eds. Peptic ulcer disease. New York: Churchill Livingstone, 1985: 45–149.
6. Sava G. Ulcerations et ulcere aigus de l'estomac. France Medicale 1967; 30:274.
7. Hunt RH, Howden CW, Jones DB, Burget DW, Kerr GD. The correlation between acid suppression and peptic ulcer healing. Scand J Gastroenterol 1986; 21:22–9.
8. Davenport HW. Salicylate damage to the gastric mucosal barrier. N Engl J Med 1967; 276:1307–12.
9. Davenport HW. Back-diffusion of acid through the gastric mucosa and its physiological consequences. In: Glass GBJ, ed. Progress in gastroenterology, Vol. II. New York: Grune and Stratton, 1970: 42–56.
10. Nagashima R, Samloff IM. Aggressive factors II: pepsin. In Brooks FP, Cohen S, Soloway RD, eds. Peptic ulcer disease. New York: Churchill Livingstone, 1985: 181–214.
11. Alphin RS, Vokac VA, Gregory RL, et al. Role of intragastric pressure, pH, and pepsin in gastric ulceration in the rat. Gastroenterology 1977; 73:495–500.

12. Robert A, Nexamis JE, Stowe DF. Production of duodenal ulcers by administration of hydrochloric acid. Gastroenterology 1971; 60:709A.

13. Lai K-H, Wyckoff JB, Samloff IM. Aspartic proteinases in gastric mucosa of the rat: absence of pepsinogen I, genetic polymorphism of pepsinogen II, and presence of slow moving proteinase. Gastroenterology 1988; 95:295–301.

14. Rovelstad RA. Continuously recorded in situ pH of gastric and duodenal contents in patients with and without duodenal ulcer. Gastroenterology 1956; 31:530–7.

15. Archambault AP, Rovelstad RA, Carlson HC. In situ pH of duodenal bulb contents in normal and duodenal ulcer subjects. Gastroenterology 1967; 52:940–7.

16. Rhodes J, Apsimon HT, Lawrie JH. pH of the contents of the duodenal bulb in relation to duodenal ulcer. Gut 1966; 7:502–8.

17. Blaser MJ. Gastric *Campylobacter*-like organisms, gastritis, and peptic ulcer disease. Gastroenterology 1987; 93:371–83.

18. Rosenthal LE, Mobley HLT. *Campylobacter pylori*: an infectious cause of peptic ulcer disease? Contemp. Gastroenterol. 1988; 1:9–13.

19. Rauws, EAJ, Langenberg W, Houthhoff HJ, Zanen HC, Tytgat GNJ. *Campylobacter pyloridis*-associated chronic active antral gastritis. Gastroenterology 1988; 94:33–40.

20. Turnberg LA. Resistance factors I: "mucus-bicarbonate" barrier. In Brooks FP, Cohen S, Soloway RD, eds. Peptic ulcer disease. New York: Churchill Livingstone, 1985: 215–32.

21. Williams SE, Turnberg LA. Retardation of acid diffusion by pig gastric mucus: a potential role in mucosal protection. Gastroenterology 1980; 79:299–304.

22. Morris GP, Wallace JL. The roles of ethanol and of acid in the production of gastric mucosal erosions in rats. Virchows Arch (Cell Pathol) 1981; 38:23–38.

23. Wallace JL. Increased resistance of the rat gastric mucosa to hemorrhagic damage after exposure to an irritant: role of the "mucoid cap" and prostaglandin synthesis. Gastroenterology 1988; 94:22–32.

24. Kurito Y, Nakazawa S, Segawa K, Tsukamoto Y. Clinical significance of gastric juice viscosity in peptic ulcer patients. Dig Dis Sci 1988; 33:1070–6.

25. Flemstrom G, Sachs G. Ion transport by amphibian antrum in vitro: 1. General characteristics. Am J Physiol 1975; 216:167–74.

26. Williams SE, Turnberg LA. Studies of the "protective" properties of gastric mucus: evidence for a "mucus-bicarbonate" barrier. Gut 1981; 22:94–6.

27. Bahari HMM, Ross IN, Turnberg LA. Demonstration of a pH gradient across the mucus layer on the surface of human gastric mucosa in vitro. Gut 1982; 23:513–6.

28. Gannon B, Browning J, O'Brien P, Rogers P. Mucosal microvascular architecture of the fundus and body of human stomach. Gastroenterology 1984; 86:866–75.

29. Ross IN, Bahari HMM, Turnberg LA. The pH gradient across mucus adherent to rat fundic mucus in vivo and the effects of potential damaging agents. Gastroenterology 1981; 81:713–8.

30. Silen W. Gastric mucosal defense and repair. In Johnson LR, ed. Physiology of the gastrointestinal tract. New York: Raven, 1987: 1056–63.

31. Wilkes JM, Garner A, Peters TJ. Mechanisms of acid disposal and acid-stimulated alkaline secretions by gastroduodenal mucosa. Dig Dis Sci 1988; 33:361–7.

32. Isenberh JI, Selling JA, Hogan DL, Thomas JF, Koss MA. Duodenal ulcer (DU) patients have impaired proximal duodenal mucosal bicarbonate secretion. Gastroenterology 1986; 90:1472.

33. Ohe K, Miura Y, Taoka Y, Okada Y, Miyoshi A. Cysteamine-induced inhibition of mucosal and pancreatic alkaline secretion in rat duodenum. Dig Dis Sci 1988; 33:330–7.

34. Chou CC, Hsieh CP, Yu YM, et al. Localization of mesenteric hyperemia during digestion in dogs. Am J Physiol 1976; 230:583.

35. Tepperman BL, Jacobson ED. Circulatory factors in gastric ulcers. In Brooks FP, Cohen S, Soloway RD, eds. Peptic ulcer disease. New York: Churchill Livingstone, 1985: 261–78.

36. Yabana T, Yachi A. Stress-induced vascular damage and ulcer. Dig Dis Sci 1988; 33:751–61.

37. Seidler U, Knafla K, Kownatzki R, Sewing K-Fr. Effects of endogenous and exogenous prostaglandins on glycoprotein synthesis and secretion in isolated rabbit gastric mucosa. Gastroenterology 1988; 95:945–51.

38. Guth PH, Paulsen G, Nagata H. Histologic and microcirculatory changes in alcohol-induced gastric lesions in the rat: effect of prostaglandin cytoprotection. Gastroenterology 1984; 87:1083–90.

38. Lacy ER, Ito S. Ethanol-induced insult to the superficial rat gastric epithelium: a study of damage and rapid repair. In Allen et al., eds. Mechanisms of mucosal protection in the upper gastrointestinal tract. New York: Raven, 1984: 49–56.

40. Robert A. Role of endogenous and exogenous prostaglandins in mucosal protection. In Allen A., et al., eds. Mechanisms of mucosal protection in the upper gastrointestinal tract. New York: Raven, 1984: 377–82.

41. Malagelada J-R. Prostaglandin metabolism in peptic ulcer disease. Scand J Gastroenterol 1986; 21:136–41.

42. Schepp W, Steffen B, Ruoff H-J, Schusdziarra V, Classen M. Modulation of rat gastric mucosal prostaglandin E_2 release by dietary linoleic acid: effects on gastric acid secretion and stress-induced mucosal damage. Gastroenterology 1988; 95:18–25.

43. Barakat M, Bounameaux A, Badawi A, El Sobki N, Kuruppachery V. Double-blinded study comparing cimetidine and two doses of a slow release formulation of trimoprostil in duodenal ulcer patients with a 6-month follow-up. Digestion 1988; 40:11–8.

44. Pruitt BA, Foley FD, Moncrief JA. Curling's ulcer: a clinical pathology study of 323 cases. Ann Surg 1970; 172:523–39.

45. Harrison AM, Gaisford JCC, Wechsler RL. Gastric secretion in the burned patient. J Trauma 1972; 12:1041–43.

46. Rosenthal A, Czafa AJ, Pruitt BA. Gastrin levels and gastric acidity in the pathogenesis of acute gastroduodenal disease after burns. Surg Gynecol Obstet 1977; 144:232–4.

47. Pruitt BA, Goodwin CW Jr. Stress ulcer disease in the burned patient. World J Surg 1981; 5:209–22.

48. McAlhany JC, Czaja AJ, Pruitt BA. Antacid control of complications from acute gastroduodenal disease after burns. J Trauma 1976; 16:645–9.

49. O'Neill JA, Ritchey CR, Mason AD Jr, Villarreal Y. Influence of thermal burns on gastric mucus production. Surg Forum 1966; 17:293–5.

50. O'Neill JA Jr, Ritchey CR, Villarreal Y. Effect of thermal burns on gastric mucus production. Surg Gynecol Obstet 1970; 131:29–33.

51. Kamaka T, Fusamoto H, Kawano S, et al. Gastrointestinal bleeding following head injury: a clinical study of 433 cases. J Trauma 1977; 17:44–7.

52. Stremple JF, Molot MD, McNamara J, et al. Posttraumatic gastric bleeding: prospective gastric secretion composition. Arch Surg 1972; 105:177–85.

53. Stremple JF. Prospective studies of gastric secretion in trauma patients. Am J Surg 1976; 131:78–85.

54. Silvoso GR, Ivey KS, Butt JH, et al. Incidence of gastric lesions in patients with rheumatic disease on chronic aspirin therapy. Ann Intern Med 1979; 91:517–20.

55. Ivey KS, Morrison S, Gray C. Effect of intravenous salicylates on the gastric mucosal barrier in man. Am J Dig Dis 1972; 17:1055–64.

56. Ivey KS, Paone DB, Krause WJ. Acute effect of systemic aspirin on gastric mucosa in man. Dig Dis Sci 1980; 25:97–9.

57. Simon LS, Mills JA. Nonsteroidal anti-inflammatory drugs. N Engl J Med 1980; 302:1179–85.

58. Caruso D, Bianchi Porro G. Gastroscopic evaluation of anti-inflammatory agents. Br Med J 1980; 1:75–8.

59. Cooke AR, Hunt JN. Absorption of acetylsalicylic acid from unbuffered and buffered gastric contents. Am Dig Dis 1970; 15:95–102.

60. Hunt JN, Smith SL, Jiang CL. Gastric bleeding and gastric secretion with sulindac and naproxen. Dig Dis Sci 1983; 28:169–73.

61. Oates PJ, Hakkinen JP. Studies on the mechanism of ethanol-induced gastric damage in rats. Gastroenterology 1988; 94:10–21.

62. Dreyling KW, Lange K, Peskar BA, Peskar BM. Release of leukotrienes by rat and human gastric mucosa and its pharmacologic modification. Br J Pharm 1986; 99:236P.

63. Meshkinpou H, Marks JW, Schoenfield LJ, et al. Reflux gastritis syndrome: mechanism of symptoms. Gastroenterology 1980; 79:1283–7.

64. Duane WC, Weigand DM. Mechanism by which bile salt disrupts the gastric mucosal barrier in the dog. J Clin Invest 1980; 66:1044–9. Cloud WG, Ritchie WP Jr. Deconjugated bile acids are more damaging to gastric mucosa than are conjugated bile acids. Surg Forum 1980; 31:115–7.

65. Duane WC, Wiegand DM, Sievert CE. Bile acid and bile salt disrupt gastric mucosal barrier in the dog by different mechanisms. Am J Physiol 1982; 242:G95-9.

66. Baum S, Ward S, Nusbaum M. Stress bleeding from the mid-duodenum: an often unrecognized source of gastrointestinal hemorrhage. Radiology 1970; 95:595–602.

67. Fiddian-Green RG, McGough E, Pittenger G, Rothman E. Predictive values of intramural pH and other risk factors for massive bleeding from stress ulceration. Gastroenterology 1983; 85:613–20.

68. Jennewien HM, Hammer R. Animal models of ulcer diseases. In: Holtermuller KH, Malagedala JR, eds. Advances in ulcer disease. Amsterdam: Excerpta Medica, 1980: 37–483.

69. Innes DL, Tansy MF. Gastric mucosal ulceration associated with electrochemical stimulation of the limbic brain. Brain Res Bull 1980; 5(Suppl 1):33–6.

70. Goto Y, Tache Y. Gastric erosions induced by intracisternal thyrotropin-releasing hormone (TRH) in rats. Peptides 1985; 6:153–6.

71. Lucas CE, Sugawa C, Riddle J, et al. Natural history and surgical dilemma of "stress" gastric bleeding. Arch Surg 1971; 102:266–73.

72. Cowan WK. Genetics of duodenal and gastric ulcer. Clin Gastroenterol 1973; 2:539–46.

73. Crean GP, Spiegelhalter DJ. Symptoms of peptic ulcer. In Brooks FP, Cohen S, Soloway RD, eds. Peptic ulcer disease. New York: Churchill Livingstone, 1985: 1–16.

74. Sonnenberg A, Sonnenberg GS. The implication of the birth-cohort phenomenon for the etiology of peptic ulcer disease. In De Mares F, Battaglia G, Viarello F, eds. Advances in gastroenterology. Padad: Picaa Nuova Libraria, 1988: 119–30.

75. Rotter JI, Rimoin DL. Peptic ulcer disease: a heterogeneous group of disorders? Gastroenterology 1977; 73:604–7.

76. Ellis A, Woodrow JC. HLA and duodenal ulcer. Gut 1979; 20:760–2.

77. Faber RG, Hobsley M. Basal secretion: reproducibility and relationship with duodenal ulceration. Gut 1977; 18:57–63.

78. Feldman M, Richardson CT, Fordtran JS. Effect of sham feeding on gastric acid secretion in healthy subjects and duodenal ulcer patients: evidence for increased basal vagal tone in some ulcer patients. Gastroenterology 1980; 79:796–800.

79. Bergegardh S, Nilsson G, Olbe L. The effect of antral distention on acid secretion and plasma gastrin in duodenal ulcer patients. Scand J Gastroenterol 1977; 73:447–52.

80. Isenberg JJ, Ippoliti AF, Maxwell VL. Perfusion of the proximal small intestine with peptone stimulates gastric acid secretion in man. Gastroenterology 1977; 73:746–52.

81. Malagelada J-R, Langstreth GF, Deering TB, et al. Gastric secretion and emptying after ordinary meals in duodenal ulcer. Gastroenterology 1977; 73:989–94.

82. Harty RF, Maico DG, McGuigan JE. Antral release of gastrin and somatostatin in duodenal ulcer and control subjects. Gut 1986; 27:652–8.

83. Brooks FP. The pathophysiology of peptic ulcer disease. Dig Dis Sci 1985; 30:15S–29S.

84. Szabo S, Reichlin S. Somatostatin in rat tissues is depleted by cysteamine administration. Endocrinology 1981; 109:2255–7.

85. Szabo S, Reichlin S. Somatostatin depletion by cysteamine: mechanism and implication for duodenal ulceration. Fed Proc 1985; 44:2540–5.

86. Achord JL. Gastric pepsin and acid secretion in patients with acute and healed duodenal ulcer. Gastroenterology 1981; 81:15–8.

87. Takeuchi K, Nishiwaki H, Okabe S. Role of local motility changes in the pathogenesis of duodenal ulcers induced by cysteamine in rats. Dig Dis Sci 1987; 32:295–304.

88. Szabo S, Pihan G, Gallagher GT, Brown A. Role of local secretory and motility changes in the pathogenesis of experimental duodenal ulcer. Scand J Gastroenterol 1984; 19(Suppl 92):106–11.

2

Epidemiology of Peptic Ulcer Disease

JOHN H. KURATA

San Bernardino County Medical Center,
San Bernardino,
and University of California, Los Angeles,
School of Medicine, Los Angeles, California

I. INTRODUCTION

Peptic ulcer disease is a chronic disease with low mortality. Yet, in the United States, the lifetime prevalence is nearly one in ten persons. This indicates a high cost in both economic and human terms.

Problems of rate assessment and interpretation of the epidemiological literature associated with ulcer disease have been discussed elsewhere [1]. One recent development may have added to these problems. The American College of Physicians' Health and Public Policy Committee has recommended initial antacid or H_2-blocker therapy for ulcerlike symptoms and that endoscopy be performed only after this regimen has failed to alleviate symptoms [2]. This may affect the validity of ulcer rate data, since many patients being treated with ulcer medications may, in fact, not have ulcer disease.

In Section II, current data on the frequency of peptic ulcer in the United States are present. Sections III−V review and summarize selected studies on ulcer risk factors.

II. FREQUENCY OF PEPTIC ULCER IN THE UNITED STATES

A. Period Prevalence

Lifetime and 1-year period prevalence data for peptic ulcer disease in the United States are available from surveys administered by the National Center for Health Statistics. The National Health and Nutrition Examination Survey (NHANES) provides esti-

31

mates of lifetime ulcer prevalence, the proportion of the U.S. population who have ever had a peptic ulcer during their lifetime. The National Health Interview Survey (NHIS) measures 1-year period prevalence, the frequency of self-reported peptic ulcer in the United States during a 1-year period.

Data from NHANES II (1976–1980) indicate that lifetime ulcer prevalence for white and black adults between the ages of 20 and 74 years is approximately 9.4% [3]. The male and female prevalence is 11.3% and 7.7%, respectively. The lifetime prevalence rate for whites is 9.6%; that for blacks is 8%.

The crude 1-year period prevalence rate for peptic ulcer is approximtely 16/1000 in 1988 based on NHIS data [4]. There are no strong sex- or race-specific patterns, although crude rates are slightly higher for whites than for blacks, but there is a strong inverse relationship between income and ulcer prevalence (Table 1) [4]. Ulcer prevalence is highest for the 45–64-year-old group (Figs. 1–3) [4]. For all ages, lower income groups consistently have higher prevalence than upper income groups (Fig. 3). It should be noted that these patterns have fluctuated between NHIS surveys. For example, in previous surveys, rates were higher for whites than for blacks for those over 64 years old.

B. Time Trends

Examination of changes in disease rates over time may provide insight into peptic ulcer etiology, efficacy of medical therapy, and health manpower needs.

Table 1   1988 Self-Reported Ulcer Disease Prevalence

Demographic factor	Rate per 1000
Sex	
Male	15.9
Female	16.0
Race	
White	16.4
Black	15.3
Family income	
<$10,000	25.2
$10,000–19,999	20.3
$20,000–34,999	13.4
$35,000+	12.4

Source: National Center for Health Statistics [4].

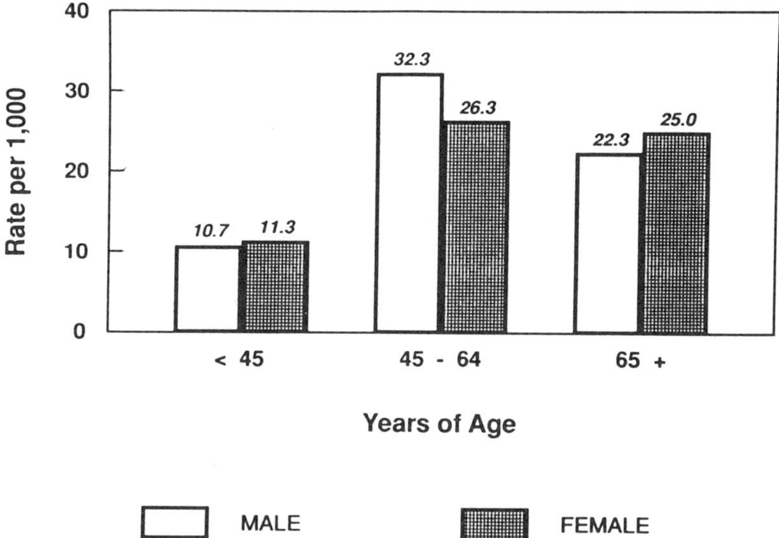

FIGURE 1 One-year period prevalence for peptic ulcer by sex and age for 1988, United States. (Source: National Health Interview Survey, National Center for Health Statistics [4].)

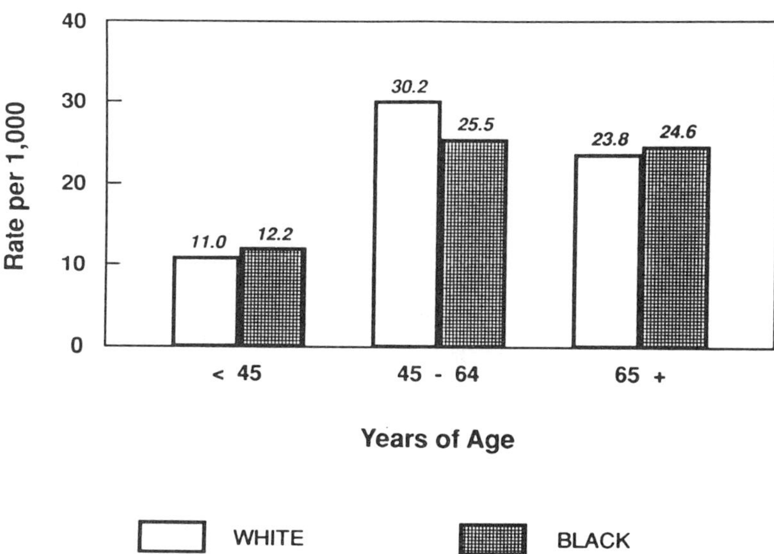

FIGURE 2 One-year period prevalence for peptic ulcer by race and age for 1988, United States. (Source: National Health Interview Survey, National Center for Health Statistics [4].)

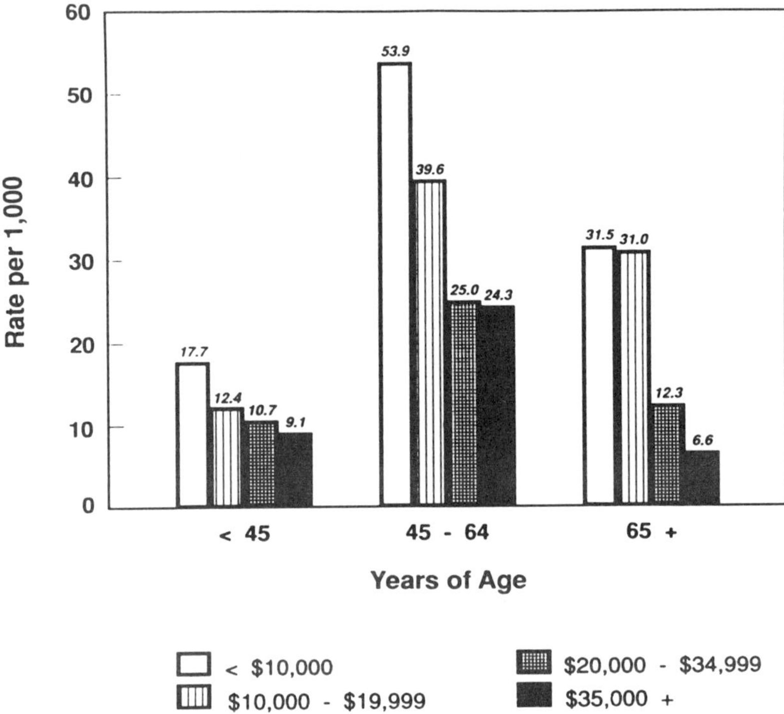

FIGURE 3 One-year period prevalence for peptic ulcer by income and age for 1988, United States. (Source: National Health Interview Survey, National Center for Health Statistics [4].)

1. Prevalence (1957–1988)

Approximately 20 years ago, the 1-year period prevalence of peptic ulcer was twice as high for males as for females based on NHIS data [5]. The number of self-reported ulcer cases for females steadily increased, however, and by 1979 the 1-year period prevalence for females exceeded that for males (Fig. 4) [4–7]. Identifying reasons for this increasing trend in ulcer prevalence for females requires further research to overcome limitations of data related to classification (data are not available by ulcer site) and self-reporting bias (susceptibility to over- and underreporting biases).

2. Hospitalizations (1970–1987)

Between 1970 and 1985, peptic ulcer hospitalizations overall decreased by about 25%, largely because uncomplicated duodenal ulcer hospitalizations declined (Fig. 5) [8]. Gastric ulcer hospitalizations rose owing to an increase in hemorrhage cases (Fig. 6). These trends continued through 1987 (Figs. 5 and 6) [8–10], the most recent year for which data were available at the time of writing. The crude hospitalization rate for

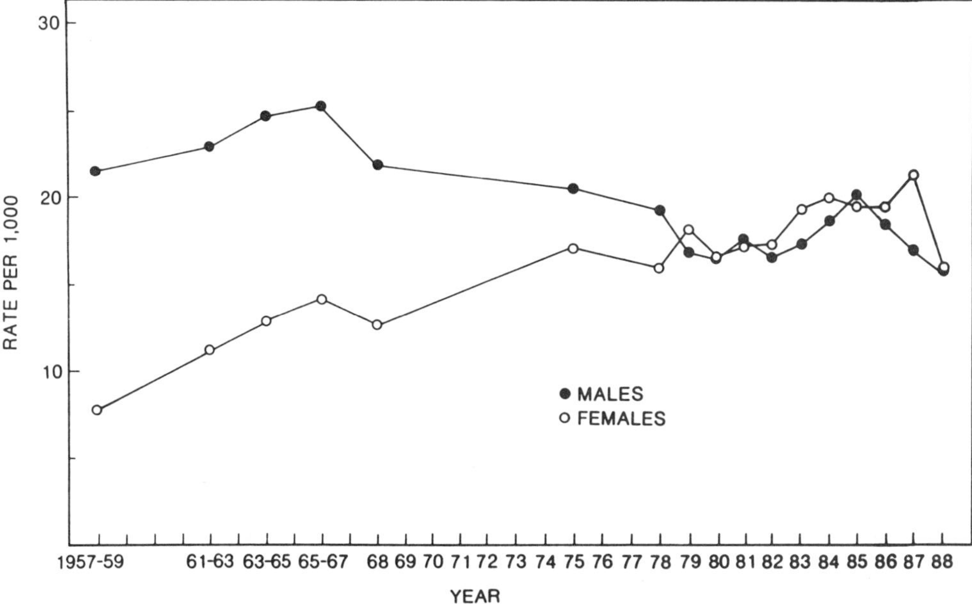

FIGURE 4   One-year period prevalence for peptic ulcer disease for 1957–1988, United States. (Source: National Health Interview Survey, National Center for Health Statistics [4–7].)

all ulcers in 1987, 118.8/100,000, was slightly below the 1986 rate [9,10]. Changing national population patterns may contribute to differences in hospitalization trends. Other factors that bear investigation are new ulcer therapies or side effects due to nonsteroidal anti-inflammatory drugs (NSAIDs).

3. Mortality (1962–1988)

Peptic ulcer mortality decreased sharply between 1962 and 1978, by 58% for gastric ulcer and 68% for duodenal ulcer [11]. Since then, crude gastric and duodenal ulcer mortality rates have stabilized at approximately one death per 100,000 for both sexes [8,12]. Age-specific mortality rates, however, have decreased noticeably over time for males under 85 years of age (Fig. 7) [8,12]. They have tended to decline only slightly or remain fairly stable for females under age 75 (Fig. 8). For the oldest age group, there has been a large increase in mortality for both sexes since 1978 (Figs. 7 and 8). In 1988, peptic ulcer was listed as the underlying cause of 6360 deaths (2.6/100,000) [13]. (1988 data are provisional estimates based upon a 10% sample of deaths.)

4. Summary

Trends for the three measures of ulcer frequency are different. Self-reported prevalence rates for males and females are now similar because of increases in female rates over

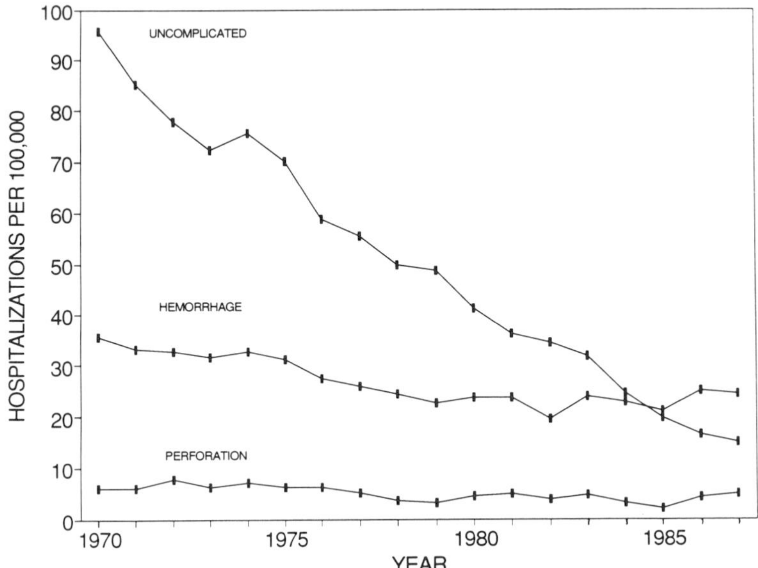

FIGURE 5 Duodenal ulcer hospitalization rates for 1970–1987, United States. (Source: National Hospital Discharge Survey, National Center for Health Statistics [8–10].)

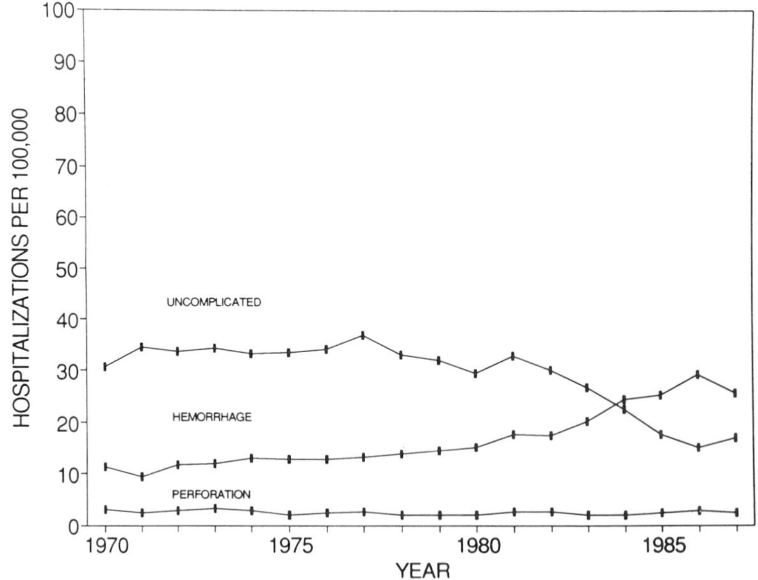

FIGURE 6 Gastric ulcer hospitalization rates for 1970–1987, United States. (Source: National Hospital Discharge Survey, National Center for Health Statistics [8–10].)

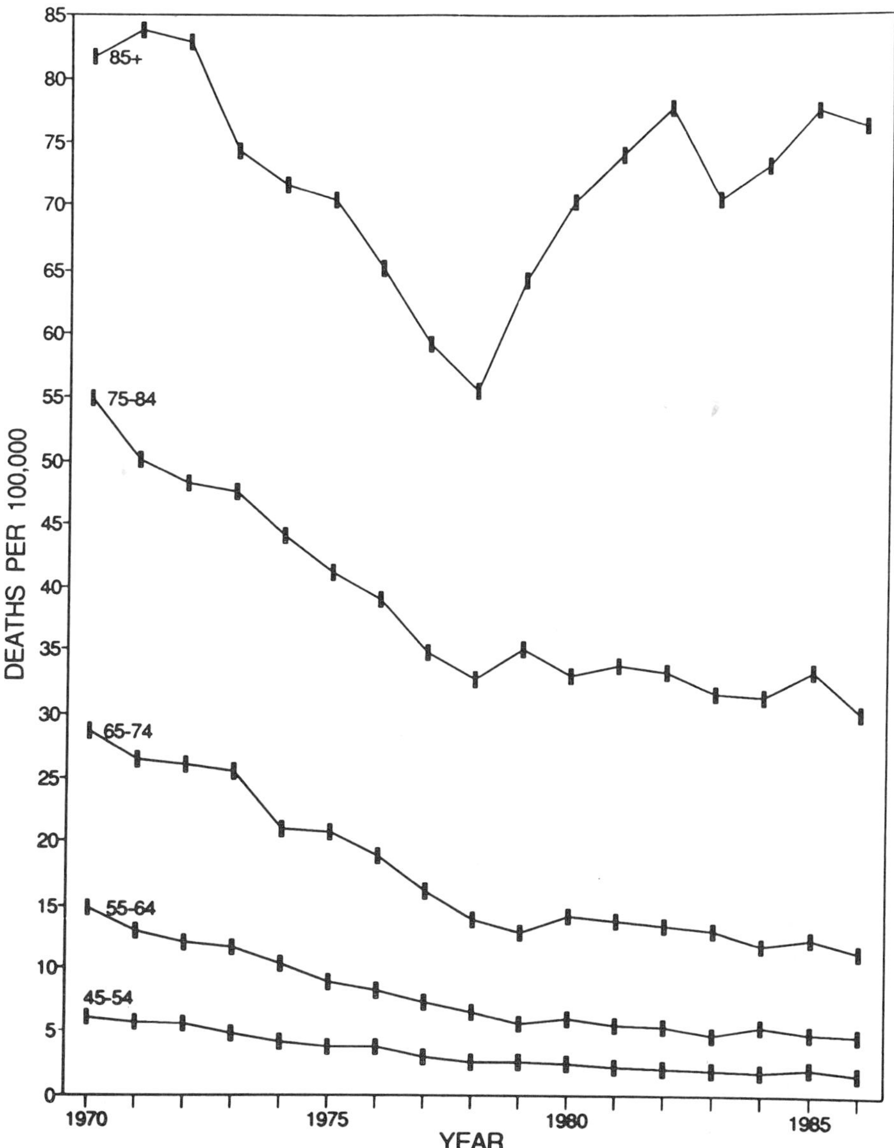

FIGURE 7 Age-specific peptic ulcer mortality rates for men, 1970–1986, United States. (Source: Vital Statistics, National Center for Health Statistics [8, 12].)

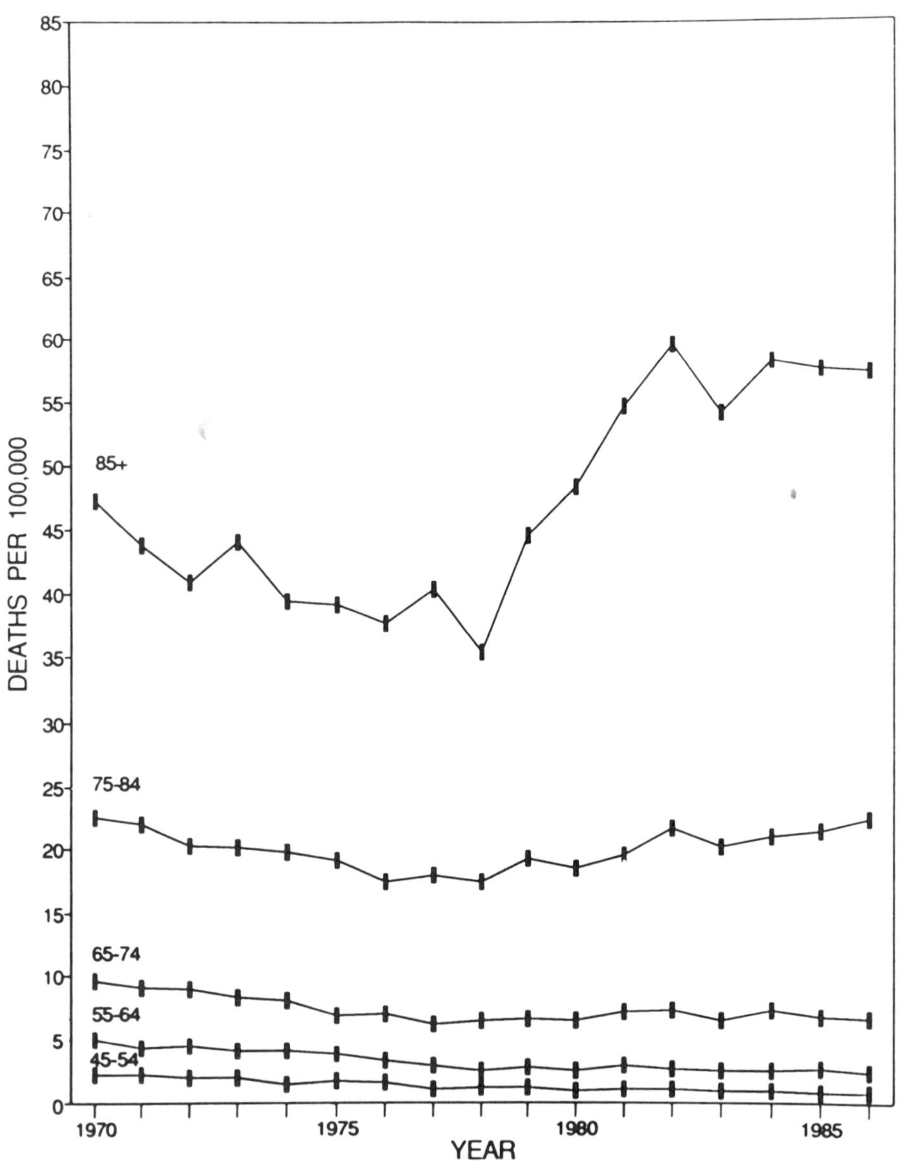

FIGURE 8 Age-specific peptic ulcer mortality rates for women, 1970–1986, United States. (Source: Vital Statistics, National Center for Health Statistics [8,12].)

time. The sharp drop in uncomplicated duodenal ulcer hospitalizations has contributed to the decline in total peptic ulcer hospitalizations despite the increasing rates for gastric ulcer hemorrhage. Gastric and duodenal ulcer mortality has remained fairly constant for both sexes since 1978. These conflicting trends do not resolve the issue of whether or not peptic ulcer disease is increasing or decreasing, but rather indicate the need for further investigation.

III. ENVIRONMENTAL FACTORS

Researchers have had a long-standing interest in the association between environmental factors and increased risk of peptic ulcer disease. The number of factors, however, for which there is strong evidence in support of such an association remains small; only cigarette smoking, aspirin, and nonaspirin NSAIDs (NANSAIDs) have been consistently associated with peptic ulcer. The link between prolonged use of corticoids and peptic ulcer will require more study. New approaches to assess the effect of psychosocial stress have shown some promising preliminary results; however, overall results are still equivocal. There is also limited evidence that dietary fiber is protective. A summary of evidence for hypothesized environmental factors is presented in Table 2 [14].

A. Smoking

There is considerable evidence for an association between smoking and peptic ulcer disease [15,16]. A variety of studies have linked mortality to smoking. Smoking increases the risk for developing ulcer disease, dose–response effects have been

Table 2 Environmental Factors for Ulcer Disease

Association with ulcer disease	Factor
Strong evidence for association	Cigarette smoking
	Regular use of aspirin and NANSAIDs
Equivocal evidence	High total doses or extensive use of corticoids
Good evidence for lack of association	Coffee
	Alcohol (except for alcoholic hepatic cirrhosis)
Not adequately studied	Psychological factors
	High-fiber diet

Source: Adapted from Grossman [14].

reported, and a high percentage of patients with complications smoke. Ulcer healing rates are lower and recurrence rates are higher for smokers than for nonsmokers.

Death certificate studies have shown that male cigarette smokers have higher peptic ulcer mortality rates than nonsmokers [17–19]. A study to determine the cause of decreased life expectancy among 779 male peptic ulcer surgery patients concluded that excess mortality was due to smoking-related disorders [20]. An analysis of time trends for cigarette smoking rates and duodenal ulcer mortality from 1920 to 1980 found a strong positive association for both males and females [21].

Both prospective and retrospective studies have demonstrated an increased risk for peptic ulcer in smokers. A prospective study of former college students, all males, found that smokers were at a one-third greater risk of developing an ulcer later in life than nonsmokers [22]. A 20-year follow-up of Japanese men enrolled in the Honolulu Heart Program reported that cigarette smoking was associated with increased risks for both gastric and duodenal ulcer [23]. Results from retrospective and cross-sectional studies suggest that cigarette smokers are about twice as likely to have ulcers as nonsmokers [15,24–26]. Australian case-control studies have reported risk ratios as high as 6.9 [27–30].

A dose–response relationship between peptic ulcer and smoking has been described by several researchers. Petitti et al. [31] found that the percentage of current regular cigarette smokers who had ever had peptic ulcer disease increased significantly with the number of cigarettes smoked but was not associated with the tar or nicotine yield of the cigarettes. A Scandinavian study reported an association between duodenal ulcer risk for men and the number of cigarettes smoked per day [25]. An American study on Japanese immigrant males found increasing risk for gastric but not duodenal ulcer with increasing pack-years of smoking [23].

Postoperative morbidity and mortality studies on peptic ulcer surgery patients reported that over 80% were smokers [20,32]. According to an editorial on this subject [16], smoking increases the risk that ulcer surgery will be hazardous, although higher rates of ulcer complications are not found for smokers.

The impact of cigarette smoking on ulcer healing is an area of ongoing research. Most studies indicate that ulcers heal more slowly in smokers than in nonsmokers, even under treatment with H_2 blockers or cytoprotective agents [33–39]. Smokers also have higher relapse rates than nonsmokers [37,40,41].

B. Drugs

1. Aspirin

Case-control studies have documented risk ratios of 3 or higher for gastric ulcer associated with aspirin use [27,29,30,42–44]. In addition, studies indicate that regular aspirin use increases the risk of duodenal and gastric ulcer bleeding and hospitalization. Case-control studies show aspirin-associated risk ratios of 3.0–9.3 for bleeding duodenal ulcer and 2.0–3.3 for bleeding gastric ulcer [45,46]. The Aspirin Myocardial Infarction Study and the Physicians' Health Study are both large-scale, randomized, double-blind, placebo-controlled trials that have found higher peptic ulcer rates in patients randomly assigned aspirin than in those assigned placebo [47–49].

In the Aspirin Myocardial Infarction Study, 4524 patients were randomly assigned to a high-dose aspirin regimen (1 g daily) or to placebo for 3 years [47]. The peptic ulcer hospitalization rate was six times higher in the aspirin group, with statistically significant adjusted relative risks of 10.7 for duodenal ulcer and 9.1 for gastric ulcer hospitalizations in males [47,48]. In the Physicians' Health Study, 22,071 physicians were randomly assigned to 325 mg of aspirin every other day or placebo for over 5 years [49]. The number of gastric and duodenal ulcer side effects was twice as high for the aspirin group as for the placebo group, although the difference was statistically significant only for duodenal ulcer.

2. Nonaspirin Nonsteroidal Anti-inflammatory Drugs

Reviews of recent epidemiological studies indicate that there is a positive association between NANSAIDs and peptic ulcer [50–53]. The wide variation in risk ratios, anywhere from 1 to 46, is due to differing study populations (e.g., nationality, advanced age, arthritis, gastrointestinal symptoms), outcome measures (e.g., severity of ulcer morbidity, mortality, ulcer site, method of diagnosis), NSAID therapy (e.g., dosage, duration, type), or study design. Risks for ulcer occurrence, complications, and mortality associated with NANSAID use are presented below.

Ulcer Occurrence.   Australian case-control studies have reported risk ratios above 3 associated with NANSAIDs for gastric ulcer but no association for duodenal ulcer [29,30,44]. An American cohort study found statistically significant risk ratios of 1.9 for duodenal ulcer and 2.8 for gastric ulcer associated with NANSAID exposure [54].

Complications.   American cohort studies of upper gastrointestinal (UGI) bleeding associated with NANSAID exposure reported risk ratios below 2, only one of which was statistically significant [55–57]. Case-control studies have yielded higher risk estimates. An international study reported a multivariate adjusted risk ratio of 9.1 for UGI bleeding associated with NANSAID use [58]. A British study found that elderly patients hospitalized with bleeding duodenal ulcer were 2.7 times as likely to have used NANSAIDs as matched hospital or community controls, and the risk ratio for gastric ulcer was between 2.8 and 3.7 [59].

Two British case-control studies concluded that NSAIDs were associated with perforated peptic ulcer in the elderly [60,61]. Both studies, however, relied solely on clinical notes to ascertain exposure, so that possible differentials in recording of past drug use may have contributed to the reported association. A more recent cohort study, which was not susceptible to this bias, failed to find evidence that NANSAID use caused gastric or duodenal perforation. Jick et al. [62] reported a statistically nonsignificant risk ratio of 1.6 between hospital admissions for perforated ulcer and concurrent use of NANSAIDs for a large, well-defined population.

Mortality.   Two North American studies reported statistically significant associations for NSAID use and gastrointestinal mortality in the elderly. An American case control study of ulcer deaths associated with current NSAID prescriptions from a state Medicaid database found adjusted odds ratios of 4.2 for gastric ulcer and 7.9 for duodenal ulcer [63]. A Canadian cohort study found that the mortality rate from UGI hemorrhage or perforation was over five times as high for elderly female NSAID users as for nonusers [64].

In summary, there is substantial evidence that NANSAID use is associated with peptic ulcer bleeding, perforation, and mortality. More studies, however, are needed to examine risk factors that predispose to ulcer and/or complications in patients on NSAIDs. For example, dosage levels, duration of NSAID therapy, and type of NSAID need further study. Smoking, *Helicobacter pylori* infection, prior history of ulcer disease, age, and sex are other possible risk factors. In the meantime, current evidence suggests that these drugs should be used cautiously in the elderly and in those with a history of ulcer disease.

3.   Corticoids

Corticoids may be implicated in ulcer formation or recurrence. A review of 50 studies concluded that corticoids can cause ulcers if they are administered at a high total dose equivalent to 1000 mg of prednisone or for more than 30 days [65]. No association was found between increased ulcer prevalence and short treatment periods (less than 30 days) or low total dose. In contrast, in a study of pooled data from 71 controlled clinical trials, a significant increase in the incidence of ulcer was observed, even for short treatment periods and total doses below 1000 mg [66]. However, these studies offer no firm conclusions with respect to either safe minimum dosage level or duration of treatment. An assessment of the role of corticoids in ulcer disease remains dependent on the combination of data from different studies. Problems associated with this methodology have been reviewed elsewhere [67–69].

C.   Coffee and Alcoholic Beverages

Although both coffee and alcoholic beverages have been shown to stimulate acid secretion in humans [70–72], there is no strong evidence that either is associated with peptic ulcer disease. Studies of coffee and ulcer disease have produced contradictory findings: Some have detected a relationship [22,73] whereas others have reported no association [24,25,74]. Many studies have demonstrated that alcohol is unrelated to increased risk for peptic ulcer disease [22,24,25,27,73,74], although a recent case-control study reported a positive association between alcohol and chronic duodenal ulcer for men when several environmental factors were assessed simultaneously [28]. Earlier studies of alcoholics, such as the frequently cited study conducted by Engeset et al. [75], showed an increased occurrence of peptic ulcer. The increased incidence of peptic ulcer disease in patients with hepatic cirrhosis, however, is probably related to the cirrhosis, not the alcohol [76].

D.   Diet

Small, bland meals and milk were once accepted treatments for peptic ulcer. The evidence does not support either dietary recommendation. Studies suggest that special bland diets are ineffective [77–81], and milk has been shown to increase gastric acid secretion levels in ulcer patients [82]. Furthermore, a recent study apparently indicates that milk inhibits duodenal ulcer healing by cimetidine [83].

Other investigators have focused on different dietary factors thought to influence peptic ulceration. A high salt diet is the common risk factor for gastric ulcer found by several studies [84,85]. Intriguing evidence exists, despite some reports to the contrary, that correlates high duodenal ulcer incidence in India and Africa with high consumption of peppers and spices [86]. In a recent randomized crossover trial of 12 healthy volunteers, however, endoscopy showed no gastroduodenal mucosal damage associated with highly spiced foods such as jalapeno peppers or pepperoni [87].

The role of dietary fiber has also been investigated. Rydning et al. [88], in a blinded study with endoscopic verification of ulcer, examined the effects of fiber on the recurrence of duodenal ulcer and found that a high-fiber diet was associated with fewer ulcer recurrences. This is the first controlled trial to support earlier work by Malhotra [89] that showed reduced ulcer recurrence for an unrefined wheat diet. Although these findings are suggestive, further research will be required to determine whether, in Rydning and Berstad's words, "it is the low-fibre diet that is harmful [or] the high-fibre diet that is beneficial" [90].

Few adequately controlled studies of dietary factors and peptic ulcer have been attempted. More are needed before recommendations can be made for anything other than a normal diet. Until such research is completed, ulcer patients should avoid food items that appear to initiate or exacerbate symptoms.

E.   Psychological Factors

Attempts to link ulcer disease to both personality type and response to stressful events have a long history. However, though a number of studies have investigated these variables, consistent evidence linking them to ulcer disease has yet to emerge.

The relationship between personality characteristics and peptic ulcer disease has been under investigation for more than 50 years [91,92]. Research in this century on the effect of emotional response on the gastric lining has noted elevated acid secretion levels associated with emotional response to stressful situations [93,94]. Relationships between psychological stress and peptic ulcer disease have also been investigated. Some studies have indicated an association [95,96]; however, most have shown no association, with recent studies tending to support this latter position [97–102].

Newer research has used multivariate models to investigate various factors of ulcer etiology. Feldman et al. [103] found that traits such as hypochondriasis, lowered ego strength, and excessive dependency were more apt descriptions of male subjects with peptic ulcer disease. Walker et al. [104] proposed a model incorporating psychosocial, behavioral, physiological, and genetic factors to explain the etiology of ulcer. Their study of 49 peptic ulcer cases and 52 controls found that psychopathology in general (hostility, irritability, hypersensitivity, and impaired coping ability) correlated significantly with serum pepsinogen concentration in ulcer patients. Depression was the best discriminator between ulcer patients and controls, but a negative perception of life events also had discriminatory value. While these results are suggestive, a deeper understanding of possible links between psychological factors and peptic ulcer awaits further investigation.

In summary, evidence for a causal role of stress in peptic ulcer disease is still lacking. It has been clearly demonstrated that emotional change can result in changes in the gastric mucosa, but there is no proof that these changes in turn result in peptic ulceration. In addition, most studies examining stressful life events and subsequent illness, including peptic ulcer disease, have found little or no differences between cases and controls. However, psychological stress should not be ruled out as a risk factor given the complex nature of this disease.

IV. *HELICOBACTER PYLORI*

The bacterium *Helicobacter pylori*, formerly called *Campylobacter pylori*, is accepted as a cause of gastritis [105]. It has been proposed as the pathogen in a wide range of gastric and duodenal conditions, including nonulcer dyspepsia, gastric carcinoma, and peptic ulcer disease [105]. Investigators have sought to establish *H. pylori* as a causal factor for peptic ulcer since it was first cultured in the early 1980s [106].

A variety of studies have shown an association, but not a cause-and-effect relationship, between *H. pylori* and peptic ulcer disease. The bacterium is present in 61–100% of peptic ulcer patients, with higher rates for duodenal ulcer [107–111]. In contrast, about a third of asymptomatic persons are infected with the bacteria [112], with higher prevalence associated with increasing age and possibly non-Caucasian race [112–114]. *Helicobacter pylori* antibody titer levels are three to five times as high for peptic ulcer patients as for healthy adults or children [115]. Duodenal ulcer healing and lower relapse rates were associated with *H. pylori* clearing in anti-ulcer trials of cimetidine, bismuth therapy, or combinations of bismuth and antibiotics [108,116–118]. There is evidence that relapse rates are lower when combined bismuth–antibiotic therapy, rather than H_2 blockers alone, is used in the healing phase [116,119]. Recent studies have produced conflicting results on whether smoking, NSAID use, and *H. pylori* infection interact as risk factors for ulcer disease [120–122].

These findings show that *H. pylori* may be associated with the pathophysiology of peptic ulcer disease. Much of the information, however, is available only in abstracts or for small samples of patients. Ulcer relapse trials indicate a role for *H. pylori*, but there is still insufficient evidence to prove ulcerogenicity. Conclusions about a causal relationship await confirmation from further studies, particularly well-designed,

properly controlled clinical trials. Follow-up studies are also needed of how interaction among *H. pylori* infection, smoking, and NSAID consumption will affect risk
for ulcer.

V.   GENETIC FACTORS

Many chronic diseases develop as the result of an interaction between genetic and
environmental factors, and peptic ulcer is no exception. While the genetic predisposi-
tion varies from individual to individual, family studies indicate that peptic ulcer
occurs more than twice as frequently among first-degree relatives of ulcer patients as
among relatives of control subjects [123]. Moreover, the risk to first-degree relatives
is restricted to the same ulcer site, either duodenal or gastric [124]. Rotter [125] and
McConnell [126] found that both twins have peptic ulcer more frequently in mono-
zygotic twins than in dizygotic twins and that twins also share ulcer location.

Additional evidence that ulceration involves genetic components comes from
studies of blood type and the secretion of blood group antigens in body fluids [125–
128]. Blood group O individuals are about 30% more likely to develop duodenal
ulcer than members of other blood groups. Individuals who do not secrete blood
group antigens into body fluids are about 1.5 times as likely to have duodenal ulcer as
secretors.

In other human genetic studies, investigators have used radioimmunoassays of
serum pepsinogen levels to assess the link between pepsinogen concentrations and
duodenal ulcer disease. High pepsinogen I levels are a recognized risk factor for
duodenal ulcer [129]. Research indicates that 30–50% of duodenal ulcer patients
have hyperpepsinogenemia I and the remainder have normopepsinogenemia I [130].
Family studies of duodenal ulcer and elevated serum pepsinogen I demonstrate
familial aggregation consistent with autosomal dominant inheritance [131–133].
Familial aggregation of duodenal ulcer in normopepsinogenemic I families is also
being investigated, as are familial duodenal ulcer associated with rapid gastric
emptying and familial hypergastrinemic duodenal ulcer [132,134–136]. Rotter
[125] has compiled a thorough review of the genetic factors implicated in peptic ulcer
disease.

VI.   SUMMARY

Major findings from the epidemiological literature covered in this chapter are summarized here. As was noted in the introduction, a complete review of the literature
was not attempted, because of the tremendous increase in the volume of literature.

In 1988, the 1-year period prevalence of ulcer disease was 1.6% for both males and
females. Over much of the period since 1979, more females than males have self-
reported ulcer. This is an important change from the rate of 20 years ago when the
prevalence of peptic ulcer was twice as high for men as for women. There has been a

steep decline in reported hospitalizations for peptic ulcer disease in the past two decades, which is attributed to an over 50% decrease in duodenal ulcer hospitalizations, mainly uncomplicated cases. Hospitalizations for gastric ulcer hemorrhages have been increasing. Although gastric and duodenal ulcer mortality rates decreased sharply between 1962 and 1978, crude site-specific rates have since remained fairly stable at about 1 death per 100,000 annually for both sexes. Age-adjusted rates have continued to fall. Approximately 6400 deaths per year are still attributable to peptic ulcer disease as the underlying cause.

The number of environmental factors for which there is strong evidence of association with peptic ulcer remains small. Only cigarette smoking and regular use of aspirin and NANSAIDs are consistently associated with peptic ulcer. Coffee and alcohol do not appear to be associated with ulcer disease. Psychological factors and high-fiber diets require further study. Some of the more complex models employed with recent psychological research suggest new means for investigating the manner in which psychological and other factors are implicated in ulcer disease. Inconclusive but promising findings are also beginning to emerge from investigations of the effects of diet, where there has been some suggestion that dietary fiber has a beneficial effect.

The presence of *H. pylori* correlates with peptic ulcer disease; however, a causal relationship has not yet been demonstrated. Genetic factors associated with ulcer disease include family history of ulceration, blood type O, and hyperpepsinogenemia I.

REFERENCES

1. Kurata JH, Haile BM. Epidemiology of peptic ulcer disease. Clin Gastroenterol 1984; 13: 289–307.
2. Health and Public Policy Committee, American College of Physicians. Endoscopy in the evaluation of dyspepsia. Ann Intern Med 1985; 102:266–9.
3. FitzSimmons SC, Guarlnick J, Everhart JE, Roth H. Self-reported peptic ulcer disease among black and white adults: prevalence and correlates in NHANES II, 1976–80. In: Health care for people or for profit? Published abstracts of the 115th annual American Public Health Association meeting. New Orleans, Oct. 18–22, 1987:26.
4. National Center for Health Statistics. Current estimates from the National Health Interview Survey, 1988. Washington, DC: US Govt. Printing Office, 1989; DHHS publication no. (PHS)89-1501. (Vital and health statistics; series 10.)
5. Kurata JH, Haile BM, Elashoff JD. Sex differences in peptic ulcer disease. Gastroenterology 1985; 88:96–100.
6. National Center for Health Statistics. Prevalence of selected chronic digestive conditions: United States, 1968, 1975. Washington, DC: US Govt. Printing Office, 1974–1979; DHEW publication nos. (HRA)74-1510, (PHS)79-1558. (Vital and health statistics, series 10.)
7. National Center for Health Statistics. Current estimates from the National Health Interview Survey, 1979, 1980, 1982–1987. Washington, DC: US Govt. Printing Office,

1981–1988; DHHS publication nos. (PHS)81-1564, (PHS)82-1567, (PHS)85-1578, (PHS)86-1582, (PHS)86-1584, (PHS)86-1588, (PHS)87-1592, (PHS)88-1594. (Vital and health statistics; series 10.)

8. Kurata JH, Corboy E. Current peptic ulcer time trends: an epidemiological profile. J Clin Gastroenterol 1988; 10:259–68.

9. National Center for Health Statistics. Detailed diagnoses and surgical procedures for patients discharged from short-stay hospitals: United States, 1977, 1979, 1983–1986. Washington, DC: U.S. Govt. Printing Office, 1979–1988; DHHS publication nos. (PHS)79-1272, (PHS)82-1274-1, (PHS)85-1743, (PHS)86-1747, (PHS)87-1751, (PHS)88-1756. (Vital and health statistics; series 13.)

10. National Center for Health Statistics. Detailed diagnoses and procedures: National Hospital Discharge Survey, 1987. Washington, DC, 1989; DHHS publication no. (PHS)89-1761. (Vital and health statistics; series 13.)

11. Kurata JH, Elashoff JD, Haile BM, Honda GD. A reappraisal of time trends in ulcer disease: factors related to changes in ulcer hospitalization and mortality rates. Am J Public Health 1983; 73:1066–72.

12. National Center for Health Statistics. Vital statistics of the United States, Vol. II: Mortality, part A, 1984–1986. Washington, DC: U.S. Govt. Printing Office, 1987–1988; DHHS publication nos. (PHS)87-1122, (PHS)88-1101, (PHS)88-1122.

13. National Center for Health Statistics. Births, marriages, divorces, and deaths for September 1989. Washington, DC: U.S. Govt. Printing Office, 1989:13. (Monthly vital statistics report, vol. 38, no. 9, Dec. 26, 1989.)

14. Grossman MI. Peptic ulcer. In: A guide to the practicing physician. Chicago Yearbook Medical Publishers, 1981:18.

15. Harrison A, Elashoff J, Grossman MI. Cigarette smoking and ulcer disease. In: The Surgeon General's report on smoking and health. US Department of Health, Education and Welfare, Public Health Service, 1979:9–21.

16. McCarthy DM. Smoking and ulcers—time to quit [Editorial]. N Engl J Med 1984; 311:726–8.

17. Hammond EC. Smoking in relation to the death rates of 1 million men and women. In: Haenszel W, ed. Epidemiological approaches to the study of cancer and other chronic diseases. National Cancer Institute Monograph No. 19. Bethesda: US Public Health Service, 1966:127–204.

18. Kahn HA. The Dorn study of smoking and mortality among U.S. veterans: report on 8½ years of observation. In: Haenszel W, ed. Epidemiological approaches to the study of cancer and other chronic diseases. National Cancer Institute Monograph No. 19. Bethesda: US Public Health Service, 1966:1–125.

19. Doll R, Peto R. Mortality in relation to smoking: 20 years' observations on male British doctors. Br Med J 1976; ii:1525–36.

20. Ross AHL, Smith MA, Anderson JR, Small WP. Late mortality after surgery for peptic ulcer. N Engl J Med 1982; 307:519–22.

21. Kurata JH, Elashoff JD, Nogawa AN, Haile BM. Sex and smoking differences in duodenal ulcer mortality. Am J Public Health 1986; 76:700–2.

22. Paffenbarger RS, Wing AL, Hyde RT. Chronic disease in former college students. Am J Epidemiol 1974; 100:307–15.

23. Stemmermann GN, Marcus EB, Buist AS, MacLean CJ. Relative impact of smoking and

reduced pulmonary function on peptic ulcer risk: a prospective study of Japanese men in Hawaii. Gastroenterology 1989; 96:1419–24.

24. Friedman GD, Siegelaub AB, Seltzer CC. Cigarettes, alcohol, coffee and peptic ulcer. N Engl J Med 1974; 290:469–73.

25. Ostensen H, Gudmundsen TE, Ostensen M, Burhol PG, Bonnevie O. Smoking, alcohol, coffee, and familial factors: any associations with peptic ulcer disease? Scand J Gastroenterol 1985; 20:1227–35.

26. Kurata J, Abbey D, Nogawa A, Phillips R. Lifestyle and peptic ulcer disease in a Seventh-Day Adventist population [Abstract]. Am J Gastroenterol 1989; 84:1164.

27. Piper DW, McIntosh JH, Greig M, Shy CM. Environmental factors and chronic gastric ulcer: a case control study of the association of smoking, alcohol, and heavy analgesic ingestion with the exacerbation of chronic gastric ulcer. Scand J Gastroenterol 1982; 17:721–9.

28. Piper DW, Nasiry R, McIntosh J, Shy CM, Pierce J, Byth K. Smoking, alcohol, analgesics, and chronic duodenal ulcer: a controlled study of habits before first symptoms and before diagnosis. Scand J Gastroenterol 1984; 19:1015–21.

29. McIntosh JH, Byth K, Piper DW. Environmental factors in aetiology of chronic gastric ulcer: a case control study of exposure variables before the first symptoms. Gut 1985; 26:789–98.

30. McIntosh JH, Fung CS, Berry G, Piper DW. Smoking, nonsteroidal anti-inflammatory drugs, and acetaminophen in gastric ulcer: a study of associations and of the effects of previous diagnosis on exposure patterns. Am J Epidemiol 1988; 128:761–70.

31. Petitti DB, Friedman GD, Kahn W. Peptic ulcer disease and the tar and nicotine yield of currently smoked cigarettes. J Chronic Dis 1982; 35:503–7.

32. Heuman R, Larsson J, Norrby S. Perforated duodenal ulcer—long-term results following simple closure. Acta Chir Scand 1983; 149:77–81.

33. Doll R, Jones F, Pygott F. Effect of smoking on the production and maintenance of gastric and duodenal ulcers. Lancet 1958; i:657–62.

34. Peterson WL, Sturdevant RAL, Frankl HD, et al. Healing of duodenal ulcer with an antacid regimen. N Engl J Med 1977; 297:341–5.

35. Lam SK, Lam KC, Lai CK, Yeung CK, Yam LYC, Wong WS. Treatment of duodenal ulcer with antacid and sulpirimide. Gastroenterology 1979; 76:315–22.

36. Gugler R, Rohner H-G, Kratochvil P, et al. Effect of smoking on duodenal ulcer healing with cimetidine and oxmetidine. Gut 1982; 23:866–71.

37. Sonnenberg A, Muller-Lissner SA, Vogel E, et al. Predictors of duodenal ulcer healing and relapse. Gastroenterology 1981; 81:1061–7.

38. Nicholson PA. A multicenter international controlled comparison of two dosage regimes of misoprostol and cimetidine in the treatment of duodenal ulcer in out-patients. Dig Dis Sci 1985; 30:171S–7S.

39. Rachmilewitz D, Chapman JW, Nicholson PA. A multicenter international controlled comparison of two dosage regimens of misoprostol with cimetidine in treatment of gastric ulcer in outpatients. Dig Dis Sci 1986; 31:75S–80S.

40. Korman MG, Hansky J, Eaves ER, Schmidt GT. Influence of cigarette smoking on healing and relapse in duodenal ulcer disease. Gastroenterology 1983; 85:871–4.

41. Sontag S, Graham DY, Belsito A, et al. Cimetidine, cigarette smoking, and recurrence of duodenal ulcer. N Engl J Med 1984; 311:689–93.

42. Levy M. Aspirin use in patients with major upper gastrointestinal bleeding and peptic ulcer disease. N Engl J Med 1974; 290:1158–62.

43. Piper DW, McIntosh JH, Ariotti DE, Fonton BH, MacLennan R. Analgesic ingestion and chronic peptic ulcer. Gastroenterology 1981; 80:427–32.

44. Duggan JM, Dobson AJ, Johnson H, Fahey P. Peptic ulcer and non-steroidal anti-inflammatory agents. Gut 1986; 27:929–33.

45. Coggon D, Langman MJS, Spiegelhalter D. Aspirin, paracetamol, and haematemesis and melaena. Gut 1982; 23:340–4.

46. Faulkner G, Prichard P, Somerville K, Langman MJS. Aspirin and bleeding peptic ulcers in the elderly. Br Med J 1988; 297:1311–3.

47. Aspirin Myocardial Infarction Study Research Group. A randomized, controlled trial of aspirin in persons recovered from myocardial infarction. JAMA 1980; 243:661–9.

48. Kurata JH, Abbey DE. The effect of chronic aspirin use on duodenal and gastric ulcer hospitalizations. J Clin Gastroenterol 1990; 12:260–6.

49. Steering Committee of the Physicians' Health Study Research Group. Final report on the aspirin component of the ongoing Physicians' Health Study. N Engl J Med 1989; 321:129–35.

50. Soll AH, Kurata J, McGuigan JE. Ulcers, nonsteroidal antiinflammatory drugs, and related matters. Gastroenterology 1989; 96:561–8.

51. Langman MJS. Epidemiologic evidence on the association between peptic ulceration and antiinflammatory drug use. Gastroenterology 1989; 96:640–6.

52. McCarthy DM. Nonsteroidal antiinflammatory drug-induced ulcers: management by traditional therapies. Gastroenterology 1989; 96:662–74.

53. Kurata JH. Ulcer epidemiology: an overview and proposed research framework. Gastroenterology 1989; 96:569–80.

54. Bloom BS. Risk and cost of gastrointestinal side effects associated with nonsteroidal anti-inflammatory drugs. Arch Intern Med 1989; 149:1019–22.

55. Carson JL, Strom BL, Soper KA, West SL, Morse ML. The association of nonsteroidal anti-inflammatory drugs with upper gastrointestinal tract bleeding. Arch Intern Med 1987; 147:85–8.

56. Beard K, Walker AM, Perera DR, Jick H. Nonsteroidal anti-inflammatory drugs and hospitalization for gastroesophageal bleeding in the elderly. Arch Intern Med 1987; 147:1621–3.

57. Jick H, Feld AD, Perera DR. Certain nonsteroidal anti-inflammatory drugs and hospitalization for upper gastrointestinal bleeding. Pharmacotherapy 1985; 5:280–4.

58. Levy M, Miller DR, Kaufman DW, et al. Major upper gastrointestinal tract bleeding: relation to the use of aspirin and other nonnarcotic analgesics. Arch Intern Med 1988; 148:281–5.

59. Somerville K, Faulkner G, Langman M. Non-steroidal anti-inflammatory drugs and bleeding peptic ulcer. Lancet 1986; i:462–4.

60. Thompson MR. Indomethacin and perforated duodenal ulcer. Br Med J 1980; 280:448.

61. Collier DStJ, Pain JA. Non-steroidal anti-inflammatory drugs and peptic ulcer formation. Gut 1985; 26:359–63.

62. Jick SS, Perera DR, Walker AM, Jick H. Non-steroidal anti-inflammatory drugs and hospital admission for perforated peptic ulcer. Lancet 1987; ii:380–2.

63. Griffin MR, Ray WA, Schaffner W. Non-steroidal anti-inflammatory drug use and death from peptic ulcer in elderly persons. Ann Intern Med 1988; 109:359–63.

64. Guess HA, West R, Strand LM, et al. Fatal upper gastrointestinal hemorrhage or perforation among users and nonusers of non-steroidal anti-inflammatory drugs in Saskatchewan, Canada, 1983. J Clin Epidemiol 1988; 41:35–45.

65. Conn HO, Blitzer BI. Medical progress: non-association of adrenocorticosteroid therapy and peptic ulcer. N Engl J Med 1976; 294:473–9.

66. Messer J, Reitman D, Sachs HS, et al. Association of adrenocorticosteroid therapy and peptic ulcer disease. N Engl J Med 1983; 309:21–4.

67. Conn HO, Poynard T. Adrenocorticosteroid administration and peptic ulcer: a critical analysis. J Chronic Dis 1985; 38:457–68.

68. Kurata JH, Elashoff JD, Grossman MI. Inadequacy of the literature on the relationship between drugs, ulcers, and gastrointestinal bleeding [Editorial]. Gastroenterology 1982; 82:373–6.

69. Kurata JH, Koch GG, Nogawa AN. Comparison of ranitidine and cimetidine ulcer maintenance therapy. J Clin Gastroenterol 1987; 9:644–50.

70. Cohen S, Booth GH Jr. Gastric acid secretion and lower esophageal-sphincter pressure in response to coffee and caffeine. N Engl J Med 1975; 293:897–9.

71. Lenz HJ, Ferrari-Taylor J, Isenberg JI. Wine and five percent ethanol are potent stimulants of gastric acid secretion in humans. Gastroenterology 1983; 85:1082–7.

72. Peterson WL, Barnett C, Walsh JH. Effect of intragastric infusions of ethanol and wine on serum gastrin concentration and gastric acid secretion. Gastroenterology 1986; 91:1390–5.

73. Kasanen A, Forsstrom J. Social stress and living habits in the etiology of peptic ulcer. Ann Med Intern Fenn 1966; 55:13–22.

74. Jorgensen TG, Gyntelberg F. Occurrence of peptic ulcer disease in Copenhagen males, age 40–59. Dan Med Bull 1976; 23:23–8.

75. Engeset A, Lygren T, Idsoe R. The incidence of peptic ulcer among alcohol abusers and non-abusers. Quart J Stud Alcohol 1963; 24:622–6.

76. Langman MJS, Cooke AR. Gastric and duodenal ulcer and their associated diseases. Lancet 1976; i:680–3.

77. Lawrence JS. Dietetic and other methods in the treatment of peptic ulcer. Lancet 1952; i:482–5.

78. Evans PRC. Value of strict dieting, drugs, and robaden in peptic ulceration. Br Med J 1954; i:612–6.

79. Truelove SC. Stilboestrol, phenobarbitone, and diet in chronic duodenal ulcer. Br Med J 1960; ii:559–66.

80. Doll R. Medical treatment of gastric ulcer. Scot Med J 1964; 9:183–96.

81. Buchman E, Kaung DT, Dolan K, Knapp RN. Unrestricted diet in the treatment of duodenal ulcer. Gastroenterology 1969; 56:1016–20.

82. Ippoliti AF, Maxwell VA, Isenberg JI. The effect of various forms of milk on gastric acid secretion. Studies in patients with duodenal ulcer and normal subjects. Ann Intern Med 1976; 84:286–9.

83. Kumar N, Kumar A, Broor SL, Vij JC, Anand BS. Effect of milk on patients with duodenal ulcers. Br Med J 1986; 293:666.

84. Sonnenberg A. Dietary salt and gastric ulcer. Gut 1986; 27:1138–42.

85. Stemmermann G, Haenszel W, Locke F. Epidemiologic pathology of gastric ulcer and gastric carcinoma among Japanese in Hawaii. J Natl Cancer Inst 1977; 58:13–9.

86. Anonymous. Diet and peptic ulcer [Editorial]. Lancet 1987; ii:80–1.

87. Graham DY, Smith JL, Opekun AR. Spicy food and the stomach: evaluation by videoendoscopy. JAMA 1988; 260:3473–5.

88. Rydning A, Berstad A, Aadland E, Odegaard B. Prophylactic effect of dietary fibre in duodenal ulcer disease. Lancet 1982; ii:736–9.

89. Malhotra SL. A comparison of unrefined wheat and rice diets in the management of duodenal ulcer. Postgrad Med J 1978; 54:6–9.

90. Rydning A, Berstad A. Dietary fiber and peptic ulcer. Scand J Gastroenterol 1986; 21:1–5.

91. Alexander F. The influence of psychologic factors upon gastrointestinal disturbances: General principles, objectives and preliminary results. Psychoanal Quart 1934; 3:501–39.

92. Weiner H, Thaler M, Reiser ME, Mirsky IA. Etiology of duodenal ulcer: relation of specific psychological characteristics to rate of gastric secretion (serum pepsinogen). Psychosom Med 1957; 19:1–10.

93. Mittlemann B, Wolff HG. Emotions and gastroduodenal function: experimental studies on patients with gastritis, duodenitis, and peptic ulcer. Psychosom Med 1942; 4:5–61.

94. Peters MN, Richardson CT. Stressful life events, acid hypersecretion, and ulcer disease. Gastroenterology 1983; 84:114–9.

95. Alp MH, Court JH, Grant AK. Personality pattern and emotional stress in the genesis of gastric ulcer. Gut 1970; 11:773–7.

96. Rose RM, Jenkins CD, Hurst MW. Air traffic controller health change study. Report to Federal Aviation Administration under contract no. FA7 3WA-3211, 1978.

97. Piper DW, Greig M, Shinners J, et al. Chronic gastric ulcer and stress: a comparison of an ulcer population with a control population regarding stressful events over a lifetime. Digestion 1978; 18:303–9.

98. Piper DW, McIntosh JH, Ariotti DE, et al. Life events and chronic duodenal ulcer: a case control study. Gut 1981; 22:1011–7.

99. Thomas J, Greig M, Piper DW. Chronic gastric ulcer and life events. Gastroenterology 1980; 78:905–11.

100. Feldman EJ, Elashoff JD, Samloff IM, Grossman MI. Psychologic stress and duodenal ulcer [letter]. N Engl J Med 1980; 302:1206.

101. McIntosh JH, Nasiry RW, McNeil D, Coates C, Mitchell H, Piper DW. Perception of life event stress in patients with chronic duodenal ulcer. Scand J Gastroenterol 1985; 20:563–8.

102. Adami H-O, Bergstrom R, Nyren O, et al. Is duodenal ulcer really a psychosomatic disease? Scand J Gastroenterol 1987; 22:889–96.

103. Feldman M, Walker P, Green JL, Weingarden K. Life events stress and psychosocial factors in men with peptic ulcer disease: a multidimensional case-controlled study. Gastroenterology 1986; 91:1370–9.

104. Walker P, Luther J, Samloff IM, Feldman M. Life events stress and psychosocial factors in men with peptic ulcer disease. II. Relationships with serum pepsinogen concentrations and behavioral risk factors. Gastroenterology 1988; 94:323–30.

105. Bartlett JG. *Campylobacter pylori*: fact or fancy? Gastroenterology 1988; 94:229–38.

106. Warren JR, Marshall B. Unidentified curved bacilli on gastric epithelium in active chronic gastritis. Lancet 1983; i:1273–5.

107. Blaser M. Gastric campylobacter-like organisms, gastritis, and peptic ulcer disease. Gastroenterology 1987; 93:371–83.

108. Eberhardt R, Kasper G, Dettmer A, Hochter W, Hagena D. Effect of oral bismuth-subsalicylate on *Campylobacter pyloridis* and on duodenal ulcer [Abstract]. Gastroenterology 1987; 92:1379.

109. Niemela S, Karttunen T, Lehtola J. Campylobacter-like organisms in patients with gastric ulcer. Scand J Gastroenterol 1987; 22:487–90.

110. Rauws EAJ, Langenberg W, Houthoff HJ, Zanen HC, Tytgat GNJ. *Campylobacter pyloridis*-associated chronic active antral gastritis. Gastroenterology 1988; 94:33–40.

111. Graham DY. *Campylobacter pylori* and peptic ulcer disease. Gastroenterology 1989; 96:615–25.

112. Dooley CP, Cohen H, Fitzgibbons P, et al. Prevalence of *Helicobacter pylori* infection and histologic gastritis in asymptomatic persons. N Engl J Med 1989; 321:1562–6.

113. Graham DY, Adam E, Klein PD, et al. Comparison of the prevalence of asymptomatic *C. pylori* infection in the United States: effect of age, gender and race [Abstract]. Gastroenterology 1989; 96:A180.

114. Dehesa M, Dooley CP, Cohen H, Fitzgibbons P, Perez-Perez GI, Blaser MJ. High prevalence of *Campylobacter pylori* in an asymptomatic Hispanic population [Abstract]. Gastroenterology 1989; 96:A115.

115. Kaldor J, Tee W, McCarthy P, Watson J, Dwyer B. Immune response to *Campylobacter pyloridis* in patients with peptic ulceration [Letter]. Lancet 1985; i:921.

116. Marshall BJ, Goodwin CS, Warren JR, et al. Prospective double-blind trial of duodenal ulcer relapse after eradication of *Campylobacter pylori*. Lancet 1988; ii:1437–42.

117. Coghlan JG, Gilligan D, Humphries H, et al. *Campylobacter pylori* and recurrence of duodenal ulcers—a 12-month follow-up study. Lancet 1987; ii:1109–11.

118. Lambert JR, Borromeo MG, Korman MG, Hansky J, Eaves ER. Effect of colloidal bismuth (DE-NOL) on healing and relapse of duodenal ulcers—role of *Campylobacter pyloridis* [Abstract]. Gastroenterology 1987; 92:1489.

119. Graham DY, Lew GM, Michaletz PA. Randomized controlled trial of the effect of eradication of *C. pylori* on ulcer healing and relapse [Abstract]. Gastroenterology 1989; 96:A181.

120. Martin DF, Montgomery E, Dobek AS, Patrissi GA, Peura DA. *Campylobacter pylori*, NSAIDs and smoking: risk factors for peptic ulcer disease. Am J Gastroenterol 1989; 84:1268–72.

121. Laine L, Marin-Sorensen M, Weinstein WM. Is *Campylobacter pylori* prevalence lower in gastric ulcers because of nonsteroidal antiinflammatory drug use? A prospective evaluation [Abstract]. Gastroenterology 1989; 96:A282.

122. Evans DJ Jr, Evans DG, Lidsky MD, et al. Is NSAID-damaged gastric mucosa more susceptible to *C. pylori* infection? [Abstract]. Gastroenterology 1989; 96:A143.

123. Doll R, Jones FA, Bukatzsch MM. Occupational factors in the aetiology of gastric and duodenal ulcers with an estimate of their incidence in the general population. Medical Research Council, Special Report Series No. 276. HRM Stationery Office, 1951:96.

124. Doll R, Kellock TD. The separate inheritance of gastric and duodenal ulcers. Ann Eugen 1951; 16:231–40.

125. Rotter JI. Peptic ulcer. In: Emery AEH, Rimoin DL, eds. The principles and practice of medical genetics, Vol. 2. Edinburgh: Churchill Livingstone, 1983:863–78.

126. McConnell RB. Peptic ulcer: early genetic evidence–families, twins, and markers. In: Rotter JI, Samloff IM, Rimoin DL, eds. The genetics and heterogeneity of common gastrointestinal disorders. New York: Academic, 1980:31–41.

127. Aird I, Bentall HH, Mehigan JA, Roberts JAF. The blood groups in relation to peptic ulceration and carcinoma of colon, rectum, breast and bronchus. Br Med J 1954; ii:315–21.

128. Langman MJS. Blood groups and alimentary disorders. Clin Gastroenterol 1973; 2:497–506.

129. Samloff IM, Stemmermann GN, Heilbrun LK, Nomura A. Elevated serum pepsinogen I and II levels differ as risk factors for duodenal ulcer and gastric ulcer. Gastroenterology 1986; 90:570–5.

130. Samloff IM, Liebman WM, Panitch NM. Serum group I pepsinogens by radioimmunoassay in control subjects and patients with peptic ulcer. Gastroenterology 1975; 69:83–90.

131. Rotter JI, Sones JQ, Samloff IM, et al. Duodenal ulcer disease associated with elevated serum pepsinogen I. An inherited autosomal dominant disorder. N Engl J Med 1979; 300:63–6.

132. Rotter JI, Petersen G, Samloff IM, et al. Genetic heterogeneity of hyperpepsinogenemic I and normopepsinogenemic I duodenal ulcer disease. Ann Intern Med 1979; 91:372–7.

133. Habibullah CM, Mujahid Ali M, Ishaq M, Prasad R, Pratap B, Saleem Y. Study of duodenal ulcer disease in 100 families using total serum pepsinogen as a genetic marker. Gut 1984; 25:1380–3.

134. Rotter JI, Rubin R, Meyer JH, Samloff IM, Rimoin DL. Rapid gastric emptying—an inherited pathophysiologic defect in duodenal ulcer? [Abstract]. Gastroenterology 1979; 76:1229.

135. Taylor IL, Calam J, Rotter JI, et al. Family studies of hypergastrinemic, hyperpepsinogenemic I duodenal ulcer. Ann Intern Med 1981; 95:421–5.

136. Lamers CBHW, Jansen JBMJ, Rotter JI, Samloff IM. Serum pepsinogen I in hereditary hypergastrinemic peptic ulcer syndromes. In: Kreuning J, Samloff IM, Rotter JI, Eriksson AW, eds. Pepsinogens in man: clinical and genetic advances. New York: Allen R. Liss, 1985:273–81.

3

Biological Rhythms in Gastrointestinal Function and Processes: Implications for Pathogenesis and Treatment of Peptic Ulcer Disease

JOHN G. MOORE

Salt Lake City Veterans Administration Medical Center,
Salt Lake City, Utah

MICHAEL H. SMOLENSKY

University of Texas, School of Public Health and
School of Medicine and Center for Medical and Public
Health Chronobiology, Health Science Center–Houston,
Houston, Texas

I. INTRODUCTION

This chapter explores the significance of biological rhythms (chronobiology) in the mechanisms and treatment of ulcer disease. During the past 20–30 years, 24-hr and seasonal rhythms have been substantiated in a multitude of biological functions and processes [1–3]. Such findings are of clinical significance not only for the diagnosis and treatment of disease, but also for the elucidation of their mechanisms. In this chapter, the basic principles and concepts of medical chronobiology are first presented. Thereafter, the chronobiology and chronotherapeutics of peptic gastroduodenal ulcer disease are discussed in detail.

II. MEDICAL CHRONOBIOLOGY

A. Definitions and Concepts

Chronobiology is that branch of science concerned with the study of biological rhythms and their mechanisms. Biological rhythms are ubiquitous in nature. From an evolutionary perspective, they are believed to represent an aspect of the genetic adaptation of ancestral organisms to predictable changes over time in the external environment resulting, for example, from the regular rotation of the earth about its axis every 24 hr and about the sun each year [2]. Although human bioperiodicities have a genetic basis, their expression may nonetheless be influenced by certain environmental factors [2,4].

Biological rhythms in plants, insects, lower animals, and human beings share several common characteristics [1–3,5]. One characteristic is *oscillatory frequency*. *Circadian* rhythms are bioperiodicities that exhibit one cycle roughly (*circa*) every 24 hr (*dian*). Oscillations that are of shorter duration (less than 20 hr), such as the 60–90-min temporal variability in the secretion of hormones from endocrine glands or in sleep stage progression during rest, are term ultradian rhythms. Finally, oscillations that are longer than 28 hr, such as those of 7, 28–30, or 365 days are termed infradian rhythms. Ultradian, circadian, and infradian rhythms are manifested at all levels of biological organization as well as by individual processes and functions.

A second characteristic of rhythms is staging, the occurrence of a peak and trough with respect to a given time scale, be it 24 hr, month (e.g., menstrual cycle), or year. Within each biological time scale there exists a precise relationship between the staging of each of the multitude of rhythmic phenomena. This constitutes a biological time structure and represents an aspect of our biological efficiency [2,6–8]. The staging of circadian rhythms is set to support day–night patterns in energy expenditure associated with the differential requirements of activity and sleep. Although the temporal alternation of activity and rest during each 24 hr does not cause circadian rhythms, the periods according to clock time during which a person sleeps and is active do determine their staging [4]. Thus, individuals who consistently work day shifts and sleep at night exhibit a nearly opposite staging of their circadian rhythms compared to those who consistently work night shifts and sleep during the day [9].

In human beings, the sleep–wake routine during the 24 hr is a powerful *zeitgeber* ("time giver") or synchronizer of circadian clocks and rhythms. In the majority of humans, the resetting of biological clocks following an abrupt change in the sleep–activity schedule is not immediate; instead, several days may be required for their complete resetting [9,10]. This fact is especially apparent in travelers transported by jet aircraft over several time zones as well as in workers on rotating shifts whose normal nocturnal sleep period is disrupted when they work the night shift. In both situations, a "jet-lag" type of phenomenon is experienced due to a disorganization of the phase relationships between circadian and perhaps other period rhythms. The synchronization schedule of patients can be ascertained by determining the clock times of activity and sleep during the 24 hr and the nature of the work routine— regular day or rotating shift work. This information is critical for correctly utilizing findings from research in medical chronobiology.

A third characteristic of biological rhythms is amplitude. *Amplitude* refers to the extent of predictable variability ascribable to rhythmicity; it is equal to the difference between the values found at the time of the peak and those at the trough of a given bioperiodicity. Some rhythms are of relatively small amplitude. This is the case for the circadian variation in body temperature and heart rate in healthy persons. Other circadian rhythms are of quite high amplitude. This is exemplified by the 24-hr change in serum hydrocortisone or adrenaline concentration and lymphocyte numbers [2,5].

Finally, a fourth characteristic of rhythms is the mesor. The *mesor* is the baseline or mean level around which predictable-in-time variation occurs with respect to a given bioperiodicity.

Differences in health status and age may be associated with differences in the characteristics of biological rhythms. The amplitude and/or mesor of the circadian rhythm in airways patency typically differs between asthmatic and nonasthmatic persons and between young and elderly individuals [11]. In asthmatic patients, the amplitude of the 24-hr bioperiodicity is generally markedly enhanced and the mean level (mesor) lowered in comparison to those with normal lung function. In patients suffering from hypertension, the 24-hr mean level and/or amplitude of the rhythm in blood pressure are increased over the reference values of healthy persons [12].

B. Biological Rhythms and Disease

Since bodily functions and processes are rather precisely organized as rhythms, it is not surprising that there are temporal patterns in when the symptoms of disease worsen and when the onset of morbid events occurs. One branch of chronobiology, chronopathology, is concerned with biological rhythms in the manifestations of illnesses and symptoms and their underlying mechanisms [2]. Some chronopathologies can be demonstrated only through population studies. This is the case, for example, for myocardial or cerebrovascular infarction [2,13,14,15], and cerebral hemorrhage [2], in which the occurrence of the attacks in a given individual may be limited generally to just one or two events per lifetime (Fig. 1). On the other hand, the symptoms and/or exacerbation of chronic diseases tend to be recurrent over time in individuals. With these diseases, temporal patterns can be tracked by means of patient diaries or patient self-assessments done several times daily over many days [16–19]. In this manner, circadian rhythms have been substantiated in the symptoms of rheumatoid arthritis (with pain and stiffness typically worse at the commencement of daily activity), osteoarthritis (with pain generally worse toward the end of daily activity), Prinzmetal's variant angina (with ST segment anomaly most frequent overnight and exercise capability most limited in the morning), allergic rhinitis (with stuffy and blocked nose typically worse upon awaking), and asthma (with exacerbation of wheezing or coughing overnight), among others [2,16–22]. The occurrence and exacerbation of some illnesses may also exhibit a menstrual rhythm in women (e.g., epilepsy and asthma [2,23,24]) and a seasonal rhythm in men and women (e.g., asthma and cardiovascular and ulcer disase [2,25,26]), in addition to a circa-

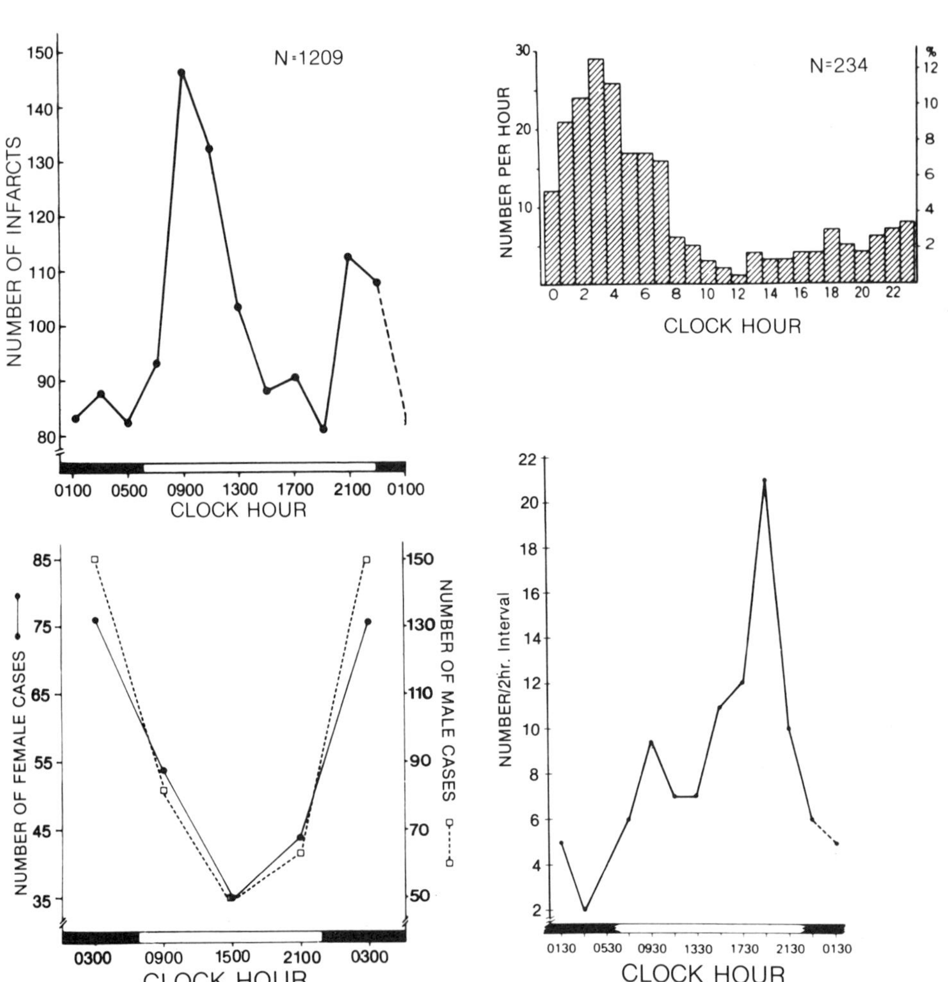

FIGURE 1 Examples of human circadian chronopathologies of diseases of the cardiovascular system. The vulnerability of populations of human beings to the morbid events of myocardial infarction (upper left), cerebral infraction (lower left), ST-segment anomaly of Prinzmetal's varient angina (upper right), and spontaneous intracerebral hemorrhage (lower right) is not random over the 24 hr. Darkened areas of abscissa in some figures indicate times of sleep in the patient samples. (Examples drawn from Reinberg and Smolensky [2], Marshall [15], and Kuroiwa [21].)

dian pattern. For certain diseases, the seasonal variation in incidence may represent, at least to some extent, environmental influences that vary over the year rather than a seasonal change in physiological status due to circannual (about 1-year) endogenous-in-origin rhythms, although this remains to be substantiated.

Bioperiodicities in the symptom intensity and morbidity of human diseases define susceptibility—resistance rhythms in patients [1,2,27,28]. These arise from rhythms in those bioprocesses and functions constituting the mechanism(s) of the given disease. For example, the noctural exacerbation of asthma in day-active patients is one example of a circadian susceptibility—resistance rhythm. The nighttime prevalence of symptoms is due to the specific staging of several 24-hr bioperiodicities in biochemical and physiological processes, such as in airways patency and airways hyperreactivity to chemical mediators (histamine and acetylcholine) and antigen (house dust) and also in adrenaline and hydrocortisone among others [29,30]. As discussed later in this chapter, the nocturnal pain and flaring of gastroduodenal ulcer disease constitutes, also, a circadian susceptibility—resistance rhythm. Overall, circadian and other temporal patterns in the susceptibility of predisposed persons to the breakthrough of disease and/or its exacerbation suggest that the requirement for medication varies in time.

C. The Chronopharmacology and Chronotherapeutics of Medications

Chronopharmacology is the study of biological rhythm influences on medications and also the effect of medications on the characteristics of biological rhythms. Chronopharmacokinetics (or chronokinetics) refers to administration-time-dependent differences in the absorption, distribution, metabolism, and elimination of medications due to rhythms in biological functions and processes [2,31–33]. Results of numerous investigations indicate that the pharmacokinetics and/or effects of various classes of medications differ, sometimes markedly, as a function of their administration time—morning, midday, or evening, for example.

A number of medications have been shown to exhibit significant variation in their pharmacokinetics with respect to the biological time of drug administration (Fig. 2). This is the case for certain theophylline drugs (especially in children) [34–36], nonsteroid anti-inflammatory drugs [37–40], antihistamines [41–43], cardiovascular drugs [22,44], and synthetic corticoid drugs [45–47], for example. The chronokinetics of medications cannot be explained by the timing or content of meals or day–night alternation in posture. In principle, chronopharmacology is concerned not only with biological rhythm-dependent influences on drug pharmacokinetics but on pharmacodynamic effects as well, whether they be desirable (in terms of chronoeffectiveness) or undesirable (in terms of chronotoxicology) [2,31,32]. The ultimate goal is to devise chronotherapies, that is, to schedule the delivery of medication in relation to biological rhythms to achieve an enhancement of desired effects and/or to control or avert undesired ones.

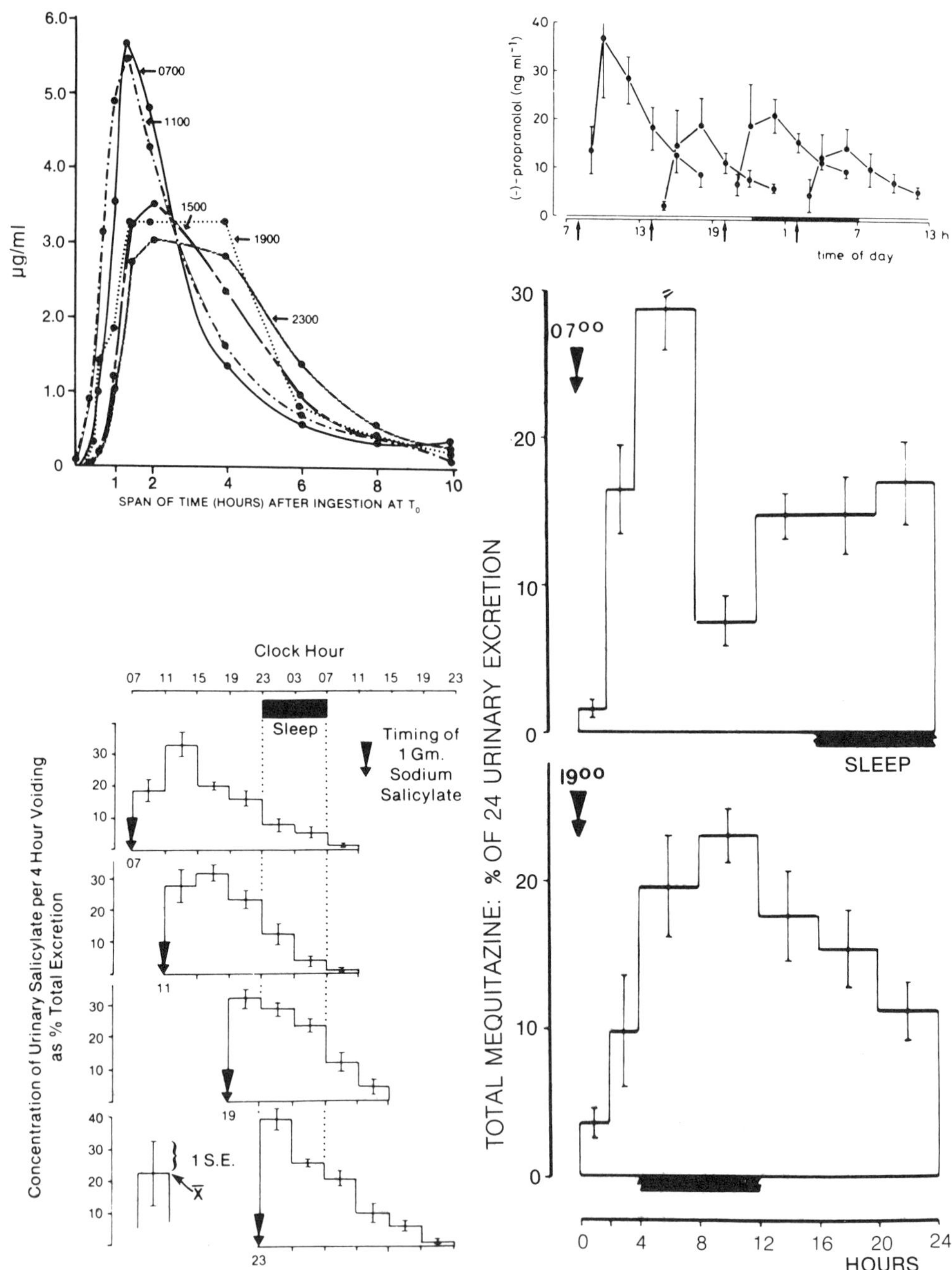
0700
1100
1500
1900
2300
µg/ml
SPAN OF TIME (HOURS) AFTER INGESTION AT T₀
(-) - propranolol (ng ml⁻¹)
time of day
h
Clock Hour
Sleep
Timing of
1 Gm.
Sodium
Salicylate
Concentration of Urinary Salicylate per 4 Hour Voiding
as % Total Excretion
1 S.E.
X̄
07
11
19
23
07°°
1900
SLEEP
TOTAL MEQUITAZINE: % OF 24 URINARY EXCRETION
HOURS

III. THE CHRONOBIOLOGY
OF PEPTIC GASTRODUODENAL ULCER DISEASE

Peptic gastroduodenal ulcer disease is a common disorder, affecting about one in ten persons at some time during their lifetime [48]. It has long been recognized that the disease is characterized by rhythmicity, with circadian and circannual patterns of symptom expression [2,49–52]. Indeed, Moynihan, an Irish surgeon, described the circadian pattern in the pain of ulcer disease by 1912 [49]. During the past two decades, an impressive body of evidence has accumulated to support the role of chronobiological factors in the pathogenesis and treatment of this disorder [52]. For example, circadian rhythms have been detected in intestinal functions in humans and animals, including blood flow to the gut [53], small intestinal mucosal function [54,55], epithelial cell turnover rate [56], susceptibility to experimentally induced upper gastrointestinal ulceration [57–62], gastric mucosal resistance to damage [62], and gastric acid secretion [62–65]. Rhythmic changes in gastrointestinal function in health and disease are ubiquitous [65]. The role of circadian rhythms in gut function as well as their alterations in disease is of intense scientific interest currently [65]. Herein, circannual and circadian variations in gut function are reviewed not only in relation to experimental and clinical ulcer disease, but also with respect to optimization of H_2-receptor antagonist medications.

A. Circannual Rhythmicity in Peptic Ulcer Disease

The seasonality of peptic ulcer disease, with either fall and winter or spring and fall peaks in frequency of newly diagnosed or recurrent ulcer craters, is a long-held belief [66]. However, evidence in support of such seasonality is conflicting, and this may be due to differences in the methods used by various investigators. The proper study of seasonality in peptic ulcer disease requires the very frequent use of fiberoptic endoscopy for ulcer verification for several consecutive years in a given cohort of participants. In a large retrospective study, no significant seasonal variation was observed over a 3-year period in 882 endoscopically diagnosed gastric and duodenal ulcer craters [67]. In a more rigidly controlled prospective study (Fig. 3), a statistically significant increase in active ulcerations was observed during the months of Septem-

---

FIGURE 2 Circadian chronokinetics of orally ingested medications in diurnally active healthy persons. In all examples, single identical doses were ingested at the designated clock hours with control of meal contents and timing. Shown are the chronokinetics of nonsustained-release indomethacin (upper right) and propranolol (upper left) based on frequent blood samplings and the chronokinetics of sodium salicylate (lower left) and the antihistamine mequitazine (lower right) based on frequent urine samplings. Darkened areas of abscissa in some figures indicate times of sleep in the participants studied. (Examples taken from Clench et al. [37], Reinberg et al. [40,43], and Lemmer and Langner [44].)

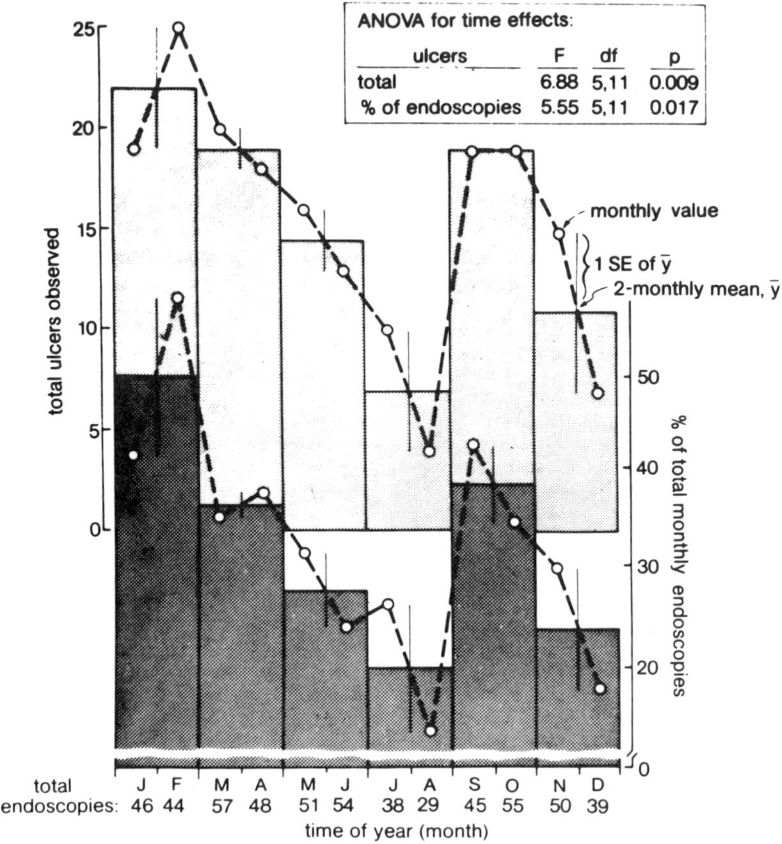

FIGURE 3 ANOVA summary of 50 ulcer patients followed for 1–5 years with serial endoscopies. An average of 5.6 endoscopies/patient were performed. Upper graph reveals total number of ulcers observed monthly. Lower graph indicates the number of ulcers observed as a percent of the total number of endoscopies performed monthly over the circannual period. Statistically significant increases in ulcer craters were observed in the months of February and September. (Reproduced and redrawn from Halberg et al. [68] with permission.)

ber and February [50]. This latter study was conducted on a group of 50 ulcer patients followed for 1–5 years with repeated examinations (average of 5.6 endoscopies per patient per year) during active and inactive phases of their disease. In addition, the same group of investigators documented significant fall and springtime recurrences of ulcer disease in a group of 10 patients subjected to routine endoscopy every 3 months during an 8-year span [51]. Larger, prospectively designed, geographically separated, and endoscopically controlled studies of the type reported by Gibinski and collaborators [51,52], with the data analyzed by appropriate objective statistical techniques designed for rhythm detection and description, are required before the seasonality of ulcer disease can be more firmly established [68]. Too, the mechanisms underlying, for example, seasonal patterns in weather, alcohol, and food consumption and/or circannual (about 1-year) rhythms in endogenous bioprocesses remains to be elucidated. Finally, the significance of seasonal patterns of ulcer disease in individual patients in terms of their clinical management remains to be explored.

B. Circadian Rhythmicity in Gastroduodenal Ulceration

Peptic gastroduodenal ulceration is conceptualized to be a result of an imbalance between those endogenous factors and exogenous agents that are aggressive and thus detrimental to the integrity of the gut and those that are protective. The most aggressive endogenous factor is gastric hydrochloric acid; its presence is considered sine qua non for the development of ulcer disease. Indeed, the no acid—no ulcer dictum, attributed to Schwarz in 1910 [69], is central to the rationale underlying medical and surgical treatment of the disorder today. Our understanding of the control of acid secretion has vastly increased over the past two decades, and much has been learned of the difference in acid secretory patterns in health and disease. Yet relatively little attention has been given to the investigation of rhythmic patterns in acid secretion, primarily because of the prolonged periods of study required. The recent introduction of H_2-receptor antagonist medications has stimulated interest in rhythmic patterns of gastric acid secretion. Current advances in the technological development of biomedical instrumentation has facilitated investigations of this nature.

1. Circadian Rhythmicity in Acid Secretion

Significant circadian variation in basal gastric acid secretion was initially documented in studies on healthy men [63–65,70–72]. Figure 4 shows the circadian pattern of acid secretion in 14 healthy men, and Figure 5 presents the pattern for 21 men with active duodenal ulcer disease. Both groups were studied in an identical and standardized manner using identical methods. All participants followed a routine of diurnal activity alternating with nocturnal sleep. During the 24-hr studies, food intake was controlled, so all data were obtained while participants were in the fasting state.

Visual inspection of the two curves reveals a remarkable similarity in the 24-hr temporal pattern of acid secretion between the groups, with evening peak and morning trough levels. Apparent, too, is the difference in the mean level of acid secretion, it being higher in the ulcer group, an expected and long-standing observation in such patients. The circadian rhythm in gastric acidity is not due to meal timings or contents, because studies were conducted on fasting participants. The data shown in Figure 4 were obtained under very precisely controlled conditions; subjects were given a control meal 8 hr before the commencement of their 24-hr study, and no nourishment (except drinking water ad libitum) was allowed during the ensuing 24

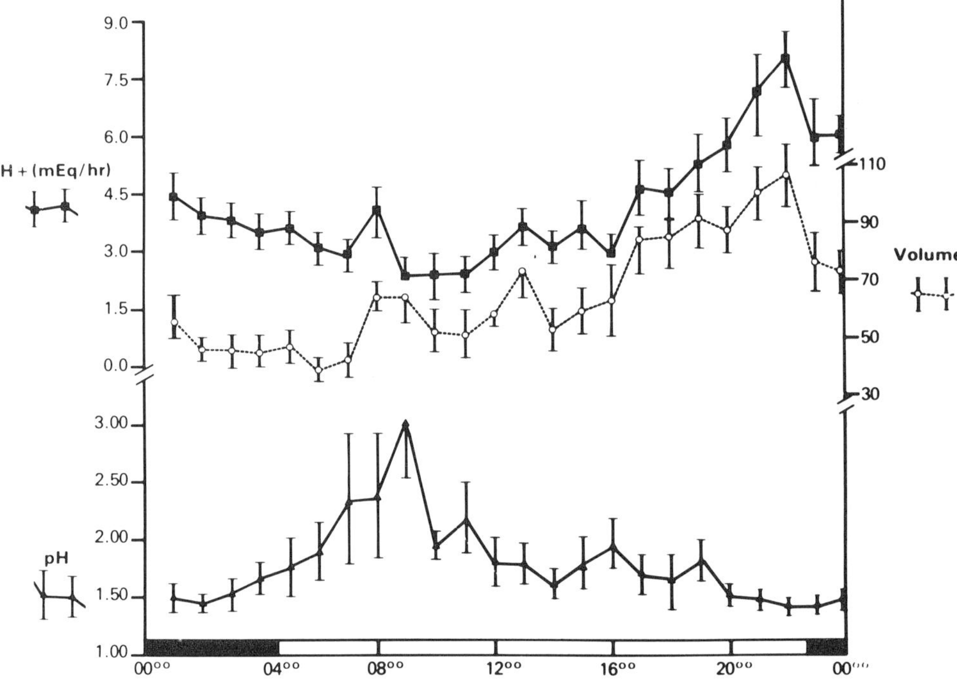

No. Subjects	Measurement	p-value	Percent Rhythm	Acrophase (95% CL)
14	H + (mEq/hr)	0.000000	25.90	-326° (-321° -331°)
14	volume(m/hr)	0.000000	22.03	-292° (-286° -298°)
14	pH, hourly	0.000000	12.31	-153° (-145° -161°)

P = probability of hypothesis amplitude = 0

Percent Rhythm = percentage of variability accounted for by cosine curse

95% CL = conservative confidence limits derived from cosine ellipse

FIGURE 4 Relationship of basal acid secretion (total H^+ in mEq/hr), volume (mL/hr), and gastric pH in relation to clock time in a group of healthy male subjects. (Reproduced with permission from Moore and Englert [63].)

hr, during which gastric contents were collected at hourly intervals and measured for pH and total acid output.

Figure 6 presents the population-mean cosinor statistical summary of the acid secretory data [5,73,74]. This statistical program allows for more precise character-ization of important rhythm parameters: the mesor (a 24-hr time series mean), acrophase (the peak time referenced to local midnight), and amplitude (one-half the

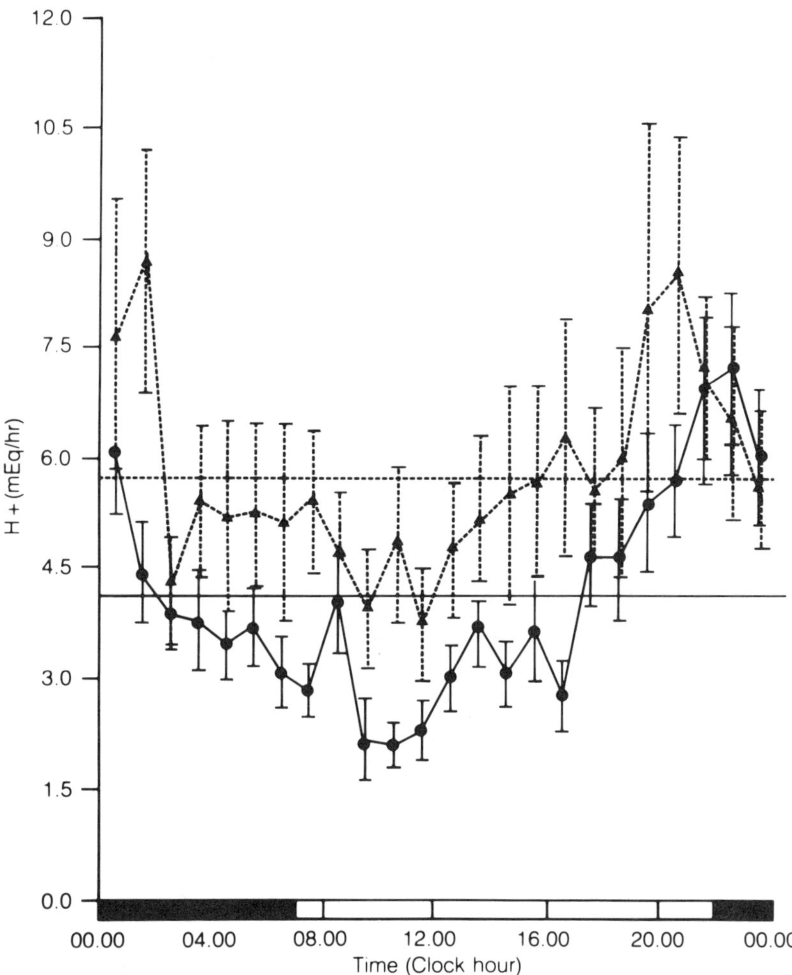

FIGURE 5 Twenty-four-hour gastric acidity (H^+) in 14 healthy male volunteers (filled circles) and 21 male patients with active ulcer disease (filled triangles). Each point represents mean ± SEM values. Note the low morning and high evening rates of secretion in both groups. Dashed line represents mean H^+ secretory rate (5.76 ± 0.98 mEq/hr) for the ulcer group; straight line represents mean H^+ secretory rate for the healthy group (4.12 ± 0.40 mEq/hr). (Reproduced with permission from Moore and Halberg [64].)

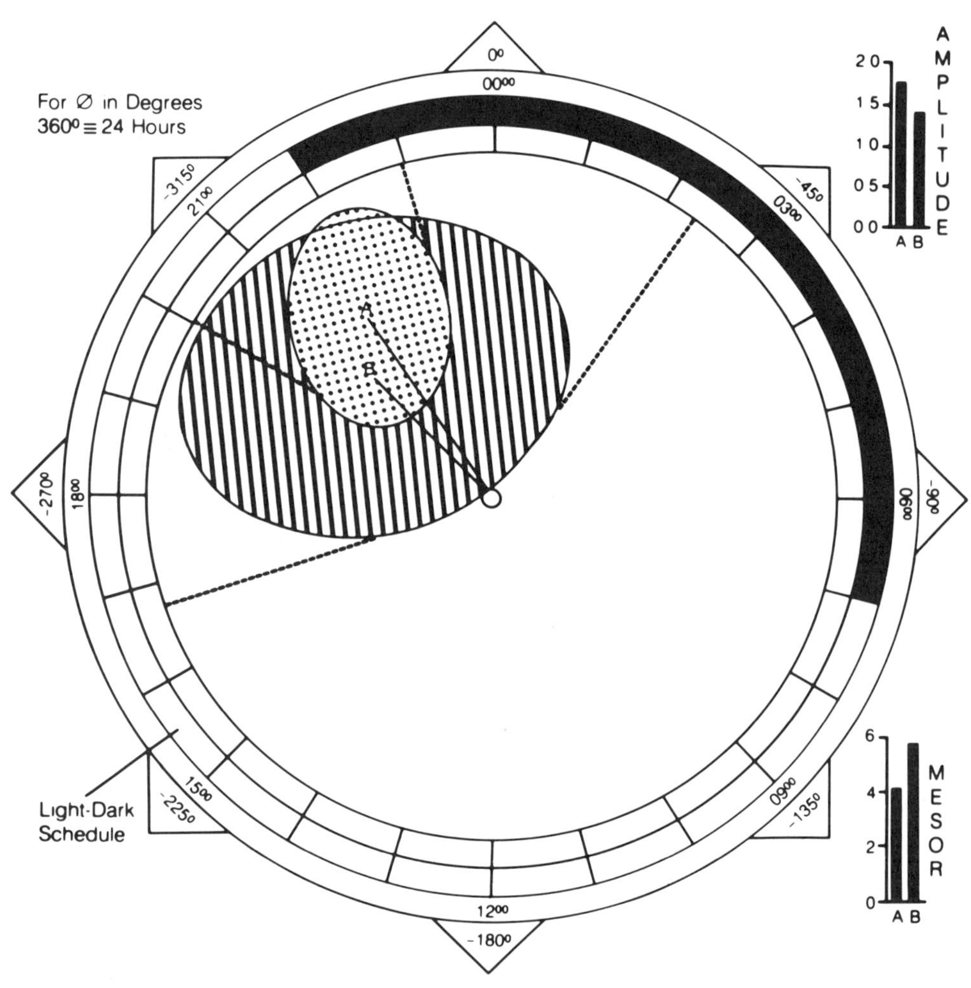

Key To Ellipses	P	PR	No. Obs.	Mesor	SE	Amplitude (95% CL)		Acrophase (∅) (95% CL)	
A. Health	<0.001	38	14	4.12	0.40	1.78	(0.97 2.61)	−326° (−300	−345)
B. Ulcer	0.034	33	21	5.76	0.98	1.38	(0.09 2.72)	−316° (−251	−35)

P = Probability of hypothesis amplitude = 0; No. Obs. = Number of observations
PR = Percent rhythm (percentage of variability accounted for by cosine curve)
95% CL = Conservative 95% confidence limits derived from cosinor ellipse

peak-to-trough variability due to bioperiodicity). These endpoints are derived by approximating the data by a cosine function with a period equal to 24.0 hr. Statistical significance of rhythm detection is determined by a test of the amplitude being nonzero in value. When rhythmicity is so documented, the mesor (M), acrophase (ϕ), and amplitude (A) are derived with 95% confidence limits [5,73,74]. The cosinor analyses reveal statistically significant circadian rhythms in basal gastric acidity in both the healthy and ulcer groups. The acrophase and amplitude values are quite similar between the two groups. The large confidence limits exhibited by the ulcer group compared to the healthy group are due to greater variability in the amplitudes and acrophases of the circadian patterns of acid secretion between the individual participants.

In the animal model, circadian rhythmicity in basal gastric acidity has also been demonstrated [59–62, 75]. For example, in the rat, Ventura et al. [62] demonstrated higher acid production during the activity span of the animals as compared to the rest span by using gastric mucosal preparations incubated ex vivo in Ussing-type chambers.

The mechanism underlying the circadian rhythmicity in basal gastric acidity is unknown. It is not associated with rhythmic alterations in serum gastrin, an endogenous hormone known to stimulate acid secretion [70]. However, integrity of the vagal nerve appears necessary, since circadian rhythmicity in basal acid secretion cannot be substantiated in postvagotomy patients exhibiting high levels of acid secretion [76].

2. Circadian Rhythmicity in Factors Affording Gastric Mucosal Protection

In recent years, attention has been directed to the role of defects in factors protective of the gastric mucosa in relation to the pathogenesis of gastroduodenal ulcer disease. Motivation for this is based on observations that more than one-half of all ulcer

---

FIGURE 6 Population-mean cosinors of 24-hr gastric acidity (H^+ in mEq/hr) in 14 healthy volunteers (group A) and 21 patients (group B) with active duodenal ulcer disease. Compare plot with the same data plotted in Figure 5. The two groups are represented by two lines (vectors) originating at center (pole) of plot. Length of vector represents rhythm's amplitude (A). Vector direction indicates rhythm's acrophase (ϕ, peak of rhythm) expressed in degrees with 360° = period of rhythm. Acrophase takes negative sign in clockwise direction. Elliptical or circular region at tip of vector portrays joint confidence region for amplitude and acrophase. Arc described by tangents to region depicts conservative 95% confidence interval for acrophase. Comparison of healthy and ulcer groups reveals significant circadian rhythms of basal gastric acid secretion with similar amplitudes and acrophases. The mean 24-hr (mesor) secretory rate for the ulcer group is significantly higher, and the confidence limits for the acrophase are wider. The outer circular regions from the outside in represent degrees (with 360° = 24 hr), clock hour, sleep–wake schedules in clock-hour and 24-hr, 60-min divisions, respectively. (Reproduced with permission from Moore and Halberg [64].)

H⁺ secretion
µeq/cm²/45min

n. 10   n. 6   n. 11   n. 10   n. 8   n. 10
01⁰⁰   05⁰⁰   09⁰⁰   13⁰⁰   17⁰⁰   21⁰⁰   HALO

single cosinor

key	rats	p°	PR	MESOR (90% CL)	amplitude (90% CL)	acrophase (90% CL)
H⁺	58	.06	31	2.23 (1.89/2.57)	.58 (.09/1.05)	-259° (-195°/324°)

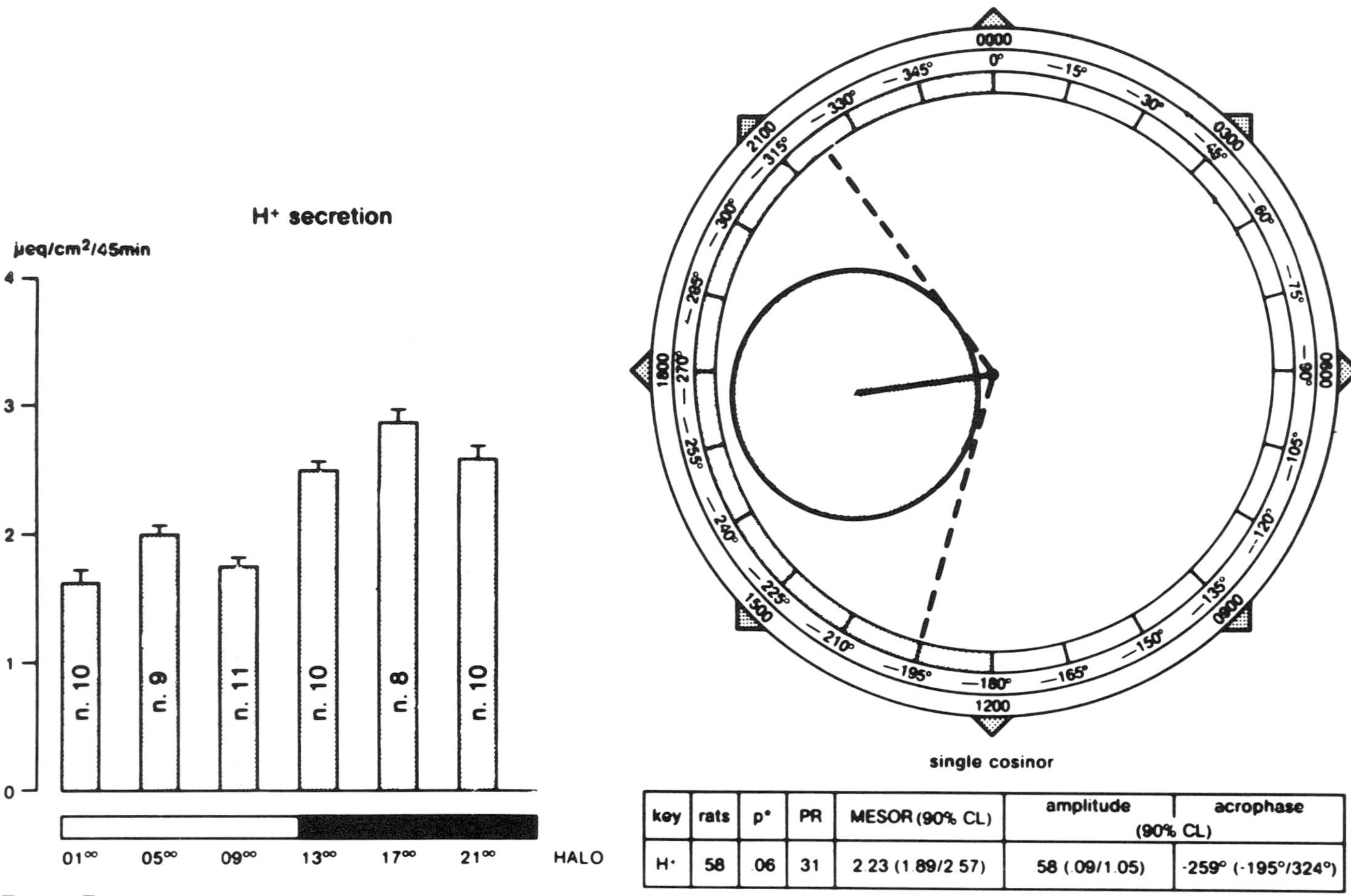

FIGURE 7

patients exhibit normal, or less than normal, gastric acid secretory rates and that a significant percentage of these patients—between 10 and 20% in some series—fail to respond to acid-inhibiting medical or surgical treatments [48]. Those "protective" factors that are currently under examination include gastric mucus and epithelial bicarbonate production; epithelial cell proliferation, migration, and integrity; gastric potential difference (PD) and electrical resistance (R) to ion movement; and gastric tissue prostaglandin concentration, among others [77].

The majority of experimental and clinical studies have examined the relationship of protective factors to the ulcerative process using investigative protocols restricted to single time-point measurements or to at most a few measurements during the daytime hours. Ventura et al. [62], on the other hand, reported day–night differences in PD and R in the rat (Fig. 7). In this study, circadian rhythmicity of nearly statistical significance ($p = .06$) in gastric transmucosal PD and R was detected that, like acid secretion in the same animal model (Fig. 8), peaked during the nocturnal span of rodent activity. These results demonstrate that, at least in the rat model, the factor of mucosal aggression (gastric acid) and protection (PD and R) are circadian rhythmic in normal animals with a common phase (i.e., peak and trough) relationship.

Investigations of factors that are protective to the gastric mucosa, surveying adequate numbers of time points over the circadian time scale, have not been reported in humans. In a limited two-time-point study, Moore and Goo [78] demonstrated that a 1300-mg dose of acetylsalicylic acid (ASA) was more damaging when administered to day-active participants in the morning at 0800 than in the evening at 2000. The endoscopic assessment of mucosal hemorrhages revealed statistically significantly more damage following the morning than the evening drug administration (Fig. 9). These findings, revealing greater morning versus evening ASA-induced mucosal damage, were related neither to a circadian difference in PD (Fig. 10) nor to tissue concentration of 6-keto-PGF$_{1\alpha}$, a metabolite of PGI$_2$ (Fig. 11) [79]. The results of this investigation are inconsistent with the general acceptance that ASA-induced damage is acid-dependent and the observation that morning gastric acid secretory rates are lower than evening ones (Figs. 4 and 5).

FIGURE 7 Basal secretion of H$^+$ in rat gastric mucosa isolated in vitro and incubated in Krebs-Henseliet solution (serosal fluid, buffered at pH 7.4; mucosal fluid, unbuffered). Left: Chronogram, n = number of rats studied at each time point; each datum represents the mean of three experiments conducted on different days. HALO = hours after light onset. Darkened band on abscissa indicates the span of nocturnal activity of the rodents; the white band indicates time of their rest during the 24 hr. Right: Single cosinor analysis. Statistical significance of rhythm detection (rejection of zero-amplitude assumption) is $P = .06$; PR = percent of variability accounted for by the fit of a 24-hr cosine curve; mesor and amplitude are in mEq/(cm^2 · 45 min). The acrophase (peak of rhythm) is given in degrees with reference to local midnight ($360° = 24$ hr; $15° = 1$ hr). (Reproduced with permission from Ventura et al. [62].)

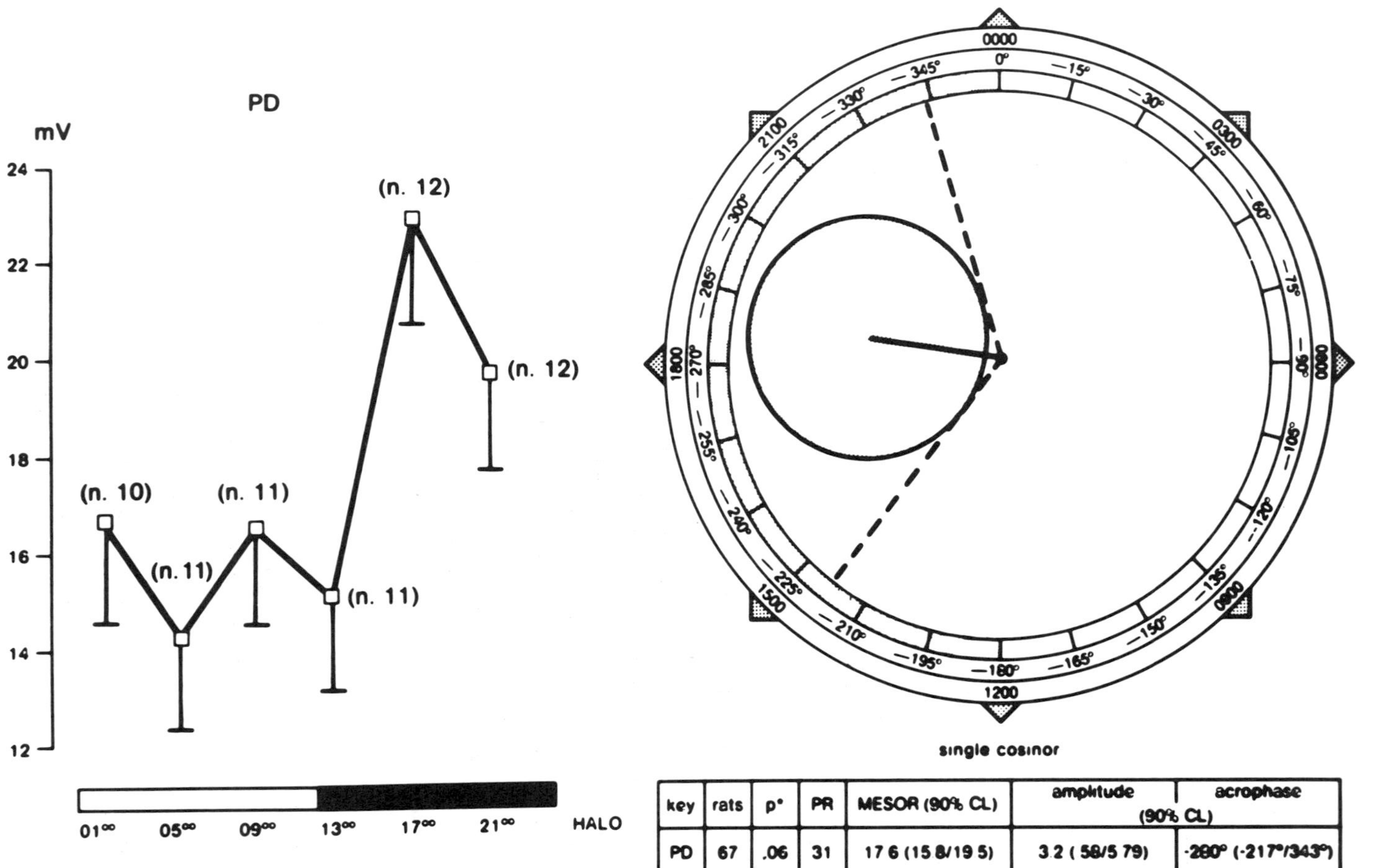

key	rats	p°	PR	MESOR (90% CL)	amplitude (90% CL)	acrophase (90% CL)
PD	67	.06	31	17.6 (15.8/19.5)	3.2 (.58/5.79)	-280° (-217°/343°)

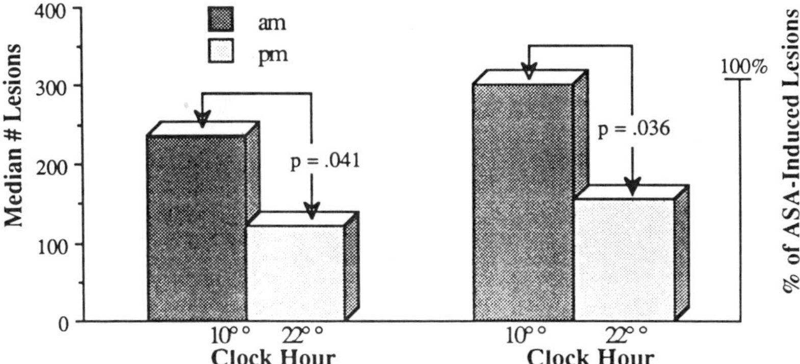

FIGURE 9 Morning and evening aspirin-induced lesions. Effect of time of day (AM: 1000; PM: 2200) on aspirin-induced gastric mucosal lesions (left) and as percent of the total number of lesions produced by the morning administration of ASA (= 100%) (right). For the group, morning administration produced more damage; evening administration produced 37% fewer lesions. Statistical significance of findings between AM and PM tests determined by Wilcoxon signed rank analysis. (Reproduced with permission from Moore and Goo [78].)

The dissociation of the circadian time of greatest acid secretion from that of maximal ASA-induced mucosal damage suggests that the presence of acid alone is not the sole determinant of tissue-induced damage. Moreover, the greater morning-time ASA damage was not correlated with delayed gastric emptying, a factor that would lead to greater contact time between ASA and the gastric mucosa. In fact, as Figure 12 depicts, human gastric emptying times are actually more rapid in the morning than in the evening hours [80]. Another factor to consider is administration-time-

---

FIGURE 8 Transmucosal potential difference (PD) of basal secreting rat gastric mucosa isolated in vitro and incubated in Krebs-Henseleit solution (serosal fluid buffered at pH 7.4; mucosal fluid unbuffered). Left: Chronogram, n = number of rats at each time point; each point is the mean of three experiments conducted on different days. HALO = hours after light onset. Right: Single cosinor analysis. Statistical significance of rhythm detection (rejection of zero-circadian amplitude assumption) is P = .06; PR = percent of variability accounted for by the fit of a 24-hr cosine curve; mesor and amplitude are shown in units of mV. Acrophase (peak of rhythm) is given in degrees with reference to local midnight (360° = 24 hr; 15° = 1 hr). The shaded portion of the abscissa in plot shown on the left-hand side indicates the nocturnal span of rodent activity. The 24-hr pattern of transmucosal electrical resistance (R) as documented in the same study (data not shown) was almost identical to that in PD. (Reproduced with permission from Ventura et al. [62].)

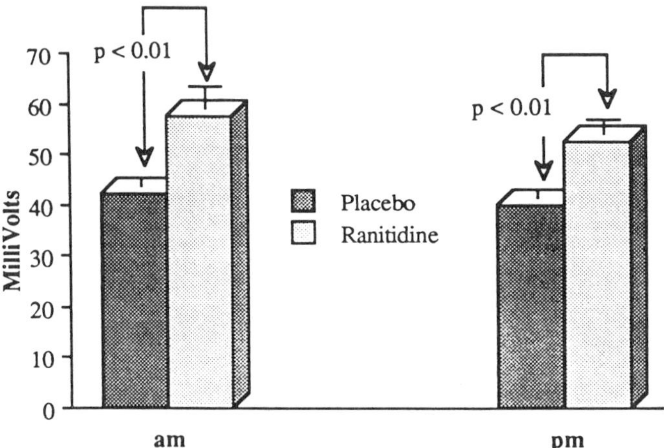

FIGURE 10 Effect of time of day (AM: 1000; PM: 2200) and ranitidine (150 mg) on gastric mucosal potential difference (PD) in 10 healthy males. The mean morning PD was 3.8 mV above the mean evening PD response. There was no correlation between ASA-induced lesions (Fig. 9) and PD level in seven subjects participating in both studies. As shown, the H_2-receptor antagonist ranitidine significantly elevated PD in both AM and PM. (Reproduced with permission from Moore et al. [79].)

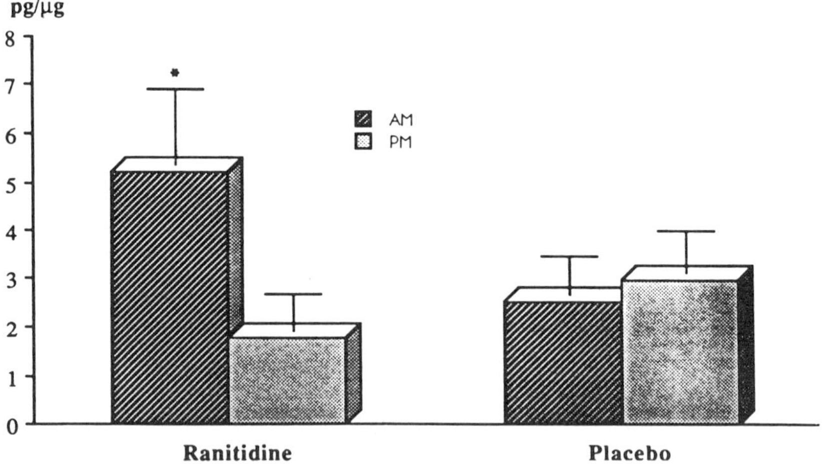

FIGURE 11 Effect of time of day (AM: 1000; PM: 2200) and ranitidine (150 mg) on prostacyclin generated by gastric biopsy tissue samples in 5 of 10 subjects participating in the gastric PD study (Fig. 10). Abscissa values represent picograms of 6-keto $PGF_{1\alpha}$ (a metabolite of PGI_2) generated per microgram of wet weight tissue in 1 hr. Morning and evening placebo levels were not significantly different. Ranitidine had no effect on PGI_2 generation in the evening but caused a significant elevation in the morning. (Reproduced with permission from Moore et al. [79].)

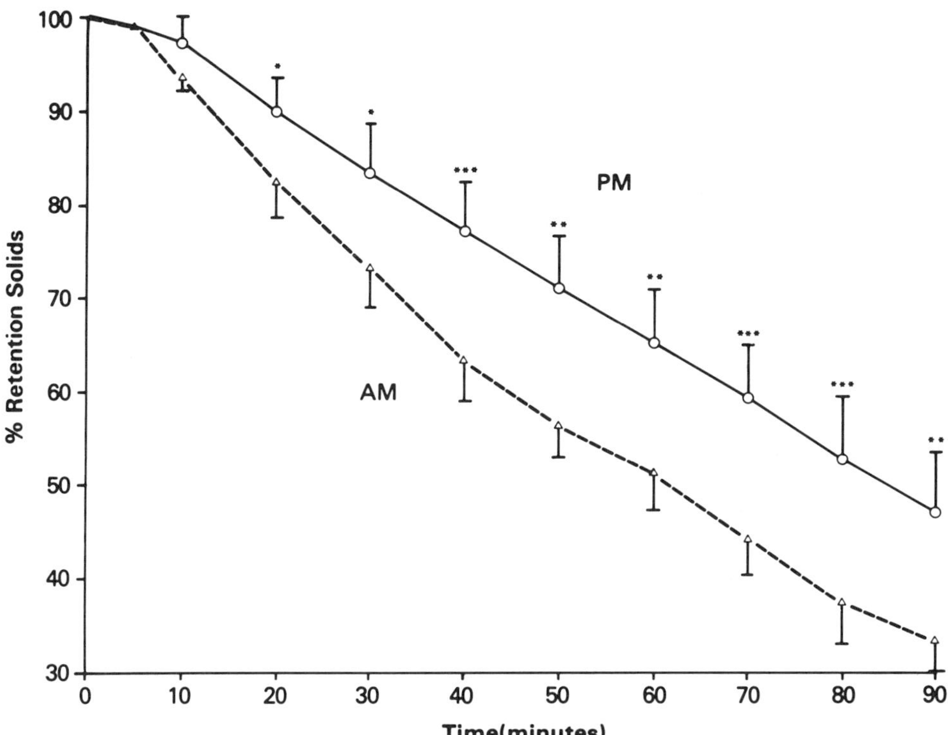

FIGURE 12 Effect of time of day (AM: 0800; PM: 2000) on gastric emptying of solids in 16 healthy male volunteers. 99-Technetium-labeled liver paté, mixed into a beef stew meal, was consumed before each test. Solid food emptying rates were monitored by a scintillation gamma camera focused on the gastric region. Meal conclusion is represented by 100% of the radionuclide marker within the stomach at 0 time. Gastric emptying of solids was significantly more rapid in the morning than in the evening (AM emptying half-time = 64 ± 6.4 min; PM emptying half-time = 95 ± 11.5 min; $p < 0.01$). Significant differences in emptying rates were recorded at every counting interval after 10 min. (Reproduced with permission from Goo et al. [80].)

dependent variation in the pharmacokinetics of ASA due to circadian rhythms in gastrointestinal function [39,81]. The dissolution of aspirin tablets and the absorption of ASA from the gut is statistically significantly more rapid when the medication is taken in the morning than in the evening [81]. Taken together, the findings suggest that other, as yet unknown, factors conferring mucosal protection, including their circadian variation, are likely to constitute important determinants of drug-induced mucosal damage.

IV. CIRCADIAN RHYTHM-DEPENDENT ATTRIBUTES OF AGGRESSIVE AND PROTECTIVE FACTORS IN THE GUT: CHRONOBIOLOGICAL MODELS OF ULCEROGENESIS

It is generally agreed that gastroduodenal ulceration in humans results from an imbalance between aggressive factors (e.g., acid, pepsin, ASA) and protective factors (e.g., mucosal blood flow, mucus and bicarbonate secretion, prostaglandin tissue concentration) acting on the gut. At any point in time, measurement of the balance between the two types of factors may be determined to be equal, positive, or negative. Ulceration does not occur unless the total of the aggressive factors exceeds the total of the protective factors. The data of Ventura et al. [62] derived from studies on rats suggest that aggressive and protective factors vary in parallel (with the same phase relationship) throughout the circadian cycle. In healthy humans, too, these factors may be in circadian synchrony with the level of safety afforded by protective factors as conceptualized in Figure 13. In gastroduodenal ulcer disease, in contrast, aggressive factors exceed the capability of host factors to protect the gastric mucosa from injury during part, or throughout all, of the circadian cycle. Because it appears that aggressive and protective factors and the mechanisms of their activities vary over the circadian time scale, several chronobiological models of ulcerogenesis are worthy of consideration.

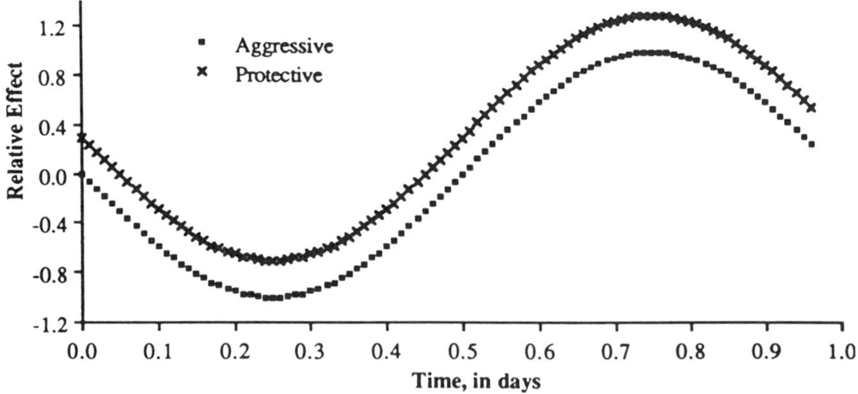

FIGURE 13 Circadian rhythm patterns in health. Hypothetical patterns of gastric protective (defensive) and aggressive (damaging) factors in health. As depicted, both types undergo circadian rhythms with similar acrophase and amplitude values. The mesor (24-hr mean) for protective factors exceeds the mesor for aggressive factors; hence the mucosa is protected from injury at all times during the 24 hr. Vertical scale equals the total effect on mucosal integrity resulting from summation of all protective and aggressive factors. Thus, a high level of aggressive factors (acid, pepsin, etc.) is balanced at all times by a higher level of protective factors (HCO_3^-, mucus, prostaglandins, blood flow, cell vitality, etc.).

In Figure 14, the absolute level of the aggressive factors (e.g., gastric acid in mmoles/hr) may be increased, normal, or even decreased, as may be the absolute level of the protective factors. The figure illustrates the case in which aggressive factors exceed the ability of the mucosa to resist injury throughout the day and night. With regard to the 24-hr time domain, ulcerogenesis may result from an alteration in the mesors (24-hr means) of the protective and aggressive factors, the former being decreased and the latter normal or increased.

Figure 15 illustrates asynchrony in aggressive and protective factors throughout the circadian cycle. Depicted is a phase difference of 12 hr between the timing of the peaks, or acrophases, of protective and aggressive factors, which produces an unfavorable (i.e., ulcerogenic) and imbalanced condition for a duration of 12 hr of each circadian cycle. Figure 16 presents the situation in which no circadian rhythmic fluctuations are observed in protective factors, while the rhythm in aggressive factors is maintained. For such a situation, an ulcerogenic potential exists for 12 of the 24 hr of each circadian cycle.

The susceptibility–resistance patterns regarding ulcerogenesis as conceptualized in Figures 14–16 are hypothetical. Such chronobiological models as these permit the investigation and testing of alternative hypotheses involving changes in the circadian mesor, amplitude, acrophase, or even period, either individually or collectively, of aggressive and protective factors. Evidence in support of a susceptibility–resistance pattern of mucosal vulnerability to injury is suggested by reports substantiating

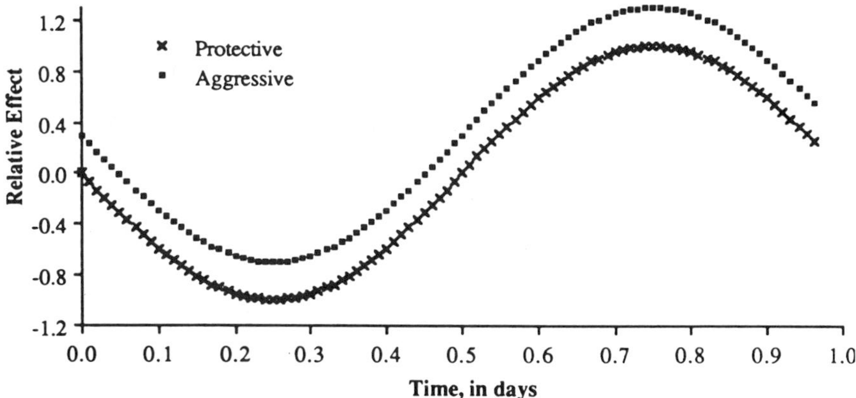

FIGURE 14 Altered mesor (24-hr mean), values in disease. Hypothetical circadian patterns of protective and aggressive factors in one postulated form of gastroduodenal rhythm dysfunction. In this case, the acrophase and amplitude values are unchanged, but the mesor values are altered such that the total level of the protective factors is not sufficient to prevent mucosal injury from the total of aggressive factors. The mucosa is subject to lesion formation throughout the circadian cycle.

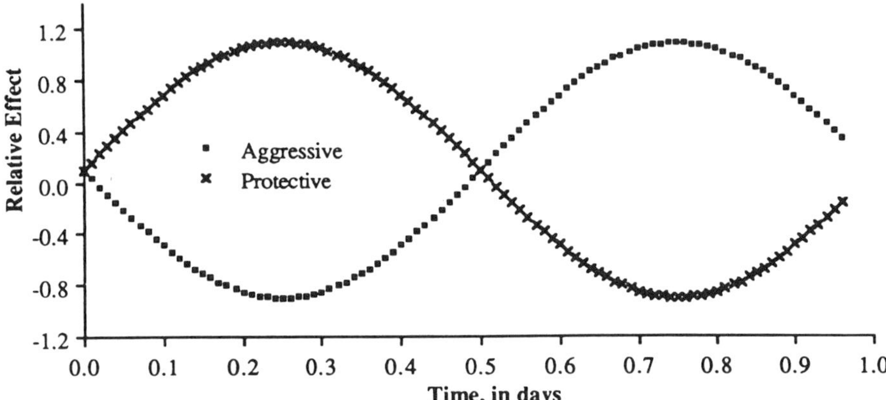

Figure 15 Circadian rhythm acrophase alteration in disease. Hypothetical circadian patterns of aggressive and protective factors as a second postulated form of gastroduodenal rhythm dysfunction. In this case, the amplitude and mesor are comparable. In fact, the mesor (24-hr mean) of protective factors could even be higher than the mesor of aggressive factors. However, the acrophase times are altered such that the aggressive factors exceed the protective factors during part of the 24 hr. In the extreme case of a 12-hr desyncrhonization illustrated here, the mucosa is protected from aggressive factors for 12 hr and unprotected for the following 12 hr.

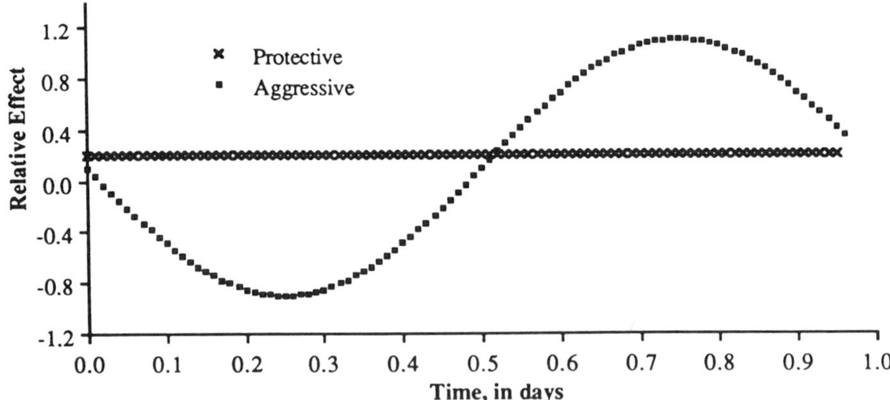

Figure 16 Circadian rhythm amplitude alteration in disease. This hypothetical pattern illustrates a third postulated type of circadian rhythm dysfunction. In this case, the mesor (24-hr mean) values may remain unchanged from the healthy pattern, but the rhythm amplitude of protective factors may be decreased or the rhythm amplitude of aggressive factors may be increased to create an ulcerogenic potential. In the extreme case illustrated here, the amplitude for the protective factors is zero, resulting in the mucosa being unprotected for one-half of the circadian cycle. This may occur despite a higher 24-hr mesor for the protective factors or a reduced 24-hr mesor for the aggressive factors.

circadian differences in the induction of experimental ulcer [57–63]. In laboratory animals, the administration time of ulcerogenic chemical and physical procedures significantly affects the results. In human beings, the circadian rhythm of acid secretion seems to be one of the most significant contributing variables. It is of interest that higher ulcer healing rates have been documented for once-daily evening or before bedtime dosing of H_2-receptor antagonist as compared to a twice-daily dosing [82–84]. The inference of these clinical findings from a rather large number of patients is that nighttime control of acid secretion is particularly critical for achieving healing of ulcer disease. Conversely, the nighttime seems to constitute a period of enhanced susceptibility to ulcer formation and aggravation in patients at risk.

V.   CIRCADIAN RHYTHMICITY IN ACID SECRETION: IMPLICATIONS FOR ORAL AND INTRAVENOUS H_2-RECEPTOR ANTAGONIST CHRONOTHERAPY

In the preceding section, the 24-hr variation in basal acid secretion was presented and characterized. The chemotherapy of peptic gastroduodenal disease is currently dominated by the use of H_2-receptor antagonists, of which cimetidine, famotidine, nizatidine, and ranitidine are popular examples. The principal physiological action of such medications is inhibition of gastric acid secretion, and presumably through this effect gastroduodenal ulcer healing ensues [85]. With reference to the nocturnal surge in gastric acid secretion as well as the circadian rhythm of the susceptibility or resistance of the gastric mucosa to injury, the matter of whether the timing of H_2-receptor antagonist medications is clinically significant deserves detailed examination.

It has been a popular belief of many practitioners that an equal-interval equal dosing of H_2-receptor antagonist medication administered every 8 or 12 hr is the most appropriate manner of modulating gastric acid secretion throughout the 24 hr. However, since the propensity for acid secretion is markedly greater during the evening hours in patients, more appropriate dosing schedules for this type of medication have been explored. In many countries worldwide, once-per-day evening (hs) administration schedules for H_2-receptor antagonists have been evaluated. Compared to the conventional (homeostatic-based) equal-interval, equal-dose treatment regimen, the hs schedule has proven to be very effective in controlling acid secretion and in healing ulcer disease, even with reduced total daily doses [82,86–88].

It is of interest to recall the rationale for the hs dosing schedule for oral H_2-receptor antagonist medications. Initially, it was based on the clinical observation that patients frequently complained about the worsening of their symptoms at night. In relation to this, it was initially hypothesized that the absence of food in the stomach overnight to buffer gastric acidity played the major role in the exacerbation of ulcer pain at this time. It was not until the conduct of chronobiological investigations on ulcer patients that evidence for circadian rhythmicity in gastric acid secretion, with the peak being at night, was published [63,64]. The significance of this and other circadian changes in gastrointestinal function are becoming better appreciated in terms of the once-at-bedtime schedule of H_2-receptor antagonist pharmacotherapy.

As a word of caution, it must be recognized that the staging, that is, the timing of peak and trough levels, of circadian rhythmic processes is determined primarily by the sleep–activity schedule of individuals. With reference to the circadian rhythm in gastric acid secretion, elevated levels can be predicted to occur during a particular span of time in the majority of patients. Generally, the increase in gastric acid begins to occur approximately 10 hr following the start of daily activity and, typically, elevated levels of gastric acid last for the ensuing 6–10 hr in persons adhering to a relatively consistent sleep–wake regimen, whether they be day workers or night workers. In persons who regularly undergo alterations in their sleep–activity schedule, which is the case for workers on rotating shifts, prediction of the span of heightened acid secretion is likely to differ from one day to the next as the circadian processes undergo phase advances and delays during the adjustment to each newly imposed sleep–activity routine associated with a given shift-work schedule [9].

It is commonly assumed that H_2-receptor antagonist drugs maintain a constant dose-response (acid-inhibiting) relationship throughout the circadian period, that is, a given dose will be equally effective throughout all hours of the day and night. However, evidence of resistance to H_2-receptor antagonist therapy during the evening hours, compared to the morning hours, has recently been detected by our group [89]. In our study, 24-hr intragastric pH measurements were obtained from 15 male subjects with healed duodenal ulcer disease. The measurements were continuously recorded by use of a tethered pH probe passed nasally and placed intragastrically. Each subject underwent three 24-hr studies separated in time by at least 1 week. Each participant received placebo intravenously (infused boluses of saline at 0800 and 2000) as well as constant-rate infusions of ranitidine in doses of 6.5 and 10 mg/hr, each dose given for 24 hr during one of three separate trials. Studies were conducted as before in the absence of meals and under conditions standardized for the elaboration of biological rhythm phenomena [63,64].

As depicted in Figure 17, circadian variation in the effect of ranitidine on intragastric pH was clearly observed for the group, with lowest pH values corresponding in time to the highest acid output observed in healthy and ulcer subjects as previously discussed (see Figs. 4 and 5). Results of preliminary analyses on these data indicate that the dose required to achieve an intragastric pH of 4 as a goal by means of the continuous infusion of ranitidine varies in a statistically significant manner according to the circadian stage of the gastric acid secretory cycle. For example, the serum concentration required to achieve a pH 4 goal for gastric acidity at 1400, a biological time of relatively low acid secretion, averages approximately 70 μg/mL compared to about 150 μg/mL at 2000, a time of high gastric acid secretion [90]. These preliminary data suggest that the clinical requirement for H_2-receptor antagonist medication is dependent on the circadian stage of the basal gastric acid secretory cycle. The drug dose-response (acid-inhibiting) relationship is not constant through

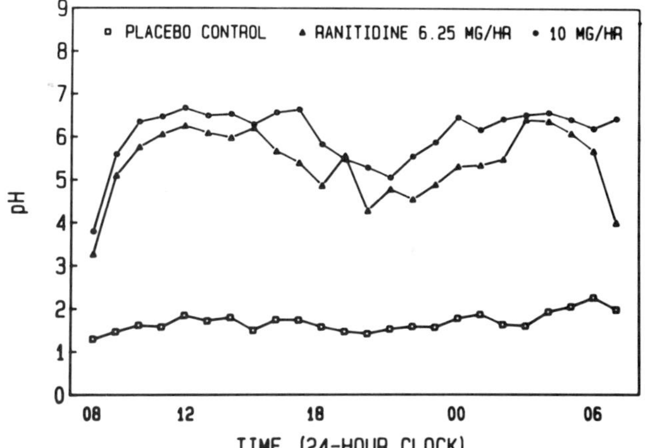

FIGURE 17 Average hourly intragastric pH levels in 15 healed duodenal ulcer patients studied over 24-hr periods. Using a randomized design, patients received intravenously (IV) a bolus infusion of placebo at 0800 and 2000 (bottom curve) as well as constant-rate IV ranitidine infusions of 6.5 mg/hr (filled triangles) and 10 mg/hr (top curve, filled circles), each treatment for 24 hr on separate occasions. Patients were fasted during each of the three study periods except for tapwater ad libitum. Note evening drop in pH, corresponding in time to the span of increased acid output observed in healthy and ulcer groups as shown in Figures 4 and 5. (Reproduced with permission from Sanders et al. [89].)

the 24 hr. Because of this, a greater dose of H_2-receptor antagonist medications appears necessary during the evening versus the morning hours to achieve an equivalent suppression of gastric acidity [89,91].

VI. CONCLUSIONS

The chronobiological investigation of ulcerogenosis is a relatively new area of scientific endeavor [52,65,92]. This chapter has reviewed pertinent clinical and experimental data relevant to circadian rhythms in gastroduodenal function and pathophysiology. Evidence for 24-hr rhythmicity in gastric acid secretion is substantial, but few data exist regarding rhythmicity in those factors that are regarded as protective against mucosal injury. Indeed, gastric mucosal protection is still largely a conceptual entity. Chronobiological models of ulcerogenesis based on changes in the rhythmic expression of those factors that are aggressive and putatively protective have been presented. They are testable in both laboratory and clinical settings. Chronobiology—the study of biological time structure—offers a new and more realistic perspective into the mechanisms and treatment of several human diseases, particularly gastroduodenal ulceration.

It is worthy of mention that the significance of chronobiology in medicine has been demonstrated for several disorders other than ulcer disease, including the nocturnal prevalence of asthma [29,30], the morning symptoms of rheumatoid arthritis [20], and the morning susceptibility of myocardial infarct [14]. In the case of allergic asthma, for example, approximately 85% of patients experience symptoms during the overnight period [93]. Indeed, the risk of asthma during the night versus the day may vary by more than 100-fold [94]! A large series of studies commencing about 30 years ago reveal the importance of circadian changes in bodily and airways function. During the daytime, circulating levels of adrenaline and corticoids are vastly elevated in comparison to those found overnight. These hormones are protective against the risk of asthma in that they promote bronchodilation via β-adrenergic stimulation and by moderation of the inflammatory process, thereby facilitating elevated airways patency and reduced airways hyperreactivity [29,30]. Identification of the day–night, resistance–susceptibility cycle of asthma has resulted in the development of more appropriate chronochemotherapeutic approaches for the management of asthma, such as the once-daily-in-the-evening ultraslow sustained-release theophylline, and β-agonist bronchodilator formulation and schedules [36,95].

From chronobiological investigations of several common chronic diseases, it appears that the mechanisms underlying their pathogenesis share susceptibility–resistance rhythms. During specific time spans over the 24 hr (and perhaps menstrual cycle and year), the vulnerability of cells, tissues, and organs to aggressive factors is markedly increased and/or the resistance compromised. Like asthma, ulcer disease also seems to exhibit a type of circadian susceptibility–resistance rhythm. It appears that in normal persons the nocturnal surge in gastric secretion is balanced by an enhanced protection of the gastric mucosa by processes that are hypothesized to be circadian rhythmic. It is known, also, based on laboratory animal [57–61] and human [78] studies that resistance and susceptibility to ulcerogenic chemicals and procedures are markedly circadian rhythmic. Investigators are just beginning to understand and appreciate the chronobiology of the gut in relation to ulcerogenesis. The extent to which rhythms and the alteration of their characteristics—mesor, amplitude, acrophase, and period—contribute to ulcerogenesis, in particular, awaits further elaboration. Nonetheless, depiction of the chronobiology of gastroduodenal function and organization has already been substantiated to be of critical importance in optimizing the therapeutic management of ulcer disease with oral H_2-receptor antagonist medications, on the one hand, and in revealing new avenues for exploring the mechanisms of ulcerogenesis, on the other.

REFERENCES

1. Halberg F. Chronobiology. Ann Rev Physiol 1975; 31:675–725.
2. Reinberg A, Smolensky MH. Biological rhythms and medicine. New York: Springer-Verlag, 1983.

3.   Moore-Ede MC, Sulzman FM, Fuller CA. The clocks that time us. Cambridge, Mass.: Harvard Univ. Press, 1982.

4.   Halberg F, Simpson H. Circadian acrophase of human 17-hydroxycorticosteroid excretion referred to midsleep rather than midnight. Human Biol 1967; 39:405–13.

5.   Halberg F, Johnson EA, Nelson W, Sothern R. Autorhythmometry—procedures for physiologic self-measurements and their analysis. Physiol Teach 1982; 1:1–11.

6.   Halberg F, Nelson W. Chronobiologic optimization of aging. In Smith HV, Capobianco S, eds. Aging and biological rhythms. London: Plenum, 1978:5–55.

7.   Ferin M, Halberg F, Richart RM, Vande Wiele RL, eds. Biorhythms and human reproduction. New York: Wiley, 1974.

8.   Reinberg A. Aspects of circannual rhythms in man. In: Pengelley ET, ed. Circannual clocks. New York: Academic, 1974:423–505.

9.   Reinberg A, ed. Chronobiological field studies of oil refinery shift workers. Chronobiologia 1979; 6(Suppl 1):1–119.

10.   Halberg F, Reinberg A, Reinberg A. Chronobiologic serial sections gauge circadian rhythm adjustments following transmeridian flight and life in novel environment. Waking Sleeping 1977; 1:259–79.

11.   Smolensky MH, Halberg F. Circadian rhythm in airway patency and lung volumes. In: McGovern JP, Smolensky MH, Reinberg A, eds. Chronobiology in allergy and immunology. Springfield, Ill.: CC Thomas, 1977:117–38.

12.   Carandente F, Halberg F. Chronobiology of blood pressure in 1985. Chronobiologia 1974; 11:189–310.

13.   Smolensky MH, Reinberg A, Prevost RJ, McGovern JP, Gervais P. The application of chronobiological findings and methods to the epidemiological investigation of the health effects of air pollutants on sentinel patients. In: Smolensky MH, Reinberg A, McGovern JP, eds. Recent advances in the chronobiology of allergy and immunology. New York: Pergamon, 1980:211–36.

14.   Muller JE, Stone PH, Turi ZG, Ruthford JD, Czeisler CA, Parker C, Poole WK, Passamani E, Roberts R, Robertson T, Sobel BE, Willerson JT, Braunwald E. The MILIS study group: circadian variation in the frequency of onset of myocardial infarction. N Engl J Med 1985; 313:1315–22.

15.   Marshall J. Diurnal variation in the occurrence of strokes. Stroke 1977; 8:230–1.

16.   Gervais P, Reinberg A. The clinical significance of chronobiological methods for allergic asthma. In: McGovern JP, Smolensky MH, Reinberg A, eds. Chronobiology in allergy and immunology. Springfield, Ill.: CC Thomas, 1977:64–78.

17.   Reinberg A, Gervais P, Ghata J. Chronobiologic aspects of allergic asthma. In: McGovern JP, Smolensky MH, Reinberg A, eds. Chronobiology in allergy and immunology. Springfield, Ill.: CC Thomas, 1977:36–63.

18.   Reinberg A, Gervais P, Ugolini C, Del Cerro L, Bicakova-Rocker A, Nicolaï A. A multicentric chronotherapeutic study of mequitazine in allergic rhinitis. Annu Rev Chronopharmacol 1986; 3:441–4.

19.   Reinberg A, Gervais P, Levi F, Smolensky MH, Del Cerro L, Ugolini C. Circadian and circannual rhythms of allergic rhinitis: an epidemiological study involving chronobiologic methods. J Allergy Clin Immunol 1988; 81:51–62.

20.   Lévi F, LeLouarn C, Reinberg A. Chronotherapy of osteoarthritic patients: optimization of indomethacin sustained release (ISR). Annu Rev Chronopharmacol 1984; 1:345–8.

21. Kuroiwa A. Symptomatology of variant angina. Jpn Circ J 1978; 42:459–76.
22. Lemmer B. The chronopharmacology of cardiovascular medications. Annu Rev Chrono-pharmacol 1986; 2:199–228.
23. Newmark ME, Penry JK. Catamenial epilepsy: a review. Epilepsia 1980; 21:281–300.
24. Wulfsohn NL, Politzer WM. Bronchial asthma during menses and pregnancy. S Afr Med J 1964; 38:173.
25. Orie NGM, Sluitter HF, Tammeling GJ, DeVries K, Wal AMVD. Fight against bronchitis. In: Orie NGM, Sluiter NJ, eds. Bronchitis: 2nd international bronchitis symposium. Springfield, Ill.: CC Thomas, 1960:352–69.
26. Smolensky MH, Halberg F, Sargent F. Chronobiology of the life sequence. In: Itoh S, Ogata K, Yoshimura H, eds. Advances in climatic physiology. Tokyo: Igaku Shoin, 1972:281–318.
27. Halberg F. Temporal coordination of physiological function. Cold Spring Harbor Symp Quant Biol 1960; 25:289–310.
28. Smolensky MH. Chronobiology and epidemiology. Pathol Biol (Paris) 1987; 3:991–1004.
29. Smolensky MH, Barnes PJ, Reinberg A, McGovern JP. Chronobiology and asthma. I. Day–night differences in bronchial patency and dyspnea and circadian rhythm dependencies. J Asthma 1986; 23:321–43.
30. Smolensky MH, D'Alonzo GE, Kunkel G, Barnes PJ. Day–night patterns in bronchial patency and dyspnea: basis for once-daily and unequally divided twice-daily theophylline dosing schedules. Chronobiol 1987; 4:303–17.
31. Reinberg A, Smolensky MH, Labrecque G. New aspects in chronopharmacology. Annu Rev Chronopharmacol 1986; 2:1–26.
32. Reinberg A, Smolensky MH. Circadian changes of drug disposition in man. Clin Pharmacokinet 1982; 7:401–20.
33. Bruguerolle B. Chronopharmacokinetics. Pathol Biol 1987; 35:925–34.
34. Smolensky MH, McGovern JP, Scott PH, Reinberg A. Chronobiology and asthma. II. Day–night differences in the kinetics and effects of bronchodilator medications. J Asthma 1987; 24:91–134.
35. Smolensky MH, Scott PH, Kramer WG. Clinical significance of day–night difference in serum theophylline concentration with special reference to TheoDur. J Allergy Clin Immunol 1986; 78:716–22.
36. Smolensky MH, Scott PH, Barnes PJ, Jonkman JHG. The chronobiology and chrono-therapy of asthma. Annu Rev Chronopharmacol 1986; 2:229–73.
37. Clench J, Reinberg A, Dziewanowska Z, Ghata J, Smolensky MH. Circadian changes in the bioavailability and effects of indomethacin in healthy subjects. Eur J Clin Pharmacol 1981; 20:359–69.
38. Guissou P, Cuisinaud G, Llorca G, Lejeune E, Sarsard J. Chronopharmacokinetic study of a prolonged form of indomethacin. Eur J Clin Pharmacol 1983; 24:667–70.
39. Reinberg A, Zagula-Mally Z, Ghata J, Halberg F. Circadian rhythms in duration of salicylate excretion referred to phase of excretory rhythms and routine. Proc Soc Exp Biol 1967; 124:826–32.
40. Reinberg A, Clench J, Ghata J, Halberg F, Abulker C, Dupont J, Zagula-Mally Z.

Rythmes circadiens des parametres de l'excrétion urinaire du salicylate (chronophamacocinétique) chez l'homme adulte sain. CR Acad Sci 1975; 280:1697–700.

41. Reinberg A, Sidi E. Circadian changes in the inhibitory effects of an antihistaminic drug in man. J Invest Dermatol 1966; 46:415–9.

42. Reinberg A, Lévi F, Guillet P, Burke JT, Nicolaï A. Chronopharmacological study of antihistamines in man with special references to terfenadine. Eur J Clin Pharmacol 1978; 14:245–52.

43. Reinberg A, Lévi F, Fourtillan JP, Peiffer C, Bicakova-Rocker A, Nicolaï A. Antihistamine and other effects of 5mg mequitazine vary between morning and evening acute administration. Annu Rev Chronopharmacol 1984; 1:57–60.

44. Lemmer B, Langner B. Daily variations in pharmacokinetics and cardiovascular effects of oral propranolol in man. Naunyn-Schmiedeberg's Arch Pharmacol 1985; 329:R60.

45. Morselli PL, Marc V, Garattini S, Zaccala M. Metabolism of exogenous cortisol in humans—diurnal variations in plasma disappearance rate. Biochem Pharmacol 1970; 19:1643–7.

46. English J, Dunne M, Marks V. Diurnal variation in prednisolone kinetics. Clin Pharmacol Therap. 1983; 33:381–5.

47. Reinberg A, Smolensky MH, D'Alonzo GE, McGovern JP. Chronobiology and asthma. III. Timing corticotherapy to biological rhythms to optimize treatment goals. J Asthma 1988; 25:219–48.

48. Boyd EJS, Wormsley KG. Etiology and pathogenesis of peptic ulcer. In: Berk JE, ed. Bockus gastroenterology. 4th ed. Philadelphia: WB Saunders, 1985; 66:1013.

49. Moynihan BGA. Duodenal ulcer. Philadelphia: WB Saunders, 1912.

50. Gibinski K, Rybicka J, Novak A, Czarnecka K. Seasonal occurrence of abdominal pain and endoscopic findings in patients with gastric and duodenal ulcer disease. Scand J Gastroenterol 1982; 17:481–5.

51. Gibinski K. A review of seasonal periodicity in peptic ulcer disease. Chronobiol Int 1987; 4:91–8.

52. Vener K, Moore J, Szabo S, eds. Chronobiology and ulcerogenesis. Chronobiol Int 1987; 4:1–22.

53. Labrecque G, Bélanger PM, Dore F, Lalande M. 24-Hour variations in the distribution of labeled microspheres to the intestine, liver and kidney. Annu Rev Chronopharmacol 1988; 5:445–8.

54. Stevenson NR, Ferrigni F, Parnicky K, Day S, Fierstein JS. Effect of changes in feeding schedule on the diurnal rhythms and daily activity levels of intestinal brush border enzymes and transport systems. Biochim Biophys Acta 1975; 406:131.

55. Markiewicz A, Kaminski M, Tarquini B, Halberg F. Circadian rhythm of enzymatic activity in human jejunum. Int J Chronobiol 1981; 7:282.

56. Scheving LE, Cardosa SS, Pauley JE, Tsai TH. Circadian variation and cell division of the mouse alimentary tract, bone marrow and corneal epithelium. Anat Rec 1978; 191:479–85.

57. Ader R. Gastric erosions in the cat: effects of immobilization at different time points in the activity cycle. Science 1964; 145:406–7.

58. Carandente F, Halberg E, Dubey DP, Beard K, Klein P, Halberg F. Chronobiology and

sex as codeterminants of gastric ulcerogenesis in loaded rats of two inbred strains. Proceedings of the XII Int. Conf., Int. Soc. Chronobiol., meeting in Washington, DC. published in Il Ponte, Italy, 1977:157–66.

59. Oishi T, Gallagher GT, Szabo S. Diurnal variation of duodenal ulcer induced by cysteamine. Gastroenterology 1982; 82:1139.

60. Szabo S, Pfeiffer S, Oishi T. The chronopharmacology of drug-induced gastric and duodenal ulcers. Annu Rev Chronopharmacol 1986; 3:383–4.

61. Olson CE, Soll AH, Guth P. Circadian variation of susceptibility to gastric mucosal injury by acidified aspirin or absolute ethanol in the rat. Gastroenterology 1986; 91:1192–7.

62. Ventura U, Carandente F, Montini E, Ceriani T. Circadian rhythmicity of acid secretion and electrical function in intact and injured rat gastric mucosa—the relation of timing to ulcerogenesis. Chronobiol Int 1987; 4:43–52.

63. Moore JG, Englert E Jr. Circadian rhythm of gastric acid secretion in man. Nature 1970; 226:1261–2.

64. Moore JG, Halberg F. Circadian rhythm of gastric acid secretion in man with active duodenal ulcer. Dig Dis Sci 1986; 31:1185–91.

65. Vener KJ, Moore JG. Chronobiologic properties of the alimentary canal affecting xenobiotic absorption. Annu Rev Chromopharmacol 1988; 4:257–82.

66. Ivy AC, Grossman MI, Bachrach WH. Peptic ulcer. Philadelphia: Blakeston, 1950.

67. Safrany L, Schott B, Portocarrero G, Krause S, Newhaus B. Zur Frage der Fruhjahrs— und Herbstdisposition des gastroduodenalen ulkus. Dtsch Med Wisssenr 1982; 107:685–9.

68. Halberg F, Moore JG, Gibinski K, Szabo S. Further chronobiologic steps in gastroenterology. Chronobiologia 1983; 10:409–21.

69. Schwarz K. Veber penetrierende magenund jejunalgeschwure. Beit Klin Chir 1910; 67:96–128.

70. Moore JG, Wolfe ME. The relation of plasma gastrin to the circadian rhythm of gastric acid secretion in man. Digestion 1973; 9:97–105.

71. Moore JG, Wolfe ME. Circadian plasma gastrin levels in feeding and fasting man. Digestion 1974; 11:226–32.

72. Moore JG. Gastric acid suppression by intravenous glucose solutions. Gastroenterology 1973; 64:1106–10.

73. Nelson W, Tong YL, Lee JK, Halberg F. Methods for cosinor-rhythmometry. Chronobiologia 1979; 6:305–23.

74. De Prins J, Cornelissen G, Malbecq W. Statistical procedures in chronobiology and chronopharmacology. Annu Rev Chronopharmacol 1986; 2:27–142.

75. Szabo S, Pihan G. Development and significance of cysteamine and proprionitrile models of duodenal ulcer. Chronobiol Int 1987; 4:31–42.

76. Moore JG. High gastric acid after vagotomy and pyloroplasty in man. Evidence for non-vagal mediation. Am J Dig Dis 1973; 18:661–9.

77. Allan A, Flemstrom G, Garner A, Silen W, Turnberg LA, eds. Mechanisms of mucosal protection in the upper gastrointestinal tract. New York: Raven Press, 1984.

78. Moore JG, Goo RH. Day and night aspirin-induced gastric mucosal damage and protection by ranitidine in man. Chronobiol Int 1987; 4:111–6.

79. Moore JG, Larsen KR, Goo RH, Bjorkman DJ. AM and PM measurements of gastric potential difference and prostacyclin production in humans: effects of ranitidine. Chronobiol Int 1988; 5:395–401.

80. Goo RH, Moore JG, Greenberg E, Alazrak NP. Circadian variation in gastric emptying of meals in humans. Gastroenterology 1987; 93:515–8.

81. Markiewicz A, Semenowicz K. Time dependent change in the pharmacokinetics of aspirin. Int J Clin Pharmacol Biopharm 1979; 17:409–11.

82. Ireland A, Colin-Jones DG, Gear P, Golding P, Romage JK, Williams JG, Leicester RJ, Smith CL, Ross G, Banforth J, De Gara CJ, Gledhill T, Hunt RH. Ranitidine 150 mg twice daily vs. 300 mg nightly in treatment of duodenal ulcers. Lancet 1984; ii:274–6.

83. Porro GB. Famotidine in the treatment of gastric and duodenal ulceration: overview of clinical experience. Digestion 1985; 32(Suppl 1):62–9.

84. Simon B, Dammann HG, Jakob G, Miederer SE, Muller P, Ottenjam R, Paul F, Scholten T, Shutz E, Seifert E, Stadleman O. Famotidine versus ranitidine for the short term treatment of duodenal ulcer. Digestion 1985; 32(Suppl 1):32–7.

85. Thomson ABR, Mahachai V. Medical management of uncomplicated ulcer disease. In: Berk JE, ed. Bokus gastroenterology. 4th ed. Philadelphia: WB Saunders, 1985:1116–54 (Chap. 68).

86. Orr WC, Allen M, Finn A, Robinson MG. Timing of evening meal and ranitidine administration on patterns of 24 hr intragastric pH. Annu Rev Chronopharmacol 1988; 5:321.

87. Cloud M, Often W. Nizatidine 300 mg h.s. compared with cimetidine 800 mg h.s. in the treatment of acute duodenal ulcer. Annu Rev Chronopharmacol 1988; 5:285.

88. Humphries TJ, Berlin RG. The suppression of nocturnal acid secretion by h.s. famotidine therapy is sufficient to heal benign gastric ulcers. Annu Rev Chronopharmacol 1988; 5:291–4.

89. Sanders SW, Moore JG, Buchi KN, Bishop AL. Circadian variation in the pharmacodynamic effect of intravenous ranitidine. Annu Rev Chronopharmacol. 1988; 5:335–8.

90. White K, Smolensky MH, Sanders S, Buchi K, Moore J. Day-night and individual differences in response to constant rate ranitidine infusion. Chronobiol. Int. (In press).

91. Merki H, Witzel L, Langman M, Kaufmann D, Neumann J, Röhmel J, Walt R. Continuous infusion of famotidine maintains high gastric pH in duodenal ulcer. Annu Rev Chronopharmacol 1988; 5:315.

92. Tarquini B, Vener KJ. Temporal aspects of the pathophysiology of human ulcer disease. Chronobiol Int 1987; 4:43–52.

93. Turner-Warwick M. Epidemiology of nocturnal asthma. Am J Med 1988; 85(1B):6–8.

94. Dethlefsen U, Repges R. Ein neues therapieprinzip bei nachtlichem asthma. Med Klin 1985; 80:44–7.

95. Smolensky MH, D'Alonzo GE, Barnes PJ, Kunkel G, eds. Circadian rhythm-adapted theophylline schedules for nocturnal asthma. Chronobiol Int 1987; 4:303–446.

4

Ulcer Disease: What Is Known and What Questions Remain

GIOVANNI GASBARRINI, PIETRO ANDREONE, STEFANO PRETOLANI, MARIO BARALDINI, and FIORENZA BONVICINI

University of Bologna, S. Orsola Hospital,
Bologna, Italy

I. INTRODUCTION

The pathogenesis of ulcer disease remains as highly disputed a question today as it was 100 years ago [1]. However, there is general agreement in the literature, which considers ulcer disease a multifactorial condition with common morphological manifestations [2–5]. Current concepts of ulcerogenesis rely on the imbalance between aggressive and protective factors in the gastroduodenal mucosa [6]. Even if it is possible to separate different populations of subjects with peptic ulcer from normal subjects on the basis of different etiological factors, no evidence exists for a universal and unifying mechanism for the development of ulcers. In this chapter we will focus on what is known and what questions remain about the pathogenesis of ulcer disease.

II. ACID-PEPTIC SECRETION

Despite numerous published studies, the role of acid in pathogenesis of peptic ulcer is unclear. Impairment of acid secretion, in both gastric and duodenal ulcer, has been reported. Patients with ulcer in the body of the stomach have lower acid secretion, which results from gastritis, probably secondary to a decrease of parietal cells [7]. In contrast, about half of the patients with prepyloric or duodenal ulcer have higher acid secretion than normal subjects, but considerable overlap exists [8].

In particular, patients with duodenal ulcer have an increase in total parietal cell mass (1.5–2 times greater than in control subjects) [9], which could be responsible for the increase in basal, maximal, nocturnal, and meal-stimulated acid secretion reported by some authors [10,11]. An important role in the determination of acid secretion alterations is carried out by gastrin. Up-to-date studies have demonstrated an increased sensibility of the parietal cells to exogenous gastrin as well as abnormalities in meal-stimulated gastrin release, but the results have not established a firm conclusion [12,13]. In addition to excessive activity of the factors stimulating acid secretion, there have also been indicated alterations of the mechanisms capable of inhibiting the acid secretion such as gastric distention, gastric and duodenal acidification, and somatostatin secretion [14,15]. These alterations have been seen in some patients only and not confirmed in successive studies [10,16].

As far as pepsin is concerned, its ulcerogenic activity has been widely demonstrated also because acid alone is less aggressive than acid plus pepsin [17,18]. Recently, Pearson and coworkers showed that pepsin I, found in higher amounts in ulcer patients, digests mucus more effectively than pepsin III [19], and their data further support the hypothesis that pepsin may induce mucosal damage by degrading the mucus gel layer. Concerning pepsinogen production, it has been demonstrated that duodenal and gastric ulcer patients have higher serum pepsinogen I and II than normal subjects and that not only patients with gastritis but also patients with peptic ulcer have a diminished ratio of pepsinogen I to pepsinogen II [20]. We do not know if these alterations constitute a pathogenetic event of the peptic disesase or if the peptic disease determines these alterations.

III. RISK FACTORS

Some alimentary habits are considered risk factors for peptic ulcer because they may favor the appearance of peptic ulcer as well as recurrence and complications.

A. Smoking

Several epidemiological studies indicate that smokers are at increased risk for both duodenal and gastric ulcers and that this risk may be proportional to the amount smoked [21,22]. Furthermore, smoking impairs the healing of ulcers, promotes recurrences, and increases the risk of complications. Numerous mechanisms have been proposed to justify this effect: increased basal and maximal acid secretion, decreased pancreatic bicarbonate secretion, induced duodenogastric reflux, increased gastric emptying, increased pepsinogen secretion, altered mucosal blood flow, and decreased mucosal prostaglandin production [23–27].

In a study on healthy volunteers, no differences were found in the 24-hr gastric acid secretion of smokers compared with nonsmokers. In contrast, the therapeutic efficacy of H_2 antagonists was significantly reduced in smokers [28].

B. Alcohol

Elevated concentrations of alcohol can bring about acute mucosal gastric damage, but there is no proof that moderate alcohol consumption during meals can favor the appearance of chronic ulcer. Drinks such as wine and beer may stimulate acid secretion [29,30], but this effect is probably due to substances other than ethanol. Several studies demonstrated that alcohol consumption is not a risk factor [21,31] and that patients with duodenal ulcer consume less alcohol than controls [32]. Furthermore, it has been shown that moderate alcohol consumption may favor the healing of duodenal ulcer [33].

C.   Dietary Habits

Alimentary habits have always been incriminated as risk factors for peptic ulcer, but this has never been clearly demonstrated. Undoubtedly some drinks (tea, coffee, cola, beer, etc.) and several spices can cause dyspepsia by stimulating acid secretion or by favoring gastroesophageal reflux [34–36], but there is no evidence of an increased risk in peptic ulcer for those patients who consume these products.

In spite of the above-mentioned data, research on experimental and clinical use of antacids, antipepsin, and mucosa-protective drugs, and even the most potent antisecretory agents (H_2 antagonists, omeprazole), has not enhanced our understanding of the pathophysiology of ulcer disease.

Although rapid healing of ulcers is now easy to achieve, the natural history of this disease remains unchanged, and recurrence within 1 year after the withdrawal of antisecretory therapy is the rule. Therefore, the acid-pepsin-oriented approach to the pathogenesis of ulcer disease receives less attention than other biochemical and morphological factors, as can be seen from recent reviews in the literature [37–41].

IV.   MUCUS SECRETION

The presence of an unstirred layer of mucus gel, together with the balance between its synthesis and degradation, has been considered a mechanical and biochemical protective factor for the gastroduodenal mucosa exposed to various damaging agents [42]. Besides the well-known lubricating and viscoelastic properties of the gastric mucus, evidence exists that an intact layer of this gel adherent to the mucosa creates a pH gradient from the lumen toward the membrane of epithelial cells [43]. This condition retards the rate of H^+ retrodiffusion [44], protecting the surface epithelium from luminal acid injury, as does HCO_3^- secretion.

The constituents of mucus are a heterogeneous mixture of proteins, glycoproteins, and lipids secreted by mucous cells (Fig. 1). The polymeric structure of mucus glycoprotein (consisting of four subunits with a protein core and carbohydrate side chains joined by disulfide bridges) prevents large molecules such as pepsins from reaching the luminal membranes of epithelial cells. Aggressive factors can directly damage the underlying mucosa either when the mucus is degraded in a monomeric soluble form by proteolytic agents or when its production is impaired by nonsteroidal anti-inflammatory drugs (NSAIDs) [45]. However, some ulcerogenic agents, such as absolute ethanol, 0.6 N HCl, 80 mM sodium taurocholate, and 1 M NaCl, do not

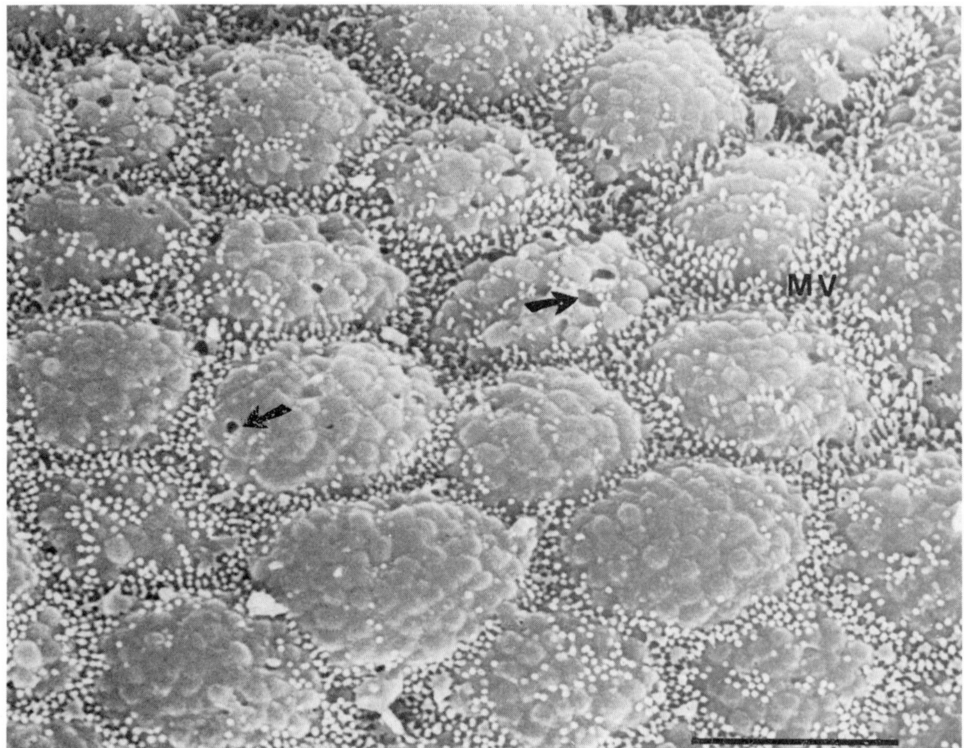

FIGURE 1 Scanning electron micrograph of human gastric mucosa. Surface mucous cells in active phase of secretion: peripheralized microvilli (MV), bulging of the apical membrane due to the underlying mucus granules. Arrows indicate holes left by secreted granules (SEM, 2700×). Bar = 10 μm.

modify the mucus structure [46]. These findings suggest that they can permeate the intact mucus layer, producing epithelial lesions, but the persistence of mucus minimizes mucosal damage and maximizes cellular repair [47].

Animal model studies demonstrate that the functional properties of mucus depend on its chemical characteristics. Glycolipids and phospholipids are more effective than proteins in H^+ retardation and determine the degree of resistance to proteolytic agents as well as enhancing mucus viscosity and hydrophobicity [48]. These lipids are more prevalent in intracellular mucus than in surface mucus. Experimental depletion of the former in rats induces much higher H^+ permeability of the gastric mucosa [49]. It has been suggested that surface mucus could represent the first line of gastric mucosal protection and the intracellular mucus a second line of defense [49]. Stimulation of mucus synthesis and secretion might be an interesting therapeutic option in ulcer disease [38], as structural mucus modification has been demonstrated in such patients [50,51]. Cholinergic agents and E-type prostaglandins are the most potent stimulants of mucus secretion. Even though recent studies demonstrate that adaptive cytoprotection in rats is not mediated by prostaglandins [52], other animal experiments confirm that PGE derivatives increase mucus synthesis and particularly the intramucosal glycoprotein content [53]. Histochemical techniques utilizing lectins—proteins of nonimmune origin that agglutinate cells and/or precipitate glycoconjugates [54]—can now be used to study the intracellular mucins because different lectins are able to bind specific glycoside components of mucus glycoproteins (Figs. 2 and 3) [55].

In a previous study we observed that patients with gastric ulcer show a different pattern of intracellular mucins in the antral mucosa, expressed by the reduction in the binding of lectins specific for neutral carbohydrates (in particular Lotus Tetragonolo-

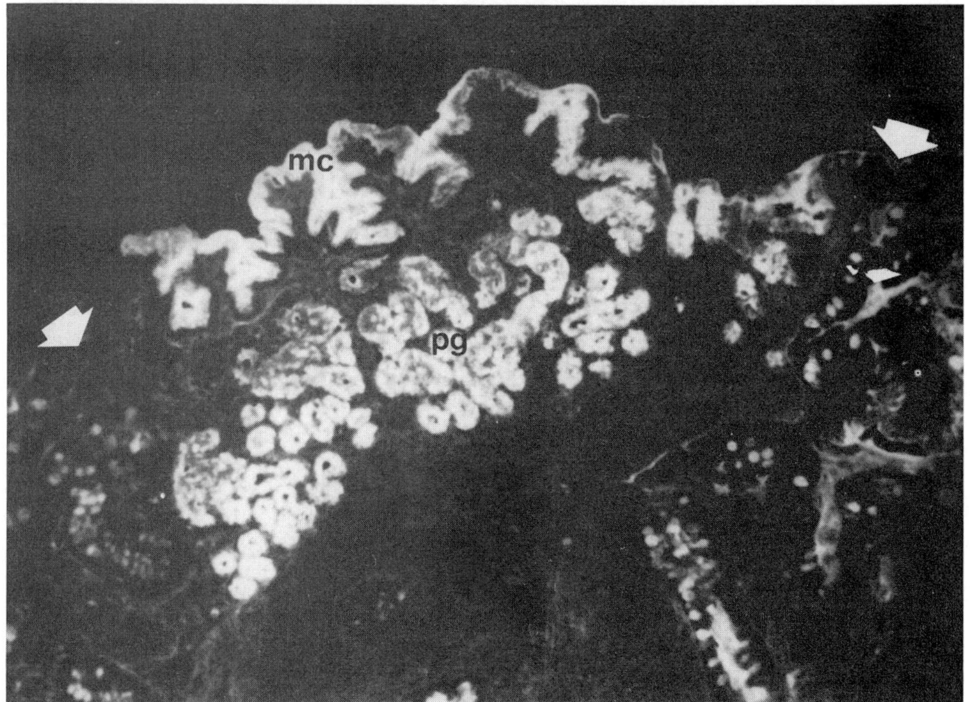

Figure 2   Histological section of human gastric mucosa (antrum) incubated with fluoresceinated Lotus Tetragonolobus lectin (LTA). A bright fluorescence is visible on surface mucous cells (mc) and on pyloric glands (pg). Arrow indicates intestinal metaplasia with fluorescent goblet cells (125×).

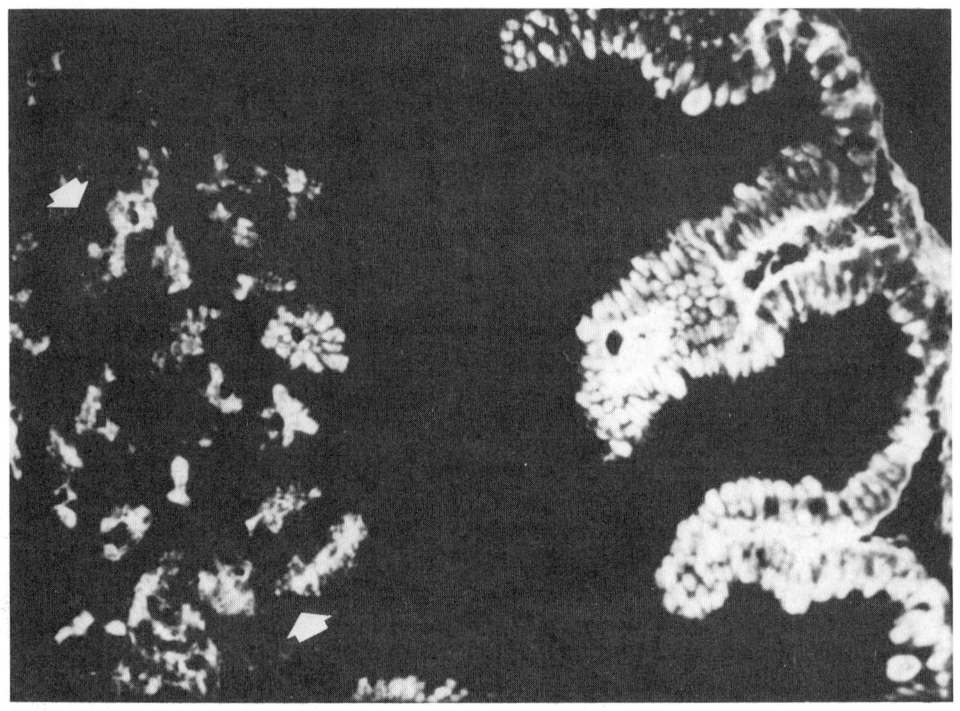

FIGURE 3 Histological section of human gastric mucosa (body) incubated with fluoresce-inated Lotus Tetragonolobus lectin (LTA). Surface mucous cells are intensely stained. In body glands (arrows), neck cells and chief cells are fluorescent too, while parietal cells are not (250×).

bus agglutinin, which binds L-fucose) [56]. Therefore it is conceivable that enhancing or modifying gastric mucus glycoprotein synthesis could be useful not only against acute drug-induced lesions but also for long-term safeguarding of gastroduodenal mucosa by other aggressive agents. In a recent preliminary study, in patients with *Helicobacter pylori* positive gastritis, we demonstrated that enprostil, a synthetic E_2 dehydroprostaglandin, not only can heal erosive antral lesions but also seems to partially restore the decreased intracellular content of neutral mucins [57].

V. BICARBONATE SECRETION

The role of alkaline secretion (the establishment of a pH gradient affording pre-epithelial gastroduodenal protection) has been reevaluated by studies that stressed the intramucosal protection of nutrient HCO_3^- delivered by blood flow [39]. This new protective mechanism is related to cellular HCO_3^- transport (intracellular pH regulation) and passive effusion after mucosal injury. This process, together with the rapid formation of a thick mucus cap and necrotic debris [52], probably facilitates the repair of the gastroduodenal mucosa. Moreover, evidence exists that cellular HCO_3^- transport is under sympathoadrenergic control [58] and that acidosis per se is a more critical factor in the development of mucosal lesions than O_2 supply during ischemia [59]. This response is mediated by short intramural neural cholinergic pathways and is independent of mucosal production of prostaglandins [60].

Interesting results are obtained by therapeutic studies in isolated gastric mucosa, where aluminum salts and aluminum content of sucralfate were able to stimulate alkali secretion by a prostaglandin-independent mechanism [61]. The mechanism of this secretion is neither electrogenic nor a passive diffusion but seems likely to be an electroneutral ion exchange, such as Cl^-/HCO_3^-. This mechanism may be activated in gastroduodenal mucosa by enkephalins and gastric inhibitory polypeptide [62].

These data may be of particular relevance to the pathogenesis and therapy of stress ulceration. In this complex condition there are multiple interrelations between vascular, neuroendocrine (central and peripheral), physicochemical, and immuno-inflammatory mechanisms that could require specific pharmacological approaches.

VI. PROSTANOIDS

In recent years many researchers have focused their attention on several lipidic substances generally called prostaglandins. In physiological conditions these molecules exert a protective action on the gastroduodenal mucosa, as they are able to influence both mechanisms of acute protection (mucosal blood flow, smooth muscle, cell renewal) and those of chronic protection (bicarbonate and mucus secretion, cell regeneration, and acid secretion) [63–67]. Their role is still not clear in the pathogenesis of peptic disease. The hypothesis that a decrease in the production of protective prostaglandins can be responsible for the appearance of peptic ulcer is attractive and is supported by the evidence that prostaglandin synthesis inhibition induced with NSAIDs may favor gastroduodenal mucosal lesions. The studies carried out to date have evaluated prostanoid synthesis in an incomplete fashion and have shown contrasting results that have not led to any firm conclusion [68–75].

To verify the role of prostanoids in peptic disease, in recent years we evaluated prostanoid synthesis (PGE_2, PGD_2, $6KPGF_{1\alpha}$, $PGF_{2\alpha}$, TXB_2) in inflammatory diseases of the upper gastrointestinal tract. We used a brief incubation, in a culture medium, of mucosal biopsy specimens taken during endoscopy at gastric and duodenal levels [76]. The results demonstrated the following:

1. In healthy subjects, synthesis of some prostanoids (PGI_2 and TXB_2) is significantly greater in the stomach than in the duodenum (Table 1).
2. In patients with chronic superficial gastritis, prostanoid synthesis is significantly greater than in normal subjects at both antrum and gastric body; the

Table 1 Prostanoid Production from Biopsy Specimens of 15 Normal Subjects after Incubation in Krebs Solution for 30 min

	Duodenal bulb	Gastric antrum	Gastric body
PGE_2	2.55 ± 0.36[a,b]	12.57 ± 2.35[a]	13.64 ± 3.17[b]
$PGF_{2\alpha}$	12.99 ± 2.73	10.74 ± 1.03	11.40 ± 2.01
$6KPGF_{1\alpha}$	12.64 ± 2.15	11.10 ± 1.63	10.35 ± 1.60
PGD_2	15.05 ± 3.79	13.71 ± 2.91	12.61 ± 2.20
TXB_2	14.16 ± 2.14[c,d]	24.96 ± 4.47[c]	22.60 ± 3.05[d]

The results (M $\pm$ SE) are expressed as ng/mg soluble proteins per 30 min. The results were analyzed by nonparametric statistics: [a]$p < .001$; [b]$p < .005$; [c]$p < .005$; [d]$p < .05$.

Table 2 Prostanoid Production from Biopsy Specimens of 21 Normal Subjects and 53 Patients with Chronic Superficial Gastritis after Incubation in Krebs Solution for 10 min*

| | Controls | Chronic superficial gastritis | |
		Quiescent	Active
PGE_2			
Antrum	2.77 ± 0.64[a]	6.07 ± 1.29[b]	14.33 ± 1.99[a,b]
Body	4.38 ± 0.66[c,d]	8.56 ± 1.49[c,e]	16.36 ± 4.51[d,e]
$6KPGF_{1\alpha}$			
Antrum	1.56 ± 0.17[f,g]	2.95 ± 0.42[f,h]	4.63 ± 0.46[g,h]
	$p < .025$	$p < .05$	
Body	2.72 ± 0.34[i,k]	4.78 ± 0.80[i]	5.08 ± 0.96[k]
TXB_2			
Antrum	8.85 ± 1.73[l]	10.81 ± 1.69[m]	20.78 ± 4.03[l,m]
Body	7.05 ± 1.08[n,o]	13.32 ± 2.38[n]	13.86 ± 2.92[o]

*Of the 53 patients, 31 had quiescent chronic superficial gastritis (16 at antral level, 15 at body level) and 22 had active chronic superficial gastritis (12 at antral level, 10 at body level).

The results (M $\pm$ SE) are expressed as ng/mg soluble proteins per 10 min. The results were analyzed by nonparametric statistics: [a]$p < .001$; [b]$p < .005$; [c]$p < .05$; [d]$p < .01$; [e]$p < .05$; [f]$p < .025$; [g]$p < .001$; [h]$p < .02$; [i]$p < .05$; [k]$p < .025$; [l]$p < .05$; [m]$p < .02$; [n]$p .05$; [o]$p < .05$.

production of these substances is influenced by the degree of gastritis activity, being particularly elevated in the mucosa with neutrophilic infiltration (Table 2).

3. In duodenal ulcer patients we found a significant rise in the production of all cyclooxygenase metabolites of the mucosal specimens taken from the ulcer crater. The synthesis of prostanoids progressively diminishes from the area around the crater toward the opposite wall, with the exception of PGD_2, which is significantly increased in all areas studied (Table 3).

4. We found the same trend for gastric ulcer as for duodenal ulcer, but PGE_2 and $6KPGF_{1\alpha}$ only are significantly increased; the latter is greater in all the examined areas (Table 4).

These observations suggest that in inflammatory diseases of the upper gastrointestinal tract the metabolization of arachidonic acid, through the cyclooxygenase pathway, is enhanced in the same manner as in inflammatory bowel disease [77–79].

In our opinion, it is of particular importance that the duodenal mucosa bordering the ulcer crater produces about a fourfold increase of PGE_2, confirming the efficiency of the cyclooxygenase metabolic pathway. Indirect support of these data is given by the evidence that synthetic prostaglandins are slightly more effective than placebo in healing peptic ulcers unless high doses are used that inhibit the acid secretion [80,81]. On the other hand, synthetic prostaglandins are effective in protecting or promoting the healing of mucosal lesions induced by NSAIDs [82–84]. The results

Table 3 Prostanoid Production from Biopsy Specimens of 15 Normal Subjects and 21 Patients with Duodenal Ulcer after Incubation in Krebs Solution for 30 min

		Duodenal ulcer		
	Controls	US	1 cm	WO
PGE_2	2.55 ± 0.36[a]	11.17 ± 1.87[a]	6.09 ± 1.91	5.05 ± 1.00
$PGF_{2\alpha}$	12.99 ± 2.73[b]	15.85 ± 1.21[b]	15.45 ± 1.64	16.13 ± 1.68
$6KPGF_{1\alpha}$	12.64 ± 2.15[c]	19.92 ± 1.95[c]	18.87 ± 2.36	18.91 ± 2.39
PGD_2	15.05 ± 3.79[d,e,f]	22.21 ± 2.38[d]	22.28 ± 3.04[e]	22.14 ± 3.36[f]
TXB_2	14.16 ± 2.14[g]	25.04 ± 2.47[g]	20.08 ± 2.28	20.11 ± 2.76

The results (M ± SE) are expressed as ng/mg soluble proteins per 30 min. US = ulcer site; 1 cm = 1 cm from ulcer site; WO = wall opposite the ulcer. The results were analyzed by nonparametric statistics: [a]$p < .002$; [b]$p < .02$; [c]$p < .025$; [d]$p < .05$; [e]$p < .05$; [f]$p < .05$; [g]$p < .005$.

Table 4 Prostanoid Production from Biopsy Specimens of 15 Normal Subjects and 11 Patients with Antral Gastric Ulcer after Incubation in Krebs Solution for 30 min

	Controls	Gastric ulcer		
		US	1 cm	WO
PGE_2	12.57 ± 2.35[a,b]	24.01 ± 3.81[a]	22.68 ± 3.93[b]	18.53 ± 3.95
$PGF_{2\alpha}$	10.74 ± 1.03	14.06 ± 2.07	12.03 ± 1.51	13.42 ± 1.48
$6KPGF_{1\alpha}$	11.10 ± 1.63[c,d,e]	19.30 ± 3.42[c]	18.19 ± 2.60[d]	17.47 ± 2.35[e]
PGD_2	13.71 ± 2.91[f]	19.07 ± 3.01	15.69 ± 2.20	19.87 ± 4.08[f]
TXB_2	24.96 ± 4.47	28.85 ± 4.64	26.83 ± 3.91	26.60 ± 4.50

The results (M $\pm$ SE) are expressed as ng/mg soluble proteins per 30 min. US = ulcer site; 1 cm = 1 cm from ulcer site; WO = wall opposite the ulcer. The results were analyzed by nonparametric statistics: [a]$p < .025$; [b]$p < .05$; [c]$p < .05$; [d]$p < .025$; [e]$p < .025$; [f]$p < .025$.

reported by other authors are difficult to interpret [69,71,72,74], because it is necessary to hypothesize the deficiency of one or more enzymatic activities (reductase, isomerase, synthetase). Since these enzymes are normally found throughout the body, their decrease should also cause a functional alteration of one or more organs or systems. In recent years several experimental data have shown that other substances such as leukotrienes and platelet-activating factor are able to produce a potent inflammatory and ulcerogenic activity in the gastroduodenal mucosa of animals [85,86]. Recent studies have demonstrated that these substances are produced in amounts significantly higher in the mucosa of patients with duodenal ulcer [87]; therefore, it is conceivable that in the pathogenesis of peptic disease the increased production of inflammatory molecules is more important than the decreased production of those with protective activity. Further supporting this hypothesis are our data indicating that during inflammatory disease of the gastroduodenal mucosa there is an increased synthesis of TXB_2 and PGD_2, particularly the latter in duodenal ulcer. The effect of TXB_2 in this site is well known, whereas we know little or nothing about the activity of PGD_2 even though it has a widely documented inflammatory effect in other tissue such as the lungs [88].

Our results, as well as those of other authors, lead us to presume that mucosal inflammatory cells might play an important role in the determination of peptic ulcer disease by synthesizing phospholipid-derived substances responsible for damaging the gastroduodenal mucosa.

VII.   STRESS ULCERS

Since the demonstration by Selye in the 1930s that physically restraining a rat can produce gastric erosions, interest has been increasing in the subject of stress-induced ulcers. These lesions are becoming more common in hospitalized patients as the number of intensive care units increases. In fact, stress ulcers occur in several acute conditions: severe trauma (particularly with cerebral and spinal cord lesions), coma, thermal burn injury, major surgery, sepsis, pulmonary and renal insufficiency, and chronic ingestion of steroids or NSAIDs. The pathophysiology of these conditions often include similar neurological, endocrine, metabolic, (micro)vascular, and coagulation defects. The selected clinical spectrum, together with histological features of stress ulcers, raised the hypothesis of a specific pathogenesis.

Many experimental studies have underlined the possible mechanisms by which stress ulcers develop. Evidence exists that demonstrates the damaging effects on the gastroduodenal mucosa of local ischemia [89], lowered intramucosal pH [90], oxygen-derived free radicals [91], NSAIDs and steroids, stimulatory activity of the central nucleus of the amygdala induced by TRH or by dopamine receptor blockers [92], and inflammatory mediators such as thromboxanes, leukotrienes, and platelet-activating factor (PAF).

Platelet-activating factor, an endogenous phospholipid, is synthesized and released by several inflammatory cells as well as by platelets and endothelial cells [93,94]. It has been implicated in many allergic and inflammatory processes [95] and is also the most potent gastric pro-ulcerogen yet described [96]. Recent studies demonstrate that PAF acts as a mediator of endotoxin-induced gastrointestinal damage in the rat [97] and that this mechanism of septic shock bowel necrosis seems to be realized by sequential release of leukotriene C_4 and norepinephrine [98]. Interestingly, the ulcerogenic effect of PAF can be inhibited by dexamethasone [99] and by specific molecular antagonists [97].

Our group studied some patients affected by ascitic cirrhosis, where there is a high prevalence of endotoxemia, and some affected by rheumatoid arthritis. These are two human pathological conditions at high risk for developing hemorrhagic gastric lesions and stress ulcers. In both conditions we demonstrated for the first time the presence of PAF activity in the gastric mucosa with hemorrhagic lesions [100,101]. In another study, we also showed that in rheumatoid arthritis patients taking NSAIDs, 1 month of treatment with misoprostol induced not only the healing of erosive lesions but also improvement of the inflammatory gastric infiltrate [102]. In addition to the treatment of stress ulcers with somatostatin [103] and prostaglandin [104] already reported, it is possible to suggest that, in the near future, therapeutic trials could also prove the clinical usefulness of free radical scavengers, PAF antagonists, and CNS peptides (β-endorphins).

VIII. *HELICOBACTER PYLORI*

Concerning the pathogenesis of peptic ulcer disease, an exponential number of scientific studies dealing with *Helicobacter pylori* previously named *Campylobacter pylori*) have been published worldwide since the mid-1980s [105]. The discovery of bacteria in the stomach, however, is not a new finding; in 1893 Bizzozero described the presence of spiral bacteria on the gastric mucosa of animals [106]. Even though for decades this observation was considered somewhat anomalous, it is now accepted that *Helicobacter pylori* is the most common and most important cause of chronic gastritis [107]. Moreover, epidemiological [108] and therapeutic [109] studies have demonstrated its importance in the pathogenesis and natural history of ulcer disease [41].

At present, identification of *Helicobacter pylori* is based on both invasive and noninvasive methods. Noninvasive methods include both serological tests and functional tests. Serological tests consist in the titration of specific IgG and IgM response to *H. pylori*. They can be used not only to diagnose *H. pylori* infection but also for the patients' follow-up after medical treatment. In fact, there is evidence that anti-*H. pylori* IgG levels decline upon the eradication of the organism and increase again upon reinfection [110]. To date, the available methods using crude *H. pylori* antigen preparations have high sensitivity but a rather low specificity. Second-generation tests using purified *H. pylori* proteins (for example, urease) as antigen are necessary to increase specificity and sensitivity [111].

Functional tests are represented by urea breath tests; both ^{13}C- and ^{14}C-urea tests [111,112] have been proven to be highly specific, sensitive, and responsive to the presence of *H. pylori* infection [111]. Moreover, in comparison to serological techniques or invasive methods, the ^{13}C-urea breath test has several advantages: It is safer, it detects lower levels of infection, permitting a scalar term of comparison between individuals, and it reflects current infection. Finally, it is probably more appropriate for in vivo drug sensitivity studies and for monitoring the outcome of therapeutic trials.

Invasive methods allow direct diagnosis of the *H. pylori* infection by the use of biopsy material obtained during upper endoscopic examination. The high endogenous urease activity of *H. pylori* led to the development of a number of in vitro rapid tests [113,114]. In our experience, a modified microtiter urease time test was useful not only to diagnose *H. pylori* infection with high concordance with histology, but also to correlate the grading of bacterial colonization with inflammatory cell counts in the mucosa [115].

The "gold standard" of *H. pylori* detection is represented by (a) microbiological culture with selective media and (b) morphological identification of *H. pylori* on biopsy with histological techniques (Warthin-Starry, Giemsa) or with electron microscopy [116]. Histology offers high sensitivity and specificity but could fail to detect scarce bacteria given the patchy distribution of *H. pylori* on the mucosa. This pattern can otherwise be easily evidenced by scanning electron microscopy (Fig. 4).

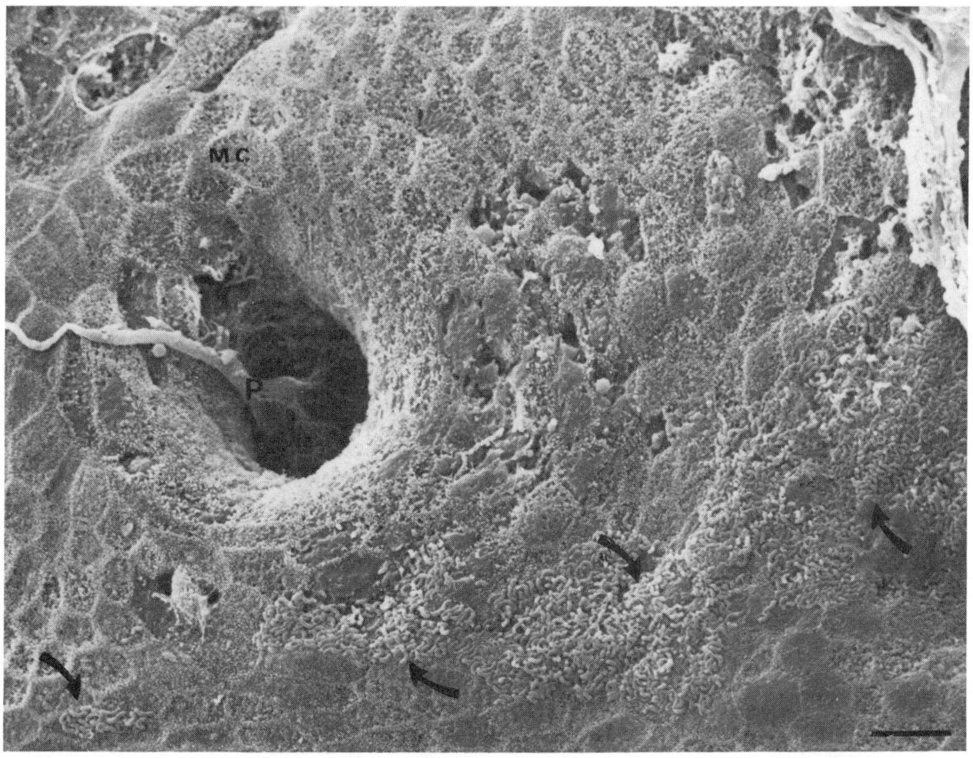

FIGURE 4 Scanning electron micrograph of human gastric mucosa. Patchy distribution of *Helicobacter pylori* on the mucosal surface (arrows). The polygonal profiles of mucous cells are evident. P = pit opening. MC = surface mucous cells. (SEM, 1000×). Bar = 10 μm.

We studied the relationships between *H. pylori* and gastric antral mucosa in patients with chronic gastritis by scanning electron microscopy [116]. Colonization of superficial epithelium does not induce any specific ultrastructural alteration (Fig. 5). Only minor modifications of the luminal membranes can be observed along with the characteristic pattern of *H. pylori* adhesion and penetration into the intercellular spaces. This feature could be the morphological expression of the recent biochemical demonstration of the presence of a glycolipidic receptor specific for *H. pylori* on the gastric epithelial cells [117]. These data confirm the hypothesis that histological modifications induced in the gastric mucosa by *H. pylori* colonization could depend on the effect of inflammatory mediators released by polymorphonuclear and lymphocytic infiltration [118]. Our previous studies showed that the entity of *H. pylori* infection is

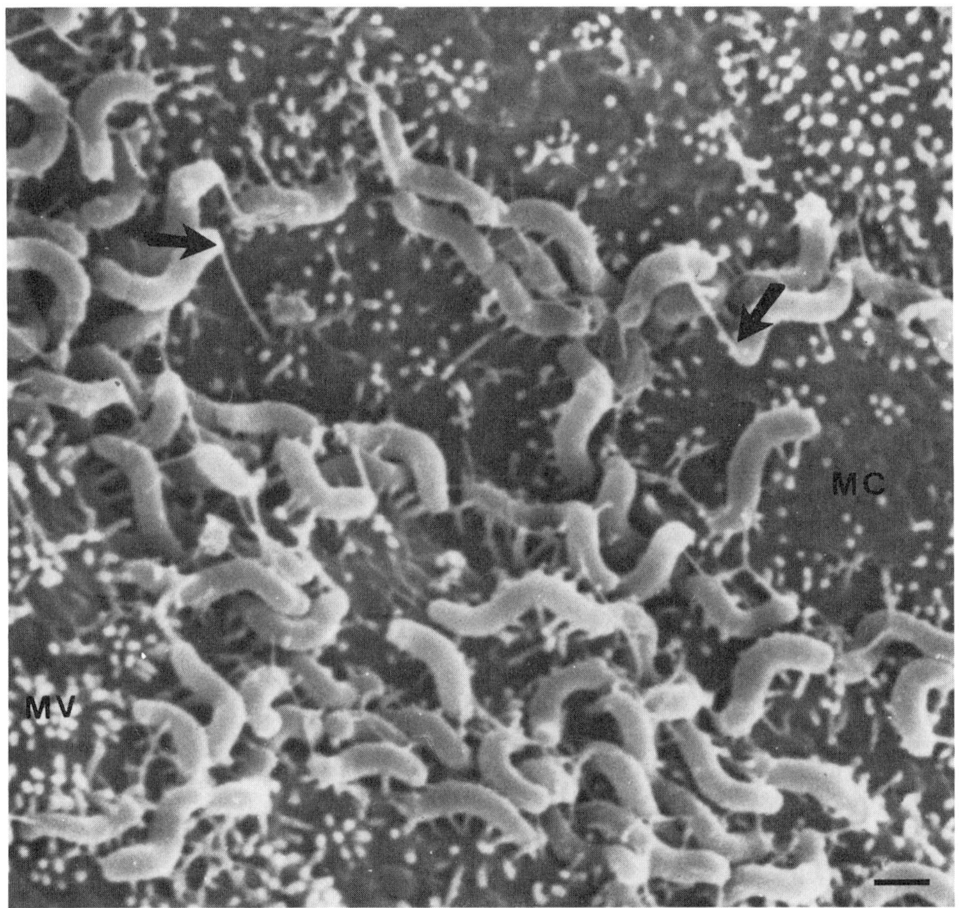

FIGURE 5 Scanning electron micrograph of human gastric mucosa colonized by *Helicobacter pylori*. Bacteria are located mainly in the intercellular junctions of surface mucous cells (MC). Arrows indicate polar flagella. MV = microvilli (SEM, 5500×). Bar = 1 μm.

significantly related to the semiquantitative counts of inflammatory cells (particularly neutrophils and eosinophils) infiltrating the gastric mucosa in chronic gastritis [119].

Treatment studies with antibiotics alone demonstrate that neutrophilic response disappears with eradication of *H. pylori* [120], suggesting that the polymorph infiltration is a specific response to the organisms.

Regarding immunohistochemical characterization of inflammatory cells, studies show that, unlike those with normal mucosa, patients with *H. pylori* gastritis express

HLA-DR antigen on the antral mucosa [121]. They also have an increase in the number of mucosal infiltrating cytotoxic suppressor T cells [122]. A small number of patients have a distinct type of histological gastritis, "lymphocytic gastritis," characterized by a dense intraepithelial T-cell (CD8-positive) infiltrate [123]. This feature could represent a modified response to *H. pylori* infection in particular types of patients with immunological abnormalities.

Other hypotheses on the pathogenic properties of *H. pylori* include the production of substances toxic for the gastric mucosa such as urease [124], endopeptidase [125], and lipase [126]. A recent study demonstrates that *H. pylori* strains producing vacuolating cytotoxin are significantly associated with ulcer disease [127]. Unexpectedly, some patients with clinical disease characterized by immunological and vascular abnormalities (cirrhosis, rheumatoid arthritis, hematological malignancies) at high risk for gastroduodenal lesions do not have a high prevalence of *H. pylori* infection. In these subjects we demonstrated the presence of detectable levels of PAF in the gastric mucosa, together with hemorrhagic lesions and *H. pylori* colonization. This could suggest a link between the immunological response induced by *H. pylori* in the stomach and the local production of inflammatory mediators that can damage the gastroduodenal mucosa [128].

Even though there is evidence for a pathogenic role of *H. pylori* in ulcer disease, many doubts remain to be elucidated:

1. Experimental inoculation with *H. pylori* produces gastritis and dyspepsia but not ulcers.
2. The prevalence of *H. pylori* gastritis increases with age, but that of ulcers does not.
3. Ulcers do not show the epidemiological characteristics of an infectious disease.
4. The causal relationship between duodenal ulcer and antral gastritis remains unclear, as gastritis is a diffuse disease whereas an ulcer is a focal one.
5. Some therapeutic agents heal ulcers without affecting *H. pylori*.
6. Prolonged randomized trials demonstrating a clear correlation between *H. pylori* eradication and ulcer healing are yet not available.

IX. SUMMARY

We have reviewed the most accepted physiopathological mechanisms for ulcer disease, giving special attention to some recently recognized but not completely elucidated points. Both researchers and practitioners have been faced for a long time with these and many other questions about the development and recurrence of ulcers. It is now clear that useful information for future clinical strategies can come only from extensive work with the new structural, biochemical, functional, and chronobiological approaches.

REFERENCES

1. Rokitansky C. Manual of pathological anatomy, Vol. 2. London: Sydenham, 1849; 22–46.
2. Baron HJ. Current views on pathogenesis of peptic ulcer. Scand J Gastroenterol 1982; 17(Suppl 80):1–10.
3. Wormsley KG. Duodenal ulcer: does pathophysiology equal etiology? Gut 1983; 24:775.
4. Szabo S. Pathogenesis of duodenal ulcer disease. Lab Invest 1984; 51:121–47.
5. Brooks FP. The pathophysiology of peptic ulcer disease. Dig Dis Sci 1985; 30(Suppl 11):15–29S.
6. Soll AH. Pathogenesis and pathophysiology of duodenal ulcer. In: Sleisenger MH, Fordtran JS, eds. Gastrointestinal disease. 4th ed. Philadelphia: WB Saunders, 1989: 823–31.
7. Johnson HD, Love AHG, Rogers NC, Wyatt AP. Gastric ulcers, blood groups and acid secretion. Gut 1964; 5:402–8.
8. Blair AJ III, Feldman M, Barnett C, Walsh JH, Richardson CT. Detailed comparison of basal and food-stimulated gastric acid secretion rates and serum gastrin concentrations in duodenal ulcer patients and normal subjects. J Clin Invest 1987; 79:582–7.
9. Cox AJ. Stomach size and its relation to chronic peptic ulcer. Arch Pathol 1952; 54:407–11.
10. Malagelada JR, Longstreth GF, Deering B, Summerskill WHJ, Go VLW. Gastric secretion and emptying after ordinary meals in duodenal ulcer. Gastroenterology 1977; 73:989–94.
11. Feldman M, Richardson CT. Total 24-hour acid gastric secretion in patients with duodenal ulcer. Gastroenterology 1986; 90:540–4.
12. Lam SK, Isenberg JI, Grossman MI, Lane WH, Walsh JH. Gastric acid secretion is abnormally sensitive to exogenous gastrin released after peptone test meals in duodenal ulcer patients. J Clin Invest 1980; 65:555–62.
13. Lam SK, Koo J. Gastrin sensitivity in duodenal ulcer. Gut 1985; 26:485–90.
14. Walsh JH, Richardson CT, Fordtran JS. pH dependence of acid secretion and gastrin release in normal and ulcer subjects. J Clin Invest 1975; 55:462–8.
15. Schoon IM, Bergegardh S, Grotzinger U, Olbe L. Evidence for a defective inhibition of pentagastrin-stimulated gastric acid secretion by antral distention in the duodenal ulcer patient. Gastroenterology 1978; 5:363–7.
16. Cooper RG, Dockray GJ, Calam J, Walker R. Acid and gastrin responses during intragastric titration in normal subjects and duodenal ulcer patients with G-cell hyperfunction. Gut 1985; 26:232–6.
17. Alphin RS, Vokak VA, Gregory LR, Bolton PM, Tawes JW III. Role of intragastric pressure, pH, and pepsin in gastric ulceration in the rat. Gastroenterology 1977; 73:495–500.
18. Joffe SN, Roberts NB, Taylor WH, Baaron JH. Exogenous and endogenous acid and pepsin in the pathogenesis of duodenal ulcers in the rat. Dig Dis Sci 1980; 25:837–41.
19. Pearson JP, Ward R, Allen A, Roberts NB, Taylor WH. Mucus degradation by pepsin: comparison of mucolytic activity of human pepsin I and pepsin III: implications in peptic ulceration. Gut 1986; 27:243–8.

20. Ichinose M, Miki K, Furihata C, Kageyama T, Hayashi R, Niwa H, Oka H, Matsushima T, Takahashi K. Radioimmunoassay of serum group I and group II pepsinogens in normal controls and patients with various disorders. Clin Chim Acta 1982; 126:183–8.

21. Friedman GD, Siegelaub AB, Seltzer CC. Cigarettes, alcohol, coffee and peptic ulcer. N Engl J Med 1974; 290:469–73.

22. McCarthy DM. Smoking and ulcers—time to quit. N Engl J Med 1984; 311:726–8.

23. Sontag S, Graham DY, Belsito A, Weiss J, Farley A, Grunt R, Cohen N, Kinnear D, Davis W, Archambault A, Achord J, Thayer W, Gillies RG, Sidorov J, Sabesin SM, Dyck W, Fleshler B, Cleator I, Wenger J, Opekun A. Cimetidine, cigarette smoking, and recurrence of duodenal ulcer. N Engl J Med 1984; 311:689–93.

24. Muller-Lissner SA. Bile reflux is increased in cigarette smokers. Gastroenterology 1986; 90:1205–9.

25. Massarrat S, Enschai F, Pittner PM. Increased gastric secretory capacity in smokers without gastrointestinal lesions. Gut 1986; 27:433–9.

26. McCreaty DR, Clark L, Cohen MM. Cigarette smoking reduces human gastric luminal prostaglandin E_2. Gut 1985; 26:1192–6.

27. Quinby GF, Bonnice CA, Burstein SH, Eastwood GL. Active smoking depresses prostaglandin synthesis in human gastric mucosa. Ann Intern Med 1986; 104:616–9.

28. Bauerfeind P, Cilluffo T, Fimmell CJ, Emde C, Von Ritter C, Kohler W, Gugler R, Gasser T, Blum AL. Does smoking interfere with the effect of histamine H_2-receptor antagonists on intragastric acidity in man? Gut 1987; 28:549–56.

29. Lenz HJ, Ferrari-Taylor J, Isenberg JI. Wine and five percent ethanol are potent stimulants of gastric acid secretion in humans. Gastroenterology 1983; 85:1082–7.

30. Peterson WL, Barnett C, Walsh J. Effect of intragastric infusions of ethanol and wine on serum gastrin concentration and gastric acid secretion. Gastroenterology 1986; 91:1390–5.

31. Paffenbarger RS, Wing AL, Hyde RT. Chronic disease in former college students. XIII. Early precursor of peptic ulcer. Am J Epidemiol 1974; 100:307–15.

32. Ostensen H, Gudmundsen TE, Burhol PG, Bonnevie O. Smoking, alcohol, coffee, and familial factors: any associations with peptic ulcer disease? A clinically and radiologically prospective study. Scand J Gastroenterol 1985; 20:1227–35.

33. Sonnenberg A, Muller-Lissner SA, Vogel E, Schmid P, Gonvers JJ, Peter P, Strohmeyer J, Blum AL. Predictors of duodenal ulcer healing and relapse. Gastroenterology 1981; 81:1061–7.

34. Cohen S. Pathogenesis of coffee-induced gastrointestinal symptoms. N Engl J Med 1980; 303:122–4.

35. McArthur K, Hogan D, Isenberg JI. Relative stimulatory effects of commonly ingested beverages on gastric acid secretion in humans. Gastroenterology 1982; 83:199–203.

36. Dubey P, Sundram KR, Nundy S. Effect of tea on gastric acid secretion. Dig Dis Sci 1984; 29:202–6.

37. Silen W. What is cytoprotection of the gastric mucosa? Gastroenterology 1988; 94:232–5.

38. Szabo S, Bynum TE. Alternatives to the acid-oriented approach to ulcer disease: does "cytoprotection" exist in man? Scand J Gastroenterol 1988; 23:1–6.

39. Starlinger M, Schiessel R. Bicarbonate (HCO_3) delivery to the gastroduodenal mucosa by the blood: its importance for mucosal integrity. Gut 1988; 29:647–54.

40. Konturek SJ. Role of epidermal growth factor in gastroprotection and ulcer healing. Scand J Gastroenterol 1988; 23:129–33.

41. Graham DY. *Campylobacter pylori* and peptic ulcer disease. Gastroenterology 1989; 96:615–25.

42. Allen A, Hutton DA, Leonard AJ, Pearson JP, Sellers LA. The role of mucus in the protection of the gastroduodenal mucosa. Scand J Gastroenterol 1986; 21(Suppl 125): 71–7.

43. Turnberg LA, Ross IN. Studies of pH gradient across gastric mucus. Scand J Gastroenterol 1984; 19(Suppl 92):48–51.

44. Pfeiffer CJ. Experimental analysis of hydrogen ion diffusion in gastrointestinal mucus glycoprotein. Am J Physiol 1981; 240:G176.

45. Rainsford KD. The effects of aspirin and other non-steroid anti-inflammatory/analgesic drugs on the gastrointestinal mucus glycoprotein biosynthesis in vivo: relationship to ulcerogenic actions. Biochem Pharmacol 1978; 27:877–82.

46. Allen A, Garner A, Kerss S. A simple method for measuring thickness of the mucus gel layer adherent to rat, frog and human gastric mucosa: influence of feeding, prostaglandin, *N*-acetylcysteine and other agents. Clin Sci 1982; 63(2):187–95.

47. Bell AE, Sellers LA, Allen A, Cunliffe WJ, Morris ER, Ross-Murphy SB. Properties of gastric and duodenal mucus: effect of proteolysis, disulfide reduction, bile, acid, ethanol, and hypertonicity on mucus gel structure. Gastroenterology 1985; 88:269–80.

48. Slomiany BL, Sarosiek J, Mizuta K, Slomiany A. Effect of acetylsalicylic acid on gastric mucus viscosity, H^+ permeability and susceptibility to pepsin. Gastroenterology 1986; 90:1638.

49. Slomiany BL, Piasek A, Sarosiek J, Slomiany A. The role of surface and intracellular mucus in gastric mucosal protection against hydrogen ion. Compositional differences. Scand J Gastroenterol 1985; 20:1191–6.

50. Allen A, Carroll NJH. Adherent and soluble mucus in the stomach and duodenum. Dig Dis Sci 1985; 30:55–62S.

51. Vatier J, Poitevin C, Mignon M. Sialic acid content and proteolytic activity in gastric juice in humans. An approach for appreciating mucus glycoprotein erosion. Dig Dis Sci 1988; 33:144–51.

52. Hawkey CJ, Kemp RT, Walt RP, Bhaskar NK, Davies J, Filipowicz B. Evidence that adaptive cytoprotection in rat is not mediated by prostaglandins. Gastroenterology 1988; 94:948–54.

53. Ishihara K, Kuwata H, Ohara S, Ohkawa H, Okabe H, Hotta K. Mucus glycoprotein and mucosal protection. J Clin Gastroenterol 1988; 10(Suppl 1):S24–7.

54. Damjanov I. Biology of disease. Lectin cytochemistry and histochemistry. Lab Invest 1987; 57:5–20.

55. Bonvicini F, Maltarello MC, Versura P, Bianchi D, Gasbarrini G, Laschi R. Correlative scanning electron microscopy in the study of human gastric mucosa. Scan Electron Microsc 1986; II:687–702.

56. Bonvicini F, Gasbarrini G. Lectin histochemistry in the study of human gastric mucins. In: Cheli R, et al., eds. Gastric protection. New York: Raven, 1988:101–8.

57. Pretolani S, Bonvicini F, Brocchi E, Funaro S, Careddu N, Cilla D, Dal Pra' ML, Gasbarrini G. Enprostil treatment in *Campylobacter pylori* gastritis. Klin Wochenschr 1989; 67(Suppl XVIII):55.

58. Fändrics L. Sympatho-adrenergic inhibition of vagally induced gastric motility and gastroduodenal HCO_3 secretion in the cat. Acta Physiol Scand 1986; 128:555–62.

59. Starlinger M, Jakesz R, Matthews JB, Yoon CH, Schiessel R. The relative importance of HCO_3 and blood flow in the protection of rat gastric mucosa during shock. Gastroenterology 1981; 81:732–5.

60. Forssell H, Olbe L. Basal and stimulated gastric bicarbonate secretion. Scand J Gastroenterol 1987; 22:627–33.

61. Crampton JR, Gibbons LC, Rees WD. Stimulation of amphibian gastroduodenal bicarbonate secretion by sucralfate and aluminum: role of local prostaglandin metabolism. Gut 1988; 29:903–8.

62. Flemstrom G, Garner A. Gastroduodenal HCO_3 transport: characteristics and proposed role in acidity regulation and mucosal protection. Am J Physiol 1982; 242:G183–93.

63. Bennett A, Hensby CN, Sanger GJ, Stamford IF. Metabolites of arachidonic acid formed by human gastrointestinal tissues and their actions on the muscle layers. Br J Pharm 1981; 74:436–44.

64. Salvati P, Whittle BJR. Investigation of the vascular actions of arachidonate lipoxygenase and cyclo-oxygenase products on the isolated perfused stomach of rat and rabbit. Prostaglandins 1981; 22:141–56.

65. Kauffman GL, Whittle BJR. Gastric vascular actions of prostanoids and the dual effect of arachidonic acid. Am J Physiol 1982:G582–7.

66. Johansson C, Kollberg B. Stimulation by intragastrically administered E_2 prostaglandins of human gastric mucus output. Eur J Clin Invest 1979; 9:229–32.

67. Domschke W, Domschke S, Hornig D, Demling L. Prostaglandin-stimulated gastric mucus secretion in man. Acta Hepato-Gastroenterol 1978; 25:292–4.

68. Schlegel W, Wenk K, Dollinger HC, Raptis S. Concentrations of prostaglandin A-, E- and F-like substances in gastric mucosa of normal subjects and of patients with various gastric diseases. Clin Sci Mol Med 1977; 52:255–8.

69. Konturek SJ, Obtulowicz W, Sito E, Olesky J, Wilkon S, Kiec-Dembinska A. Distribution of prostaglandins in gastric and duodenal mucosa of healthy subjects and duodenal ulcer patients: effects of aspirin and paracetamol. Gut 1981; 22:283–9.

70. Ahlquist DA, Duenes JA, Madson TH, Romero JC, Dozois RR, Malagelada JR. Prostaglandin generation from gastroduodenal mucosa: regional and species differences. Prostaglandins 1982; 24:115–25.

71. Wright JP, Young GO, Klaff LJ, Lweers LA, Price SK, Marks IN. Gastric mucosal prostaglandin E levels in patients with gastric ulcer disease and carcinoma. Gastroenterology 1982; 82:263–7.

72. Sharon P, Cohen F, Zifroni A, Karmeli F, Ligumsky M, Rachmilewitz D. Prostanoid synthesis by cultured gastric and duodenal mucosa: possible role in the pathogenesis of duodenal ulcer. Scand J Gastroenterol 1983; 18:1045–9.

73. Moore SC, Shorter RG, Barham SS, Duenes JA, Zinsmeister AR, Malagelada JR. Interrelationships among gastric mucosal morphology and prostaglandin (PG) synthesis, luminal pH, and motility in ulcer disease. Gastroenterology 1984; 86:1188.

74. Hillier K, Smith CL, Jewell R, Arthur MJP, Ross G. Duodenal mucosa synthesis of prostaglandins in duodenal ulcer disease. Gut 1985; 26:237–40.

75. Racz I, Teri N, Javor T. Gastric mucosal potential difference and prostaglandin E_2 levels in gastric ulcer patients. It J Gastroenterol 1986; 18:324–8.

76. Baraldini M, Andreone P, Cursaro C, Micaletti E, Saggioro A, Bortoluzzi F, Miglio F, Gasbarrini G. Sintesi di prostanoidi nella mucosa gastrica e duodenale di soggetti sani. Bol Soc It Biol Sper 1988; LXIV(11):985–92.

77. Sharon P, Ligumsky M, Rachmilewitz D, Zor U. Role of prostaglandins in ulcerative colitis. Enhanced production during active disease and inhibition by sulphasalazine. Gastroenterology 1978; 75:638–40.

78. Rampton DS, Sladen GE, Youlten LY. Rectal mucosal prostaglandin E_2 release and its relation to disease activity, electrical potential difference and treatment in ulcerative colitis. Gut 1980; 21:591–6.

79. Ligumsky M, Karmeli F, Sharon P, Zor U, Cohen F, Rachmilewitz D. Enhanced thromboxane A_2 and prostacyclin production by cultured rectal mucosa in ulcerative colitis and its inhibition by steroids and sulphasalazine. Gastroenterology 1981; 81: 444–9.

80. Brand DL, Roufail WM, Thomson ABR, Tapper EJ. Misoprostol, a synthetic PGE_1 analog in the treatment of duodenal ulcers: a multicenter double-blind study. Dig Dis Sci 1985; 30(Suppl):147–58S.

81. Agrawal NM, Saffouri B, Kruss DM, Callison DA, Dajani EZ. Healing of benign gastric ulcer: a placebo-controlled comparison of two dosage regimens of misoprostol, a synthetic analog of prostaglandin E_1. Dig Dis Sci 1985; 30(Suppl):164–70S.

82. Lanza FL. A double-blind study of prophylactic effect of misoprostol on lesions of gastric and duodenal mucosa induced by oral administration of tolmetin in healthy subjects. Dig Dis Sci 1986; 31:131–6S.

83. Silverstein FE, Kimmy MB, Saunders DR, Levine DS. Gastric protection by misoprostol against 1300 mg of aspirin: an endoscopic study. Dig Dis Sci 1986; 31:137–41S.

84. Graham DY, Agrawal NM, Roth SH. Prevention of NSAID-induced gastric ulcer with misoprostol: multicentre, double-blind, placebo-controlled study. Lancet 1988; ii: 1277–80.

85. Whittle BJR, Oren-Wolman N, Guth PH. Gastric vasoconstrictor actions of leukotriene C_4, $PGF_{2\alpha}$, and thromboxane mimetic U-46619 on rat submucosa microcirculation in vitro. Am J Physiol 1985; 248:G580–6.

86. Whittle BJR, Kauffman GL, Wallace JL. Gastric vascular and mucosal damaging actions of platelet-activating factor in the canine stomach. In: Samuelsson B, Paoletti R, Ramwell RW, eds. Advances in prostaglandin, thromboxane, and leukotriene research. New York: Raven, 1987; 17A:285–92.

87. Ackerman Z, Karmeli F, Ligumsky M, Rachmilewitz D. Pathogenesis of duodenal ulcer: enhanced gastroduodenal formation of platelet-activating factor (PAF) and leukotrienes (LT). Gastroenterology 1989; 96(5):A2.

88. Peters SP, MacGlashan DW, Schulman ED, Schleimer RP, Hayes EC, Rokach J, Adkinson NF, Lichtenberger LM. Arachidonic acid metabolism in purified human lung mast cells. J Immunol 1984; 132:1972–9.

89. Murakami M, Lam SK, Inada M, Miyake T. Pathophysiology and pathogenesis of acute gastric mucosal lesions after hypothermic restraint stress in rats. Gastroenterology 1985; 88:660–72.

90. Kivilaasko E. Pathogenetic mechanisms in experimental gastric stress ulceration. Scand J Gastroenterol 1985; 20(Suppl 110):57–62.

91. Itoh M, Guth PH. Role of oxygen-derived free radicals in hemorrhagic shock-induced gastric lesions in the rat. Gastroenterology 1985; 88:1162–7.

92. Henke PG. Recent studies of the central nucleus of the amygdala and stress ulcers. Neurosci Biobehav Rev 1988; 12:143–50.

93. Mencia-Huerta JM, Benveniste J. Platelet-activating factor (PAF-acether) and macrophages. II. Phagocytosis associated release of PAF-acether from rat peritoneal macrophages. Cell Immunol 1981; 57:281–92.

94. Camussi G, Aglietta M, Coda R, Bussolino F, Piacibello W, Tetta C. Release of platelet-activating factor (PAF) and histamine. II. The cellular origin of human PAF: monocytes, polymorphonuclear neutrophils and basophils. Immunology 1981; 42:191–9.

95. Braquet P, Touqui L, Shen TY, Vargaftig BB. Perspectives in platelet activating factor research. Pharmacol Rev 1987; 39:97–145.

96. Rosam AC, Wallace JL. Potent ulcerogenic actions of platelet-activating factor on the stomach. Nature 1986; 319:54–6.

97. Wallace JL, Steel G, Whittle BJR, Lagente V, Vargaftig BB. Evidence for platelet-activating factor as a mediator of endotoxin-induced gastrointestinal damage in the rat. Effects of three platelet-activating factor antagonists. Gastroenterology 1987; 93:765–73.

98. Hsueh W, Gonzalez-Crussi F, Arroyave JL. Sequential release of leukotrienes and norepinephrine in rat bowel after platelet-activating factor. A mechanistic study of platelet-activating factor-induced bowel necrosis. Gastroenterology 1988; 94:1412–8.

99. Wallace JL, Whittle BJR. Gastrointestinal damage induced by platelet-activating factor. Inhibition by the corticoid, dexamethasone. Dig Dis Sci 1988; 33:225–32.

100. Pretolani S, Bonvicini F, Brocchi E, Paul-Eugène N, Mencia-Huerta JM, Braquet P, Miglio F, Gasbarrini G. Gastrite ipertensiva ed emorragia digestiva nella cirrosi epatica: possibile ruolo del fattore di attivazione piastrinica (PAF). Atti LXXXIX Congresso Nazionale Societa' Italiana Medicina Interna. Bologna, 3–6 novembre 1988.

101. Pretolani S, Bonvicini F, Brocchi E, Paul-Eugène N, Mencia-Huerta JM, Braquet P, Frizziero L, Gasbarrini G. Platelet-activating factor (PAF) activity in gastric biopsies of patients with rheumatoid arthritis (RA). 3rd Interscience World Conference on Inflammation: Antirheumatics, analgesics, immunomodulators. Monte Carlo, 1989: 394.

102. Pretolani S, Bonvicini F, Baraldini M, Brocchi E, Careddu N, Frizziero L, Miglio F, Gasbarrini G. Effetto del misoprostol sulla gastrite e sul *Campylobacter pylori* nell'artrite reumatoide in trattamento con FANS. Atti LXXXIX Congresso Societa' Italiana di Medicina Interna. Bologna 3–6 novembre 1988.

103. Kayasseh I, Keller U, Gyr K, Stadler GA. Somatostatin and cimetidine in peptic ulcer hemorrhage: a randomized controlled trial. Lancet 1980; i:844–8.

104. Zinner MJ, Rypins EB, Martin LR, Jonasson O, Hoover EL, Swabb EA, Fakouhi TD. Misoprostol versus antacid titration for preventing stress ulcers in postoperative surgical ICU patients. Ann Surg 1989; 210:590–5.

105. Marshall BJ. The *Campylobacter pylori* story. Scand J Gastroenterol 1988; 23(Suppl 146):58–66.

106. Bizzozero G. Ueber die schlauchfoermigen Drüsen des Magendarmkanals und die Beziehungen ihres Epithels zu dem Oberflächenepithel der Schleimhaut. Ark Mikr Anat 1893; 42:82–152.

107. Dooley CP, Cohen H. The clinical significance of *Campylobacter pylori*. Ann Intern Med 1988; 108:70–9.

108. Graham DY, Klein DP, Opekun AR, Boutton TW. Effect of age on the frequency of active *Campylobacter pylori* infection diagnosed by the (^{13}C)urea breath test in normal subjects and patients with peptic ulcer disease. J Infect Dis 1988; 157:777–80.

109. Marshall BJ, Goodwin CS, Warren JR, Murray R, Blincow ED, Blackbourn SJ, Phillips M, Waters TE, Sanderson CR. Prospective double blind trial of duodenal ulcer relapse after eradication of *Campylobacter pylori*. Lancet 1988; ii:1437–42.

110. Van Bohemen CG, Langenberg ML, Rauws EAJ, Oudbier J, Weterings E, Zanen HC. Rapidly decreased serum IgG to *Campylobacter pylori* following elimination of *Campylobacter* in histological chronic biopsy *Campylobacter*-positive gastritis. Immunol Lett 1989; 20:59–62.

111. Evans DG Jr, Evans DG, Graham DY, Klein PD. A sensitive and specific serologic test for detection of *Campylobacter pylori* infection. Gastroenterology 1989; 96:1004–8.

112. Marshall BJ, Surveyor I. Carbon-14 urea breath test for diagnosis of *Campylobacter pylori* associated gastritis. Clin Sci 1988; 29:11–26.

113. McNulty CAM, Wise R. Rapid diagnosis of *Campylobacter* associated gastritis [Letter]. Lancet 1985; i:1443–4.

114. Marshall BJ, Warren JR, Francis GJ, Langton SR, Goodwin CS, Blincow ED. Rapid urease test in the management of *Campylobacter pyloridis*-associated gastritis. Am J Gastroenterol 1987; 82:200–10.

115. Pretolani S, Bonvicini F, Baraldini M, Micaletti E, Brocchi E, Caletti GC, Gasbarrini G. The value of microtiter urease test in grading of *Campylobacter pylori* gastric colonization and associated gastritis. In: Gasbarrini G, Stefanini GF, Desideri D, eds. Attualita' in gastroenterologia. Bologna: Editrice Compositori, 1988: 503–6.

116. Bonvicini F, Versura P, Pretolani S, Gasbarrini G, Laschi R. Scanning electron microscopy in the study of *Campylobacter pylori* associated gastritis. Scanning Microsc 1989; 3(1):355–68.

117. Lingwood CA, Law H, Pellizzari A, Sherman P, Drumm B. Gastric glycerolipid as a receptor for *Campylobacter pylori*. Lancet 1989; ii:238–41.

118. Taha AS, McKinlay AW, Upadhyay R, Kelly R, Russell RI. Prostaglandins and *Campylobacter pylori*. Lancet 1989; ii:800–1.

119. Gasbarrini G, Bonvicini F, Baraldini M, Andreone P, Pretolani S, Cursaro C, Cheli R, Saggioro A, D'Errico A, Grigioni WF. *Campylobacter pylori*, inflammatory infiltration and prostanoid synthesis in gastric mucosa. Acta Endoscop 1988; 18(1):XXVI.

120. Rauws EAJ, Langenberg W, Houthoff HJ, Zanen HC, Tytgat GNJ. *Campylobacter pyloridis*-associated chronic antral gastritis. Gastroenterology 1988; 94:33–40.

121. Engstrand L, Scheynius A, Pahlson C, Grimelius L, Schwan A, Gustavsson S. Association of *Campylobacter pylori* with induced expression of class II transplantation antigens on gastric epithelial cells. Infect Immun 1989; 57:827–32.

122. Papadimitriou CS, Ioachim-Velogianni EE, Tsianos EB, Moutsopoulos HM. Epithelial HLA-DR expression and lymphocyte subsets in gastric mucosa in type B chronic gastritis. Virchows Arch A Pathol Anat 1988; 413:197–204.

123. Haot J, Delos M, Wallez I. Intraepithelial lymphocytes in inflammatory gastric pathology. Acta Endoscop 1986; 16:61–7.

124. Barer MR, Elliott TSJ, Berkeley D, Thomas JE, Eastham EJ. Cytopathic effects of *Campylobacter pylori* urease. J Clin Pathol 1988; 41:597.

125. Slomiany BL, Bilski J, Sarosiek J, Murty VLN, Dvorkin B, Vanhorn K, Zielenski J, Slomiany A. *Campylobacter pylori* degrades mucins and undermines gastric mucosal integrity. Biochem Biophys Res Commun 1987; 144:307–14.

126. Sarosiek J, Slomiany A, VanHorn K, Zalesna G, Slomiany BL. Lipolytic activity of *Campylobacter pylori*: effect of sofalcone. Gastroenterology 1988; 94:A399.

127. Figura N, Gugliemetti P, Rossolini A, Barberi A, Cusi G, Musmanno RA, Russi M, Quaranta S. Cytotoxin production by *Campylobacter pylori* strains isolated from patients with peptic ulcers and from patients with chronic gastritis only. J Clin Microbiol 1989; 27:225–6.

128. Pretolani S, Bonvicini F, Brocchi E, Paul-Eugène N, Mencia-Huerta JM, Braquet P, Gasbarrini G. *Campylobacter pylori* and the platelet-activating factor in the development of gastroduodenal erosive lesions. Klin Wochenschr 1989; 67(Suppl XVIII):56.

PRESENTATIONS

5

Clinical Presentation of Ulcer Disease

T. Edward Bynum

Harvard Medical School, Boston, Massachusetts

I.   INTRODUCTION

Disease presents as one or more symptoms or is diagnosed at the patient's death. Fortunately, ulcer disease is not often fatal; in epidemiological jargon, it is a disease of low mortality [1–4].

II.   SYMPTOMS AND SIGNS OF ULCER DISEASE

The classic symptom of nonmalignant gastroduodenal ulcer disease is epigastric discomfort or pain (often of a burning or gnawing character) [5] that occurs 2 hr or more after a meal, when one skips a meal, late at night (perhaps wakening the patient from sleep), or upon arising in the morning. Typically, it is relieved by the ingestion of milk, food, or a dose of antacid. Rarely it may radiate to the midback. Since the days when almost everyone believed that the sole cause of ulcer was excess acid (and pepsin) secretion, the symptoms (and the disease) have been called peptic: peptic ulcer disease, peptic ulcer symptoms. One suspects that an effort to shorten and classicize the phrase "peptic ulcer symptoms" led to the term dyspepsia. In recent years, the flexible fiberoptic endoscope has allowed us to recognize with considerable confidence that a patient can have dyspeptic symptoms without having an ulcer: non-ulcer dyspepsia [6,7]. An effort is being made to distinguish classic ulcer symptoms from the symptoms more frequently recognized in patients with non-ulcer dyspepsia: general abdominal discomfort that is more often cramping or aching, discomfort occurring immediately after a meal, intolerance to food, abdominal bloating and distention, burping, and weight gain (in spite of purported food intolerance and symptoms being triggered by a meal). I would estimate that approximately 15% of patients with classic symptoms would be found by endoscopy to have no ulcer and that 10% of patients with dyspeptic symptoms would be found to have an ulcer if endoscopy were performed.

It is difficult to know by what mechanism pain occurs in ulcer disease. A large biopsy instrument can create a tissue defect in the stomach or duodenum equal in diameter and depth to the average ulcer, yet no pain is felt when the crater is made or while it heals. Traditionally teaching acknowledges that gastric and duodenal mucosa is insensitive to direct trauma but attributes pain to a combination of motor activity in the region of inflammation that surrounds an ulcer (motor activity + inflammation = pain). That explanation is less than totally satisfactory, however. At least 20% of ulcer patients who present with a major complication (bleeding, perforation, obstruction) have had no classic ulcer symptoms or dyspepsia prior to the complication [8]. Furthermore, if a classically symptomatic ulcer is treated by either an H_2-receptor antagonist [9,10] or a cytoprotective agent [11–13], pain disappears long before the ulcer heals or even diminishes in size [9,14]. If a patient with ulcer and classic symptoms is healed by the H_2-receptor antagonist cimetidine and therapy is stopped after complete healing, when the ulcer recurs (often the same size, in the same location) [15], up to 40% of the time the patient has no pain or any other symptoms. (When ulcers are healed by cytoprotective therapy, only about 10% or fewer of the patients have no symptoms when the ulcer recurs—a difference that remains unexplained [14,16,17].)

Because the gross appearance of an ulcer is that of an open sore, it is easy to imagine that gastric acid getting on that sore would cause pain. Nevertheless, the relationship of acid to ulcer pain [18] is at least as difficult to understand as other aspects of ulcer pain. For example, cytoprotective therapy that has no effect on gastric acid or its access to the ulcer crater relieves pain just as quickly, and just as well, as the most potent H_2-receptor antagonist therapy [12]. Over 30 years ago, one clinical investigator (considered by many of his colleagues at the time to have become bereft of his sanity) randomly assigned symptomatic duodenal ulcer patients to one of two groups; one group had liquid antacid dripped constantly on the ulcer by means of a nasogastric (or nasoduodenal) tube, and the other group had 0.1 N hydrochloric acid (comparable to human gastric acid) dripped constantly on the ulcer. There was no difference in alleviation of pain between the two groups. When healthy volunteer patients are started on aspirin or other nonsteroidal medication in rheumatological doses and are then followed clinically and endoscopically, 20% will develop peptic/dyspeptic symptoms but have no ulcer or erosion, and over 40% with endoscopically identified ulcer or erosions will have no symptoms at all.

III. EPIDEMIOLOGY

Some clinical facets of ulcer disease reside in its epidemiology [19–21]. Approximately 30 years ago, duodenal ulcer disease attained its peak incidence. At that time, figures for male/female sex ratios among patients ranged from 3/1 up to 5/1. By the mid-1980s, duodenal ulcer incidence had fallen markedly in males (to about a third of what it was at its peak) and moderately in women, and the sex ratio had become almost 1/1. Over the same time, the incidence of gastric ulcer showed no change, and it has increased slightly in females in recent years. The precipitous decline in the incidence of duodenal ulcer began two decades before the introduction of H_2-receptor antagonists or modern cytoprotective therapy; the sharply declining slope of plotted incidence was not accelerated when H_2-receptor antagonists became available. If anything, the rate of decline became somewhat less (the slope began to level off somewhat) after 1975.

What accounts for the decline in duodenal ulcer? That is not known. Nevertheless, there has been no dearth of speculation. Some have focused on parts of the story for women. If one says that the incidence in women is equal to what it is in men, the interpretation is that women are more stressed now, having become liberated, having entered traditionally male occupations outside the home. (That interpretation assumes that toiling inside the home is not stressful, or at least that it is less stressful.) However, the incidence of duodenal ulcer in women has not risen in the last 30 years; it has declined. It just started its decline at a lower point and declined less rapidly than in men, until the ratio became almost equal. For men, one speculation attributes the decline in duodenal ulcer to a decline in cigarette smoking. If smoking plays a role in this decline, it must do so selectively in men; in recent decades smoking has increased among women (as attested by a dramatic increase in lung cancer in women), yet duodenal ulcer has declined in women.

A larger view indicates that duodenal ulcer was probably uncommon in the late 19th and early 20th centuries. The incidence appears to have increased progressively after World War I until it reached its peak in the late 1950s. Epidemiological and experiment evidence identifies that this represents a cohort phenomenon [22]. By this theory, a cohort of fetuses or young children were exposed to some influence or insult in the first decade or two of this century, which event was expressed as duodenal ulcer some three decades later. (An analogy is Parkinson's disease, where older adults express a neurological disease that was caused by exposure or infection during the influenza epidemic when they were children or young adults.)

In the last 30 years, there have been numerous published reports about upper gastrointestinal bleeding, including several in the past decade. All of these reports, from decade to decade, including the most recent, record the same proportion of bleeding from duodenal ulcer; approximately 20–25% of all patients with upper gastrointestinal bleeding are found to be bleeding from a duodenal ulcer. As mentioned above, over the same 30-year era the incidence of duodenal ulcer declined markedly. This implies that now relatively more patients with duodenal ulcer have bleeding as a complication [23]. If this implication is correct, it then becomes difficult to understand why it should be so.

IV. RISK FACTORS

Cardiologists have developed a list of risk factors for myocardial infarction and death from coronary artery disease. Taking that cue, gastroenterologists have identified risk factors for duodenal ulcer recurrence [3,20,24]. The strongest of these is cigarette smoking [25–30]. The others are male sex, onset of ulcer disease after age 50, previous recurrence, complication (bleeding, perforation, obstruction), family history, low socioeconomic level, and high rate of acid secretion. Interestingly, the following do not increase risk: alcohol consumption, coffee or tea consumption, type of diet, occupational stress, and personality profile. When this information was first available, it caused considerable surprise. Although some adverse role of cigarette smoking had been suspected for several decades, it had not been given such singular importance. More surprising was the evidence that diet was not a factor.

Ulcers are a disease of the system that handles food; common sense would appear to dictate that certain foods, especially if they caused a burning sensation in the mouth the way ulcers cause a burning sensation in the epigastrium, would contribute in some way to the formation or recurrence of an ulcer. Most surprising, because it runs directly counter to long and widely held lay and medical belief, was that personality and life stress do not stand out as risk factors for recurrence [31–34]. The most deeply entrenched notion is that the pathophysiological sequence for developing an ulcer runs singularly and linearly as follows: A person encounters stress somewhere in his or her life (at work, in marriage, with money, with adolescent children, etc.); the stress is processed in the brain in such a way that messages are sent from frontal lobe cortex to vagal nuclei in the midbrain; activation of vagal nuclei generates efferent activity in the vagus nerves, which release acetylcholine at their terminals in the gastric mucosa; the acetylcholine attaches to cholinergic (muscarinic) receptors on parietal cells, which results in acid secretion. Excess acid secretion thus generated by life stress overwhelms what is perceived to be an entirely normal and essentially passive duodenal (or gastric) mucosa, causing the formation of an ulcer. Other aspects of a busy and stressful life are given roles exacerbating or augmenting this sequence: irregular eating and skipped meals fail to maximize food's buffering of acid; the ingestion of improper or spicy food is believed to stimulate more acid than "proper," blander food; cigarettes and alcohol are seen as stimulators of acid secretion; late nights and inadequate sleep increase the brain activity that stimulates the vagal nuclei, and so forth.

The last decade has provided information that allows some students of ulcer disease to conclude that most of the events in that pathophysiological sequence are at least naive and probably incorrect [35–39]. Certain pieces of information fail to support stress as a cause of ulcer. In England during World War II, through the Blitz of London, the incidence of duodenal ulcer in London and the rest of England did not increase as medical experts had expected. It is hard to imagine a more stressful time for an entire community than the Blitz was for London. (Interestingly, although there was no increase in duodenal ulcers during that time, proportionately more of the ulcers that did occur were complicated by perforation [40], implying that although stress may not have contributed to the genesis of an ulcer, if one formed from other causes it was more likely to perforate under such intense and prolonged stress.) In the United States, duodenal ulcer incidence peaked in the 1950s and declined markedly by the 1980s. Does anyone imagine that the 1950s was a *more* stressful era in the United States than the 1980s? (Most people recall the 1950s as a relatively idyllic period.)

A recent paper evaluated stress assessment and personality profiles in duodenal ulcer patients compared to age- and sex-matched controls; although the theme of the paper and the conclusion by the author were that ulcer patients were indeed different from controls with regard to stress (particularly in that ulcer patients *processed* stress in a way that was more deleterious to them), the actual objective data in the paper showed no statistically significant difference between ulcer patients and controls by any of the methods used to assess stress and personality [31]. Certainly, I believe that stress plays *some* role in ulcer disease. If a person has a cold, or pneumonia, or a urinary tract infection, stress will augment symptoms, will make the person feel worse, and may even prolong the duration of the disease. Stress plays this adverse role in most diseases, perhaps all disease. However, the issue here is whether stress (or personality type) has a primary causative (etiological) role in the formation of an ulcer. On the basis of available information of several types, one is forced to recognize that there is a paucity of evidence that psychosocial/environmental stress alone causes ulcer in humans, and there are even several points suggesting that it does not do so— established pathophysiological tradition notwithstanding.

During the long era when stress was believed to be the main risk factor and causative agent in ulcer disease, the role of cigarette smoking was uncertain. Every now and then over the years, a suspicion emerged that cigarette smoking might not be good for ulcer patients, but there was no solid information. Believing so strongly in the adverse role of stress, many physicians recommended that patients with an active ulcer *not* try to give up smoking, at least until the ulcer healed, because smokers report that smoking gives them a sense of relaxation (alleviation of stress) whereas giving up (or trying to give up) smoking generates severe sensations of stress. Now the best data indicate that the coin should be flipped over: stress is not a major factor, and cigarette smoking has emerged as the most prominent adverse agent ever identified. Not only is it the strongest risk factor for ulcer recurrence, recent epidemiological evidence has identified it as strongly associated with the initial development of an ulcer. Additionally, continued smoking severely blunts the therapeutic effectiveness of H_2-receptor antagonists [30] but has less effect on cytoprotective agents [27]. In fact, cessation of smoking alone results in a higher healing rate for duodenal ulcer than if a smoker with ulcer continues to smoke and takes full doses of the most potent H_2 blocker.

The mechanism responsible for smoking's adverse effect in ulcer disease is not yet known but does not appear to be mediated by increased acid secretion. Reports have varied, but most show no change in acid secretion with cigarette smoking or administration of nicotine. One good study showed a 15% decline in acid secretion during cigarette smoking. Smoking does inhibit pancreatic bicarbonate secretion [25] and endogenous prostaglandin generation in gastroduodenal mucosa [28,29]; both may play some role in ulcer formation or recurrence.

V.   RECURRENCE

Both duodenal and gastric ulcer [41] have a high rate of recurrence [42], around 70–80% at 1 year and around 95% by 2 years. The recurrence rate and the slope of the recurrence curve are the same whether an ulcer originally healed spontaneously (or under placebo therapy) or was healed by active ulcer therapy (such as an antacid or H_2-receptor blocker). Maintenance therapy with an active agent will significantly reduce the recurrence rate at 1 year and at 2 years; when maintenance therapy is stopped, the subsequent slope of the recurrence curve is the same as the slope of recurrence after initial ulcer healing, when no maintenance was given [43]. This indicates that our favorite therapy does little if anything to alter the natural course of the disease. If sucralfate is used to accomplish initial ulcer healing, and there is no maintenance therapy, the time to recurrence is significantly longer (compared to antacid or H_2-blocker therapy) but the ultimate recurrence rate is the same at 2 years. This implies that cytoprotective therapy does alter the natural course, but not for very long. When an ulcer that was originally symptomatic recurs after initial H_2-blocker therapy, 40% of endoscopically documented recurrences are without symptoms. When initial therapy is the cytoprotective agent sucralfate, only 10% are asymptomatic. The reason for this discrepancy is not apparent. Cimetidine is remarkably effective therapy for relieving the severe pain of corneal ulcers in herpes ophthalmia; the mechanism for this benefit is not known, and any relationship between this and duodenal or gastric ulcer pain is speculative at best.

VI.   INDICATION FOR SURGERY

Two to three decades ago, one learned and memorized the indications for surgery in ulcer disease: perforation, obstruction, hemorrhage, and intractibility. With the passage of time, a combination of clinical experience and specific clinical trials led to erosion of the absoluteness of those surgical indications. Hemorrhage had to be persistent and require five to six units of transfusion. Recent efforts have raised the potential that endoscopic therapy may stop bleeding and obviate surgery. Obstruction had to be unrelenting after 72 hr of medical management consisting of effective nasogastric suction, intravenous fluids, and an H_2 blocker. Even treatment of perforation [44], which in the United States was longest perceived as an absolute indication for urgent surgery, has been modified by recent experience in England indicating that a majority of patients can reasonably avoid surgery when treated medically with nasogastric suction, intravenous fluids, antibiotics, and an H_2 blocker.

The fourth indication for surgery, intractability, has become almost a conceptual embarrassment; experts are highly reluctant to even use the term any longer. It was always difficult to define [45]; speculations about its definition involved questions as to whether it was intractability of the disease, of the patient, or of the surgeon. Looking back at that earlier time, it seems obvious that one aspect meant to be covered was ulcer recurrence [24]. If an ulcer recurred even once, it was labeled intractable. Now there is wide recognition, even in the United States, that recurrence is a central characteristic of the disease, with 80% recurrence of duodenal ulcer at 1 year and more than 95% recurrence by 2 years.

Another facet of intractability was what was referred to as "failure of medical therapy." Distinctions here are difficult to depict sharply; occasionally *recurrence* was seen as a form of failure of medical therapy. But more specifically it referred to the patient who failed to achieve initial ulcer healing during appropriate medical therapy. Now we possess a large quantity of data, endoscopically verified, that give a remarkably consistent average of 20% (range 10–30%) of duodenal ulcers that fail to heal after "gold standard" H_2-blocker therapy administered for 8 weeks. This approximately 20% residual who fail to heal are now most often placed in the refractory ulcer category. A great deal of effort has been directed at this group of patients, effort that has been rewarded by separating out a small number who have a readily understandable reason for refractoriness of their ulcer. Isolated individuals turn out to have Zollinger-Ellison syndrome; some others have failed to take their medication.

It is biologically intriguing that despite intensive scrutiny, most refractory ulcers occur in persons who cannot be distinguished from their "garden-variety" cohorts who healed uneventfully on the same program. The therapeutic strategy for this largest group with refractory ulcer disease is variable. Some will respond to a change of therapy, either to another H_2 blocker or to a cytoprotective agent. Some will respond to a higher dose of the same therapy or to longer duration of therapy. Perhaps future clinical trials may show that some patients benefit from antibiotic therapy that eradicates *Helicobacter pylori* [46,47]. Ultimately, some will require surgery, but it is interesting to note that this group has the highest incidence of unsatisfactory results postoperatively (vomiting, bloating, dyspepsia, weight loss, diarrhea) even when surgery has cured the ulcer.

VII.   SUMMARY

This chapter has, necessarily and naturally I believe, meandered from the strictly defined category of "clinical presentation" into other areas, particularly epidemiology and therapy [11,48]. Those categories will be discussed at greater length in other chapters, but some of these "adjacent" concepts are helpful in filling out and giving perspective to the presenting clinical aspects of ulcer disease.

In summary, ulcer disease presents with upper abdominal symptoms that have a broad (and rather clinically disturbing) overlap with the symptoms of essential dyspepsia, a mysterious disorder that is characterized by little that is definite other than *not* having an ulcer, or it presents with complications of bleeding, perforation, or obstruction. With regard to clinical presentation, pertinent questions for future investigation have to do with the mechanisms of ulcer pain, the relationship of therapy to symptoms, why more ulcers seem to bleed, and better definition and pathophysiological understanding of essential dyspepsia.

REFERENCES

1.   Bonnevie O. Causes of death in duodenal and gastric ulcer. Gastroenterology 1977; 73:1000–4.

2.   Bonnevie O. Survival in peptic ulcer. Gastroenterology 1978; 75:1055–60.

3.   Bynum TE. Clinical interpretation of recurrence data. J Clin Gastroenterol 1987; 9:31.

4.   Schiller LR, Fordtran JS. Ulcer complications during short term therapy of duodenal ulcer with active agents and placebo. Gastroenterology 1986; 90:478–81.

5.   Bynum TE. Abdominal pain. In: Stein JH, et al., eds. Internal medicine, 2nd ed. Boston: Little Brown, 1987.

6.   Bynum TE, Branch WT. Chronic dyspepsia and upper abdominal pain. In: Branch WT, ed. Office practice of medicine, 2nd ed. Philadelphia: WB Saunders, 1987.

7.   Read L, et al. Diagnosis and treatment of dyspepsia. Med Decis Making 1982; 2:415–38.

8.   Hirschowitz BI. Natural history of duodenal ulcer. Gastroenterology 1983; 85:967–70.

9.   Archambault AP, et al. Omeprazol vs. cimetidine in duodenal ulcer healing and pain relief. Gastroenterology 1988; 94:1130–4.

10.   Lauritsen K, et al. Effect of omeprazol and cimetidine on duodenal ulcer. N Engl J Med 1985; 312:958–61.

11.   Bynum TE. Sucralfate in duodenal ulcer patients. Curr Concepts Gastroenterol 1984; 9:18.

12.   Martin F, et al. Comparison of the healing capacities of sucralfate and cimetidine in the short term treatment of duodenal ulcer. Gastroenterology 1982; 82:401–5.

13.   Sutton DR. Gastric ulcer healing with tripotassium dicitrato bismuthate. Gut 1982; 23:621–4.

14.   Bynum TE, Koch GG. Multicenter Study Group: Sucralfate tablets 1 gm twice a day prevent duodenal ulcer recurrence. Am J Med 1989; 86:127–32.

15.   Kirk RM. Can the singularity of chronic peptic ulcers be described by catastrophe theory and explained by biofeedback? Gastroenterology 1977; 73:608–10.

16. Korman MG, et al. Relapse rate of duodenal ulcer after cessation of long term cimetidine treatment. Dig Dis Sci 1980; 25:88–91.

17. Martin DF, et al. Difference in relapse rates of duodenal ulcer after healing with cimetidine or tripotassium dicitrato bismuthate. Lancet 1981; i:7–10.

18. Bendtsen F, et al. Duodenal bulb acidity in patients with duodenal ulcer. Gastroenterology 1987; 93:1263–9.

19. Ivy AC, Grossman MI, Bachrach WH. Peptic ulcer. Philadelphia: Blakiston, 1950.

20. Sonnenberg A. Predictors of duodenal ulcer healing and relapse. Gastroenterology 1981; 81:1061–7.

21. Sonnenberg A. Changes in physician visits for gastric and duodenal ulcer in the United States. Dig Dis Sci 1987; 32:1–7.

22. Sonnenberg A. Appearance of a cohort phenomenon in peptic ulcer mortality. Gastroenterology 1984; 86:389–401.

23. Elashoff JD, et al. Long-term follow-up of duodenal ulcer patients. J Clin Gastroenterol 1983; 5:509–15.

24. Stabile BE, Passaro E. Recurrent peptic ulcer. Gastroenterology 1976; 70:124–35.

25. Bynum TE, Solomon TE, Johnson LR, Jacobson ED. Inhibition of pancreatic secretion in man by cigarette smoking. Gut 1972; 13:361.

26. Korman MG, et al. Influence of cigarette smoking on healing and relapse in duodenal ulcer disease. Gastroenterology 1983; 85:871–74.

27. Lam SK, et al. Sucralfate overcomes adverse effect of cigarette smoking on duodenal ulcer healing and prolongs subsequent remission. Gastroenterology 1987; 92:1193–1201.

28. McCready DR, Clark L, Cohen MM. Cigarette smoking reduces human gastric luminal prostaglandin E_2. Gut 1985; 26:1192–6.

29. Quimby GF, et al. Active smoking depresses prostaglandin synthesis in human gastric mucosa. Ann Intern Med 1986; 104:616–9.

30. Sontag S, et al. Cimetidine, cigarette smoking, and recurrence of duodenal ulcer. N Engl J Med 1984; 311:689–93.

31. Feldman M, et al. Life events, stress and psychosocial factors in men with peptic ulcer disease. Gastroenterology 1986; 91:1370–9.

32. Piper DW, et al. Personality pattern of patients with chronic gastric ulcer. Gastroenterology 1977; 73:444–6.

33. Thomas J, Greig M, Piper DW. Chronic gastric ulcer and life events. Gastroenterology 1980; 78:905–11.

34. Walker P, et al. Life events, stress and psychosocial factors in men with peptic ulcer disease. Gastroenterology 1988; 94:323–30.

35. Isenberg JI, et al. An apparent exception to Schwartz's dictum, "no acid, no ulcer." N Engl J Med 1971; 285:620.

36. Mannier JW, Beltaos E. Benign gastric ulcer in a patient with pernicious anemia. Gastroenterology 1975; 69:744–5.

37. Reid J, et al. Benign gastric ulceration in pernicious anemia. Dig Dis Sci 1987; 25:148–9.

38. Szabo S. Pathogenesis of duodenal ulcer disease. Lab Invest 1984; 2:121–47.

39. Szabo S, Bynum TE. Alternatives to the acid-oriented approach to ulcer disease: does "cytoprotection" exist in man? Scand J Gastroenterol 1988; 23:1.

40. Illingworth CFW, et al. Acute perforated peptic ulcer. Br Med J 1944; 2:617–20.

41. The Veterans Administration cooperative study on gastric ulcer. Gastroenterology 1971; 61:567–654.

42. Fry J. Peptic ulcer: a profile. Br Med J 1964; 2:809–12.

43. Tovey FI, et al. Comparison of relapse rates and of mucosal abnormalities after healing of duodenal ulceration and after one year maintenance with cimetidine or sucralfate. Gut 1989; 30:586–93.

44. Crofts TJ, et al. A randomized trial of non-operative treatment for perforated peptic ulcer. N Engl J Med 1989; 320:970–3.

45. Bynum TE, Hartsuck J, Jacobson ED. Gastric ulcer. Gastroenterology 1972; 62:1052–60.

46. Blaser MJ, Brown WR. Campylobacters and gastroduodenal inflammation. Adv Intern Med 1989; 34:21–42.

47. Dooley CP, Cohen H. The clinical significance of *Campylobacter pylori*. Ann Intern Med 1988; 108:70–9.

48. Bynum TE. Peptic ulcer therapy. Consultant 1978; 18:121.

49. Whitaker JA, Cooke AR. Achlorhydria and benign gastric ulcer. Acta Hepato-Gastroenterol 1979; 26:417–8.

50. Wormsley KG, Grossman MI. Maximal histalog test in control subjects and patients with peptic ulcer. Gut 1965; 6:427–35.

<h1 style="text-align:center">6</h1>

Nonsteroidal Anti-inflammatory Drug Gastropathy: Old Disease, New Name

SANFORD H. ROTH

Humana Hospital and Arthritis Center,
Phoenix, Arizona

RALPH E. BENNETT

Arthritis Center, Phoenix, Arizona

I. INTRODUCTION

Nonsteroidal anti-inflammatory drug (NSAID) gastropathy was born into medical nosology in the late 1980s [1]. By no coincidence, this was the era of "key words" and MEDLAR data retrieval. And this was the "era of the NSAIDs"—among the most widely used drugs in the world, popular primarily for safe pain relief and inflammation control in arthritis. But this was also that period of years when unprecedented attention was focused by regulatory authorities upon the issue of safety. NSAIDs were for the first time withdrawn from the market and regulatory hearings held because of gastrointestinal bleeding and death, primarily gastric in origin. Yet the literature of the times reflected that NSAIDs were "better tolerated" than aspirin [2,3], and aspirin, warned the Arthritis Foundation brochures of this period, "might cause gastric irritation" [4].

Thus, this was not an easy birth by any means. The terminology was iatrogenic in focus. The pathophysiology was called to question. Furthermore, "peptic ulcer disease," or "acid peptic disease," was the well-established terminology used for the lesions and ulcers of the upper gastrointestinal tract, wasn't it?

And therein lies the rub as well as the answer. For peptic ulcer disease by ths time had been efficiently suppressed, if not ablated, by the ubiquitous use of H_2-receptor blockade agents throughout the world [5]. Whole legions of Billroth surgeons sought other employment while happy patients returned to normal healthy productivity, their duodenal ulcers healed, their symptoms effectively suppressed.

At this same time, thoughtful medical authorities and epidemiologists, first in Britain, began reflecting upon the rising incidence of ulcer disease, bleeding, perforation, and death in elderly women [6,7]. This was not the target population of classic peptic ulcer disease. This was also prone to be that aging population with arthritis and long-term NSAID use [8,9].

This was also the era of the common use of endoscopy. No longer regarded as an invasive procedure, fiberoptics had extended its use into all gastrointestinal problems, with dramatic documentation on film and videotape. In the case of NSAID gastropathy, those films documented a range of gastric lesions—from erosions into the capillary bed to microbleeding, to ulcer crater disease with the ultimate potential for major vascular bleeding and perforations. Thus, nomenclature directed toward gastritis, gastric ulcers, or the generic peptic ulcer proved to be inadequate to describe the evolution of problems at hand.

This chapter will review those historic events that led to our present understanding of this disorder. We will then consider the basic pathophysiology as we now understand it that makes this disorder unique and separate. On the basis of these understandings, we will consider the putative consequences of present-day NSAID therapy as used in relation to the evolution of NSAID gastropathy, the treatment of this problem, and its prophylaxis. Finally, we will consider defensive measures that can be taken in response to NSAID gastropathy. This will provide a rationale for appropriate therapeutic management and prevention of NSAID gastropathy, especially in the face of the need to safely continue such NSAID therapy in the chronic treatment of arthritis.

II. EVOLUTION OF A CONCEPT

Salix derivatives are the hoary legacy of modern-day anti-inflammatory therapy. At the turn of the century, sodium salicylate could have been heir to modern-day NSAIDs were it not for its unpalatable taste in solubilized form as initially produced [10]. This prototype of nonacetylated salicylate, which we now recognize as gastro-sparing and even cytoprotective, translated as intolerant, while the acetylated form, aspirin, became the most-used NSAID in modern times and certainly the most gastrotoxic! Yet even at the turn of the century when aspirin was first popularized, the literature reflects awareness of gastric distress associated with its use [11].

In the face of the phenomenal success of aspirin in the modern era, a plethora of nonsteroidal molecules have been developed (Table 1), none of which has proved to be clearly superior to aspirin in analgesic and anti-inflammatory efficacy [12]. All have claimed (usually inadequately documented) increased safety as well as less gastric intolerance [13–15]. Through the refinements of upper gastrointestinal fluoroscopic studies and, ultimately, the age of endoscopy, we have come to a more realistic assessment of those claims. Although we had forewarned of the gastropathy of NSAIDs in the early 1970s [16] on the basis of a large clinical study of the serious mucosal toxicity associated with both aspirin and nonsalicylate NSAIDs (and subsequent studies have reinforced that information), it was not until 15 years later that the FDA finally came to serious terms with the problem. The NSAID package insert no longer described the "gastric irritation" of aspirin and NSAID use but rather "ulcers, bleeds and perforations" as well as identifying those most at risk (Table 2) [17].

By this time it was also clear that thousands were dying annually of this iatrogenic

Table 1 Molecular Classification of Nonsalicylate NSAIDs

Proprionic acids	Anthranitic acids (fenamates)
Ibuprofen[a]	Flufenamic acid
Flubiprofen	Methanamic acid[a]
Ketoprofen[a]	Meclofenamic acid[a]
Naproxen[a]	Niflumic acid
Indoprofen[a]	Pyrazolones
Tiaprofenic acid	Phenylbutazone[a]
Carprofen	Azapropazone
Nabumetone	Biprazone
Etodolac[a]	Benzothiazines (Oxicams)
Diclofenac	Piroxicam[a]
Fenclofenac	Nonacetic agents
Fentiazic	Proquazone
Heterocarboxyindole acetic acid	Fluproquazone
Indomethacin[a]	Tiaramide
Sulindac[a]	Bufexamac
Tometin[a]	Flunizole
Clopirac	Epirazole
	Tinoridine

[a]Available in the United States.
Source: Roth [12].

Table 2 At-Risk NSAID Gastropathy Population

Age: elderly
Sex: female
Combination NSAID therapy
History of ulcers and/or gastric bleeding
Large ulcers

Source: Roth and Bennett [13].

disorder and that hundreds of millions of U.S. dollars were being expended on hospitalization and disability from the consistent consequences of such use and, at times, abuse [12,18,19].

To understand how almost a century could elapse without recognition of the dangers of this problem, a number of parallel events should be revisited.

1. Through this same time period, peptic ulcer disease had been recognized as a major health disorder whose pathophysiology was associated with hyper-acidity. Effective antisecretory pharmacological agents had been synthesized to respond to this pathophysiology. Those responses were so effective by the time of the H_2 blockers, so well known to readers of this text, that classic acid peptic disease had become almost a historical footnote. In fact, pharmaco-logically a whole group of drugs directed toward mucosal protective therapy were in search of a new disorder, as it were. NSAID therapy at this time was the most pervasive single form of drug therapy [20]. One could argue that because of selfish concerns there was no real interest in endoscopic studies to better confirm the reports of NSAID-associated clinical gastrotoxicity and ulcers. An incidence of ulcers of less than 2% was reported from research and development studies of each of those NSAIDs [15]. Separately, antisecre-tory and cytoprotective drugs, now without a disease, entered in force into endoscopic documentation of NSAID-associated mucosal disease. Those study results are riveting and persuasive. We will visit them in perspective throughout this chapter as we come to understand the problems that had confounded epidemiological and clinical interpretation.

2. In the 1940s, corticoids were discovered and, because of the hormonal toxicity associated with their use, were also quickly stigmatized for their safety problems though respected for their incredible potential for anti-inflammatory efficacy and immunoregulation [21]. Aside from the issue of ulcerogenicity—put to rest at lower dosages, which appear to be cyto-protective in investigational studies—corticoids are not a central part of the story. Rather, through comparison with aspirin use in arthritis, was the classical documentation that aspirin (and ultimately NSAIDs) could be anti-inflammatory in high doses compared to the common analgesia susceptible to usual ad libitum low-dosage use [14]. From this turning point toward anti-inflammatory therapy, with its noteworthy potential to increase function in arthritis through suppression of inflammation as well as reduce symptomatol-ogy, was to come the unavoidable legacy of NSAID gastropathy.

3. In this age of key word data retrieval, peptic ulcer disease can be separated from what we have since described as NSAID gastropathy (Table 3). Those differences can be importantly distinguished in this table on the basis of anatomical location (duodenal versus antral/prepyloric/gastric), demographic (old women versus young men), and pathophysiology (cyclooxygenase inhibi-

Table 3 Parameters for NSAID Gastropathy and
Classic Peptic Ulcer Disease

NSAID gastropathy	Classic peptic ulcer disease
Antral, prepyloric	Duodenal
NSAID-associated	Unknown etiology
Prostaglandin E_2	Acid-mediated
Cytoprotection	Acid suppression prescription
Women/older	Men/younger

Source: Roth and Bennett [13].

tion versus acid hypersecretion), and therefore on the basis of important differential response and lack of response to H_2-blockage therapy [13]. Until this nosological difference is appreciated, the literature will continue to be confounded when mucosal lesional disease is not uniquely differentiated when associated with NSAID therapy.

4. The NSAID therapy itself must be more precisely defined as long-term and administered in anti-inflammatory doses. Small-animal studies and, more important, studies in humans of normal mucosal response to acute NSAID exposure have not been successfully bridged to the gastropathy seen in anti-inflammatory arthritis studies. Accordingly, epidemiological case control studies that have not controlled for these factors as well as such other critical cofactors as length of use of drugs, combinations of drugs, codisease, and other cofactors so important clinically (previous history of NSAID gastropathy, ulcers, bleeding, intolerance) will remain difficult to interpret in relation to the risk ratios they seek to confirm [17].

5. Finally, NSAID gastropathy is further complicated by the documented experience that it is often silent. In fact, as important as the relief of gastric distress is to successful arthritis therapy, it is not related to lesional degree or the degree of lesional disease. Furthermore, it appears that variable periods of exposure to NSAIDs are required before natural cytoprotective adaptation is fatigued and fails [14]. Those data are not yet complete, but the picture of a chronic iatrogenic disorder that often silently pursues its pathophysiology in the face of sustained NSAID therapy over potentially long periods of time presents a dilemma not unlike the "time bomb" of essential hypertension. This clinical analogy extends to the previous arguments that early clinical hypertension without clinical complications may not justify pharmacological therapy because of the expense of that therapy and the usual toxicity ratios

common to all pharmacological interventions. We now know that cerebro-vascular accidents can be avoided in many cases through early prophylactic intervention. Thus, sustained pathophysiology should be interdicted when-ever clinically reasonable and feasible. Not until recent times was it accepted that NSAID gastropathy, even without proven active lesions or bleeding, may require prophylactic response [22].

6. Most recent data have now confirmed that approximately one of five patients on sustained NSAID therapy will experience ulcer crater disease [14]. Many large series of over 100 to many hundreds of NSAID users have found 20% or more with ulcer craters at baseline endoscopic screening, whether of rheuma-toid or osteoarthritis cohorts [16,22–25]. In fact, such ulcer findings with NSAIDs are so common that at first many questioned their clinical impor-tance, arguing that they could be reversed by cytoprotective adaptation [26].

7. Ulcer crater disease is deep to the muscularis mucosa, threatening the vascula-ture. Bleeding from that vasculature is fatal in 10% of cases and is especially common in the elderly [7,27]. Those data are in marked contrast to the less than 2% acute incidence of ulcers found in clinical studies with NSAIDs. This could best be accounted for on the basis of the difficulty of recognizing often silent gastropathy without endoscopy (which was previously uncom-monly pursued in clinical NSAID studies).

8. We finally come full circle to the physicians who must identify and respond to this disorder. NSAIDs have been a boon to rheumatology. They have pro-vided what has been perceived as a useful, relatively safe response to the symptoms and inflammation of our common arthritides. Sir John Vane [28] helped us understand that blockade of cyclooxygenase was central to that effect. We therefore focused upon prostaglandin products as the "enemy camp" to be subdued for control of pain and inflammation, but we find almost a decade later that prostaglandin products are indeed pro- and anti-inflammatory. The mechanisms are far too complex to explain on the basis of a single mediator substance. Through this same time period, gastroenterolo-gists had been attracted to the elegant cytoprotection theory of Robert [29]. Within this theory was the central role of prostaglandins propelling gastro-defensive events in relation to adherent mucus production, bicarbonate secre-tion, and especially vascularization. Within this framework, prostaglandins were "desirable."

9. We are an aging society. Whereas mean survival was age 39 at the beginning of the century, it entered the 80s in the 1980s. In lock step with a graying population is our improved understanding of NSAID pharmacokinetics (Fig. 1) [12]. As drug handling differs and is compromised late in life, aged patients have increasing difficulty metabolizing and excreting drugs, espe-cially drugs with longer half-lives ($T_{1/2}$) [30]. They are more sensitive to drug dosage. They commonly have atrophic gastritis with decreased vasculariza-

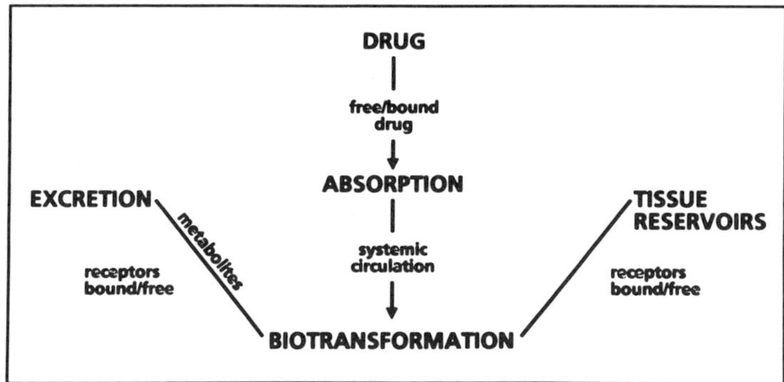

FIGURE 1   NSAID pharmacokinetics. (Reprinted from Roth [12].)

tion. Vascularization is critical to restoration of the mucosa and buffering of acidity (intravascular pH 7.4 versus gastric luminal pH 1.5). Gastrointestinal bleeding occurs in the elderly over seven times as often as in younger patients [6,7]. The risk of deaths from such bleeding may be five times greater in this group [31]. And yet those over 60 probably represent a major segment of the population that commonly consumes NSAIDs. As we come to grips with these risk factors, we will ultimately have a basis of response to this disorder that is so difficult to recognize and prevent.

III. CLINICAL–PATHOPHYSIOLOGICAL CORRELATIONS

Endoscopic documentation of NSAID toxicity was first demonstrated by Douthwaite and Lintott [32] over 50 years ago. Yet no systematic attempts were made to determine the prevalence of gastrointestinal mucosal lesions in a population of patients taking NSAIDs until recent years. Only recently has there been constructive debate over the significance of some of the lesions in the spectrum of NSAID gastropathy [33].

Although the academic issues with respect to the prevalence and importance of gastrointestinal lesions continue to generate controversy, these issues are of pragmatic importance to the practicing clinician. Between 9 million and 18 million kg of aspirin are consumed annually in the United States [34]. NSAIDs represent over 4% of all prescription sales, with over 67 million prescriptions each year in the United States [19]. In an epidemiological study of NSAID use in a Michigan and Minnesota Medicaid population [35], 8.3% of the study population were dispensed prescription NSAIDs. Because NSAIDs are so commonly used in the general population, and to an even greater extent in the older population, it has often been the practicing clinician who developed initial insights into NSAID gastropathy.

We documented a prevalence of serious gastropathy associated with NSAID use in 28% in our endoscopic series of 140 rheumatoid arthritis patients in 1974 [16]. The Boston Collaborative Drug Study Program demonstrated this in a large group of patients without any illnesses predisposed to bleeding [36]. It was estimated that 50–70% of patients taking 1 g of aspirin three times a day (a dose routinely used in rheumatoid arthritis) will lose several extra milliliters of blood in the feces daily [37]. This is equivalent to a loss of 2 L of blood per year per patient, or an iron loss of more than 1 g per year. A recent study done at the Long Beach Veterans Administration Hospital demonstrated multiple gastrointestinal ulcers "as a result of one 2600 mg dose of aspirin taken one day before endoscopy" [38].

With the advent of fiberoptic endoscopy in routine clinical practice, short-term and more recently long-term studies have demonstrated the frequency of gastropathic lesions with NSAID use. Silvoso et al. [39] conducted a prospective study of 82 symptomatic patients without any history of peptic ulcer disease. These patients were examined after they ingested at least 2400 mg of aspirin per day for 3 months or more. Of these 82 patients, 75% had erythema, 40% had gastric erosions, and 20% had gastric ulcers. Only 5% of normal controls had erythema, while none had erosions or ulcers. Only two-thirds of those patients with ulcers admitted to any gastrointestinal symptoms, even in retrospect. Of further interest was that only 2 of 36 patients who took enteric-coated aspirin had ulcers, though the same percentage of these patients did suffer from erythema and erosions. O'Laughlin et al. [40] observed five healthy volunteers endoscopically after they had ingested 650 mg of aspirin over 15-min intervals for 1 hr, and then at 4 and 24 hr, and observed multiple subepithelial hemorrhages in the gastric antrum and fundus, which were worst at 60″. Hoftiezer et al. [41] found an average of 14 antral lesions in all patients after nine volunteers took 2.6 g of aspirin per day for 2 weeks, with one patient developing active bleeding.

Some longer term studies are also available. Caruso and Bianchi-Porro [23] followed 12 rheumatoid paients without any endoscopic lesions at entry for 3 months. Half the patients received less than 3 g of aspirin per day, and half received more. In the lower-dose group, two patients had lesions at 1 month and four were noted to have lesions at 3 months. In the higher dose group, all had lesions at 1 month but only one had lesions at 3 months, thereby suggesting the possibility that the gastric mucosa adapted to aspirin-induced injury.

We studied 104 patients taking NSAIDs for a variety of rheumatic disorders over the course of 1 year [25]. The study demonstrated the inefficacy of cimetidine in the treatment and prophylaxis of NSAID gastropathy. It also demonstrated the natural history of NSAID gastropathy in that 50% (7/14) of placebo-treated and 42% (5/12) of cimetidine-treated patients showed progression of their gastropathic lesions over the course of 10 months; seven patients from each group progressed to grade IV ulcer lesions.

While the endoscope has shed a great deal of light on the effects of NSAIDs on the gastrointestinal mucosa under protocol conditions, its role in daily clinical practice remains problematic. Though it is obviously not practical to perform an endoscopy on every patient taking NSAIDs, numerous studies have demonstrated the poor correlation between symptoms and endoscopic findings with these patients. The reason for this poor correlation is unclear. Because most rheumatic disease patients must deal with pain on a daily basis, they may not pay as much attention to a new minor discomfort. Furthermore, in one study, nearly 15% of patients complaining of dyspepsia were receiving placebo NSAIDs [42]. The Silvoso et al. study [39] described above demonstrated that even patients with ulcer craters were often unaware of any problem. Also, Lanza [42] was unable to demonstrate any clinical correlation between symptoms and gastric and duodenal lesions in patients taking aspirin or any of a variety of NSAIDs. Of the cases of complicated ulcerations reported by Armstrong and Blower [27], 60% had no symptoms prior to hemorrhage and perforation. Caruso and Bianchi-Porro [23] found that 24 of 41 patients (59%) without gastrointestinal symptoms had endoscopic lesions within 3 and 6 months of NSAID treatment; 108 of 136 patients (79%) who experienced gastrointestinal symptoms were endoscopically noted to have lesions. Using these numbers, Butt et al. [34] calculated the predictive value of dyspepsia as a test for gastric lesions as only 0.58. They noted that a careful physical examination with the finding of epigastric tenderness could increase this predictive value to 0.90.

Though NSAID gastropathy is being increasingly accepted as a major public health hazard [18,19], because of differences in methodology it has been difficult to demonstrate this consistently in the epidemiological data. Carson et al. [35] performed a retrospective cohort study using 1980 billing data from all Medicaid patients in the states of Michigan and Minnesota. Of the 47,136 patients exposed to NSAIDs within the previous 30 days, there was an increased risk of 1.5 of developing clinical upper gastrointestinal bleeding compared to 44,634 patients not exposed to NSAIDs. This population, however, which includes many younger patients taking NSAIDs for a short term only (e.g., women taking NSAIDs for dysmenorrhea) does not accurately reflect the population at risk in the typical rheumatic disease clinic. The Group Health Cooperative Study of Puget Sound [44] examined the risk of patients over 64 years of age who had filled a prescription for an NSAID in the study period of 90 days and also found this to only be approximately 1.5 times the risk of hospitalization from upper gastrointestinal bleeding compared to nonusers. Because this large study population (84,654 prescriptions filled between 1977 and 1983) was obtained by linking pharmacy records to hospital records, the authors estimated a 20% error in linkage; it is also difficult to control for aspirin usage in both users and nonusers of NSAIDs in this type of study.

Other studies that have focused on patients admitted to the hospital for ulcer disease and upper gastrointestinal bleeding have found a strong relationship between aspirin and/or NSAID use and hospital admission. Bartle et al. [45] found that 24 of 57 (42.1%) of patients with occult upper gastrointestinal bleeding were taking NSAIDs compared with 23 of 181 (18.1%) control subjects. Levy [46] surveyed

25,000 consecutive hospital admissions and found that 15.9% of patients used aspirin at least 4 days per week, compared to only 6.9% of the control group ($p \leq 0.05$). Somerville et al. [7] found that 406 hospital inpatients with bleeding ulcers took NSAIDs twice as often as hospital or community-based controls.

In a 36-month study examining 235 consecutive patients who either died or required surgery as a result of peptic ulceration [27], 60% were found to be taking an NSAID compared with 9.9% of a hospital control group. Eighty percent of ulcer-related deaths occurred in patients taking NSAIDs ($p < 0.0001$). Other authors [6,7] estimated a 10% mortality among the elderly who suffer NSAID-induced hemorrhage.

How is it that NSAIDs disrupt the natural defense mechanisms of the gastric mucosa, and what can be done to pharmacologically manipulate these natural mechanisms? Possible mechanisms of gastric mucosal damage include disruption of the mucosal barrier, inhibition of mucus and bicarbonate secretion, inhibition of prostaglandin synthesis, and disruption of the mucosal blood flow.

Acidic compounds such as aspirin damage the mucosa by both their systemic and local effects. The un-ionized portion of aspirin easily passes through the mucosal cellular membrane, causing damage and allowing hydrogen ion diffusion that leads to further damage [47]. Enteric-coated and intravenously administered compounds still cause damage because of their systemic effects, but their lesser toxicity is evidence of the damage of local contact [39,48]. Many of the traditional measures used to treat gastrointestinal distress and ulcers are aimed at reducing this local acidic damage.

Antacids neutralize acid secretion, and H_2-receptor blockade diminishes acid production. However, gastric ulcer patients have been shown to have reduced levels of acid secretion. Antacids and H_2 blockers may still be useful in treating gastric ulcer patients, especially with respect to symptomatic relief, if it is possible to discontinue use of the offending agent (e.g., NSAID), but, as will be further discussed, because of the difference in pathogenesis, acid reduction should not be the mainstay of gastric ulcer therapy.

The mucus–bicarbonate layer adjacent to the gastric mucosa has long been considered another natural defense mechanism. This layer has been credited with maintaining the pH gradient. Yet a similar layer in the duodenum does not maintain this gradient. In fact, administration of N-acetylcysteine can decrease the thickness of the gastromucosal layer without affecting the pH gradient. Studies by Robert et al. [49] and McQueen et al. [50] have shown that the mucus layer is not a barrier to absorption of ethanol, hypertonic saline, or indomethacin. The mucus layer remains intact despite absorption of these substances and subsequent damage.

Szabo and Pihan [51] effectively argued that preservation of the microcirculation is the most important element in mucosal protection. By injecting the vasculature of rats with monastral blue and then exposing the animals to ethanol, they were able to demonstrate endothelial damage within 1 min. The lesions progressed to increased vascular permeability and finally to complete stasis in superficial capillaries in the gastric mucosa. These lesions were completely prevented by pretreatment with sucralfate.

Epithelial cell regeneration is also an important defense mechanism, as the gastromucosa is capable of rapid regeneration. If these superficial cells are damaged by a toxic agent such as dilute alcohol, reepithelialization will occur within 60 min if the vasculature remains intact. If the integrity of the mucosal blood flow is not maintained, then reepithelialization proceeds at a much slower rate. If 100% ethanol is administered, a rapid decrease in blood flow is seen in superficial capillaries within 1–2 min. Pretreatment with prostaglandin prevents the reduction in blood flow, presumably by preservation of the endothelium [52].

Cytoprotection is defined as the ability of an agent to protect the upper gastrointestinal mucosa from damage from a variety of noxious insults such as absolute alcohol or indomethacin. To be considered cytoprotective, an agent should not directly decrease the presence of the noxious agent as antacids or H_2 blockers decrease the amount of luminal acid, but rather, through some unknown mechanism, confer upon the deeper mucosa the ability to withstand injury from a variety of agents.

Prostaglandins may be cytoprotective for a variety of reasons. Initial studies examined their ability to decrease gastric acid secretion. Various analogues have shown different properties in regard to acid secretion [53,54], which has resulted in different conclusions regarding prostaglandin antisecretory properties. There have also been conflicting reports on whether or not prostaglandins' cytoprotective properties can be separated from their antisecretory properties in humans [54–56], and some believe that this may not be possible [57].

Carbenoxolone and deglycyrrhizinated licorice have also been found to be cytoprotective. They stimulate the release of mucus, stimulate epithelial renewal, and stabilize cellular membranes [53]. Because of these properties, it is postulated that they act through the inhibition of prostaglandin inhibition.

Other authors have attributed cytoprotection to paracetomol and sulfhydryl compounds, and some have shown that sodium salicylate, aminosalicylic acid, and a low concentration of ethanol, HCl, or NaOH are cytoprotective because they slightly irritate the gastric mucosa and stimulate it to increase the synthesis of cytoprotective prostaglandins. This protection elicited by mild irritants is called "adaptive cytoprotection" [58].

Chemicals that contain or modify sulfhydryl groups also protect against acute gastric mucosal injury. Unlike adaptive cytoprotection, which can be completely inhibited by indomethacin, mucosal protection provided by cysteamine or dimercaprol (BAL) was only 50% reduced by pretreatment with indomethacin [59,60].

Sucralfate has been used for many years for the treatment of both gastric and duodenal ulcers. Its effectiveness was thought to be due to its ability to act as a physical barrier to pepsin, acid, and bile salts. Because the drug adheres to proteins, it can bind selectively to ulcers and erosions [61–63]. Studies have, in fact, demonstrated this selective binding to acute gastric mucosal lesions caused by ethanol and anti-inflammatory drugs [64]. However, sucralfate has recently been shown to do far more than act as a physical barrier for the denuded gastric mucosa. When it was demonstrated that it could be effective against ulcers, the question was asked if this was a cytoprotective drug. Tarnowski et al. [65] demonstrated this cytoprotective quality against induced gastric necrosis in rats. Because of the cytoprotective abilities, these investigators wondered if they were observing a prostaglandin-mediated effect. It was found that pretreatment with indomethacin abolished the cytoprotection [66], and increased ulcerogenic PGE_2 levels were found in rats treated with sucralfate. Tesler and Lim [67] demonstrated that 8 of 12 patients who developed erosions while taking aspirin did not develop erosions following pretreatment with sucralfate despite the same salicylate levels.

Other authors [68] have also confirmed that sucralfate can stimulate endogenous prostaglandin formation. However, Coleman et al. [69] could find evidence of this stimulation only at 15″ and 30″ after dosing with sucralfate, whereas its cytoprotective effects are most potent at 6 hr. Thus, the authors consider that sucralfate may only transiently affect gastric mucosal production of PGE_2.

Various studies have been accomplished with sucralfate in normal volunteers with NSAIDs. The only long-term endoscopy-controlled study was one we reported in which sucralfate 1 g four times a day was compared with placebo for a 4-week interval [70]. The 143 arthritis patients were divided into two groups based on the presence or absence of mucosal lesions but not ulcers at baseline endoscopy. Those with such lesions were reevaluated in 4 weeks. There was within-group improvement in the sucralfate group, but because the mean lesional scores were not comparable to the placebo group, no statistical difference between group comparison was found. However, the placebo group had progressed over the double-blinded at 4 weeks. A subsequent 6-month open-label extension was performed in 93 patients who completed the double-blinded phase. All patients were maintained on sucralfate and showed endoscopic improvement overall compared to baseline in the open-label experience. This, however, does not provide either a conclusive double-blind experience against placebo or a basis for evaluating ulcer treatment in such an arthritis population.

Therefore, clinical–pathophysiological correlations appear to be tenuous and troubled by the inability to clearly bridge laboratory and acute animal models to the clinically documented events of usual NSAID gastropathy. Yet it is those very events that require better understanding and effective response.

IV. NSAID EXPERIENCES

We have reported endoscopy-controlled long-term studies demonstrating differences between NSAIDs. The studies suggest that nonacetylated salicylate is, indeed, gastric-sparing, and in one study comparing it to naproxen we were able to demonstrate a statistically significant difference in the treatment of rheumatoid arthritis between salsalate 3 g daily (18 patients) and naproxen 1500 mg daily (21 patients) [71]. Eight naproxen patients developed ulcers, whereas no ulcers developed in the salsalate group, which demonstrated no significant gastropathy beyond one patient with erosions over the 3-month double-blinded study. Both groups responded with appropriate efficacy to NSAID therapy, and no other significant differences in adverse drug reaction events developed. Consistent with this is a clinical trial with choline magnesium trisalicylate 3 g daily versus piroxicam 20 mg daily in elderly patients (defined as over 65 years of age) with rheumatoid arthritis (Purdue-Frederick, unpublished). In this 2-month endoscopy-controlled trial, 6 of 11 piroxicam patients developed ulcer craters with one major hemorrhage whereas no ulcers developed in the nonacetylated salicylate group. Efficacy was similar in both groups, although tinnitus was a problem in the those who used salicylate.

Some have suggested that nonacetylated salicylates, by virtue of prostaglandin sparing, might be less effective in treating arthritis. A national multicenter study of salsalate versus naproxen in the treatment of rheumatoid arthritis has been now reported that found no such differences, with clinical outcome efficacy favoring the salsalate group [72].

Our endoscopy-controlled experience with a prostaglandin-sparing new NSAID carprofen versus ibuprofen conducted over 3 months in 40 patients demonstrated a single ulcer in the carprofen group versus multiple ulcers and significant gastropathy in the ibuprofen group [43]. We have also reported a significant difference in observed clinical outcomes in nabumetone versus naproxen in the treatment of rheumatoid arthritis and osteoarthritis for up to 4 years [73]. Almost all naproxen patients dropped out of the study at 4 years because of gastropathy and/or confirmed ulcer disease, whereas 13 patients remained in the nabumetone group without significant gastropathy. The latter is a prodrug that appears to have prostaglandin-sparing properties. Finally we should note that over-the-counter (OTC) ibuprofen (200 mg) is considered to be the safest OTC product in FDA history [17,74]. This argues for the importance of low-dose short-half-life drug therapy as a safety consideration.

Case-control studies using large databases provide, through sheer weight of numbers, a basis for assessing probable risk factors related to NSAID use and such outcome events as ulcers, bleeding, perforation, and death. Thus Griffin et al. [31] found that elderly NSAID users have up to 4.8 times the risk of bleeding and death associated with such NSAID use. That article emphasizes the problems of underappreciating confounding factors in other case-control studies. In the Griffin study, NSAID use is defined as at least 180 days and prescriptions filled within 30 days.

By contrast, Carson et al. [35] found a 1.5 risk factor limited to infrequent NSAID use associated with bleeding. Jick et al. do not control for long-term NSAID use, salicylate use, or other disease associated with gastrointestinal bleeding such as gastroesophageal varices and cancer. Yet from this same database they conclude in separate report [75] that "hospitalization for gastroesophageal bleeding is some five times greater in persons over 64 years of age," with the highest prevalence of NSAID use "three times higher" in the 65-year-old group. This is consistent with Collier [76] and Langman [6], who have associated those 65 and older with perforated ulcers or bleeding, respectively.

We have suggested that population studies are generally flawed in one way or another, lacking a depth of data on such confounding cofactors as codisease, co-therapy, and uncontrolled clinical patterns of NSAID use alone or in combinations [17]. Thus, epidemiology or case control of clinical studies as well as spontaneous adverse drug reporting must be buttressed by rigorous, carefully controlled, longitudinal, blinded endoscopic studies to ultimately understand which NSAIDs at what specific doses can be taken with greater safety in particular at-risk populations.

Now that regulatory agencies such as the U.S. FDA have taken positions on NSAID warnings of "GI ulcerations, bleeding, and perforation" rather than simply "gastric irritation," the practice of medicine is joined by medicolegal and ethical implications of long-term NSAID use in at-risk populations. This implies determining which particular NSAIDs may be safer than other NSAIDs (prostaglandin-sparing such as nonacetylated salicylated, carprofen, nabumetone, etc.) on the basis of endoscopy-controlled documentation.

We have conducted a study of rheumatoid arthritis patients receiving aspirin [21]. After 4 weeks of aspirin therapy (650–1300 mg qid), 270 patients underwent endoscopy. Of these, 239 were randomized to receive misoprostol (200 μg qid) or placebo for 8 weeks. Aspirin therapy was continued. Antacids were permitted for epigastric pain. Endoscopy was repeated at 4 and 8 weeks. Rheumatoid arthritis activity was assessed on entry and prior to and during administration of misoprostol or placebo.

Of patients randomized to misoprostol or placebo, erosive gastritis or ulcers were detected in 188 (79%) and gastric intramucosal hemorrhage was found in 51 (21%). In addition, 54 patients (24%) had duodenal ulcers or erosive duodenitis, and 19 (8%) had significant duodenal intramucosal hemorrhage. Success rates (disappearance of ulcers or erosions, or marked reduction in intramucosal hemorrhage) for the evaluable cohort are reported in Table 4.

Misoprostol was also numerically superior to placebo in preventing gastric and duodenal ulcer. Misoprostol failed to prevent ulcer in 9% of patients, whereas placebo was associated with such failure in 20% of patients ($p = .066$). After 4 and 8 weeks, misoprostol were significantly superior to placebo in healing duodenal lesions detected after lead-in aspirin therapy.

Rheumatoid arthritis activity did not differ between the two groups throughout the study. Although the incidence of diarrhea in the misoprostol group (14%) was greater than that in the placebo group (6%), there were no dropouts due to this effect.

The conclusions taken from this study are the following:

1. Serious mucosal injury was not only observed in 79% of rheumatoid arthritis patients after 4 weeks of aspirin therapy but continued on in almost all of the

Table 4 Healing of Aspirin-Induced Gastropathy, Misoprostol vs. Placebo

	Misoprostol	Placebo	Significance
All gastric lesions			
4 weeks	84/122 (69%)	36/116 (31%)	$P < .001$
8 weeks	85/122 (70%)	29/116 (25%)	$P < .001$
Gastric and duodenal ulcers			
4 weeks	20/36 (56%)	8/34 (24%)	$P = .006$
8 weeks	24/36 (67%)	9/34 (26%)	$P < .001$

Source: Roth et al. [21].

nongastroprotected placebo group (and some of the prostaglandin-treated group) in the face of the subsequent 2 months of aspirin therapy. This demonstrated the failure of cytoprotective adaptation in such a cohort. The implications here were profoundly important:

(a) Adaptation, as Szabo and Pihan [50] state, is an evanescent, acute mechanism.

(b) Adaptation in the face of chronic NSAID therapy can be commonly fatigued and fails as that putative therapy continues in the face of mucosal lesional disease.

2. Coadministration of misoprostol is highly effective in healing aspirin-induced gastric and duodenal lesions in patients with rheumatoid arthritis.

3. Coadministration of misoprostol appears to be effective in preventing aspirin-induced gastric and duodenal ulceration.

4. Misoprostol does not interfere with the beneficial effects of aspirin on rheumatoid arthritis activity.

We have separately reported a 420-patient study in osteoarthritis in which ibuprofen, piroxicam, or naproxen were used for arthritis therapy for 3 months [77]. Half the patients were additionally randomly assigned to misoprostol 200 µg qid (139 patients) or 100 µg qid (143 patients) for additional gastroprotection. The remaining 138 patients were randomly assigned to match placebo four times daily. Endoscopy was accomplished monthly in addition to routine clinical examinations. Forty-three gastric ulcers developed over this interval: 30 of 138 (22%) in the placebo group, 10 of 143 (7%) in the 100-µg misoprostol dosage group, and 3 of 139 (2%) in the 200-µg misoprostol group. This produced statistically significant differences in the misoprostol group as compared to the placebo group ($p \leq .001$). Because of the high development of ulcers without gastroprotection, the FDA terminated the study at this time because of the ethical problem of not gastroprotecting patients on usual NSAID therapy when serious ulcer disease was silently developing. This has produced a change in attitude toward the significance of mucosal lesional disease in the face of high-dose putative common NSAID therapy in arthritis. It has led to the FDA proposing strong warnings of serious complications of ulcers and bleeding from such therapy.

The literature is confounded by references to the importance of adaptation and even an "invisible callus" that protects the stomach in the face of gastric irritation [26]. In animal models and normal human mucosa, this is apparently well documented. Longitudinal endoscopy-controlled studies confirm that such adaptive cytoprotection fails on sustained anti-inflammatory doses of NSAIDs in arthritis therapy. This lesional progression should not be confused with "superficial ulcerations" commonly seen as "cosmetic changes" after trivial exposure to NSAID therapy. Superficial ulcerations are more appropriately described as erosions. They are common with NSAID therapy. When they are diffuse, they can be associated with profuse capillary microbleeding. In the misoprostol/aspirin study described earlier, 19% of these erosions actually progressed to ulcer craters with 3 months of aspirin exposure (and even in the prostaglandin-protected population, 9% progressed). Ulcer craters are, by definition, deep to the muscularis mucosa in anatomical proximity to the major vasculature. Ten percent of such vascular hemorrhages are fatal.

Aspirin and at least some NSAIDs (indomethacin, piroxicam) have been demonstrated to have a direct toxic effect on the "mucosal barrier," resulting in significant back-diffusion of hydrogen ions with consequent potential for gastrodamage and bleeding [78]. This acute mechanism is separate from the chronic consequences of all NSAID therapy based upon degrees of chronic ablation of prostaglandin synthetase activity. This apparently accounts for the defeat of the gastroprotective mechanisms with which prostaglandins are closely associated (adherent gastric mucin production, bicarbonate secretion, maintenance of the protective vasculature). The vasculature at pH 7.4 presents a significant potential buffering effect upon the potential for back-diffusion of hydrogen ions against a gastric lumen with an average pH of 1.5. This might better explain the potential for bleeding with gastrodamage in the elderly who already have an atrophic vascular bed [73].

From the rheumatologist's point of view, the exquisite efforts of gastroenterologic research to reconstruct the network of gastrodefenses is as inspiring as it is confusing. Perhaps the best clarification of the inconsistencies within the theory of cytoprotection are offered by Szabo, who suggests that cytoprotection be thought of as an overview concept primarily directed toward the protection of the deep vasculature [51]. The mucosal barrier in this framework comes and goes with common forms of acute irritation, and restitution is rapid and impressive. Thus, in the face of sustained repression of these gastrodefenses, as with chronic NSAID therapy in arthritis, we see that failure and the clinical consequences that have been described.

Szabo and Bynum [79] impressively argue that "failure or disease of a system" is rarely "cured by depression of its basic physiological functions." Thus, a gastroprotective approach with prostaglandin analogues or stimulation of prostaglandin production (i.e., sucralfate) versus the antagonist approach of H_2 blockade or neutralization of acid production makes more teleological sense for the amassed toxicity of sustained putative NSAID therapy.

In order to sustain chronic gastroprotection with prostaglandin analogues, we can anticipate an expected effect on smooth muscle. This leads to some degree of bowel hypermotility and even diarrhea in some patients and the potential for uterotonic effects in the face of pregnancy. The former appears to be a dose-related and clearly reversible effect that can be easily countered. The latter can be prevented by proper communication, with the avoidance of such agents in the face of potential or existing pregnancy.

By contrast, oxidizing agents that produce mild mucosal stimulation such as heavy metals (aluminum in antacids, sucralfate) and nonacetylated salicylate may offer a basis for prophylactic gastroprotection. This would especially be a boon to demonstrate for any nonacetylated salicylate that could normally be used in arthritis in lieu of the usual NSAIDs. As weak prostaglandin synthetase inhibitors, nonacetylated salicylates offer less chance of compromising mucosal defenses while they stimulate a local protective response in addition to their usual role in analgesia and anti-inflammatory therapy. Sucralfate has proven desirable as a topical protectant because it does not have systemic bioavailability or the concomitant systemic toxicities or interactions. Antioxidants such as free sulfhydryl substances can, by free radical scavenging and other mechanisms, offer the potential for gastric protection.

V. RATIONALE FOR RESPONSE

We have indicated that NSAID therapy is the single most pervasive form of pharmacological therapy today. It also accounts for more spontaneous reports of serious adverse drug reaction to the FDA than all other alternative forms of medical therapy. Gastropathy constitutes the primary adverse drug reaction associated with NSAID therapy.

The cost/benefit consequences of our therapies in practice will drive the direction of use of those therapies in the future [12]. Figure 2 indicates that in the case of NSAID therapy, risk clearly accounts for the costs that must be weighed against the benefits. Those risks include the dollars lost from death and disability and the costs of complications and hospitalizations that ultimately interrupt productivity. This, of course, must be weighed against the cost of not effectively treating a particular disease such as arthritis in order to weigh the ultimate benefit. In the case of NSAIDs, it is an anti-inflammatory outcome based upon dose and particular response to NSAIDs.

We therefore require risk management of these factors to satisfactorily answer our equation. Table 5 weights the particular NSAID and how it is used based upon its pharmacokinetics in each particular host responder and the often confounding consideration of cotherapy for codiseases in that host.

When the risk is unacceptable we might not use the NSAID therapy or we might either modify the dose of that therapy or consider prophylactic concomitant gastro-

$$\textbf{RISK} = \text{ADRs} \rightarrow \text{\$/death/disability/disease/discomfort}$$

$$\textbf{BENEFIT} = \text{AIF} \leftarrow \Delta\text{dose}/\Delta\text{NSAID}$$

$$\frac{\textbf{RISK} \rightarrow \textbf{COST}}{\textbf{BENEFIT}}$$

FIGURE 2   NSAID risk/benefit vs. cost/benefit. (Reprinted from Roth [23].)

Table 5   Risk/Benefit and Cost/Benefit Cofactors

Drug dose/duration
Drug pharmacokinetics (half-life, bioavailability,
    storage, excretion, ADRs, etc.)
Host factors (age, codisease, etc.)
Cotherapy (drug–drug interactions)

ADR = adverse drug reaction.
Source: Roth [23].

protective therapeutic measures with the attendant costs and separate adverse reactions associated with yet another therapy. But our choice must be balanced against not treating the particular suffering patient effectively, taking into consideration the resulting pain and loss of function.

And so we come to trade-offs. To achieve the ultimate good in terms of long-term suppression of disease expression, there is no medication without potential for adverse drug reactions. Yet the reduction of risk/benefit ratio will allow more appropriate use of safer products over longer periods of time in chronic diseases such as arthritis, and it is the long road to arthritis therapy that is key to providing quality-of-life controls and suppression of disease expression.

To achieve our goals, we must defensively reexamine the manner in which NSAID therapy is used for particular problem populations. For those populations most at risk of gastropathy or with demonstrable gastropathy, we must consider those gastroprotective interventions, acute and chronic, that are most appropriate.

Although the literature reflects otherwise, our present state of knowledge argues against continuing NSAIDs in the face of active ulcer crater disease [14]. In the presence of inflammatory joint disease, anti-inflammatory measures are requisite to prevent exacerbation. Therefore low-dose corticoids can temporarily be introduced or parenteral corticoids superimposed in place of NSAID therapy. Whether such steroids are cytoprotective or not is still a moot question, but certainly they appear to be well tolerated compared to NSAID therapy. This is separate from the argument concerning their use in combination with NSAID therapy.

In nonsystemic inflammatory disorders such as common osteoarthritis and primary fibrositis, NSAID therapy can safely be stopped and alternative analgesia provided, where necessary, along with physical therapy and joint protection procedures. After the acute ulcer has healed, the former NSAID approach may be reinstated, weighed against going back to prostaglandin-sparing nonacetylated salicylate or low-dose short-half-life NSAID therapy.

In the case of systemic inflammatory arthritis such as rheumatoid arthritis, the possibility of disease-modifying antirheumatic drug intervention or adjustment might mitigate against or modulate the need for further NSAID therapy. In the past we were driven toward a "steroid-sparing effect" to avoid the hazards of hormonal therapy. Now we should consider whether "NSAID-sparing effect" is desirable in the face of the ever-present chronic hazard of gastropathy.

Finally, some NSAIDs appear to be more gastrotoxic and some safer than others. That comparative information is just emerging. We have found newer agents such as carprofen and nabumetone to be more gastrosparing [43,73]. Longer half-life NSAIDs such as piroxicam appear to be more gastrotoxic in our endoscopy-controlled experience (Purdue-Frederick, unpublished). High-dose long-term aspirin is especially gastrotoxic when there are gastropathy risk factors [22,31,80].

Clinical research continues to identify those agents more appropriately gastroprotective for the unique problems of NSAID gastropathy. These are not clearly hyperacidity-driven problems, and therefore H_2-blockade drugs, though symptomatically useful, have not been found to moderate mucosal lesional disease as putative NSAID therapy is continued once gastropathy has been established [25]. To date, this also applies to antacid therapy.

Sucralfate therapy has been found useful and is cytoprotective [70], yet no pivotal clinical research study has yet confirmed its gastroprotective role in humans. It does have the advantage, however, that sucralfate is a nonabsorbable and therefore nonsystemic agent with minimal toxicity beyond occasional constipation.

On the other hand, the most persuasive studies yet accomplished in NSAID gastropathy suggest a central role for prostaglandin analogues as a rationale for replacement therapy in the face of NSAID blockade of cyclooxygenase driving the pathogenesis of that chronic disorder. Those pivotal misoprostol studies of the use of aspirin in rheumatoid arthritis and of NSAIDs in osteoarthritis have previously been described [22,24]. Agrawal et al. [81] demonstrated clear superiority of misoprostol over sucralfate in preventing gastric ulcer formation in osteoarthritis patients taking NSAIDs over a 3-month period. Because prostaglandins normally stimulate smooth muscle, the diarrhea and uterotonic effects seen with this agent must be weighed against the clinical efficacy potential.

At present sucralfate and H_2-blocker agents (cimetidine, ranitidine, famotidine) are frequently used in combination. This probably reflects the lack of faith in the possibility of reversing NSAID gastropathy with either agent alone. This is certainly not a cost-effective rationale for long-term therapy with expensive drugs.

By contrast, prostaglandin analogue therapy as in the case of misoprostol is used at antisecretory doses in addition to its known cytoprotective properties. This appears to be a more cost-effective approach. In addition, other contributory cofactors such as cigarette smoking, alcohol abuse, and uncontrolled problems with stress can all be responded to in a more effective effort to counter NSAID gastropathy [82].

Indeed, we continue to face an iatrogenic dilemma. NSAID use is pervasive, but gastropathy is all too common—it is often difficult to recognize, because symptoms are either asynchronous with severity of mucosal lesional disease or completely lacking. Endoscopy can be an expensive, not readily available, procedure for large populations at risk. But the substantiated outcomes of ulcers—bleeding and even perforation and death—as well as the cost/benefit considerations of hospitalization and disability argue for a response based upon what we already know. Such discrimination should be founded in the pharmacokinetics of drug half-life (short half-life, more rapid elimination), differential prostaglandin-sparing properties, dosage decisions, and finally, whether the NSAID should be used in the clinical circumstances at all. According to the degree of risk associated with the patient, potentially prophylactic gastroprotective choices can also be considered with agents such as sucralfate and appropriate prostaglandin analogues as well as symptomatic use of H_2 blockers and antacids. Such an individualized decision-making process can lead to mitigation of the hazards of NSAID gastropathy while research works toward even better answers to the present dilemma.

VI. SUMMARY

We have reviewed NSAID gastropathy as a recently recognized old problem presenting enormous clinical challenges. It is difficult to recognize and certainly difficult to prevent. We have reviewed those known pathophysiological mechanisms that explain the development and perpetuation of this mucosal disease in the face of NSAID therapy. Spontaneous adverse drug reporting, epidemiological and case-control studies, and postmarketing surveillance of drugs are now identifying risk ratios for this disorder. But large long-term, carefully controlled endoscopic studies of longitudinal models are providing requisite data as to which NSAIDs at which doses appear either safer or more gastrotoxic than others. Gastroprotective agents are similarly weighed in such studies. The data from that experience are already persuasive and helpful. The problem has been defined. The effort has been joined. The answers, though neither definitive nor conclusive, form a basis for a rationale for response. This is an iatrogenic disorder, and it requires responsible decision making in the use of NSAIDs. The FDA has seen the regulatory need to propose serious warnings to drive that caution.

Finally, gastroprotective interventions based upon demonstrable pathology and chronic risk factors for prophylaxis must be individually weighed. New prostaglandin analogue experience appears most promising, and sucralfate has provided alternative cytoprotective potential. Therapy with H_2 blockers and antacids in combination has been used, and research continues on other promising agents.

REFERENCES

1. Roth SH. NSAID gastropathy. We started it—can we stop it? Arch Intern Med 1986; 146:1075–6.
2. Paulus HE. Pharmacological considerations. In: Roth SH, ed. Handbook of drug therapy. Littleton, Mass.: PSG, 1985:39–78.
3. Ward JR. Nonsteroidal (nonsalicylate) anti-inflammatory drugs. In: Roth SH, Calabro JJ, Paulus HE, Willkens RF, eds. Rheumatic therapeutics. New York: McGraw-Hill, 1985:383–96.
4. Arthritis Foundation. Basic facts brochure. 1986:7.
5. Semble EL, Wu WC. Antiinflammatory drugs and gastric mucosal damage. Semin Arthritis Rheum 1987; 16:271–86.
6. Langman MJS. Antiinflammatory drug intake and the risk of ulcer complications. Med Toxicol 1986; 1(Suppl 1):34–8.
7. Somerville K, Faulkner G, Langman M. NSAIDs and bleeding peptic ulcer. Lancet 1986; i:462–4.
8. McHardy G. Ulcer disease in the elderly. In: Cytoprotection: proceedings of a symposium. New York: Medical Information Services, 1985:10–3.
9. Clinch D, Banerjee AK, Ostick G, et al. Non-steroidal anti-inflammatory drugs and gastrointestinal adverse effects. J Roy Coll Physicians Lond 1983; 17:228–30.
10. Roth SH. Salicylates revisited: are they still the hallmark of anti-inflammatory therapy? Drugs 1988; 36:1–6.
11. Balz E. Salicylsaure, salicylsaures, natron and thymol in ihren einfluss auf krankheiten. Arch Heilkd 1877; 1:1106–8.
12. Roth SH. Pharmacologic approaches to musculoskeletal disorders. Clin Geriatr Med 1988; 4(2):441–61.
13. Roth SH, Bennett RE. Nonsteroidal anti-inflammatory drug gastropathy: recognition and response. Arch Intern Med 1987; 147:2093–100.
14. Roth SH. Nonsteroidal anti-inflammatory drugs: gastropathy, deaths, and medical practice. Ann Intern Med 1988; 109(5):353–4.
15. Paulus HE. Concepts and targets for drug treatment of chronic rheumatic diseases. In: Paul H, Furst D, Dromgoole S, eds. Drugs for rheumatic therapy. New York: Churchill & Livingston, 1987:1–8.
16. Sun DC, Roth SH, Mitchell CS, et al. Upper gastrointestinal disease in rheumatoid arthritis. Am J Dig Dis 1974; 19:405–10.

17. Roth SH. Antiulcer therapy in NSAID gastropathy: a rheumatologist's perspective. Drug Inf J 1988; 22:419–24.

18. Wolfe E, Kleinheksel SM, Spitz PW, Lubeck DP, Fries JF, Roth SH, et al. A multi-center study of hospitalization in rheumatoid arthritis: frequency, medical-surgical admissions, and costs. Arthritis Rheum 1986; 29(5):614–9.

19. Roth SH. Endoscopic comparison of the tolerance and safety of carprofen and ibuprofen in patients with rheumatoid arthritis. IXth Pan American Congress of Rheumatology, Buenos Aires, Argentina, Nov. 17–22, 1986.

20. Baum D, Kennedy DL, Forbes MB. Utilization of nonsteroidal antiinflammatory drugs. Arthritis Rheum 1985; 28:686–92.

21. Roth SH. Corticosteroid therapy. In: New directions in arthritis therapy. Littleton, Mass.: PSG, 1980:43–51.

22. Roth SH, Agrawal N, Mahowald M, et al. Misoprostol heals gastroduodenal injury in patients with rheumatoid arthritis receiving aspirin. Arch Intern Med 1989; 149(4): 775–9.

23. Caruso I, Bianchi-Porro GB. Gastroscopic evaluation of anti-inflammatory agents. Br Med J 1980; 280:75–8.

24. Roth SH. NSAIDs: risk benefit versus cost benefit. Drug Inf J 1988; 22:477–81.

25. Roth S, Bennett R, Mitchell C, Hartman R. Cimetidine therapy in nonsteroidal anti-inflammatory drug therapy: double blind long term evaluation. Arch Intern Med 1987; 147:1798–1801.

26. Graham DY, Smith JL. Aspirin and the stomach. Ann Intern Med 1986; 104:390–8.

27. Armstrong CP, Blower AL. NSAIDs and life threatening complications of peptic ulceration. Gut 1987; 28:527–32.

28. Vane J. The evolution of nonsteroidal antiinflammatory drugs and their mechanism of action. Drugs 1987; 33(Suppl):18–27.

29. Robert A. Cytoprotection by prostaglandins. Gastroenterology 1979; 77:761–7.

30. Roth S. The new look in drugs: is longer lasting better? Arch Intern Med 1984; 144:472–3.

31. Griffin MR, Ray WA, Schaffner W. Nonsteroidal anti-inflammatory drug use and death from peptic ulcer in elderly persons. Ann Intern Med 1988; 109:359–65.

32. Douthwaite AH. Some recent advances in medical diagnosis and treatment. Br Med J 1939; 1:1143.

33. Trenby EN. Drug-induced peptic ulcer and upper gastrointestinal bleeding. Br J Hosp Med 1980; 23(2):185–90.

34. Butt JH, Barthel JS, Moore RA. Clinical spectrum of the upper gastrointestinal effects of NSAIDs. Am J Med 1988; 84(Suppl 2A):5–14.

35. Carson JL, Strom BL, Soper KA, West SL, Morse ML. The association of nonsteroidal anti-inflammatory drugs with upper gastrointestinal tract bleeding. Arch Intern Med 1987; 147:85–8.

36. Jick H. Effects of aspirin and acetaminophen in gastrointestinal hemorrhage. Results from the Boston Collaborative Drug Surveillance Program. Arch Intern Med 1981; 141:316–21.

37. Baskin WN, Ivey KJ, Krause WJ, et al. Aspirin induced ultrastructural changes in human gastro mucosa: correlation with potential difference. Ann Intern Med 1976; 85(3):299–303.

38. Hoftiezer JW, O'Laughlin JC, Ivey KJ. Effects of 24 hours of aspirin, Bufferin,

paracetamol, and placebo on normal human gastroduodenal mucosa. Gut 1982; 23(8): 692–7.

39. Silvoso GR, Ivey KJ, Butt JH, et al. Incidence of gastric lesions in patients with rheumatic disease on chronic aspirin therapy. Ann Intern Med 1979; 91(4): 517–20.

40. O'Laughlin JC, Hotiezer JW, Ivey KJ. Effect of aspirin in the stomach in normals: endoscopic comparison of damage produced one hour, 24 hours, and 2 weeks after administration. Scand J Gastroenterol 1981; 16(Suppl):211–4.

41. Hoftiezer JW, Silvoso GR, Burbs M, Ivey KJ. Comparison of the effect of regular and enteric-coated aspirin on gastroduodenal mucosa in man. Lancet 1980; ii:609–12.

42. Aspirin Myocardial Infarction Study Research Group. A randomized, controlled trial of aspirin in persons recovered from myocardial infarction. JAMA 1980; 243:661–9.

43. Lanza FL. Endoscopic studies of gastric and duodenal injury after the use of ibuprofen, aspirin, and other nonsteroidal antiinflammatory agents. Am J Med 1984; 77:19–24.

44. Beard K, Walker AM, Perera DR, Jick H. NSAIDs and hospitalization for gastro-esophageal bleeding in the elderly. Arch Intern Med 1987; 147:1721–3.

45. Bartle WR, Gupta K, Labor J. NSAIDs and gastrointestinal bleeding. Arch Intern Med 1986; 146:2365–7.

46. Levy M. Patients with major upper gastrointestinal bleeding and peptic ulcer disease. N Engl J Med 1974; 290:1158–62.

47. McQueen S, Hutton D, Allen A, et al. Gastric and duodenal surface mucus gel thickness in rats: effects of prostaglandins and damaging agents. Am J Physiol 1983; 245:G388–93.

48. Levy KJ, Morrison S, Cray C. Effect of intravenous salicylates on the gastric mucosal barrier in man. Am J Dig Dis 1972; 17(12):1055–64.

49. Robert A, Lancaster C, Davis JP, et al. Cytoprotection by prostaglandins occurs in spite of penetration of absolute alcohol into the gastric mucosa. Gastroenterol 1985; 88:328–33.

50. McQueen S, Allen A, Garner A. In: Allen A, Flextröm, Garner A, Silen W, Turnberg L., eds. Mechanism of mucosal protection in the upper gastrointestinal tract. New York: Raven, 1984:215–9.

51. Szabo S, Pihan G. Mechanisms of gastric cytoprotection. J Clin Gastroenterol 1987; 9(Suppl 1):8–13.

52. Pihan G, Majzabi D, Haudenschild C, Trier J, Szabo S. Early microcirculatory stasis in acute gastric mucosal injury in the rat and prevention by 16,16-dimethyl prostaglandin E_2 or sodium thiosulfate. Gastroenterology 1986; 91(6):1415–26.

53. Karim SM, Carter DC, Bhana D, et al. Effect of orally and intravenously administered prostaglandin $15(R)15$-methyl PGE_2 on gastric secretion in man. Adv Biosci 1973; 9:254–64.

54. Bennett A, Stamford F, Unger WG. PGE_2 and gastric acid secretion in man. Adv Biosci 1973; 9:265–9.

55. Konturek SJ, Brzozowski T, Piastucki I, et al. Role of locally generated prostaglandins in adaptive gastric cytoprotection. Dig Dis Sci 1982; 27:967–71.

56. Yik KY, Dreidger AA, Watson WC. Prostaglandin E_2 prevents aspirin and indomethacin damage to human gastric mucosa. Dig Dis Sci 1982; 27:972–5.

57. Wilson DE. Antisecretory and mucosal protective actions of misoprostol. Am J Med 1987; 83(Suppl 1A):2–8.

58. Robert A, Nezamis JE, Lancaster C, Davies JP, Field SQ, Hanchar AJ. Mild irritants

prevent gastric necrosis through adaptive cytoprotection mediated by prostaglandins. Am J Physiol 1983; 245:6113–21.

59. Robert A, Eberle D, Kaplowitz N. The role of glutathione and gastric mucosal cytoprotection. Am J Physiol 1984; 247:G296–304.

60. Szabo S, Maull EA, Movabedi S. Sulfhydryl drugs: a new type of gastric cytoprotective agent. Gastroenterology 1981; 80:1298.

61. McHardy G. A multicenter, double-blind trial of sucralfate and placebo in duodenal ulcer. J Clin Gastroenterol 1981; 3(Suppl 2):147–52.

62. Hollander D. Duodenal ulcer, gastric ulcer: sucralfate, a new therapeutic concept. In Caspary WF, ed. Proceedings, sucralfate symposium of the 11th international congress of gastroenterology, Hamburg, June 1980. Urben and Schwarzanburg, 1981:45–53.

63. Marks IN, Lucke W, Wright JP, et al. Ulcer healing and relapse rates after initial treatment with cimetidine or sucralfate. J Clin Gastroenterol 1981; 3(Suppl 2):163–5.

64. Harrington SJ, Schlegal JF, Code CF. Protective effects of sucralfate on gastric mucosa of rats. J Clin Gastroenterol 1981; 3(Suppl 2):153–7.

65. Tarnowski A, Hollander D, Krause WJ, et al. Sucralfate protection of gastric mucosa against alcohol injury: morphologic, ultrastructural, and functional time sequence analysis. [Abstract] Gastroenterology 1983; 84:1331.

66. Hollander D, Tarnowski A, Gergely A, et al. Sucralfate protection of the gastric mucosa against ethanol-induced injury: a prostaglandin-mediated process? Scan J Gastroenterol 1984; 101(Suppl):97–102.

67. Tesler MA, Lim ES. Protection of gastric mucosa by sucralfate from aspirin-induced erosions. J Clin Gastroenterol 1981; 3(Suppl 2):175–9.

68. Crampton JR, Gibbons LC, Ries W. Effects of sucralfate on gastroduodenal bicarbonate secretion and prostaglandin E_2 metabolism. Am J Med 1987; 83(Suppl 3B):14–8.

69. Coleman JC, Lacz JP, Browne RK, et al. Sucralfate or mild irritants on experimental gastritis and prostaglandin production. Am J Med 1987; 83(Suppl 3B):24–30.

70. Caldwell JR, Roth SH, Wu WC, et al. Sucralfate treatment of nonsteroidal antiinflammatory drug-induced gastrointestinal symptoms and mucosal damage. Am J Med 1987; 83(Suppl 3B):74–82.

71. Roth S, Bennett R, Caldron P, et al. Reduced risk of NSAID gastropathy (GI mucosal toxicity) with nonacetylated salicylate (salsalate): an endoscopic study. Sem Arthritis Rheum 1990; 19(4 Suppl 2):11–9.

72. April P, Abeles M, Baraf H. Does the acetyl group of aspirin contribute to the antiinflammatory efficacy of salicylic acid in the treatment of rheumatoid arthritis? Sem Arthritis Rheum 1990; 19(4 Suppl 2):20–8.

73. Roth SH. Endoscopy-controlled study of the safety of nabumetone compared with naproxen in arthritis therapy. Am J Med 1987; 83(Suppl 4B):25–30.

74. Harter JG. The FDA, new anti-rheumatic drugs, and you. Anti-rheumatic Drug Study Group meeting held at the 51st American Rheumatism Association meeting, Washington DC, June 9–13, 1987 (S Roth Chairman/Moderator) [unpublished].

75. Jick SS, Perera DR, Walker AM, Jick H. Non-steroidal anti-inflammatory drugs and hospital admission for perforated peptic ulcer. Lancet 1987; ii:380–2.

76. Collier DS, Pain JA. Nonsteroidal anti-inflammatory drugs and peptic ulcer perforation. Gut 1985; 26:359–63.

77. Graham DY, Agrawal NM, Roth SH. Prevention of NSAID-induced gastric ulcer with

misoprostol: multicentre, double-blind, placebo-controlled trial. Lancet 1988; ii(8623): 1277–80.

78. Davenport HW. Back diffusion of acid through the gastric mucosa and its physiological consequences. In: Glass GBJ, ed. Progress in gastroenterology, Vol. 2. New York: Grune & Stratton, 1970:42–56.

79. Szabo S, Bynum T. Alternatives to the acid-oriented approach to ulcer disease: does "cytoprotection" exist in man?

80. Roth SH. NSAIDs and gastropathy: a rheumatologist's review. J Rheum 1988; 15:912–9.

81. Agrawal N, Stromatt S, Brown J. Comparative study of misoprostol and sucralfate in the prevention of NSAID-induced gastric ulcers. Submitted for publication.

82. MacIntosh JH, Byth K, Piper DW. Environmental factors in aetiology of chronic gastric ulcer: a case control study of exposure variables before the first symptoms. Gut 1985; 26(8):789–98.

7

Hemorrhage from Gastric or Duodenal Ulceration

JEFFREY B. RASKIN

University of Miami School of Medicine,
Miami, Florida

I. INTRODUCTION

The severity of upper gastrointestinal hemorrhage is reflected in its approximate 10% mortality rate [1,2]. An ulceration is identified as the source of this hemorrhage in 50% of most large series [3–6]. If one understood the etiological considerations in the initiation of ulcer hemorrhage, then the next logical step would be to appropriately design clinical therapeutic trials that prevent or arrest the initial bleeding episode and prevent rebleeding once initial hemorrhage is controlled.

As will be discussed, ulcer hemorrhage results from the ulcer's inflammatory process eroding into and disrupting a blood vessel wall. What is not completely known is why some ulcers bleed whereas most present with dyspeptic symptoms or are "silent." Unfortunately, not all factors responsible for this initiation of ulcer hemorrhage are known. In spite of modern developments in intensive care and surgery with its accompanying high technological support, the mortality from upper gastrointestinal hemorrhage has remained around 10% for the past 40 years [1,7,8]. It is important to discuss and identify those patients at high risk for bleeding so appropriately designed clinical trials of pharmacological agents can be accomplished, in the obvious hope of reducing the associated morbidity and mortality. Pharmacological management of upper gastrointestinal bleeding through the years has been mainly empirical without the benefit of controlled trials. Over the past decade we have begun to see the results of controlled clinical trials of some agents. The agents used in these trials have attempted to address the two suspected components of ulcer pathogenesis: (a) by countering the aggressive factors of acid and pepsin or (b) by improving or stimulating mucosal defensive mechanisms. It is the purpose of this chapter to review the processes involved in ulcer hemorrhage, the patient population at risk, those factors responsible for an adverse patient outcome, and the clinical pharmacological trials directed at arresting initial ulcer hemorrhage and preventing rebleeding once this initial hemorrhage is controlled.

II.   ULCER HEMORRHAGE

A.   Etiology

It comes as no surprise, and is well documented in many pathological series, that the cause of significant bleeding from ulcer disease is an exposed and eroded vessel within the ulcer floor [9–11]. Also well documented is a high correlation of rebleeding (40–100%) with subsequent high mortality when a visible vessel is identified in an ulcer with evidence of recent hemorrhage [11–16]. Understanding the physical characteristics of these exposed vessels (pathology, size, and site) could help explain the results of pharmacological therapy directed at the cessation of bleeding or help in the design of newer trials. Additional evidence is also accumulating that demonstrates a high correlation of ulcer hemorrhage in patients ingesting certain medications.

III.   BLEEDING VESSEL

A.   Pathology

Pathological changes of arteritis are frequently seen in the bleeding artery. Older references refer to an obliterative endarteritis of small vessels in pathological specimens from patients with bleeding ulcers [17,18]. Recent studies in resected specimens of patients operated on for recurrent hemorrhage frequently show an arteritis (83%), which is usually focal and seen more severely on the wall of the artery closest to the base of the ulcer [11]. This arteritis, probably chemically induced, is associated with necrosis and disruption of the wall. There may be inflammation of the opposite wall, but the vessel usually remains intact at this point. Aneurysmal dilation of the artery has also been found in conjunction with this focal necrotizing arteritis and can be frequently seen protruding into the ulcer crater. These pathological changes could explain why some ulcers cease bleeding while others continue or recur. An obliterative endarteritis would lead to vessel occlusion with cessation of hemorrhage. This is usually found in smaller vessels. Normal hemostatic mechanisms may be altered when focal necrosis and disruption of the vessel wall occur in association with the inability of the vessel to contract, as is frequently found with significant ulcer hemorrhage. The ability of small vessels to contract is a major mechanism involved in the cessation of bleeding from ruptured vessels. Any potential intravascular clot that may form and help in arresting hemorrhage would also be exposed to acid and enzyme digestion because of the exposed nature of the vessel in the ulcer base. The formation of an intravascular clot is hindered in an acid medium [19].

As will be discussed later, elderly patients have an increased mortality associated with upper gastrointestinal hemorrhage. Age-related vascular changes, if present, could explain this excessive age-related mortality. It has also been suggested that excessive or recurrent bleeding could be age-related, in that older patients may have atheromatous changes in their vessels that would preclude contraction and subsequent cessation of bleeding. Two pathologic studies have failed, however, to demonstrate atheroma in bleeding vessels, and age-related changes appear unimportant in excessive or recurrent hemorrhage [10,11]. Additionally, the incidence of rebleeding appears to be unrelated to age [20]. Recurrent bleeding could be explained by the finding of a recanalized thrombus, which was frequently found in one study of resected specimens from patients with recurrent gastric ulcer bleeding [11]. One could postulate that an initial thrombus would lead to cessation of bleeding followed by recurrence when recanalization occurs. Recurrent bleeding could also develop when the aneurysm ruptures or if the aneurysmal clot becomes dislodged.

B. Vessel Size

It seems logical that the erosion of larger vessels would lead to excessive or recurrent bleeding because of the failure of normal hemostatic mechanisms. Ulcers may extend only into the submucosa (acute) or deeper into the serosa (chronic). In a series of resected stomach with recurrent gastric ulcer bleeding, the mean external artery diameter was 0.7 mm (0.1–1.8 mm) [11]. It is of interest that 45% of the ulcers in this series penetrated to and involved serosal vessels. These serosal vessels are larger [mean diameter of 0.88 mm (0.23–1.82 mm)] than the submucosal vessels [0.50 mm mean diameter (0.11–1.09 mm)].

C. Ulcer Site

It has been shown that severe initial or recurrent bleeding from ulcers usually occurs at two specific anatomic sites in the stomach and duodenum. These sites are related to the anatomic location of the largest arteries supplying blood to the stomach (left gastric) and duodenum (gastroduodenal). Ulcers in the high posterior lesser curvature of the stomach and proximal inferoposterior bulb frequently erode into these main trunks, with subsequent excessive or recurrent bleeding. The gastroduodenal artery is large (3–6 mm in diameter) [21].

IV. ASSOCIATED MEDICATIONS

It has been generally taught that the etiology of peptic ulceration is an imbalance between aggressive (acid and pepsin) and defensive (mucosal resistance) factors. Two additional factors seem to be gaining support in the pathogenesis of ulcer disease. Recent studies have suggested that a high percentage of gastric or duodenal ulcers are found in association with *Helicobacter pylori* or in patients taking nonsteroidal anti-inflammatory drugs (NSAIDs) [22]. Ingested medications (especially the NSAIDs) have been associated with a higher frequency of ulcer hemorrhage and adverse patient outcome (increased mortality).

A. Steroids

In one large prospective study on upper gastrointestinal bleeding, patients taking steroids had a significantly higher mortality rate (22.9% vs. 9.9%) than those not on steroids [1]. This higher mortality may have been related to a higher transfusion need (>5 units), and therefore a more severe bleeding episode, in patients taking steroids than in those not taking steroids (36.3% vs. 25.7%, respectively). There was no significantly increased complication rate or surgical requirement, however, associated with the bleeding episode in patients taking steroids.

B. Nonsteroidal Anti-inflammatory Drugs (NSAIDs)

1. Aspirin

A review of the literature reveals that aspirin use is associated with significant upper gastrointestinal bleeding. Acute hemorrhagic gastritis comprises 10–25% of all cases of upper gastrointestinal bleeding, and recent aspirin use is found in approximately 50% of these cases [23–25]. In one study, a significant increase in hemorrhage compared to controls was found in patients taking aspirin and acetaminophen within the week prior to admission [26]. In this study, the long-term use of aspirin was associated with a 9.3 bleeding risk ratio for duodenal ulcer and a 3.3 risk ratio for gastric ulcer. Significant mucosal damage (ulcers) can be found in patients taking large daily doses of aspirin [27,28]. In one study, heavy use of aspirin (15 or more tablets weekly) was found in 53% of patients with gastric ulcers [29]. In another study, regular aspirin use (at least 4 days per week) was associated with significant gastric ulcer bleeding (19% vs. 6.9% in controls) but was not associated with a significant difference in duodenal ulcer bleeding [30]. A higher proportion of patients hospitalized for gastrointestinal bleeding is also found with the daily consumption of more than 2.4 g of aspirin (1.9% vs. 0.5%) [31]. Of additional interest is the observation that aspirin use in patients hospitalized for upper gastrointestinal hemorrhage is associated with a significantly greater risk of developing complications, but mortality rates and the need for surgical intervention are significantly less in these patients [1].

2. Non-Aspirin

In the past decade, NSAID use for arthritis and pain control has gained in popularity. These agents have been associated with a high incidence of gastric mucosal damage (ulcers) and major upper gastrointestinal hemorrhage. Ulceration has been estimated to develop in 25% of patients on long-term non-aspirin NSAID therapy, with an almost equal distribution of incidence between gastric and duodenal ulceration [32]. Bleeding associated with NSAID-induced ulceration is frequently seen in the elderly and may be the initial presenting event in a patient with an existing "silent" ulcer. In one study, 87% of patients presenting with ulcer hemorrhage had recent symptoms (pain), but 87% of the symptom-free patients who bled were on NSAIDs [33]. Of a group of 235 ulcer patients presenting with a life-threatening ulcer complication (bleeding in 41%), 60% were taking NSAIDs, and in 58% the bleeding complication was the first presentation of the ulcer [34]. Of the ulcer-related deaths in this study, 80% were of patients taking NSAIDs. In a conflicting report, NSAIDs did not appear to mask ulcer pain, but NSAID use in the previous 4 weeks was seen in 58% of bleeding ulcers [35]. Ulcers that bled in this study tended to be large (>20 mm), with bleeding found in a significantly older patient population than those with abdominal pain as the initial presenting complaint (66 years vs. 51 years, respectively). There appears to be a twofold increase in ulcer hemorrhage in those patients over the age of 60 on NSAIDs [36]. This increase in NSAID-induced ulcer bleeding appears to be directly related to NSAID dosing [37]. At higher dose levels of NSAIDs, bleeding was found to occur twice as frequently as at the lower dose levels. This bleeding incidence was seen to peak after 4–5 months of treatment. Data from the United Kingdom and Germany have demonstrated a rising mortality rate in elderly women associated with ulcer hemorrhage and perforation. This appears to be related to increasing NSAID use in this population [38,39]. Another study showed no increase in mortality rates for patients with upper gastrointestinal bleeding who were taking non-aspirin NSAIDs but an increased need for blood transfusions (>5 units) during the acute bleeding episode [1].

V. ADVERSE PROGNOSTIC FACTORS

Additional adverse prognostic factors related to the patient and the severity of the initial hemorrhage have been identified that have the effect of increasing mortality rates in certain situations. These factors need to be discussed as well as considered in the design of pharmacological trials aimed at the cessation of ulcer hemorrhage and in the interpretation of trial results.

A. Age

As previously mentioned, increasingly large numbers of elderly patients are presenting with severe ulcer complications including hemorrhage seemingly related to the increased use of NSAIDs. Even before the introduction of NSAIDs, reported series in the 1970s showed that the percentage of patients over age 60 presenting with upper gastrointestinal hemorrhage had been increasing, from 2% to 48% over the previous five decades [7,8]. In the largest prospective U.S. study of upper gastrointestinal bleeding, the mean age was 57 ± 17.5 years [1]. The mortality rate for patients over 60 in this study was 13.4%, compared with 8.7% for those younger than 60. Studies from the early and late 1970s report 16.4% and 25.12% mortality rates, respectively, in patients over 60 years of age [7,40].

B. Severity of Initial Bleeding Episode

It seems logical that the more severe the initial bleeding episode, the more likely that a large vessel has been eroded. Data have been presented showing that chronic large ulcers more than likely penetrate and erode the large serosal vessels with significant hemorrhage. The more acute superficial ulcers are less likely to present with significant bleeding. Large-volume blood loss has been associated with an increased mortality in acute upper gastrointestinal bleeding. Significant mortality of 30–32% has been reported in patients presenting with shock compared to 7–9% mortality in those patients without shock [1,7]. Mortality rates of 26–70% have been associated with transfusions of more than 10 units [1,7,40,41]. When emergent surgery was required to control hemorrhage, up to a threefold increase in mortality was found compared to deaths among those undergoing elective surgery [1,8,42].

C. Associated Disease Processes

In the national prospective study on upper gastrointestinal bleeding conducted by the American Society for Gastrointestinal Endoscopy (ASGE), eight categories of disease history and specific disease states were reviewed relative to outcome [1]. Earlier studies had shown that, besides age over 60 years, a history of cardiac (especially congestive heart failure), hepatic, and renal disease were high risk factors leading to increased mortality [41,43]. The findings of the ASGE study on associated disease states revealed new and interesting data related to mortality, transfusion requirements, frequency of complications, and need for surgical intervention to control bleeding. Having this information available allows the physician to rapidly identify those patients at high risk so a more vigorous diagnostic and therapeutic approach can be initiated. Future studies on the therapeutic efficacy of older or newer treatment modalities will need to address the high-risk patients.

The eight disease categories showed the following results:

(1) *Cardiac.* Overall, there was no significant increased mortality, need for transfusions greater than 5 units, or surgery with a cardiac history. Patients with a cardiac history, however, had a significant increase in complications. Myocardial infarction, arrhythmias, and congestive heart failure were associated with increased mortality. Angina was associated with an increase in transfusion requirement of greater than 5 units of blood.

(2) *Central nervous system.* There was a significant increase in mortality and complications but not in transfusions or surgery in these patients. Acute and chronic encephalopathy or a history of stroke was associated with greater mortality and complications.

(3) *Gastrointestinal.* Interestingly, a previous history of gastrointestinal disease was associated with a decrease in mortality. A previous history of duodenal ulcer (but not gastric ulcer) and previous upper gastrointestinal bleeding was associated with a significant decrease in mortality. A duodenal ulcer history was also associated with a

significant decrease in transfusion requirement. Significant surgical intervention was needed with a previous history of duodenal ulcer or a previous upper gastrointestinal bleeding episode.

(4) *Hepatic.* Hepatic disease was associated with increased mortality, higher incidence of complications, and transfusion requirement of more than 5 units. There was no increase in the need for surgical intervention. Cirrhosis, jaundice, portal hypertension, and a history of known varices were significantly associated with a transfusion requirement of more than 5 units.

(5) *Pulmonary.* Significant mortality, increased incidence of complications, and greater transfusion requirements were found with a history of pulmonary disease. Chronic obstructive lung disease (COPD) and pneumonia were associated with a high mortality, but only COPD was associated with increased transfusion requirement (>5 units).

(6) *Renal.* An increase in mortality and transfusion requirement was found in patients with renal disease. Acute and chronic renal failure were associated with increased mortality, and acute renal failure with increased transfusion requirements.

(7) *Stress-related history.* A possible relationship of bleeding related to stress (especially sepsis and major surgery within 1 month) was associated with increased mortality, increased incidence of complications, and transfusion requirement greater than 5 units. A recent surgical procedure and a diagnosis of rheumatoid arthritis were associated with an increased surgical need to control the bleeding episode.

(8) *Neoplasm.* A history of neoplastic disease was associated with an increased mortality but not an increase in complications, surgical need, or transfusions greater than 5 units.

In reviewing these eight categories of disease history, a previous history of cardiac disease was the only disease category not associated with an overall increase in mortality. The only decrease in mortality was found with a previous gastrointestinal history (duodenal but not gastric ulcer and previous gastrointestinal bleeding). The only associated finding leading to an increase in surgical intervention to control hemorrhage was a previous gastrointestinal bleeding episode or a history of duodenal ulcer. Increased transfusion requirement (> 5 units) was found in those patients with a previous history of hepatic, pulmonary, or renal disease. A stress-related bleeding episode was also found to have an increased transfusion requirement. Newer therapeutic trials will need to consider these factors as they relate to study design and the interpretation of study results.

VI. THERAPEUTIC PHARMACOLOGICAL TRIALS IN ULCER HEMORRHAGE

Over the past two decades, a burgeoning number of pharmacological agents have been developed and shown to speed the healing of gastric or duodenal ulceration. Most of these agents neutralize or inhibit acid secretion at the cellular level. Other agents have the ability to maintain or stimulate mucosal defensive mechanisms. These agents, directed at the two-component theory of ulcer pathogenesis, have also been used in clinical trials directed at the cessation or recurrence of ulcer hemorrhage.

A.   H$_2$ Antagonists

Although effective in the healing of gastric and duodenal ulcers and in the prophylaxis of stress-related bleeding, H$_2$ antagonists have been disappointing in the clinical trials directed at the cessation of acute upper gastrointestinal (nonvariceal) hemorrhage. There are also data suggesting that the widespread use of these agents has not had an impact on decreasing hospital admissions for ulcer hemorrhage. In one study, hospital admissions for duodenal ulcer bleeding increased 8% between observation periods of 1972–1976 and 1977–1984, although the use of H$_2$ antagonists rose 3.7-fold during the study period [44]. In the largest prospective placebo-controlled, multicenter U.S. trial, involving 285 patients, there was no difference in the cessation of hemorrhage between the cimetidine or placebo groups [45]. Cimetidine, given intravenously, was successful in the cessation of bleeding in 71.2% of patients compared with 77.2% treated with placebo. There was also no difference seen between the different etiologies of bleeding, including gastric or duodenal ulcer, or any significant benefit in the prevention of rebleeding after initial cessation (23.5% rebleeding with cimetidine vs. 26% with placebo). The negative results of this intravenous use of cimetidine were confirmed by a similar European study of 213 patients [46]. In this study, no significant reduction in transfusion requirements, cessation of hemorrhage, length of hospital stay, or mortality rates was found in the cimetidine group. A previous study using oral cimetidine found no significant efficacy over placebo in the cessation of bleeding [47]. Rebleeding incidences, in this study, were 21.5% in the cimetidine group versus 24% in the patients receiving placebo. There also was no difference in surgical need to control hemorrhage. These three studies clearly demonstrate no significant efficacy in the cessation of bleeding or recurrent bleeding whether the cimetidine was given orally or intravenously.

In a study comparing ranitidine to cimetidine in acute bleeding, no difference was seen between the treatment groups related to the number of transfusions, surgery, days in the hospital, or mortality [48]. The data from this study are difficult to interpret, as there was no placebo treatment group, but they do suggest no difference in efficacy between the H$_2$ antagonists. In a study reviewing 27 clinical trials (2670 patients), no significant difference in the cessation of active hemorrhage or recurrent bleeding was found in the H$_2$-antagonist treatment group compared to assigned controls [49]. Thus it appears that the data support the conclusion that H$_2$-antagonist therapy in upper gastrointestinal bleeding is of no benefit in stopping acute bleeding or in preventing rebleeding.

When the authors of this review looked at other parameters in the combined data (mortality rates, the need for surgery, or the specific etiology of bleeding), they did find some significance. Equivocal significance was found for decreasing the need for surgery to control initial hemorrhage in patients treated with H$_2$-antagonist therapy over assigned controls. A significantly reduced mortality rate (30%) was seen with H_2-antagonist therapy. However, in these combined data, slightly over one-third of the deaths reported came from a single center. In this center, a 22% mortality rate occurred in a group of patients who were withdrawn from the study but were included in the combined analysis. If these patients are excluded from the combined analysis, there is no significant difference in mortality rates between H_2-antagonist therapy and placebo controls. When the etiological subgroups were evaluated, there was no difference in the treatment groups in relation to bleeding duodenal ulcers. There was, however, a significant difference found in favor of H_2-antagonist therapy for gastric ulcer hemorrhage with respect to arresting persistent or recurrent bleeding, the need for surgery, and mortality rates. No single study reviewed showed this significance for gastric ulcer hemorrhage. The combined data are difficult to interpret because of the wide differences in assessing efficacy and in selecting patients and the fact that some of the studies collected data retrospectively.

B.   Prostaglandin Analogues

A number of clinical trials have been completed or are presently ongoing to define a possible therapeutic role for prostaglandin analogues in upper gastrointestinal bleeding. These analogues have the dual properties of being antisecretory and capable of increasing mucosal defensive mechanisms. This combination of properties has led to them being enthusiastically tried in this difficult clinical situation. These trials were initiated after the publication of isolated case reports implying the benefit of the prostaglandin analogues in controlling hemorrhage from gastritis or refractory stress ulcer hemorrhage [50–52].

In a multicenter placebo-controlled trial of $15(R)$-15-methyl PGE_2 for upper gastrointestinal bleeding (erosive and ulcerative lesions), no significant difference was found in cessation of bleeding (PGE_2 78% vs. 68%), prevention of recurrent bleeding (PGE_2 17% vs. 23%), or need for surgery (PGE_2 10% vs. 11%) [53]. In this study, no significant difference was found either in the specific etiologies of the bleeding episode, but there was a trend toward cessation of bleeding from duodenal ulcers. In another trial using the PGE_1 analogue, misoprostol versus antacid in nonvariceal hemorrhage, no difference was found in cessation of bleeding in the misoprostol group (83%) compared with antacid (83%) [54]. In a multicenter study comparing misoprostol with placebo in acute upper gastrointestinal bleeding, cessation of bleeding was found in 91.9% of the misoprostol group versus 88.6% in the placebo controls [55]. No difference was found in the cessation of duodenal or gastric ulcer hemorrhage between the two groups, but it took slightly over twice as long for the duodenal ulcers to stop bleeding as for the gastric ulcers. A companion study showed no significant difference between misoprostol and placebo in preventing recurrent bleeding during a 7-day observation period (81.2% vs. 83.1%, respectively) [56]. No difference was seen with either duodenal or gastric ulcers in this study or if a visible vessel was found in the ulcer base during the initial bleeding episode. Additional trials are presently ongoing with different analogues.

C.   Somatostatin

The use of somatostatin in acute upper gastrointestinal hemorrhage is attractive because of its ability to decrease acid secretion, increase gastric mucus, reduce serum gastrin, and decrease splanchnic blood flow. In an early small trial of somatostatin versus cimetidine in controlling ulcer hemorrhage, somatostatin was more efficacious in controlling severe, persistent hemorrhage, but no difference was found between the two groups in the initial cessation of bleeding, transfusion requirements, or mortality rates [57]. Since this early encouraging report on the potential benefits of somatostatin in controlling hemorrhage, a number of clinical trials have been reported that claim significantly successful cessation of hemorrhage by somatostatin compared to placebo or H_2 antagonist [58–61]. Other studies have claimed that somatostatin was not significantly better than either an H_2 antagonist or placebo [62–65]. These data are difficult to interpret because of the wide variability in patient selection as well as the different efficacy criteria used in the studies. Another problem is the small patient accrual in most of these series. The larger multicenter trials have not shown any significant differences when somatostatin was compared to placebo. In a series of 630 patients, there was no difference in cessation of bleeding, rebleeding incidences, need for surgery, or mortality rates (64]. This study, however, had a limited number of patients with mucosal erosive disease. In a recent multicenter trial involving 273 patients, somatostatin therapy resulted in no significant difference over placebo in stopping the initial bleeding episode (69.6% vs. 70.6%, respectively) or in preventing rebleeding (18.2% vs. 11.9%, respectively) [65]. Nor was any difference found in duodenal or gastric ulcer hemorrhage. There was a difference in cessation of bleeding when there was arterial spurting (somatostatin 53.8%, placebo 23.1%). Additional studies will be necessary to resolve conflicting data on the potential use of somatostatin in the cessation of ulcer hemorrhage.

D.   Tranexamic Acid

Tranexamic acid (an antifibrinolytic agent) is similar in action to aminocaproic acid. In an early study, tranexamic acid was better than placebo in the cessation of all etiologies of upper gastrointestinal hemorrhage [66]. In this study, not only was there poor endoscopic control in assessing the etiology of the hemorrhage but also only 50% of the total study population received blood transfusions. Excluding variceal hemorrhage, in this study, there was a significant decrease in treatment failures (continued bleeding, recurrence, continued transfusions, or surgery) in those patients receiving tranexamic acid (11%) compared with those receiving placebo (27%). In a large study comparing cimetidine, placebo, and tranexamic acid, mortality rates were reduced in those receiving cimetidine (7.7%) or tranexamic acid (6.3%) compared with those on placebo (13.5%) [67]. Specific etiologies were not addressed in relation to the acute bleeding episode, but there were no significant differences in the rebleeding rates of duodenal or gastric ulcers in this study. In a study of gastric or duodenal hemorrhage from "benign" lesions, tranexamic acid was significantly better than placebo in reducing the need for emergency surgery (4.2% vs. 18.3%) [68]. The transfusion requirement in the group treated with tranexamic acid was also significantly lower than for the placebo-treated patients. Additional studies will be necessary before any conclusions can be drawn related to this agent's effectiveness in ulcer hemorrhage.

VII. SUMMARY

Ulcer hemorrhage results from the disruption of the wall of a vessel lying in the ulcer base. From the data presented, we can draw some conclusions about the severity of the bleeding episodes and the reasons for the recurrence of some ulcer hemorrhages. Ulcers that have hemorrhage as a complication can develop acutely (stress, medications, etc.) as superficial ulcers or penetrate deeper into the submucosa and serosa. The depth of penetration of these ulcers seems to dictate the size of the vessel involved in the bleeding event. The smaller vessels are located in the submucosa, and the larger vessels traverse the serosa of the bowel wall. The finding that most ulcers are superficial or only penetrate into the submucosa may explain why most ulcers do not bleed, or bleed subclinically, and why, if clinical hemorrhage is apparent, the bleeding is usually minor and self-limiting (80% of ulcer hemorrhages cease spontaneously).

If logic prevails with respect to ulcer hemorrhage, then one can assume that most ulcers are superficial or penetrate only to the submucosa with a low incidence of bleeding. This conclusion appears sound on the basis of pathological findings in resected specimens containing ulcers in which bleeding continued or recurred and required surgical intervention. These ulcers were usually large, penetrated to the serosa, and involved the larger vessels. Such large ulcers frequently have a "visible" vessel exposed in a hostile environment of acid and pepsin, which may interfere with normal hemostatic mechanisms and lead to continued bleeding or rebleeding.

On reviewing the pathology of the bleeding ulcer, it is not surprising that pharmacological treatment trials, using agents that are predominantly antisecretory, have been disappointing when directed at the cessation of significant ulcer hemorrhage. It is also difficult to interpret the data from a number of these trials, as frequently no placebo control group was included, patient selection criteria vary, and the ulcer hemorrhage may have been either just oozing or arterial spurting. These agents do not address the pathological events leading to clinically significant hemorrhage. They may address the suppression of acid, which may help in clot formation, but obviously this benefit is of no significance with larger vessel hemorrhage or the prevention of rebleeding from these vessels. Trials of agents that predominantly stimulate or maintain mucosal defensive mechanisms have demonstrated similar negative results.

On the basis of existing data, it appears fruitless to begin newer trials with similar agents. We have been looking for a magic pharmacological "bullet" without success. Perhaps we should not give up, but newer pharmacological trials seem justified only if the active agent selected has some effect on the bleeding vessel and its rebleeding potential after initial control is established. As mentioned above, certain patient characteristics have been identified that are associated with higher mortality rates, transfusion requirements, and surgical need. These will obviously also have to be considered in the design of newer trials as well as in the interpretation of the results of these trials.

Pharmacological trials will need to demonstrate cost effectiveness over existing radiological, surgical, or endoscopic modalities. Endoscopic techniques in the control of ulcer hemorrhage are developing rapidly and are proving to be efficacious. These techniques, as well as selective radiological procedures, directly address the eroded vessel. The results of these endoscopic techniques are discussed in Chapter 16.

REFERENCES

1. Silverstein FE, Gilbert DA, Tedesco FJ, et al. The national ASGE survey on upper gastrointestinal bleeding. II. Clinical prognostic factors. Gastrointest Endosc 1981; 27:80–93.
2. Allan RN. History, epidemiology and mortality. In: Dykes PW, Keighley MRB, eds. Gastrointestinal haemorrhage. Bristol: Wright PSG, 1981:3–20.
3. Gilbert DA, Silverstein FE, Tedesco FJ, et al. The national ASGE survey on upper gastrointestinal bleeding. III. Endoscopy in upper gastrointestinal bleeding. Gastrointest Endosc 1981; 27:94–102.
4. Palmer ED. The vigorous diagnostic approach to upper gastrointestinal tract hemorrhage. JAMA 1969; 207:1477.
5. Cotton PB, Rosenberg MT, Waldram RP, et al. Early endoscopy of oesophagus, stomach and duodenal bulb in patients with haematemesis and melaena. Br Med J 1973; 2:505.
6. Graham DY, Davis RE. Acute upper gastrointestinal hemorrhage: new observations on an old problem. Am J Dig Dis 1978; 23:76–84.
7. Schiller KFR, Truelove SC, Williams DG. Hematemesis and melena with special reference to factors influencing the outcome. Br Med J 1970; 12:7.
8. Allan R, Dykes P. A study of the factors influencing mortality rates from gastrointestinal hemorrhage. Q J Med 1976; 180:533.
9. Chalmers TC, Zamcheck N, Curtens GW. Fatal gastrointestinal hemorrhage. Clinicopathological correlations in 101 patients. Am J Clin Pathol 1953; 22:634–45.
10. Osborn GR. The pathology of gastric arteries with special reference to fatal haemorrhage from peptic ulcer. Br J Surg 1954; 41:585–94.
11. Swain CP, Storey DW, Bown SG, et al. Nature of the bleeding vessel in recurrently bleeding gastric ulcers. Gastroenterology 1986; 90:595–608.
12. Griffiths WJ, Neumann DA, Welsch JD. The visible vessel as indicator of uncontrolled or recurrent gastrointestinal haemorrhage. N Engl J Med 1979; 300:1173–7.
13. Storey DW, Bown SG, Swain CP, et al. Endoscopic prediction of recurrent bleeding in peptic ulcers. N Engl J Med 1981; 305:915–6.
14. Vallon AG, Cotton PB, Laurence BH, et al. Randomised trial of endoscopic argon laser photocoagulation in bleeding peptic ulcer. Gut 1981; 22:228–33.

15. Macleod IA, Mills PR. Factors identifying the probability of further hemorrhage after acute upper gastrointestinal haemorrhage. Br J Surg 1982; 69:256–8.

16. Wara P. Endoscopic prediction of major rebleeding—a prospective study of stigmata of haemorrhage in bleeding ulcer. Gastroenterology 1985; 88:1209–14.

17. Hurst AF, Stewart MJ. Gastric and duodenal ulcer. London: Oxford Medical Publications, University Press, 1929.

18. Anderson WAD. Pathology. London: Henry Kempton, 1948.

19. Green FW, Kaplan MM, Curtis LE, et al. Effect of acid and pepsin on blood coagulation and platelet aggregation. Gastroenterology 1978; 74:38–43.

20. Northfield TC. Factors predisposing to recurrent haemorrhage after acute gastrointestinal bleeding. Br Med J 1971; 1:26–8.

21. Michels NA. Blood supply and anatomy of upper abdominal organs. Philadelphia: Lippincott, 1955.

22. Martin DF, Montgomery E, Dobek AS, et al. *Campylobacter pylori,* NSAIDs and smoking: risk factors for peptic ulcer disease. Am J Gastroenterol 1989; 84:1268–72.

23. Ivey KJ. Acute hemorrhagic gastritis: modern concepts based on pathogenesis. Gut 1971; 12:750–4.

24. Alvarez AS, Summerskill WHJ. Gastrointestinal haemorrhage and salicylates. Lancet 1958; ii:920–5.

25. Dagradi AE, Lee ER, Bosco DI, et al. The clinical spectrum of hemorrhagic erosive gastritis. Am J Gastroenterol 1973; 60:30–46.

26. Langman MJS, Coggon D, Spielgelhalter D. Analgesic intake and the risk of acute upper gastrointestinal bleeding. Am J Med 1983; 74:79–82.

27. Graham DY, Smith JL. Effects of aspirin and an aspirin-acetaminophen combination on the gastric mucosa in normal subjects. Gastroenterology 1985; 88:1922–5.

28. Silvosa G, Ivey K, Butt J, et al. Incidence of gastric lesions in patients with rheumatic disease on chronic aspirin therapy. Ann Intern Med 1979; 91:517–20.

29. Cameron AS. Aspirin and gastric ulcer. Mayo Clin Proc 1975; 50:565–70.

30. Levy M. Aspirin use in patients with major upper gastrointestinal bleeding and peptic ulcer disease. N Engl J Med 1974; 290:1158–62.

31. Miller R, Jick H. Acute toxicity of aspirin in hospitalized medical patients. Am J Med Sci 1977; 274:271–9.

32. McCarthy DM. Nonsteroidal anti-inflammatory drug-induced ulcers: management by traditional therapies. Gastroenterology 1989; 96:662–74.

33. Mellen H, Stave R, Myren J, et al. Symptoms in patients with peptic ulcer and hematemesis and/or melena related to the use of non-steroid anti-inflammatory drugs. Scand J Gastro 1985; 20:1246–8.

34. Armstron CP, Blower AL. Non-steroidal anti-inflammatory drugs and life-threatening complications of peptic ulceration. Gut 1987; 28:527–32.

35. Matthewson K, Pugh S, Northfield TC. Which peptic ulcer patients bleed? Gut 1988; 29:70–4.

36. Somerville K, Faulkner G, Langman M. Non-steroidal anti-inflammatory drugs and bleeding peptic ulcer. Lancet 1986; i:462–4.

37. Carson JL, Strom BL, Soper KA, et al. The association of non-steroid anti-inflammatory drugs with upper gastrointestinal tract bleeding. Arch Intern Med 1987; 147:85–8.

38. Walt R, Katschinski B, Logan R, et al. Rising frequency of ulcer perforation in elderly people in the United Kingdom. Lancet 1986; i:489–92.

39. Sonnenberg A, Fritsch A. Changing mortality of ulcer disease in Germany. Gastroenterology 1983; 84:1553–7.

40. Himal HS, Watson WW, Jones CW, et al. The management of upper gastrointestinal hemorrhage: a multiparametric computer analysis. Ann Surg 1977; 185:367.

41. Thorne FL, Nyhus LM. Treatment of upper gastrointestinal hemorrhage: a ten-year review. Am Surg 1965; 31:413.

42. Dronfield MW, Atkinson M, Langman MJS. Effect of different operation policies on mortality from bleeding peptic ulcer. Lancet 1979; i:1126.

43. Morgan AG, McAdam WAF, Walmsley GL, et al. Clinical findings, early endoscopy and multivariate analysis in patients bleeding from the upper gastrointestinal tract. Br Med J 1977; 12:237.

44. Bardhan KD, Cust G, Hinchliffe RF, et al. Changing pattern of admissions and operations for duodenal ulcer. Br J Surg 1989; 76(3):230–6.

45. Zuckerman G, Welch R, Douglas A. Controlled trial of medical therapy for active gastrointestinal bleeding and prevention of rebleeding. Am J Med 1984; 75:361–6.

46. McColl KE, MacKay C, Murray GD, et al. A double-blind randomized trial of cimetidine in acute upper gastrointestinal bleeding. Scand J Gastroenterol 1984; 19:885–8.

47. Lebrooy SJ, Misiewicz JJ, Edwards J, et al. Controlled trial of cimetidine in upper gastrointestinal hemorrhage. Gut 1979; 20:892–5.

48. Thomson ABR, Maquire T, Wensel RH, et al. Ranitidine versus cimetidine in the management of acute upper gastrointestinal tract bleeding. J Clin Gastroenterol 1984; 6:295–9.

49. Collins R, Langman M. Treatment with histamine H_2 antagonists in acute upper gastrointestinal hemorrhage. N Engl J Med 1985; 313:660–6.

50. Neil G, Jeejeebhowy KN. Successful treatment of hemorrhagic gastritis with misoprostol. Gastroenterology 1986; 90:1357.

51. Weiss J, Peskin G, Isenberg J. Treatment of hemorrhagic gastritis with 15(R)-15 methyl prostaglandin E_2: report of a case. Gastroenterology 1982; 82:558–60.

52. Groeger J, Dazza S, Carlon G, et al. Prostaglandin therapy in a case of refractory stress ulcer bleeding. Crit Care Med 1982; 10:486–7.

53. Raskin J, Camara D, Levine B, et al. Effect of 15(R)-15-methyl prostaglandin E_2 on acute upper gastrointestinal hemorrhage. Gastroenterology 1985; 88:1550.

54. Bright-Asare P, Giannikipoulos I, Blackstone M, et al. Double-blind controlled pilot trial of misoprostol (Cytotec) compared with antacids in subjects with acute UGI bleeding. Gastroenterology 1986; 90:1357.

55. Personal communication. Data on file: G.D. Searle and Company. Skokie, Ill.

56. Personal communication. Data on file: G.D. Searle and Company. Skokie, Ill.

57. Kayasseh L, Keller U, Gyr K. Somatostatin and cimetidine in peptic ulcer hemorrhage. Lancet 1980; i:844.

58. Coraggio F, Scarpati O, Spina M, et al. Somatostatin and ranitidine in the control of iatrogenic hemorrhage of the upper GI tract. Br Med J 1984; 289:224.

59. Magnusson I, Ihre T, Johansson C, et al. Randomized double blind trial of somatostatin in the treatment of massive upper GI hemorrhage. Gut 1985; 26:221–6.

60. Basile M, Celi S, Parisi A, et al. Somatostatin in the treatment of severe gastrointestinal bleeding from peptic origin. A multicentric controlled trial. Ital J Surg Sci 1984; 1:31–5.

61. Torres AJ, Landa I, Hernandez F, et al. Somatostatin in the treatment of severe upper gastrointestinal bleeding: a multicentre controlled trial. Br J Surg 1986; 73:786–9.
62. Galmiche JP, Cassigneul J, Faivre J, et al. Somatostatin in peptic ulcer bleeding—results of a double-blind controlled trial. Int J Clin Pharmacol Res 1983; 5:379–87.
63. Basso N, Bagarani M, Bracci F, et al. Ranitidine and somatostatin. Their effects on bleeding from the upper gastrointestinal tract. Arch Surg 1986; 121:833–5.
64. Somerville KW, Henry DA, Davies JG, et al. Somatostatin in treatment of haematemesis and melaena. Lancet 1985; i:130–2.
65. Christiansen J, Ottenjann R, von Arx F, et al. Placebo-controlled trial with the somatostatin analogue SMS 201-995 in peptic ulcer bleeding. Gastroenterology 1989; 97:568–74.
66. Cormack F, Jouhar AJ, Chakrabarti RR, et al. Tranexamic acid in upper gastrointestinal haemorrhage. Lancet 1973; i:1207–8.
67. Barer D, Ogilvie A, Henry D, et al. Cimetidine and tranexamic acid in the treatment of acute upper gastrointestinal tract bleeding. N Engl J Med 1983; 308:1571–5.
68. von Holstein CC, Eriksson SB, Källén R. Tranexamic acid in gastric and duodenal bleeding. Scand J Gastroenterol 1987; 137:71–4.

THERAPIES

8

Antacid Therapy of Ulcer Disease

FRED HALTER
University Hospital, Inselspital, Bern, Switzerland

SHIU-KUM LAM
University of Hong Kong Queen Mary Hospital,
Hong Kong

I. INTRODUCTION

The introduction of the histamine H_2-receptor antagonist has revolutionized peptic ulcer therapy, and the efficacy and acceptability of both new and old ulcer drugs are now critically compared with this "gold standard." Antacid therapy has successfully withstood this test with respect to healing for both duodenal and gastric ulcers (Tables 1 and 2).

Efficacy during short-term treatment, albeit of prime importance, is only one of the many criteria that have to be fulfilled to allow any drug to find or maintain its place in modern ulcer therapy. To be acceptable to both the physician and the patient, a lack of significant subjective and objective side effects and a dose regimen favoring compliance are of utmost importance. A solid knowledge of the mechanisms of action make a preparation better acceptable to the physician, although this is not the major concern of the patient as long as the preparations relieve his or her symptoms without unwanted secondary effects. Not enough consideration is generally given to the cost of the treatment, but this is of particular importance in a condition that is characterized by a benign course and a high spontaneous remission rate. Of particular interest in the validation of any ulcer drug is the degree to which it influences the subsequent relapse rate. This review comprehensively discusses these points with regard to the question of whether antacids have a place in modern ulcer therapy.

Table 1 Antacid Trials in Duodenal Ulcer

Study	Antacid form	Daily dose	Daily neutralizing capacity (mmol)	Treatment duration (wk)	Antacid			Placebo			H_2 Antagonists			P Value
					n	Healed	%	n	Healed	%	n	Healed	%	
Peterson et al. [1]	Liquid	15 mL 5×	1008	4	36	28	78	38	17	45	—	—	—	0.005
Lam et al. [2]	Tablet	2 tab 7×	175	4	26	20	77	24	8	33	—	—	—	0.005
Berstad et al. [3]	Tablet	2 tab 7×	280	4	37	81	38	38	9	24	—	—	—	0.001
Kumar et al. [4]	Liquid	7.5 mL 6×	103	4	26	12	46	—	—	—	—	—	—	NS
		15 mL 6×	206	4	27	23	85	24	7	29	—	—	—	0.001
		30 mL 6×	412	4	24	21	87	—	—	—	—	—	—	0.001
Faizallah et al. [5]	Liquid	30 mL 7×	1050	4	19	6	32	15	2	13	—	—	—	0.05
		10 mL as needed	107	4	18	12	67	17	6	35	—	—	—	0.05
Weberg et al. [6]	Tablet	1 tab 4×	120	4	38	28	74	38	11	29	—	—	—	0.001
Ippoliti et al. [7]	Liquid	30 mL 7×	861	4	32	19	59	—	—	—	33	21	64	NS
Fedeli et al. [8]	Liquid	30 mL 7×	560	4	24	18	75	—	—	—	27	21	78	NS
Lauritsen et al. [9]	Liquid	10 mL 7×	600	4	25	21	84	—	—	—	28	25	89	NS
Lux et al. [10]	Liquid	10 mL 4×	280	4	86	69	80	—	—	—	85	63	75	NS
Bianchi Porro et al. [11]	Liquid	15 mL 5×	Unknown	4	39	28	72	—	—	—	39	26	67	NS
Becker et al. [13]	Liquid	10 mL 7×	595	4	34	28	83	—	—	—	33	23	69	NS
Weberg et al. [14]	Tablet	1 tab 4×	120	4	76	54	71	—	—	—	74	58	78	NS
Totals					567	468	69	194	60	30	319	237	74	NS

Table 2 Antacid Trials for Gastric Ulcer

Study	Antacid form	Daily dose	Daily neutralizing capacity (mmol)	Treatment duration (wk)	Antacid			Placebo			H_2 Antagonists			P Value
					n	Healed	%	n	Healed	%	n	Healed	%	
Hollander and Harlan [15]	Tablet	2 tab/hr awake	"Good"	4	8	8	100	8	4	50	—	—	—	0.04
Rydning et al. [16]	Tablet	1 tab 4×	12	6	42	28	67	44	11	25	—	—	—	0.001
Isenberg et al. [17]	Liquid	15 mL 4×	320	8	33	23	70	33	19	58	36	31	86	NS
Pace et al. [18]	Liquid	12 mL 6×	120	8	65	49	76	—	—	—	60	53	89	NS

II. MODE OF ACTION

Antacids, particularly in the form of calcium carbonate originating from limestone and coral, have been used for relief from symptoms of dyspepsia since ancient times, long before scientific investigations into the principle of action. The use of antacids for peptic ulcer, aimed at neutralizing gastric acid, began in America with the work of Bertram Sippy in 1915 [19] following the pronouncement by Schwartz in 1910 of his famous dictum "no acid no ulcer" [20].

Over the years, several additional modes of action were elaborated. Since pepsin is not active at high pH levels, antacids also reduce peptic activity. In addition, antacids are inclined to absorb pepsin and to inactivate bile acids. More recently, their possible action by the principle of cytoprotection has gained considerable interest.

A. Acid Neutralization

1. In Vitro Reactivity

The most frequently used components of antacids and their principal reactions with acid are illustrated by the following equations:

$$NaHCO_3 + \quad HCl \rightarrow \quad NaCl + H_2O + CO_2$$
$$Mg(OH_2) + 2\,HCl \rightarrow MgCl_2 + 2\,H_2O$$
$$Al(OH_3) + 3\,HCl \rightarrow \quad AlCl_3 + 3\,H_2O$$
$$CaCO_3 + 2\,HCl \rightarrow \quad CaCl_2 + H_2O + CO_2$$

Because of its too rapid reaction with acid and the tendency to induce metabolic alkalosis, sodium bicarbonate is rarely used in modern antacids, except in small quantities in the form of baking soda in effervescent antacid tablets. Calcium carbonate has also come into disrepute; many arguments against it, especially with respect to the so-called acid rebound, are only partially substantiated [21]. Today magnesium hydroxide and/or aluminum hydroxide are the basis of most antacid preparations.

Theoretically, the acid-neutralizing capacity of magnesium hydroxide or aluminum hydroxide can be calculated from its in vitro composition, but such calculations tend to overestimate the potency of individual preparations because the solubility and reactivity of these hydroxides vary according to the method used in manufacturing the antacid [22]. In addition, the reactivity of these cation-based antacids is considerably more complex than the above equations might indicate, because they can react reversibly with acid at physiological pH. With magnesium hydroxide, a significant hydrolysis reaction can occur, leading to the production of 1 mole of acid per mole of divalent magnesium. This reaction leads to the formation of magnesium mono-hydroxide, dimagnesium hydroxide, and tetramagnesium complexes. For magnesium, this reaction is only of theoretical importance because it occurs only at pH $>$ 8.5. However, for aluminum hydroxide, it is of considerable relevance because it occurs at a pK_a of 4.98. During this hydrolysis reaction, large octahedral macromolecules form. Several anions present in food can stabilize these aluminum hydroxide aggregates, and the complexes react only slowly with acid. This lag phase is theoretically beneficial for therapeutic application of antacids, because it allows aluminum hydroxide to react with newly formed intragastric acid in a protracted manner.

2. In Vivo Reactivity

Pioneer studies of Fordtran and coworkers [23–25] revealed that large volumes of liquid antacids are necessary to substantially neutralize intragastric acidity. These studies led to the recommendation that the standard antacid regimen should consist of application of 30 mL of a liquid magnesium/aluminum hydroxide preparation 1 and 3 hr after a meal. Postprandial medication was favored because antacids leave the empty stomach very rapidly. The therapeutic efficacy of the Fordtran antacid regimen was verified in the first controlled antacid trial in duodenal ulcer disease performed by Peterson et al. [1]. In this study a total of 210 mL of a liquid magnesium/aluminum hydroxide preparation (30 mL 1 and 3 hr after each meal and an additional dose at bedtime) led to significantly more rapid healing than placebo treatment. In this and in most subsequent ulcer trials, the so-called Fordtran in vitro test [23] was used to convert the volume of antacid used into millimoles of total neutralizing capacity (see also Tables 1 and 2). This method determines the neutralizing capacity in aqueous solutions by measuring the amount of 0.1 M HCl necessary to maintain the pH of 1 mL of a liquid antacid constant at a preset level of 3. Such studies have produced lists of the potency of various preparations [25].

Results of acid secretory studies with prolonged measurements of intragastric pH and experience from controlled ulcer trials suggest that the Fordtran test only partly allows prediction of the ulcer-healing potential of an antacid dose. It is now well established that even with the aggressive antacid regimen used in the Peterson study, intragastric acidity cannot be reduced to the same degree as with a histamine H_2 antagonist [26–29]. The main reason for the limited in vivo reactivity is interaction of food contents and transpyloric loss of antacid (Table 2) [22,26,30]. This in turn decreases the rate at which antacids interact with acid, leading to a substantial transpyloric loss of unutilized antacid. Indeed, antacids can more effectively neutralize a high intragastric acid load in the absence of food [29], but only for a limited time owing to the rapid gastric emptying (Fig. 1). Similarly, antacids exert their neutralizing capacity better in the presence of greater postprandial acid production [31]. Antacid studies in normal subjects may therefore underestimate the neutralizing capacity of antacids. The limitations of acid neutralization by antacids is, however, most obvious from intragastric pH measurements where antacid reactivity was studied during the night period. After midnight, intragastric pH was similar or, in two studies, even lower than in placebo-treated subjects when the last dose was administered 3 hr after the evening meal. The latter observation leads to the suspicion that antacids induce an acid rebound in the early morning hours (Blum [32]; Merki,

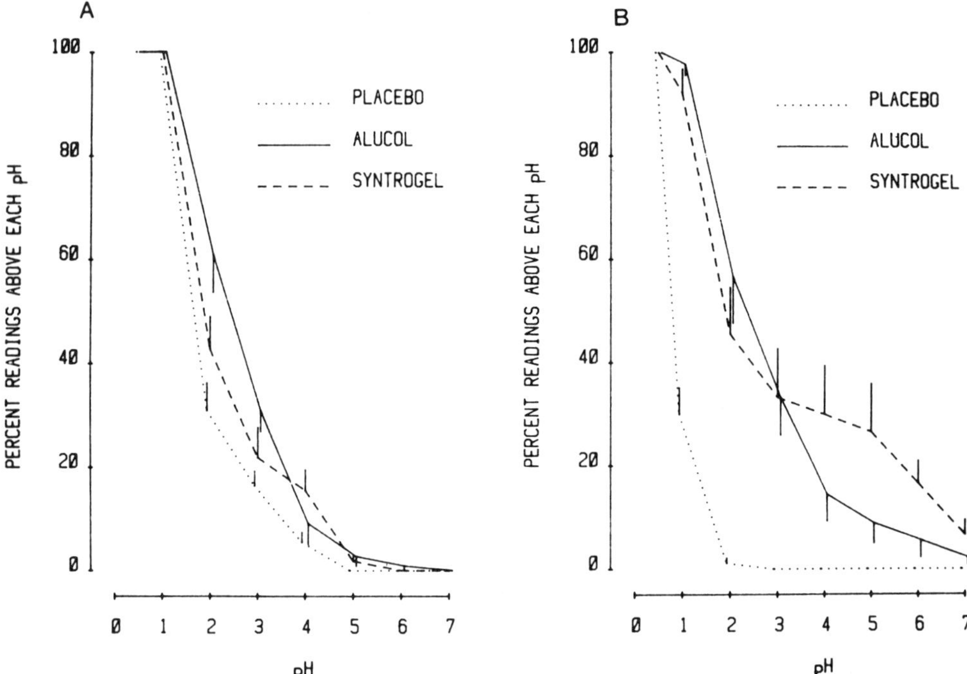

FIGURE 1   Effects of Alucol and Syntrogel Plus on intragastric pH values during stimulation of acid secretion with food on the H_2 antagonist impromidine. For the pH range 1–7, the mean percent readings ±SEM above each pH are recorded throughout (a) the 12-hr food study and (b) the 4-hr impromidine study. Per milliliter, liquid solution Alucol contains 75 mg of aluminum hydroxide and 35 mg of magnesium hydroxide, and Syntrogel Plus contains 44 mg of a codried gel of aluminum hydroxide and magnesium carbonate, 20 mg of magnesium hydroxide, and 40 mg of calcium carbonate. The neutralizing capacity of Alucol is 3.9 mEq/mL, and that of Syntrogel Plus, 1.6 mEq/mL, when tested in vitro in aqueous solution at pH 3.5. (From Berchtold et al. [29].)

unpublished observation). Consequently, antacids did not fit into the model of Hunt et al. [33], where a direct correlation was found for duodenal ulcer disease healing rates and the decrease in nocturnal acid inhibition.

Despite the obvious limitations in intragastric acid neutralization, antacids undoubtedly accelerate ulcer healing, even with doses that in vitro exert a neutralization capacity approximately 10 times smaller than that used in the Peterson study (Tables 1 and 2). These observations cast doubts on whether acid neutralization is the prime mechanism through which antacids heal ulcers. Unfortunately, in none of these recent therapeutic studies was the in vivo neutralizing capacity of the antacid measured. We also do not know to what extent intragastric pH has to be elevated to induce healing. It is likely, however, that the long-held theory that to induce peptic ulcer healing pH must be elevated above the pH level that guarantees pepsin inactivation (pH 3.5) is incorrect. Cimetidine, for example, elevates median 24-hr pH values only from 1.4 to 1.7 [34], and during treatment with muscarinic antagonists, intragastric pH is only marginally elevated [35], but healing of duodenal ulcers can be achieved in the majority of patients with either of these two drugs, and we generally agree that they heal ulcers solely by interference with acid. One has also to consider that pH-metry studies give no indication of the volume of gastric contents and their discharge rate into the duodenum. Both factors could additively contribute to an underestimation of the reduction of the duodenal acid load.

Even if antacids are not capable of greatly changing the intragastric acid milieu, their propensity to block spikes of acid excess or, in other words, to stabilize the pH of the intragastric milieu near the range of the secretion of healthy subjects, may be sufficient to trigger the healing mechanism.

B.   Bile Acid Binding

It is well established that antacids can bind conjugated bile, and it has been speculated that antacids heal peptic ulcers by inactivating the noxious effects of bile acids on the gastric mucosa [36]. The attraction of this theory is diminished by the fact that it is likely that duodenogastric reflux is a normal phenomenon that is not increased in peptic ulcer disease [37]. Furthermore, no studies are available to suggest that peptic ulcer healing can be enhanced solely by bile acid binding.

C. Cytoprotection

Prostaglandins have been shown to reduce the damage to the gastric mucosa induced by various noxious agents, such as concentrated ethanol, and this phenomenon has been named *cytoprotection* [38]. The term is misleading, because application of prostaglandins prior to exposure of the gastric mucosa to noxious agents cannot prevent the destruction of the superficial epithelial cells; however, it can reduce or eliminate the areas of necrotic lesions by minimizing deep mucosal congestion [39,40]. Because it has been claimed that prostaglandins are cytoprotective to the gastric mucosa, the term *cytoprotective* has been applied to many drugs, often in an uncritical manner. One has to consider that cytoprotection is much better established in experimental animals than in humans and that any result obtained in animals needs confirmation in humans, especially with regard to the application of "cytoprotection" to peptic ulcer healing. However, in recent years, some interesting data have been accumulated that suggest that it is reasonable to consider that cytoprotection could be one of the ways in which antacids increase the resistance of the gastric mucosa.

1. Studies in Experimental Animals

Szelenyi and his group [41–43] were the first to establish that in the rat intragastric instillation of large amounts of Al(OH)$_3$ induces a release of prostaglandins into the gastric juice for more than 24 hr. Such an effect could not be induced by Mg(OH)$_2$, CaCO$_3$, Al$_2$O$_3$, or AlCl$_3$.

Several groups have shown that Al(OH)$_3$, Al$_2$(SO$_4$)$_3$, and AlPO$_4$ can protect the gastric mucosa against noxious effects induced by absolute ethanol in a dose-dependent manner similar to sucralfate [41–46]. It is possible that aluminum crystals induce superficial damage of the gastric mucosa as observed in histological studies by Tarnawski et al. [47], which may be responsible for antacid-induced prostaglandin release. It can thus not be excluded that the prostaglandin release represents a consequence of gastric mucosal damage.

Studies by Domschke et al. [46] revealed that cytoprotective effects of antacids in experimental animals are mainly confined to the gastric glands, while the damage to the surface epithelium is not significantly lessened. Accordingly, integrity parameters of the superficial epithelial layer (potential difference, mucus secretion, cell desquamation) do not indicate protective action of antacids against damage by necrotizing agents. In contrast, significantly diminished microbleeding rates suggest that protection by antacids works at a deeper level within the mucosa. These actions of antacids very closely resemble those of protective prostaglandins. Antacids also significantly diminish the rate of gastric microbleeding induced by aspirin. It is therefore likely that antacids may additionally or alternatively act through factors other than prostaglandin synthesis within the gastric mucosa. This is also supported by the observation that antacids appear to act in opposite ways with respect to some prostaglandin effects, for example, on gastric mucus secretion [46].

Various animal experiments have thus unanimously shown that the Al(OH)$_3$ components of antacids can induce prostaglandin release in the gastric mucosa.

Of special interest is the recent observation that aluminum-containing antacids retain their cytoprotective activity when made nonbuffering by acidification ex vivo [48]. This observation clearly shows that antacids fulfill the definition of a cytoprotective agent, because they can protect the gastric mucosa in the absence of an antisecretory effect. Indomethacin did not block the protective effect of acidified aluminum, thus suggesting that prostaglandin induction is not involved. It has indeed been shown that antacids can induce cytoprotection by a nonprostaglandin process because the sulfhydryl alkylating agent N-ethylmaleimide can significantly diminish the protection evoked by aluminum hydroxide [49,50].

2. Studies in Humans

Studies performed in humans are very preliminary and have resulted in inconclusive results. While Berstad and Szelenyi (personal communication) could not confirm the data obtained from rat studies in humans, Reimann et al. [51] found that Al(OH)$_3$ but not CaCO$_3$ can stimulate ex vivo prostaglandin synthesis in biopsy samples from the human stomach. This was confirmed by Preclik et al. [52] during prolonged application of Maalox 70, a preparation containing 600 mg of $Mg(OH)_2$ and 900 mg of $Al(OH)_3$ per milliliter of the liquid solution (neutralizing capacity 7.0 mEq/L).

These data do not, however, clarify whether prostaglandin release is involved in ulcer healing or whether it only represents an epiphenomenon. In particular, one has to consider that endogenous prostaglandins do not inhibit acid secretion and that there is no evidence available from the vast literature on the role of synthetic prostaglandin analogues in peptic ulcer healing to demonstrate that prostaglandins heal peptic ulcers in doses that do not inhibit acid secretion [53]. On the other hand, it needs to be pointed out that the cytoprotective effects of prostaglandins, such as enhancement of bicarbonate secretion and mucosal blood flow, are dose-dependent phenomena [17].

The only indirect evidence that mucosal protection might be involved in peptic ulcer healing comes from studies on ulcer healing obtained with sucralfate or colloidal bismuth [54]. It is quite obvious that, at least in the animal model, $Al(OH)_3$ protects the gastric mucosa in a fashion similar to sucralfate, a preparation that also contains negatively charged aluminum, which exerts no influence on gastric acid. It appears, however, that it is the octasulfate and not the aluminum component of sucralfate that protects the acid-exposed esophageal epithelium in the rabbit [55]. Nevertheless, we cannot exclude that antacids heal peptic ulcers through pathways similar to those of sucralfate, such as by coating the ulcer ground, changing mucus viscosity, increasing mucosal bicarbonate secretion, or maintaining gastric blood flow [54]. At present, however, it is still easier to defend the acid-neutralizing hypothesis. It is also not fully excluded that acid neutralization and cytoprotection additively contribute to the phenomenon that even small doses of antacids can heal duodenal ulcers.

III. THERAPEUTIC EFFICACY

A. Duodenal Ulcers

There are now a total of 13 double-blind controlled trials that clearly show that antacids can heal duodenal ulcers either better than placebo or at the same rate as cimetidine (Table 1). In the placebo-controlled trials the mean healing rate was 75% in 4 weeks and 73% in the group where the histamine H_2 antagonist was the standard. The positive healing rate under antacid treatment occurred in doses that range in their in vitro neutralizing capacity (as established in the Fordtran test) between 1008 and 120 mEq. The lowest dose seems to be the optimal dose; symptomatic release was at least as good and was achieved with virtually no side effects.

B. Gastric Ulcers

Evidence in support of antacid efficacy in gastric ulcers is less convincing (Table 2). Of four studies, only three yielded an unequivocally positive result; in the fourth the healing rate was in an intermediate range between that of cimetidine and placebo. This situation much resembles the results with the early trials on the activity of cimetidine in gastric ulcers, where studies with larger groups and of longer duration eventually clearly established the validity of this treatment [56].

C. Combination with Other Anti-Ulcer Drugs

Before cimetidine was introduced, an antacid–anticholinergic combination was the prescriber's favorite, and the basis for the use of this combination was entirely empirical. Only recently has this question been addressed in a scientifically acceptable way, but the few studies are restricted to the treatment of duodenal ulcer disease. Strom et al. [57] did confirm that the combination approach (seven doses of antacid per day with a neutralizing capacity of 600 mmol plus 0.6 mg of L-hyoscyamine twice a day) was superior to placebo and equivalent to cimetidine (1 g/day) in the healing of duodenal ulcer. Such combined treatment seems to prolong the remission rate (see Section III.F).

Liquid antacid 1 and 3 hr after meals and at bedtime plus 300 mg of cimetidine with meals and at bedtime was more effective than cimetidine alone in the reduction of daytime gastric acidity [58]. This observation is probably of more interest in the understanding of the pharmacological control of acid secretion than in its application to clinical practice. Daytime-intensive antacid plus bedtime cimetidine resulted in healing of duodenal ulcer similar to that achieved with mealtime and bedtime cimetidine [59]. In another study, however, ranitidine (150 mg twice daily) appeared better than a combination of antacid (480 mmol/day neutralizing capacity) and anticholinergic drug (glycopyrronicum bromide 2 mg three times daily) in the healing of duodenal ulcer (91% vs. 76% in 4 weeks); follow-up results unfortunately were not reported [60]. Finally, combination with sulpiride (a hypothalamic neuroleptic and dopamine antagonist) did not offer significant additional healing efficacy over antacid alone [2].

Thus, daytime antacid may replace daytime H_2-receptor antagonists, and this may be important in countries where antacids can be obtained cheaply and where cost is a decisive factor in treatment selection. Furthermore, combination with anticholinergics is effective and may lead to longer remission than H_2-receptor antagonists alone.

D. Antacid Treatment and Cigarette Smoking

In most studies cigarette smoking consistently delays duodenal ulcer healing by placebo, and the effect is highly significant when the results are pooled [61]. An adverse effect on duodenal ulcer healing has also been observed in patients treated with antacids, and the effect is also highly significant by meta-analysis (Table 3). In this respect, therefore, antacids behave like other acid-reducing agents such as H_2-receptor antagonists and omeprazole, in which the adverse smoking effect is less

Table 3 Healing Rates of Duodenal Ulcer in Smokers and Nonsmokers
with Antacids

	Smokers		Nonsmokers	
	n	% healed	n	% healed
Peterson et al. [1]	28	75	8	89
Lam et al. [2]	17	59	34	91
Korman et al. [62]	13	39	12	67
Strom et al. [57]	16	100	8	88
Massarat and Eisenmann [63]	56	48	24	75
Totals	130	61	86	83

The studies included are those that reported the actual data in their communications.

consistently seen than with placebo but becomes highly significant when results of various studies are pooled [61].

Only one study has examined the effect of cigarette smoking on gastric ulcer healing by antacids and observed harmful effects [16]. Generally speaking, it appears that smoking does not exert any ill effect on the healing of gastric ulcers by drugs [65]. The effect of smoking on posttreatment relapse and relapse during maintenance treatment with antacids is not known.

E. Ulcer Relapse after Healing by Antacids

The relapse rates following initial healing by carbenoxolone sodium, colloidal bismuth, and sucralfate have been found to be less than those following healing by H_2-receptor antagonists [66–69]. How do antacids behave in this respect? Since aluminum antacids may be cytoprotective, do antacids behave similarly to these other cytoprotective compounds? Or do antacids act more like other acid-reducing agents?

Table 4 shows the results of three available studies that compared the duodenal ulcer relapse rates following initial healing with antacids and with H_2-receptor antagonists. The relapse rates were closely similar. In this respect, it is interesting to note that the relapse rates following initial healing with omeprazole or H_2-receptor antagonists are also closely similar [9,72–74].

Of high interest are two independent observations [57,75] that the time to relapse during the subsequent 12 months follow-up was significantly shorter with cimetidine than with the antacid–anticholinergic combination. Because, as discussed above, antacid alone does not differ from cimetidine in posttreatment relapse (Table 4), it would appear that the use of anticholinergic may contribute to the longer remission.

Table 4 Duodenal Ulcer Relapse Rates Following Initial Healing with Antacids and Histamine H$_2$-Receptor Antagonists

| | Antacids | | | | H$_2$-Receptor antagonists | | | |
| | Relapse rate (%) | | | | Relapse rate (%) | | | |
	n	3 mo	6 mo	12 mo	n	3 mo	6 mo	12 mo
Ippoliti et al. [70]	55	29	56	67	59	36	54	71
Bytzer et al. [71]	35	17	31	57	36	17	31	50
Becker et al. [13]	28	18	36	54	28	18	36	39
Totals	118	77	55	39	123	74	56	41

There were no significant differences in relapse rates between the two groups.

F. Maintenance Treatment with Antacids

Can antacids prevent ulcer recurrence? The answer is yes. Two studies have formally addressed this question in duodenal ulcer disease. In a study by Bianchi Porro [12], antacid tablets, one taken 1 hr after meals and one at bedtime (total neutralizing capacity, 100 mmol/day), were found to be as effective and as safe as cimetidine 400 mg at night as maintenance therapy for healed duodenal ulcer for a period of up to 1 year. In a multicenter study directed by Bardhan [76], which was extended to 1 year, 251 healed duodenal ulcer patients were studied. The antacid used was the aluminum/magnesium hydroxide preparation Maalox in tablets (neutralizing capacity per tablet, 162 mmol). From the 176 patients that could be evaluated, 62 patients were treated with placebo, 65 received three Maalox tablets at bedtime, 60 received three Maalox tablets twice daily, and 64 received cimetidine 400 mg at bedtime. Maalox twice daily and cimetidine at bedtime gave equally positive results, with relapse rates of 23% and 25%, compared to 57% in the placebo group. The benefit was also significant for smokers. Treatment with Maalox at bedtime gave an intermediate result (relapse rate 39%).

Does demand antacid prevent ulcer recurrence? The answer appears to be no. In a 24-month study, taking antacids only for pain relief was inferior to maintenance treatment with ranitidine, cimetidine, or pirencepine for the prevention of duodenal ulcer recurrence [77].

G. Stress Ulcer Prophylaxis

The question of whether antacids play a role in preventing stress ulcer lesions in critically ill patients is still being debated. Their application is logical because several studies suggest that the risk of developing gastroduodenal stress lesions and bleeding correlates positively with the fraction of time that the intragastric pH is below approximately 4 [78–81]. On the other hand, it has been suggested that the pH within the gastric mucosa is considerably more important than the pH of the gastric contents [82]. Positive evidence that high-dose antacid treatment prevents gastric bleeding in critically ill patients was found a decade ago in two studies published by the group of Silen in Boston [80,83]. In these studies, doses of up to 30 mL of a magnesium/aluminum preparation were administered hourly to elevate pH above 3.5.

In a placebo-controlled study on a total of 100 patients, 24.5 out of 49 placebo-treated patients bled, while a hemorrhage occurred in only 3.9% of antacid-treated patients [80]. Similar favorable results for antacid treatment were obtained in a study where 75 critically ill patients were randomized to the antacid regimen described above or to cimetidine 300 mg ever 6 hr [83]. Upper gastrointestinal tract bleeding occurred in 7 of 38 cimetidine-treated patients but in none of 37 subjects treated with antacids. Some of the antacid-treated patients had diarrhea or hypermagnesemia. The efficacy of a similar antacid regimen was, however, not confirmed in a more recent placebo-controlled study by Pinilla et al. [84] despite very high antacid dosing with attempts to keep intragastric pH above 5. In their study the visible bleeding rate was close to 12% in both groups. No patient developed severe hemorrhage in either group.

The considerably better placebo results of the latter study may be explained by either differences in the severity of the underlying disease or optimization of intensive care treatment in the last decade. These differences may also account for the very low complication rate observed in an endoscopy-controlled study at our own laboratories [85]. Only 1 of 33 patients treated with antacid (10 mL of a magnesium/aluminum hydroxide preparation every 4 hr) experienced a hemorrhage, while no significant bleeding occurred in the other 32 patients or in the 34 control patients who received ranitidine, 50 mg intravenously every 8 hr, in addition to the low-dose antacid treatment. The incidence of endoscopically visible stress lesions was similar in the two groups. This study points to the possibility that small-dose antacid treatment may not be less efficacious than a large-dose antacid regimen or profound acid blockade in preventing gastroduodenal stress lesions. This suggestion is indirectly supported by observations made with sucralfate. This aluminum sucrose octasulfate preparation, which is devoid of any important influence on gastric pH, did prevent stress ulcers at least as well as high doses of antacids or histamine H_2 antagonists [84–91]. A similar or even high efficacy was obtained, however, with a lower incidence of side effects. Of special importance is the considerably smaller incidence of nosocomial infections such as pneumonia [87–89]. Because these infections are attributed to increases in gastric pH, and small antacid doses protect the stomach even in the acidified form [48], stress ulcer studies on large patient groups with small antacid doses should be encouraged. In this context, however, attention should be drawn to the fact that all the sucralfate studies are based on small numbers of patients, and that none of these studies has had a placebo group included. It can thus not be fully excluded that all these observations present only a placebo effect. Since placebo-controlled studies in such critically ill patients are ethically questionable, it is likely that the value of antacids or other drugs in this day and age in stress ulcer prophylaxis will never be determined in a scientific way and will continue to be a controversial issue.

IV. SIDE EFFECTS AND INTERACTION WITH OTHER DRUGS

A. Side Effects

1. Magnesium

Diarrhea is the most disturbing side effect of magnesium hydroxide. Since modern antacid preparations usually also contain aluminum hydroxide, changes in bowel habit are less of a problem because the constipating effect of aluminum levels out this side effect of magnesium. Although magnesium hydroxide is generally classified as a systemic antacid, 5–10% of it is absorbed. This can induce life-threatening complications in patients with renal insufficiency, because magnesium absorption is increased in such patients. In addition, nephrolithiasis may rarely occur due to magnesium-induced lowering of the urinary pH [92]. It is unlikely that any of the side effects of magnesium are relevant in short-term low-dose antacid treatment, but caution is mandatory with large doses in patients with renal insufficiency.

2. Aluminum Hydroxide

Aluminum can hyperpolarize smooth muscle cells and reduce contractility of the gut, and this is an important factor in the constipating tendency of this cation [93,94]. A further contributing factor to severe constipation is the tendency of aluminum to form complexes with dietary phosphates. With large-dose treatment this can lead to formation of fecaliths, which can lead to intestinal obstruction and colonic perforation [94]. This phosphate binding effect of aluminum hydroxide is taken advantage of in patients with renal insufficiency to normalize serum phosphates, and intestinal obstruction is less likely to occur in nonuremic patients, where the laxative side effect of magnesium prevents extreme forms of constipation. However, phosphorus depletion may also occur on standard high-dose antacid treatment once urinary daily phosphorus reaches levels below 300 mg/day [95]. This can lead to osteoporosis, osteomalacia, and spontaneous bone fracture. Such changes have not been described during short-term low-dose or high-dose antacid treatment but should be considered during long-term treatment.

A special concern with prolonged aluminum hydroxide treatment is central nervous system damage due to aluminum absorption. Indeed, the dialysis encephalopathy syndrome, including symptoms such as speech disorder, apraxia, myoclonus, and progressive dementia, is considered to be due to aluminum absorption [96]. A large proportion of dialysis patients regularly ingest aluminum hydroxide, but the question is at debate whether aluminum content of the drinking water is the causative factor [97–99] of dialysis encephalopathy. Additionally, aluminum content has been found to be increased in the brain of patients with Alzheimer's disease [100]. In a recent British survey, a direct correlation was found between incidence of Alzheimer's disease and aluminum content of drinking water [101].

Aluminum blood levels increase even in healthy volunteers with medium-dose antacid treatment [102]. Absorption is enhanced when aluminum-containing antacids are ingested with orange juice or citric acid [103]. Aluminum levels were slightly and transiently elevated in one of the two published antacid maintenance studies [76]. Even if no evidence is available today that antacid treatment may induce Alzheimer's disease, the lesson from uremic patients indicates that great caution is warranted in this patient group. Indeed, potential brain toxicity of aluminum is the main reason long-term treatment with antacids is seldom applied outside controlled clinical studies.

B.   Interaction with Drugs

Aluminum hydroxide can adsorb several drugs in addition to bile acids and pepsin, and consequently decrease their bioavailability. This is also influenced by the delivery rate into the small bowel, because aluminum hydroxide delays gastric emptying [104,105]. Changes in gastric and small-bowel pH values may in turn diminish or enhance drug absorption [95]. Drug bioavailability is diminished for tetracyclines, digitalis, chlorpromazine, phenobarbital, carbenoxolon, and cimetidine. Enhanced renal elimination diminishes the bioavailability of salicylates. In contrast, the absorption of sulfonamides and some anticoagulants is enhanced and chinidine bioavailability increases owing to decreased renal elimination. Interaction of antacid with other drugs can be largely neglected when antacids are given no sooner than 1 hr after other medications. Since antacids are commonly administered 1 hr after meals, whereas other drugs are mostly given before meals, antacid interaction with drugs is by and large of importance only in intensive care patients treated with so-called antacid titration.

V.   CONCLUSION

With the development of histamine H_2 antagonists and more recently of omeprazole, the treatment and prophylaxis of peptic ulcer disease has become extremely simple and efficacious. This "gold standard" allows the control of healing of almost any peptic ulcer with a simple one-tablet-a-day regimen. Antacid treatment cannot fully compete with these drugs, especially since no data are available on healing of so-called therapy-resistant ulcers. Another handicap for antacid treatment is the more complicated treatment regimen, although it is now well established that four to six antacid tablets can match the healing rates obtainable with histamine H_2 antagonists and are as efficacious as the earlier high-dose treatment using daily doses of liquid antacid in volumes of up to 240 mL/day. Considerations on the superiority of modern acid blockers do not, however, generally acknowledge the fact that most peptic ulcers respond very well to modern antacid regimens with an application and dosage form that is well accepted by most patients. Since the prices of acid blockers are almost prohibitive in many highly populated countries, the much less expensive antacid treatment still has a huge potential. Since short-term, low-dose treatment is well tolerated, efficacious, and almost devoid of side effects, antacid medication can still be recommended as first choice even to a population who can afford the "gold standard" treatment. The practical and economic potential of antacids can even be expected to widen if preliminary observations are confirmed that antacids in combination with anticholinergics lead to a better quality of healing with lower recurrence rates than are commonly observed with potent acid blockers. More caution with antacids is necessary, however, in both the prevention of stress ulcers and the maintenance treatment of patients with healed ulcers until more data are available on both their efficacy and their safety.

REFERENCES

1. Peterson WL, Sturdevant AL, Frankl HD, Richardson CT, Isenberg JI, Elashoff JD, Stones JQ, Gross RA, McCallum RW, Fordtran JS. Healing of duodenal ulcer with an antacid regimen. N Engl J Med 1977; 297:341–5.
2. Lam SK, Lam KC, Lai CL, Yeung CK, Yam LYC, Wong WS. Treatment of duodenal ulcer with antacid and sulpiride. A double-blind controlled study. Gastroenterology 1979; 76:315–22.
3. Berstad A, Rydning A, Aaland E, Kolstad B, Frislid K, Asseth J. Controlled clinical trial of duodenal ulcer healing with antacid tablets. Scand J Gastroenterol 1982; 17:953–9.
4. Kumar N, Vij JC, Karol A, Anand BS. Controlled therapeutic trial to determine the optimum dose of antacids in duodenal ulcer. Gut 1984; 25:1199.
5. Faizallah R, De Haan HA, Krasner N, Walker RJ, Morris AI, Calam MJ, Budgett DA. Is there a place in the United Kingdom for intensive antacid treatment for chronic peptic ulceration? Br Med J 1984; 289:869–71.
6. Weberg R, Berstad A, Lange O, Schulz T, Aubert E. Duodenal ulcer healing with four antacid tablets daily. Scand J Gastroenterol 1985; 20:1041–5.
7. Ippoliti AF, Sturdevant RAL, Isenberg JI, Wintroub RH. Cimetidine versus intensive antacid therapy for duodenal ulcer. A multicenter trial. Gastroenterology 1978; 74:393–5.
8. Fedeli G, Anti M, Rapaccini GL, De Vitis I, Butti A, Civelo IM. A controlled study comparing cimetidine treatment to an intensive antacid regimen in the therapy of uncomplicated duodenal ulcer. Dig Dis Sci 1979; 24:758–62.
9. Lauritsen K, Bytzer P, Hansen J, Bekker C, Rask-Madsen J. Comparison of ranitidine and high-dose antacid in the treatment of prepyloric or duodenal ulcer. A double-blind controlled trial. Scand J Gastroenterol 1985; 20:123–8.
10. Lux G, Henschel H, Rohner HG, Brunner H, Schütze K, Lederer PC, Rösch W.

Treatment of duodenal ulcer with low-dose antacids. Scand J Gastroenterol 1986; 21:1063–8.

11. Bianchi Porro G, parente F, Lazzaroni M, Baroni S, Panza E. Medium-dose antacids versus cimetidine in the short-term treatment of duodenal ulcer. J Clin Gastroenterol 1986; 8:141–54.

12. Bianchi Porro G, Lazzaroni M, Pace F, Petrillo M. Long-term low dose antacid versus cimetidine therapy in the treatment of duodenal ulcer recurrence. Scand J Gastroenterol 1986; 21:1144–6.

13. Becker U, Lindorff K, Andersen C, Randlov PJ. Antacid treatment of duodenal ulcer. Acta Med Scand 1987; 221:1181–5.

14. Weberg R, Aubert E, Dahlberg O, Dybdahl J, Ellekjaer E, Farup PG, Hovdenak N, Lange O, Melsom M, Stallemo A, Vetvik KR, Berstad A. Low dose antacids or cimetidine for duodenal ulcer? Gastroenterology 1988; 95:1465–9.

15. Hollander D, Harland J. Antacids vs. placebos in peptic ulcer therapy. A controlled double-blind investigation. JAMA 1973; 226:1181–5.

16. Rydning A, Weberg R, Lange O, Berstad A. Healing of benign gastric ulcer with low-dose antacids and fiber diet. Gastroenterology 1986; 91:56–61.

17. Isenberg JI, Hogan DL, Selling JA, Koss MH. Duodenal bicarbonate secretion in humans: role of prostaglandins. Dig Disc Sci 1986; 31(Suppl):919–15.

18. Pace F, Broker HJ, Caspary W, Feuerle G, Fimmel CJ, Hackenberg K, Hammer B, Holtermüller KH, Hotz J. Therapy of stomach ulcer with low-dose antacid gel and cimetidine. A multicenter double-blind study. Dtsch Med Wochenschr 1985; 110:283–7.

19. Sippy BW. Gastric and duodenal ulcers, medical cure by efficient removal of gastric juice corrosion. JAMA 1915; 64:1625.

20. Schwarz K. Ueber penetrierende magen- und jejunalgeschwüre. Beitr Klin Chir 1910; 67:95.

21. Texter EC. A critical look at the clinical use of antacids in acid-peptic disease and gastric acid rebound. Am J Gastroenterol 1989; 84:97–108.

22. Carlson GL, Malagelada JR. Chemistry of the antacids: its relevance to antacid therapy. In: Halter F, ed. Antacids in the eighties. Baltimore: Urban & Schwarzenberg, 1982:7–16.

23. Fordtran JS, Collyns JAH. Antacid pharmacology in duodenal ulcer. N Engl J Med 1966; 274:922–7.

24. Fordtran JS. Reduction of acidity by diet, antacids and anticholinergic agents. In: Sleisinger MH, Fordtran JS, eds. Gastrointestinal diseases. Philadelphia: WB Saunders, 1973:718–42.

25. Fordtran JS, Morawski SG, Richardson CT. In vivo and in vitro evaluation of liquid antacids. N Engl J Med 1973; 288:923–8.

26. Halter F, Huber R, Häcki WH, Varga L, Bachmann C. Effect of food on antacid neutralizing capacity in man. Eur J Clin Invest 1982; 12:209–17.

27. Milton-Thompson GJ. Monitoring of 24 hour acid secretion during antacid treatment. In: Halter F, ed. Antacids in the eighties. Baltimore: Urban & Schwarzenberg, 1982:72–5.

28. Bauerfeind P, Cilluffo T, Emde C, Müller-Duysing W, Blum AL. Antacids revisited: how do they interact with food in vivo? Gastroenterology 1984; 90:1340.

29. Berchtold P, Reinhart WH, Niederhäuser U, Koller U, Halter F. In vitro tests overestimate in vivo neutralizing capacity of antacids in presence of food. Dig Dis Sci 1985; 30:522–8.

30. Gibaldi M, Kanic JL, Amsel L. Critical in vitro factors in evaluation of gastric antacids II. J Pharm Sci 1964; 53:1375–7.

31. Schürer-Maly CC, Varga L, Halter F. Influence of circadian rhythm and meal composition on the effect of antacids. Manuscript in preparaton. 1990.

32. Blum AL. Ziele bei der Therapie der Ulkuskrankheit. Schweiz Med Wochenschr 1984; 114:679–82.

33. Hunt R, Howden CW, Jones DB, Burget DW, Kerr GD. The correlation between acid suppression and peptic ulcer healing. Scand J Gastroenterol 1986; 21(Suppl 12):522–9.

34. Walt RP, Gomes MD, Wood EC, Logan LH, Pounder RE. Effect of daily oral omeprazole on 24 hour intragastric activity. Br Med J (Clin Res) 1983; 2(287):12–4.

35. Etienne A, Bron B. The effect of pirencepine on gastric pH: continuous recording for the selection of the optimal therapeutic dose. In: Dotevall G, ed. Advances in gastroenterology with the selective antimuscarinic compound pirenzepine. Princeton: Excerpta Medica 1982:81–2.

36. Clain JE, Malagelada JR, Chadwick VS. Binding properties in vitro of antacids for conjugated bile acids. Gastroenterology 1977; 73:556–9.

37. Müller-Lissner SA, Fimmel CJ, Sonnenberg A, Will N, Müller-Duysing W, Heinzel F, Müller R, Blum AL. Novel approach to quantify duodenogastric reflux in healthy volunteers and in patients with type I gastritis. Gut 1983; 24:510–8.

38. Robert A, Nezamis JE, Lancaster C, Hanchar AJ. Cytoprotection by prostaglandins in rats. Prevention of gastric necrosis produced by alcohol, HCl, NaOH, hypertonic NaCl, and thermal injury. Gastroenterology 1979; 77:433–43.

39. Lacy ER, Ito S. Microscopic analysis of ethanol damage to rat gastric mucosa after treatment with a prostaglandin. Gastroenterology 1982; 83:619–25.

40. Wallace JL, Morris GP, Krousse EJ, Graeves SE. Reduction by cytoprotective agents of ethanol-induced damage to the rat gastric mucosa: a correlated morphological and physiological study. Can J Physiol Pharmacol 1982; 60:1686–99.

41. Szelenyi I, Postius S, Engler H. Evidence for a functional cytoprotective effect produced by antacids in the rat stomach. Eur J Pharmacol 1983; 88:403–6.

42. Szelenyi I, Postius S. Functional cytoprotection by certain antacids and sucralfate in the rat stomach. Gastroenterology 1985; 88:1604.

43. Lanz R, Postius S, Szelenyi I, Brune K. PGE_2 release from cultured macrophages induced by antacids and sucralfate. Gastroenterology 1985; 88:1464.

44. Tarnawski A, Hollander D, Gergely H, Stachura J. Comparison of antacid, sucralfate, cimetidine and ranitidine in protection of the gastric mucosa against ethanol injury. Am J Med 1985; 79(Suppl 2C):19–23.

45. Hollander D, Tarnawski A, Gergely H. Protection against alcohol-induced gastric mucosal injury by aluminum-containing compounds—sucralfate, antacids and aluminum sulphate. Scand J Gastroenterol 1986; 21(Suppl 125):151–3.

46. Domschke W, Hagel J, Ruppin H, Kaduk B. Antacids and gastric mucosal protection. Scand J Gastroenterol 1986; 21(Suppl 125):144–9.

47. Tarnawski A, Hollander D, Cummings D, Krause WJ, Gergely H, Zipser RD. Are antacids acid neutralizers only? Histologic, ultrastructural and functional changes in

normal gastric mucosa induced by antacids. Gastroenterology 1984; 86:1276.

48. DiJoseph JF, Borella LE, Nabimir G. Activated aluminum complex derived from solubilized antacids exhibits enhanced cytoprotective activity in the rat. Gastroenterology 1989; 96:730–5.

49. Szelenyi I, Brune K. Possible role of sulfhydryls in mucosal protection induced by aluminum hydroxide. Dig Dis Sci 1986; 31:1207–10.

50. Dupuy O, Szabo S. Protection by metals against ethanol-induced gastric mucosal injury in the rat: Comparative biochemical and pharmacological studies implicate protein sulfhydryls. Gastroenterology 1986; 91:966–74.

51. Reimann HJ, Schmidt U, Wendt P, Dorsch W, von Sanden H, von der Ohe M, Lewin J, Ultsch B. Die wirkung von antazida auf den gehalt von gewebshistamin und prostaglandinen (PGE$_2$) in der magenmukosa. Fortschr Med 1984; 102:47–50.

52. Preclik EF, Stange G, Gerber K, Tetze H, Horn H, Ditschuneit H. Stimulation of endogenous prostaglandin synthesis by antacids in human gastric and duodenal mucosa. Gastroenterology 1987; 92:2579.

53. Hawkey CJ, Walt RP. Prostaglandins for peptic ulcer, a promise unfulfilled. Lancet 1986; ii:1084–6.

54. Koelz HR. Protective drugs in the treatment of gastroduodenal ulcer disease. Scand J Gastroenterol 1986; 21(Suppl 125):156–63.

55. Orlando RC, Turjman NA, Tobey NA, Schreiner VJ, Powell DW. Mucosal protection by sucralfate and its components in acid-exposed rabbit esophagus. Gastroenterology 1987; 93:352–61.

56. Bauerfeind P, Stalder P, Koelz HR, Blum AL, et al. Peptische Làsìonch: therapeutische fortschritte 1988. Therapiewoche 1988; 38:867–90.

57. Strom M, Gotthard R, Bodemar G, Walan A. Antacid anticholinergic, cimetidine and placebo in the treatment of active peptic ulcers. Scand J Gastroenterol 1981; 16:593–602.

58. Peterson WL, Barnett C, Feldman M, Richardson CT. Reduction of twenty-four hour gastric acidity with combination drug therapy in patients with duodenal ulcer. Gastroenterology 1979; 77:1015–20.

59. Berstad A, Bjerke K, Carlsen E, Aaland E. Treatment of duodenal ulcer with antacids in combination with trimipramine or cimetidine. Scand J Gastroenterol 1980; 15(Suppl): 46–52.

60. Miettinen P, Anttonen V, Aukee S, et al. Ranitidine versus anticholinergic/antacid for duodenal ulcer: a randomized, endoscopically controlled, single-blind multicentre trial. Scand J Gastroenterol 1985; 20:701–5.

61. Lam SK. The stomach. In: Gitnick GL, ed. Current gastroenterology. Chicago: Year Book Medical Publishers, 1986:33–62.

62. Korman MG, Shaw RG, Hansky J, Schmidt GT, Stern AI. Influence of smoking on healing rate of duodenal ulcer in response to cimetidine or high-dose antacid. Gastroenterology 1981; 80:1451–3.

63. Massarrat S, Eisenmann A. Factors affecting the healing rate of duodenal and pyloric ulcers with low-dose antacid treatment. Gut 1981; 22:97–102.

64. Lam SK, Lau WY, Choi TK, Lai CL, Lok ASF, Hui WM, Ng MTT, Choi SKY. Prostaglandin E$_1$ (misoprostol) overcomes the adverse effect of chronic cigarette smoking on duodenal-ulcer healing. Dig Dis Sci 1986; 31:68–74S.

65. McIntosh JH, Byth K, Piper DW. Environmental factors in aetiology of chronic gastric ulcer: a case control study of exposure variables before the first symptoms. Gut 1985; 26:789–98.

66. Cook PJ, Vincent-Brown A, Lewis SI, et al. Carbenoxolone (Duogastrone) and cimetidine in the treatment of duodenal ulcer—a therapeutic trial. Scand J Gastroenterol 1980; 15(Suppl 65):93–101.

67. Martin DF, Hollanders D, May SJ, Ravenscroft MM, Tweedle DEF, Miller JP. Difference in relapse rates of duodenal ulcer after healing with cimetidine or tripotassium dicitrato bismuthate. Lancet 1981; i:7–10.

68. Coghlan JG, Gilligan D, Humphries H, McKenna D, Dooley C, et al. *Campylobacter pylori* and recurrence of duodenal ulcers—12-months follow-up study. Lancet 1987; ii:1109–11.

69. Lam SK, Hui WM, Lau WY, Branicki FJ, Lai CL, Lok ASF, Ng MMT, Fok PJ, Poon GP, Choi TK. Sucralfate overcomes adverse effect of cigarette smoking on duodenal ulcer healing and prolongs subsequent remission. Gastroenterology 1987; 92:1193–1201.

70. Ippoliti A, Elashoff J, Valenzuela J, Cano R, Frankl H, Samloff M, Koretz R. Recurrent ulcer after successful treatment with cimetidine or antacid. Gastroenterology 1983; 85:875–80.

71. Bytzer P, Lauritsen K, Rask-Madsen J. Symptomatic recurrence of healed duodenal and prepyloric ulcers after treatment with ranitidine or high dose antacid. A one year follow-up study. Scand J Gastroenterol 1986; 21:765–8.

72. Lauritsen K, Rune SJ, Bytzer P, et al. Effect of omeprazole and cimetidine on duodenal ulcer. A double-blind comparative trial. N Engl J Med 1985; 312:958–61.

73. Bardhan KD, Bianchi Porro G, Bose K, Daly M, Hinchliffe RFC, et al. A comparison of two different doses of omeprazole versus ranitidine in treatment of duodenal ulcers. J Clin Gastroenterol 1986; 8:408–13.

74. Hui WM, Lam SK, Lau WY, Branicki FJ, Lai CL, Lok ASF, Ng MTT, Poon GP, Fok PJ. Omeprazole (OME) vs ranitidine (RAN) for duodenal ulcer (DU)—one-week, low-dose regimens and factors affecting healing. Gastroenterology 1987; 92:1443.

75. Tomasetti P, Stanghellini E, Bonorag G, Vezzadini P, Labo G. Comparative trial on healing and relapse of duodenal ulcer treated with trithiozine or cimetidine. Curr Ther Rev 1981; 29:517–24.

76. Bardhan KD, Hunter JO, Miller JP, Thomson ABR, Graham DY, Russell RI, Sontag S, Hines C, Martin T, Gaussen L, van Thiel D, Achord J, Butler JK. Antacid maintenance therapy in the prevention of duodenal ulcer relapse. Gut 1988; 29:1748–54.

77. Bresci G, Carpria A, Federici G, Rindi G, Geloni M. Prevention of relapse with various antiulcer drugs. Scand J Gastroenterol 1986; 21(Suppl 121):58–62.

78. Friedman CJ, Oblinger MH, Suratt PM, Bowers J, Goldberg SK, Sperling MH, Blitzer AH. Prophylaxis of upper gastroduodenal hemorrhage in patients requiring mechanical ventilation. Crit Care Med 1982; 10:316–9.

79. Weigelt JA, Aurbakken CM, Gewertz BL, Snyder WH III. Cimetidine vs antacid in prophylaxis for stress ulceration. Arch Surg 1981; 116:597–601.

80. Hastings PR, Skillman JJ, Bushnell LS, Silen W. Antacid tritration in the prevention of acute gastrointestinal bleeding. N Engl J Med 1978; 298:1041–5.

81. Stothert JC Jr, Dellinger EP, Simonowitz DA, Schilling JA. Gastric pH monitoring as a

                                                    187

prognostic indicator for the prophylaxis of stress ulceration in the critically ill. Am J Surg 1980; 140:761–3.

82. Fiddian-Green RG, McGough E, Pittenger G, Rothman E. Predictive value of intramural pH and other risk factors for massive bleeding from stress ulceration. Gastroenterology 1983; 85:613–20.

83. Priebe HJ, Skillman JJ, Bushnell LS, Long PC, Silen W. Antacid versus cimetidine in preventing acute gastrointestinal bleeding. A randomized trial in 75 critically ill patients. N Engl J Med 1980; 302:426–30.

84. Pinilla JC, Oleniuk FH, Reed D, Malik B, Laverty WH. Does antacid prophylaxis prevent upper gastrointestinal bleeding in critically ill patients? Crit Care Med 1985; 13:646–50.

85. Koelz HR, Aeberhard P, Hassler H, Kunz H, Wagner HE, Roth F, Halter F. Prophylactic treatment of acute gastroduodenal stress ulceration. Scand J Gastroenterol 1987; 22:1147–52.

86. Borrero E, Bank S, Margolis I, Schulman WD, Chardavoyne R. Comparison of antacid and sucralfate in prevention of gastrointestinal bleeding in patients who are critically ill. Am J Med 1985; 79(Suppl 2c):62–4.

87. Tryba M. Risk of acute stress bleeding and nosocomial pneumonia in ventilated intensive care unit patients: sucralfate vs antacids. Am J Med 1987; (Suppl 3B):117–24.

88. Tryba M, Zevounou F, Torok M, Zeuz M. Prevention of acute stress bleeding with sucralfate, antacids or cimetidine. Am J Med 1985; 79(Suppl 2c):55–61.

89. Driks MR, Craven DE, Celli BR, McCabe WR. Nosocomial pneumonia in intubated patients given sucralfate as compared with antacids or histamine type 2 blockers. N Engl J Med 1987; 317:1376–82.

90. Bresalier RS, Grendell JH, Cello JR, Meyer AA. Sucralfate suspension versus titrated antacid for the prevention of acute stress-related gastrointestinal hemorrhage in critically ill patients. Am J Med 1987; 83(Suppl 3B):110–6.

91. Cannon LA, Heiselman D, Gardner W, Jones J. Prophylaxis of upper gastrointestinal tract bleeding in mechanically ventilated patients. Arch Intern Med 1987; 147:2101–6.

92. Spencer H, Lesniak M, Gatza CA, Osis D, Lender M. Magnesium absorption and metabolism in patients with chronic renal failure and in patients with normal renal function. Gastroenterology 1980; 79:26–34.

93. Wienbeck M, Erckenbrecht J, Strohmeyer G. Wirkung von antazida auf die darmmotilität. Z. Gastroenterol 1983; 21(Suppl):111–6.

94. Potyk D. Intestinal obstruction from impacted antacid tablets. N Engl J Med 1970; 283:134.

95. Holtermüller KH, König U. Safety of antacids. In: Bianchi Porro G, Richardson CT, eds. Antacids in peptic ulcer disease. Perspectives in digestive disease, Vol. 3. New York: Cortina International-Verona/Raven, 1988:41–52.

96. Alfrey AC, Mishell JM, Burks J, Contiguglia SR, Randolph H, Lewin E, Holmes JH. Syndrome of dyspraxia and multifocal seizures associated with chronic hemodialysis. Trans Am Soc Artif Intern Organs 1972; 18:257–61.

97. Dunea G, Mahurkar SD, Mamdani B, Smith EC. Role of aluminium in dialysis dementia. Ann Intern Med 1978; 88:502–4.

98.   Mahrkar SD, Smith EC, Mamdani BH, Dunea G. Dialysis dementia. The Chicago experience. J Dialysis 1978; 2:447–58.

99.   Rozas VV, Port FK, Rutt WM. Progressive dialysis encephalopathy from dialysate aluminium. Arch Intern Med 1978; 138:1375–7.

100. Alfrey AC, Le Gendre G, Kaehne WD. The dialysis encephalopathy syndrome and dialysis dementia. Lancet 1976; ii:1255.

101. Martyn CN, Osmond C, Edwardson JA, Barker DJP, Harris EC, Lacey RF. Geographical relation between Alzheimer's disease and aluminum in drinking water. Lancet 1989; i:59–62.

102. Herzog P, Schmitt KF, Grendahl T, van der Linden J, Holtermüller KH. Evaluation of serum and urine electrolyte changes during therapy with a magnesium-aluminum-containing antacid: results of a prospective study. In: Halter F, ed. Antacids in the eighties. Baltimore: Urban & Schwarzenberg, 1982:123–35.

103. Weberg R, Berstad A. Gastrointestinal absorption of aluminium from single doses of aluminium containing antacids in man. Eur J Clin Invest 1986; 16:428–32.

104. Hurwitz A. Antacid therapy and drug kinetics. Clin Pharmacokin 1977; 2:269.

105. Hurwitz A, Robinson RG, Vats TS, Whitter F, Herrin WF. Effects of antacids on gastric emptying. Gastroenterology 1967; 71:268–73.

9

The Histamine H_2-Receptor Antagonists

COLIN W. HOWDEN

University of Glasgow, Western Infirmary,
Glasgow, Scotland

RICHARD H. HUNT

McMaster University Medical Centre,
Hamilton, Ontario, Canada

I.   INTRODUCTION

Since the introduction of cimetidine in 1976, the histamine H_2-receptor antagonists have proven to be an enormous therapeutic and commercial success. These drugs now constitute the most widely used treatments for acid-peptic disease, and there has been a wealth of pharmacological and clinical experience with them.

II.   HISTORICAL ASPECTS AND BASIS FOR HISTAMINE ANTAGONISM

Histamine has been known to stimulate gastric acid secretion, since the first demonstration by Popielski in 1920 [1]. However, histamine also has a variety of other actions in the body, not all of which are blocked by conventional antihistamines such as mepyramine. This observation led to the recognition of at least two subclasses of histamine receptors. H_1 receptors are distributed throughout the body and are blocked by low concentrations of traditional antihistamines [2]. Most of the effects of histamine are mediated via H_1 receptors. Receptors of the second type, termed H_2, are also widely distributed in tissue, but their only known physiological action is stimulation of acid secretion by parietal cells in the stomach. H_2 receptors were formally identified and specific antagonists developed by Sir James Black and colleagues [3]. Structural analogues of histamine help to distinguish these two subtypes of receptors. 2-Methylhistamine binds to the H_1 receptor with an affinity about 17% of that seen with histamine but binds to the H_2 receptor with only about 2% of the affinity of histamine. Conversely, 4-methylhistamine binds to the H_2 receptor with 40% of the affinity of histamine but binds to the H_1 receptor with only about 0.2% of the affinity of histamine [3–5].

The central role of histamine in the control of gastric acid secretion in humans has recently been comprehensively reviewed [6]. In humans, histamine is probably released from gastric mast cells, binds to the parietal cell H_2 receptor, and stimulates the cell by increasing the intracellular production of adenosine cyclic $3',5'$-phosphate (cAMP). Ultrastructurally, the H_2 receptor is closely linked with the enzyme adenylate cyclase, which catalyzes the conversion of ATP to cAMP. Specific cAMP-dependent protein kinases are then activated, and these, in an as yet undefined way, initiate the alteration of the structure of the tubulovesicles, which enlarge and coalesce under stimulation to form the secretory canaliculi with membrane-bound molecules of H^+-ATPase, known as the proton pump.

Currently available histamine H_2-receptor antagonists are, pharmacologically, competitive antagonists for histamine at the H_2 receptor. However, in addition to reducing acid secretion in response to histamine stimulation, they reduce acid secretion in response to other stimuli [7], including pentagastrin, which acts through a gastrin receptor, and insulin-induced hypoglycemia, which stimulates acid secretion via vagal release of acetylcholine, which acts on parietal cell muscarinic receptors. Histamine therefore occupies a central role in the modulation and control of acid secretion in humans.

Burimamide was the first H_2-receptor antagonist to be investigated in animals [3] but was not used clinically. The first agent to be extensively investigated was metiamide, which was able to reduce overnight gastric secretion and to reduce stimulated gastric acid secretion in humans [8,9]. However, the development of metiamide was halted while it was still in clinical trials because of unexpected bone marrow toxicity [10], probably due to a sulfhydryl moiety in the side chain of the molecular structure. Cimetidine was the first H_2-receptor antagonist to be introduced into clinical practice [11]; it was licensed in the United Kingdom in 1976 and in the United States in 1978. Unlike metiamide, cimetidine was synthesized without the sulfhydryl group in its side chain in an attempt to prevent the adverse hematological effects of metiamide.

III. CURRENTLY AVAILABLE HISTAMINE H_2-RECEPTOR ANTAGONISTS

In chronological order of licensing, the currently available histamine H_2-receptor antagonists are cimetidine, ranitidine, famotidine, nizatidine, and roxatidine. All are relatively short-acting competitive antagonists for histamine at the H$_2$ receptor. They reduce gastric acid secretion in response to all known secretagogues including the ingestion of food but have their greatest effect on basal acid secretion. They reduce both the acidity and the volume of gastric juice.

The H$_2$-receptor antagonists were the first specific pharmacological agents to be introduced for the treatment of peptic ulcer. All have been shown in clinical trials to be highly effective in alleviating the pain of peptic ulceration and in promoting ulcer healing. They also have an impressive and enviable record of safety. Since the pharmacological and clinical effects of these drugs are similar, it has recently been argued [12] that we already have too many agents in this therapeutic class.

A.   Cimetidine

Cimetidine (Tagamet) was the first H$_2$-receptor antagonist to be introduced into widespread use. Its chemical structure is, like histamine, based on an imidazole ring.

1.   Metabolism and Pharmacokinetics

Following administration to humans, cimetidine is mostly excreted from the body in an unchanged state. Between 69 and 95% of an oral dose is excreted in the urine within 24 hr, mostly as unchanged drug [13]. A small proportion of the absorbed dose is metabolized to a sulfoxide. Over a wide range of plasma concentrations, cimetidine is only weakly (18–26%) bound to plasma proteins.

Cimetidine is highly water-soluble and has a high total systemic clearance of 500–600 mL/min [14]. Its volume of distribution is about 1 L/kg, and its elimination half-life about 2 hr.

Since cimetidine is excreted mainly by the kidneys, the plasma concentration may rise in patients with renal impairment. Renal excretion of cimetidine is by glomerular filtration and tubular secretion. It probably competes with creatinine for tubular secretion sites, because serum creatinine levels are often slightly raised during cimetidine treatment. This does not reflect any nephrotoxicity of cimetidine, because there is no permanent impairment of renal function.

2.   Pharmacodynamics

The principal pharmacological action of cimetidine is inhibition of gastric acid secretion. The reduction of intragastric acidity over the 24-hr period or at night is dependent upon the dose given and, to some extent, the time of dosing. Cimetidine 400 mg twice daily reduces mean 24-hr acidity in duodenal ulcer patients by 37% and mean nocturnal acidity by 54% (see ref. 15). If the same total daily dose of cimetidine, 800 mg, is given as a single bedtime dose, the mean reduction in 24-hr acidity is 48%, but there is a much greater reduction in mean nocturnal acidity of 79%. Therefore, when cimetidine is given at bedtime, most of its acid-suppressing effect occurs overnight. Even very large nocturnal doses of cimetidine (e.g., 2400 mg) have only a very minor effect on daytime food-stimulated acid secretion [16].

Table 1 Percentage Suppression of 24-hr, Nocturnal, and Daytime Acidity by Various Doses of H_2-Receptor Antagonists

	24-hr	Nocturnal	Daytime
Cimetidine			
300 mg qid	65	68	63
400 mg bid	37	54	23
600 mg bid	67	71	64
800 mg hs	48	79	23
Ranitidine			
150 mg bid	68	70	66
300 mg hs	68	90	50
Famotidine			
40 mg hs	64	95	39

Source: Jones et al. [15], with permission.

The percentage reductions in 24-hr nocturnal and daytime acidity produced by different dosage regimens of cimetidine and other H_2-receptor antagonists are listed in Table 1.

3. Clinical Use

In standard doses, cimetidine is significantly superior to placebo in healing duodenal and gastric ulcers. In a maintenance dose, it is superior to placebo in preventing ulcer relapse.

For the acute treatment of duodenal ulcer, cimetidine is usually prescribed for 4–8 weeks, whereas treatment for benign gastric ulcer may require up to 12 weeks. In a review of published controlled clinical trials [15], 8 weeks of treatment with cimetidine in optimum dosage was found to heal over 95% of duodenal ulcers. In the treatment of gastric ulcers [17], cimetidine given for 12 weeks achieves healing rates of 90–95%.

Cimetidine has been prescribed in a number of different dosage schedules, which include 300 mg four times daily, 600 mg or 400 mg twice daily, 200 mg three times daily plus 400 mg at bedtime, and 800 mg at bedtime. The popularity of the different dosage schedules varies between countries. Recently, much attention has been paid to the use of the 800 mg at bedtime regimen [18]. In addition to being simple, and therefore most easily complied with, this dose provides the highest duodenal ulcer healing rates for cimetidine in controlled trials [15] and gives at least as good symptom relief as other dose regimens.

4. Adverse Effects

Although a number of different adverse reactions have been reported with cimetidine, it must be stressed that side effects are very infrequent, are usually trivial, and are virtually always reversible on stopping treatment.

Cimetidine is weakly antiandrogenic in humans. It can bind to androgen receptors, displacing dihydrotestosterone and resulting in a number of effects including loss of libido, impotence, and, rarely, gynecomastia. During cimetidine use, there is an increase of about 20% in serum estradiol levels in males [19]. Spermatogenesis may be temporarily impaired during cimetidine treatment, with sperm counts decreased by up to 43% [20,21]. When given intravenously, cimetidine causes a 2.5-fold increase in circulating prolactin levels within 15 min [22], but this is not sustained with prolonged oral administration.

Cimetidine may cause reversible mental confusion. This has usually been reported in sick elderly patients receiving intravenous cimetidine in high doses and is more frequent in the presence of renal or hepatic impairment. Since these conditions may be associated with disturbed mental function, it has not been possible always to show a definite causal role for cimetidine.

In a retrospective analysis of over 260,000 prescriptions of H$_2$-receptor antagonists [23], the rate of gastrointestinal side effects for cimetidine was 94 per 10,000. This compared favorably with the reported rate for ranitidine, which was 121.8 per 10,000. The rates of central nervous system adverse effects were not significantly different for these two drugs.

A detailed meta-analysis of 24 placebo-controlled clinical trials of cimetidine found an overall rate of reported adverse events for cimetidine of 10.9%, while that for placebo was 10.1% [24].

Intravenous cimetidine has been reported to cause acute, potentially life-threatening cardiac dysrhythmias. Although the mechanism is unclear, it may be at least partly mediated through a reflex release of histamine [25].

5. Drug Interactions

By virtue of its inhibiting effect on the P$_{450}$ hepatic mixed function oxidase drug-metabolizing enzyme system, cimetidine has the potential to interact with many different drugs. β-adrenoceptor antagonists, including propranolol and metoprolol, and benzodiazepine sedatives, including diazepam and chloridazepoxide, all show a significant prolongation in plasma elimination half-life and a reduction in systemic clearance when administered with cimetidine. However, in view of the wide therapeutic indices of these drugs and the fact that their plasma levels do not necessarily reflect their pharmacological effect, such interactions are not clinically important.

Cimetidine does have important interactions with three drugs that are extensively metabolized by the liver, and that have narrow therapeutic indices. These are warfarin [26], phenytoin (diphenylhydantoin) [27], and theophylline [28]. If a patient is on a stable maintenance dose of one of these agents and is subsequently prescribed cimetidine, the steady-state plasma levels of the index drug will be increased and toxic side effects may be produced. This is particularly likely to occur with phenytoin, because its metabolic enzymes are saturable and zero-order kinetics govern its elimination. Therefore, where adequate facilities for therapeutic drug monitoring are not available, cimetidine is best avoided in patients receiving warfarin, phenytoin, or theophylline. Alternatively, cimetidine may be safely prescribed, provided that the daily dose of the index drug is reduced and steady-state plasma levels can be monitored. For warfarin, it is not necessary to measure plasma levels, because the therapeutic effect can be assessed by measuring various parameters of coagulation. Drug interactions with cimetidine have been comprehensively reviewed elsewhere [29].

6.   Contraindications

There are few contraindications to the use of cimetidine. Insufficient data are available regarding its safety during pregnancy, and cimetidine is also probably best avoided by sick elderly patients, particularly those with significant renal or hepatic impairment or those who are on multiple drug therapy.

B.   Ranitidine

Ranitidine (Zantac) was the second of the H_2-receptor antagonists to be made available by prescription. Unlike cimetidine, whose ring structure is an imidazole, the ranitidine molecule has a furan ring. Its clinical pharmacology has been reviewed elsewhere [30,31]. The clinical indications for ranitidine are broadly similar to those for cimetidine.

1.   Metabolism and Pharmacokinetics

Ranitidine is rapidly absorbed following oral administration, reaching peak plasma concentrations in 1–3 hr. It undergoes some degree of first pass metabolism in the liver; only about 30% of an oral dose is recovered unchanged in the urine compared with 70% of an intravenous dose. Its bioavailability is around 50%, and its apparent volume of distribution is 1.2–1.4 L/kg. Its elimination half-life is 2–3 hr in individuals with normal renal function [31–33]. In patients with chronic renal impairment, the elimination half-life of ranitidine is prolonged to 5–9 hr and reflects the degree of impairment [34]. The disposition of ranitidine in patients with well-compensated cirrhosis is not substantially affected [35].

2.   Pharmacodynamics

Like cimetidine, the only important pharmacological action of ranitidine is suppression of gastric acid secretion. Ranitidine 150 mg twice daily reduces mean 24-hr acidity in duodenal ulcer patients by 68% and nocturnal acidity by 70% (see Table 1) [15]. The single bedtime dose of 300 mg has a similar effect on mean 24-hr acidity, reducing it by 68%, but suppresses mean nocturnal acidity by 90%. Like cimetidine, ranitidine is more effective in suppressing basal (i.e., nocturnal) acid secretion than in suppressing food-stimulated acid secretion during the day. Ranitidine 150 mg four times daily was no more effective in suppressing daytime acidity in a group of duodenal ulcer patients than a conventional dose of 150 mg twice daily [36]. Very large doses of ranitidine, such as 300 mg four times daily, are required to produce a substantial inhibition of daytime acid secretion. Ranitidine 300 mg four times daily reduced median 24-hr acidity by 90% [37]. The duration of the suppression of acidity produced by ranitidine in the evening and during the night can be prolonged if the dose is taken in the early evening following the main meal of the day. Ranitidine 300 mg at 6 p.m. raised median intragastric pH from 1.45 to 3.55, whereas the same dose taken at 10 p.m. only raised it to 2.55 [38].

3. Clinical Use

Ranitidine 150 mg twice a day heals around 79% of duodenal ulcers after 4 weeks, increasing to 93% at 8 weeks [15]. Ranitidine 300 mg at bedtime produces duodenal ulcer healing rates of 84% at 4 weeks and 95% at 8 weeks [15].

In gastric ulcer, ranitidine 150 mg twice a day produces healing rates of 62% after 4 weeks and 90% after 8 weeks. Corresponding figures for ranitidine 300 mg at bedtime are 66% and 91% [39].

4. Adverse Effects

Ranitidine is more selective than cimetidine in terms of receptor binding. It therefore lacks the reported antiandrogenic effects of cimetidine [40,41]. Ranitidine in intravenous doses of 200 mg or greater can, like cimetidine, stimulate prolactin release. A twofold rise in circulating prolactin levels was seen within 10 min of intravenous ranitidine 200 mg [42], whereas repeated intravenous injections of 50 mg had no effect on prolactin levels [43]. Although there have been isolated reports of impotence in patients receiving ranitidine [44], these have largely not been substantiated. Like cimetidine, ranitidine may produce reversible mental confusion [45,46]. It may also induce cardiac dysrhythmias following rapid intravenous bolus injections.

There have been sporadic reports of drug-induced hepatitis with ranitidine [47–49], although a definite causal relationship with ranitidine was not always established.

5. Drug Interactions

Ranitidine binds weakly to the hepatic P$_{450}$ microsomal enzyme system and is a weak inhibitor, but to date there have been no convincing reports of clinically important drug interactions with ranitidine. This topic has recently been extensively reviewed [50], and interactions with ranitidine and cimetidine compared [51].

6. Contraindications

There are no absolute contraindications to ranitidine, although, like cimetidine, its safety during pregnancy has not been adequately assessed.

C. Famotidine

Famotidine (Pepcid) was the third H_2-receptor antagonist to be introduced into the United States. Its structure is based on a thiazole ring. It was granted a product license in the United States in 1986 and is also available in Japan, Australia, South America, and most European countries.

1. Metabolism and Pharmacokinetics

Following oral administration, peak plasma concentrations of famotidine occur within 2 hr. Its plasma elimination half-life is around 3.8 hr, and about 25% of the administered dose is recovered unchanged in the urine [52]. The renal clearance of famotidine is about 320 mL/min, and clearance is not dependent on dose. The kinetics of famotidine are not altered by repeated dosing.

2. Pharmacodynamics

Famotidine was initially introduced with a recommended dosage regimen of 40 mg at bedtime. In patients with duodenal ulcer, this produces about 64% suppression of mean 24-hr intragastric acidity but 95% suppression of nocturnal acidity [15]. Early evening administration of famotidine after the main meal is associated with some prolongation of its antisecretory effect [53].

3. Clinical Use

Famotidine 40 mg at night heals 82% of duodenal ulcers after 4 weeks of treatment [15]. In the treatment of gastric ulcer, famotidine 40 mg at night has produced healing rates of 50% after 4 weeks and 82% after 8 weeks [39].

4. Adverse Effects

To date, there have been no serious adverse reactions reported with famotidine. However, there is currently much less clinical experience with this drug than with either cimetidine or ranitidine. Clearly, increased vigilance is necessary for any new drug in the period following its introduction.

5. Drug Interactions

Famotidine does not appear to interfere with hepatic drug metabolism to any appreciable extent [54,55], and to date there have been no reported drug interactions with famotidine.

6. Contraindications

There are no definite contraindications to famotidine, although, like the other H_2-receptor antagonists, it should be avoided during pregnancy.

D. Nizatidine

Nizatidine (Axid) was the fourth H_2-receptor antagonist to receive a license in the United States, although it was launched just prior to famotidine in the United Kingdom.

1. Metabolism and Pharmacokinetics

Following oral administration, peak plasma concentrations of nizatidine are achieved by about 1 hr. The systemic bioavailability of nizatidine is about 90%, and its elimination half-life is 1.3 hr. Nizatidine is mainly excreted unchanged in the urine; 16 hr after an oral dose in healthy volunteers, 65% of the dose was recovered unchanged in the urine [56]. The elimination of nizatidine is reduced in patients with renal impairment.

2. Pharmacodynamics

In healthy volunteers, nizatidine 150 mg and 300 mg at bedtime reduced mean nocturnal intragastric acidity by 69% and 80%, respectively [57]. Nizatidine 300 mg taken at 9 p.m. had no significant effect on intragastric acidity during the following day [57].

Like famotidine, the duration of the antisecretory effect of nizatidine can be prolonged by giving it in the early evening together with the main meal of the day [58].

3. Clinical Use

In a multicenter clinical trial in Europe [59], nizatidine 300 mg at bedtime healed 81.2% of duodenal ulcers after 4 weeks and 91.8% after 8 weeks. The corresponding figures for ranitidine 300 mg at bedtime were 80.3% and 92.6%. The differences between the two treatments were not significant.

In the treatment of gastric ulcer, nizatidine 300 mg at bedtime healed 65.2% of ulcers after 4 weeks and 86.5% after 8 weeks [60]. The corresponding healing rates for ranitidine 150 mg twice daily were 66.3% and 86.7%. Again, the differences were not statistically significant.

4. Adverse Effects

No specific adverse effects have been reported. High-dose nizatidine for 2 weeks did not affect a variety of hormone levels in a group of normal healthy males [56]. There was no effect of nizatidine 150 mg twice daily on hypothalamic-pituitary-gonadal function or on sperm count in a small group of healthy men [61].

5. Drug Interactions

Nizatidine binds only very weakly to hepatic cytochrome P$_{450}$ as judged by in vitro studies using rat liver microsomes [62]. Studies in healthy human volunteers has shown no evidence of nizatidine interactions with a variety of commonly used drugs. Since its launch, no unexpected drug interactions have been reported.

E. Roxatidine

At the time of writing, this drug was at an advanced stage of the clinical trials program but had not been licensed in either the United States or the United Kingdom. Roxatidine has a quite different chemical structure from that of existing H$_2$-receptor antagonists, but like them it is a competitive antagonist.

1. Metabolism and Pharmacokinetics

Roxatidine is administered as roxatidine acetate. Following oral administration this compound is rapidly absorbed, being about 95% bioavailable, and rapidly converted to roxatidine. Using a granulated capsule formation, peak plasma levels of roxatidine are achieved within 3 hr. About 91% of an administered dose is recovered from the urine in 24 hr. The elimination half-life of roxatidine is 4 hr [63].

2. Pharmacodynamics

Roxatidine 150 mg given at 9 p.m. significantly reduced overnight gastric acidity in a group of healthy volunteers [64]. Three days after a 2-week course, intragastric acidity had returned to baseline levels. In a separate study [65], roxatidine 150 mg at night inhibited nocturnal intragastric acidity by 76% and daytime acidity by 41%. Using intragastric pH-metry, the effects of roxatidine 150 mg given at 9 p.m. on intragastric pH were very similar to those of ranitidine 300 mg [65].

3. Clinical Use

Roxatidine 75 mg twice a day was compared with ranitidine 150 mg twice a day in the treatment of duodenal ulcer [66]. After 6 weeks, the respective healing rates were not significantly different at 93.5% and 89.2%. In a separate study, roxatidine 75 mg twice a day was compared with 150 mg at bedtime in the treatment of duodenal ulcer [67]. After 4 weeks treatment, the respective healing rates were 89.0% and 87.6%, a nonsignificant difference.

In the treatment of gastric ulcer, roxatidine 75 mg twice a day healed 86.5% of ulcers after 8 weeks compared with 88.2% for ranitidine 150 mg twice a day [68]. In a separate trial [69], roxatidine 150 mg at night was as effective as the 75 mg twice daily regimen with 8-week gastric ulcer healing rates of 86% and 83.7%, respectively.

4. Adverse Effects

To date, there has been very little clinical experience with roxatidine, but no serious adverse effects have been reported. A review of safety and tolerance data from clinical trials [65] showed roxatidine to be safe in the short term. There has been no evidence of any antiandrogenic activity.

5. Drug Interactions

Roxatidine has very low affinity for hepatic cytochrome P_{450} both in vitro and in vivo. Specific studies in human volunteers have found no evidence for interaction between roxatidine and a variety of other drugs including antipyrine, diazepam, warfarin, and theophylline [70].

IV. SHORT-TERM THERAPY WITH H$_2$-RECEPTOR ANTAGONISTS

A. Duodenal Ulcer

As a group, the H$_2$-receptor antagonists have been very successful in the management of patients with duodenal ulcer [71,72]. Initially, these drugs were prescribed in doses that aimed to suppress gastric acid secretion to as great a degree and for as much of the 24-hr day as possible. Examples of early dose regimens for cimetidine were 200 mg three times a day and 400 mg at bedtime in the United Kingdom and 300 mg four times daily in the United States. However, it became apparent that the H$_2$-receptor antagonists were more successful at suppressing basal, unstimulated acid secretion than acid secretion in response to meals [73]. The nighttime period represents the longest period of basal secretion when acidity is usually high and unbuffered by food. It was subsequently shown that the whole daily dose taken as a single dose at bedtime provided the same degree of suppression of 24-hr acidity as the more complicated earlier regimens [18]. Furthermore, the use of a single large nighttime dose produces a greater degree of suppression of acidity at night than the earlier regimens while leaving acid secretion during the day relatively unaffected. Single nighttime doses of H$_2$-receptor antagonists have become accepted as standard treatment for duodenal ulcer (cimetidine 800 mg, ranitidine 300 mg, famotidine 40 mg, or nizatidine 300 mg).

In a detailed meta-analysis of various antisecretory drugs in duodenal ulcer [15], single nighttime dosing with H$_2$-receptor antagonists was found to be the most efficacious means of administration. Furthermore, this analysis showed that the effective suppression of nocturnal acidity was the single most important factor in determining ulcer healing rates by these drugs and that the suppression of daytime acidity contributed less than 1% to overall healing rates.

Four weeks of treatment with an H$_2$-receptor antagonist given as a single bedtime dose gives duodenal ulcer healing rates of 80–84% [15]; if treatment is extended to 8 weeks, healing rates of 95–96% are possible.

The actual time of administration of the H$_2$-receptor antagonist is probably of less importance than the temporal relationship between the dose and the last meal of the day. Early drug administration at 6 p.m. followed by a late meal has been shown to reduce the nocturnal antisecretory effect of ranitidine [74], famotidine [53], and nizatidine [58]. Patients should therefore be advised not to eat anything further between the times of taking their last dose of an H$_2$-receptor antagonist and retiring. Even small snacks taken after the dose can substantially reduce the degree of suppression of acidity [75]. Early evening administration of ranitidine at the end of a meal leads to higher peak plasma concentrations and greater ranitidine absorption as judged by the area under the concentration–time curve [38].

Although earlier evening administration of ranitidine produced slightly higher duodenal ulcer healing rates at 2 weeks than bedtime administration, there was no difference between these two treatments after 4 weeks of treatment. Ranitidine 300 mg at 6 p.m. healed 74% of duodenal ulcers after 2 weeks of treatment compared with 50% on ranitidine 300 mg given at 10 p.m. [76]. However, after 4 weeks of treatment, the healing rates on either regimen were similar at 100% and 94%, respectively. A clinical trial from France using the same protocol produced very similar results [77].

B.   Gastric Ulcer

Unlike the situation with duodenal ulcer, gastric acid secretion is usually normal or lower than normal in patients with gastric ulceration [78]. However, acid is certainly necessary for the formation of gastric ulcers, and the healing of these ulcers is accelerated by the suppression of acid secretion as evidenced by the superiority of the H_2-receptor antagonists over placebo. The doses of H_2-receptor antagonists and other antisecretory drugs used in the treatment of gastric ulcer are identical to those prescribed for duodenal ulcer. This may not be entirely appropriate, particularly as the degree of suppression of acidity that such doses produce in patients with gastric ulcer is generally not known.

The efficacy of the H_2-receptor antagonists in the treatment of benign gastric ulcer has recently been reviewed [17,39]. Unlike the situation in duodenal ulcer, there is a less clear relationship between the suppression of nocturnal acidity and gastric ulcer healing rates with the H_2-receptor antagonists. Healing rates after 4 weeks of treatment range from 55 to 66%; these extend to 82 to 91% by 8 weeks [39].

C.   Gastroesophageal Reflux Disease (GERD)

In contrast to their undoubted success in the short-term healing of duodenal or gastric ulcer, the H_2-receptor antagonists have been relatively disappointing in the treatment of patients with GERD. Experience with H_2-receptor antagonists in GERD has recently been reviewed [79,80]. These drugs do not influence lower esophageal sphincter (LES) pressure or the rates of esophageal clearance or gastric emptying, so their effect in GERD depends upon the suppression of the acidity and particularly the volume of gastric juice. The prolonged suppression of nocturnal acid secretion that can be achieved with H_2-receptor antagonists is important in reducing symptoms of reflux at night.

Cimetidine in total daily doses of up to 2 g given for 6–8 weeks provides some symptomatic improvement in over two-thirds of patients with GERD [80]. Improvement or healing of the lesions of esophagitis seen at endoscopy occurs in only about half the patients treated. In a review of clinical trials of cimetidine in GERD, Tytgat [81] found that around 63% of patients on cimetidine four times daily healed or improved after 6–8 weeks compared with 36% on placebo. Results with ranitidine are, broadly, similar [80,82]. At the time of writing, neither famotidine nor nizatidine was licensed for the treatment of GERD.

V.   FAILURE TO RESPOND TO H$_2$-RECEPTOR ANTAGONISTS

Most patients treated with H$_2$-receptor antagonists for peptic ulceration respond satisfactorily, at least in the short term. In controlled clinical trials, up to 95% of duodenal ulcers [15] and up to 90% of benign gastric ulcers [39,83] are healed by 8 weeks. However, some patients appear to be genuinely refractory to treatment despite good compliance [84] and satisfactory drug absorption [85].

The term "refractory duodenal ulcer" has been used since the introduction of the H$_2$-receptor antagonists [85–88] and probably reflects the severe end of the spectrum of disease. Several extensive reviews of the clinical aspects have been undertaken [87,89–96]. A refractory duodenal ulcer should be considered an ulcer that does not heal following 3 months of full-dose treatment with an H$_2$-receptor antagonist or recurs within 1 year despite maintenance treatment [96].

After initial healing and continued maintenance therapy, between 20 and 35% of duodenal ulcers recur in 1 year [71,97], although this figure underestimates the true rate of recurrence because of the variability in time interval for endoscopies [98].

The reasons for this failure are unclear, and there is no general agreement about the importance of acid hypersecretion in these patients or about whether a reduction in acidity or total acid output is more important [99].

The evidence for hypersecretion in nonresponders is conflicting with some studies showing an increase in acid secretion [85,100] or no change [89,101–103], and there is an overlap between patients and healthy volunteers [104]. More recently, Collen and coworkers [100,105] have claimed that patients with nonhealing ulcers all have a basal acid output greater than 10 mmol/hr. However, since their patients had all been taking H$_2$-receptor antagonists in variable doses for a long duration, there is a possibility that they were studied during a period in which rebound hypersecretion occurred.

The various observations of failure to suppress nocturnal acidity [83,85,86,88] and of increased basal acid output [100] and concerns about rebound acid hypersecretion have led to extensive studies into the possible mechanisms involved [96,106].

Increased parietal cell sensitivity after treatment with the H$_2$-receptor antagonists cimetidine or ranitidine has been reported in controlled studies in which stimulation was undertaken with either pentagastrin [107–110], histamine [108], or the specific H$_2$-receptor agonist impromidine [111]. These studies showed a decreased effect of the H$_2$-receptor antagonist in inhibition of pentagastrin-stimulated acid secretion in patients on long-term H$_2$-receptor antagonists and circumstantial evidence for H$_2$-receptor up-regulation in the impromidine stimulation study [111].

Tolerance may also occur with a decreased response to repeated doses of the H$_2$-receptor antagonist when it is given orally or intravenously. A reduced suppression of intragastric acidity is seen over a time period of 1–4 weeks [112–115], and this can also occur acutely [116]. Because H$_2$-receptor antagonist treatment is associated with some increase in the 24-hr plasma gastrin profile [117,118] and the meal-stimulated gastric response [119], it has been suggested that this rise may be responsible for the decreased efficacy of the H_2-receptor antagonist and a single study would support this [114].

No consistent pattern of rebound hypersecretion was reported in early studies of basal or pentagastrin-stimulated acid output following H_2-receptor antagonist treatment, although this had been considered a possibility [94,120]. However, an increase in intragastric acidity and a marked increase in overnight acid output have been reported in duodenal ulcer patients [121] and healthy volunteers [115].

The clinical significance of these observations is difficult to determine. The H_2-receptor antagonists are extraordinarily effective drugs that have had a dramatic impact on the treatment of duodenal ulcer disease. These pharmacophysiological observations are especially interesting from the mechanistic point of view and remain to be further elucidated.

Furthermore, if hypersecretion of gastric acid is the sole explanation for poor pharmacological response, the problem should be overcome by increasing the dose of H_2-receptor antagonist, although this has only a modest effect [89], probably because of the very flat dose response of duodenal ulcer healing to suppression of intragastric acidity [15]. Some patients with a poor pharmacological response to H_2-receptor antagonists have nocturnal hypersecretion of gastric acid secondary to parasympathetic overactivity. This can be corrected by combining the H_2-receptor antagonist with an anticholinergic agent [85], although the results of clinical trials with an H_2-receptor antagonist combined with an anticholinergic agent have been equivocal [122]. Highly selective vagotomy produces a marked reduction in intragastric acidity in cimetidine nonresponders when studied 6 months after surgery [85], although the results have been controversial, with clinical improvement claimed by some [123] and disputed by others [89,124,125], while yet others [126] found no difference.

Cigarette smoking has been shown consistently to impair ulcer healing with all classes of anti-ulcer drugs including the H_2-receptor antagonists by about 10% [127]. There is no evidence to confirm that the adverse effect of smoking is due to interference with the pharmacological action of any ulcer-healing drug, because the same differences between smokers and nonsmokers are seen for placebo healing. Furthermore, studies of intragastric acidity in smokers taking H_2-receptor antagonists show no consistent changes [106]. The presence of *Helicobacter pylori* does not appear to alter the efficacy of H_2-receptor antagonists on ulcer healing but may be associated with earlier ulcer relapse after healing, although the mechanisms of action are not yet explained. The H_2-receptor antagonists do not eradicate or suppress this organism. Patients who are refractory to H_2-receptor antagonists may respond to treatment with bismuth salts [102,103], which are toxic to *Helicobacter pylori*.

VI.   USE OF H_2-RECEPTOR ANTAGONISTS IN CRITICALLY ILL PATIENTS

Critically ill patients in the intensive care unit have a high incidence of gastric and duodenal mucosal erosive lesions. One prospective endoscopic study found that 74%

of patients had erosions at first endoscopy but only about half had evidence of bleeding [128]. Bleeding from stress-related mucosal lesions increases the morbidity and mortality of critically ill patients, so various measures have been adopted in an attempt to prevent or reduce the incidence.

Gastric acid is an important factor involved in initiating bleeding from these lesions, and titration of intragastric pH to above 3.5 with antacids or intravenous administration of H$_2$-receptor antagonists may be effective in halting mild bleeding from stress-related lesions [129,130]. In one comparative trial, antacid given via a nasogastric tube was more effective than intravenous cimetidine in preventing bleeding from stress-related lesions [131].

In patients with fulminant hepatic failure, cimetidine reduces the incidence of bleeding from acute erosions but does not reduce overall mortality [132,133].

Although treatment with H$_2$-receptor antagonists reduces the incidence of bleeding from stress ulcer [128,130], there is less evidence to suggest that these agents are effective in preventing the development of lesions. However, they may prevent progression and initiate healing of stress ulcers.

Appropriate doses of H$_2$-receptor antagonists for use in critically ill patients would be cimetidine 300 mg every 4 hr or ranitidine 50 mg every 6 hr intravenously [130]. Care must be taken when administering these agents intravenously in view of the possible occurrence of cardiac dysrhythmias. Continuous intravenous infusion may be a more effective means of administration of H$_2$-receptor antagonists than intermittent intravenous boluses. In a recent study [134], continuous infusion of ranitidine produced greater control of intragastric pH with less interindividual variability than ranitidine 100 mg given every 12 hr.

A further potential hazard of the use of acid-suppressing drugs in critically ill patients is that they may be associated with an increase in the incidence of nosocomial infection, by permitting gastric bacterial overgrowth leading to subsequent pneumonia [135–137]. However, the role of H$_2$-receptor antagonists in stress ulcer remains highly controversial. A recent ICU study showed equivalent benefit for sucralfate in protecting from stress ulcer compared to antacids and H$_2$-receptor antagonists [138]. However, the authors also claimed a significantly lower rate of pneumonia in the sucralfate group than in the control group, in which they had combined for analysis the two groups of patients taking antacids or H$_2$-receptor antagonists. When these two groups are analyzed separately, the pneumonia rate in the H$_2$-receptor antagonist group is half that in the sucralfate group, whereas the antacid group had twice the number of cases of pneumonia as the sucralfate group. Clearly more studies are required for this important indication.

VII. USE OF H$_2$-RECEPTOR ANTAGONISTS IN BLEEDING PEPTIC ULCER

There have been numerous clinical trials of H$_2$-receptor antagonists to prevent rebleeding from peptic ulcer. Unfortunately, nearly all have included inadequate numbers of patients to be confident of demonstrating a useful effect [139]. A meta-analysis of 27 published randomized trials in which 1670 patients had been entered [140] suggested that H_2-receptor antagonists might reduce the incidence of ulcer rebleeding, emergency surgery, and death by around 10%, 20%, and 30%, respectively. Large-scale multicenter trials would be necessary to examine these possibilities accurately.

The increased use of H_2-receptor antagonists has not, however, altered the in-hospital mortality for bleeding peptic ulcer, which remains at about 8–10% [141]. This is at least partly due to the fact that the mean age of patients admitted to hospital with bleeding ulcers has been progressively rising for over a decade.

Conventional doses of currently available H_2-receptor antagonists do not have a major effect on intragastric pH. Cimetidine 1 g/day raises median pH from 1.4 to 1.7; ranitidine 300 mg/day, to 2.4 [142]. A much greater rise in intragastric pH to above 6 would be necessary to completely inactivate pepsinogen and so prevent further acid-peptic digestion of clot and to optimize platelet aggregation [143]. Omeprazole 30 mg/day has been shown to raise median intragastric pH to 5.3 [144], which might have a potentially useful effect in bleeding ulcers. Large-scale clinical trials of high-dose potent H_2-receptor antagonists and omeprazole in bleeding peptic ulcer are currently in progress. However, it has recently been argued pessimistically that a pharmacological approach to the treatment of bleeding ulcers is unlikely to be of major benefit [145].

VIII. USE OF H_2-RECEPTOR ANTAGONISTS IN THE TREATMENT OR PREVENTION OF GASTRODUODENAL DAMAGE DUE TO NONSTEROIDAL ANTI-INFLAMMATORY DRUGS

Up to 50% of patients on nonsteroidal anti-inflammatory drugs (NSAIDs) complain of dyspeptic symptoms. It is debatable whether or not NSAIDs actually cause the ulceration, but they do appear to increase the chances of hemorrhage or perforation from an ulcer. There has, however, been some inconsistency in attempting to calculate overall risk [146]. In a recent review [147], the relative risks of gastric and duodenal ulceration in patients on NSAIDs were estimated at 46 and 8, respectively.

A. Treatment of Gastroduodenal Damage

Peptic ulcers in patients on NSAIDs can be effectively healed by H_2-receptor antagonists given in conventional doses [148–151] whether or not treatment with NSAIDs is discontinued.

When NSAIDs were continued, 83% of duodenal ulcers and 50% of gastric ulcers were successfully healed within 9 weeks using either ranitidine or sucralfate [151]. In patients from whom NSAIDs had been withdrawn, corresponding ulcer healing rates were 92% and 86%, respectively, for ranitidine and sucralfate. The differences were not statistically significant. Overall, ranitidine healed ulcers in 84% of patients on NSAIDs within 9 weeks, suggesting that ulcers associated with NSAIDs may take longer to heal.

B.   Prevention of Gastroduodenal Damage

There are few adequate studies of prevention by H$_2$-receptor antagonists of damage to the mucosa of the upper alimentary tract induced by NSAIDs. Cimetidine reduces the fecal blood loss in patients with arthritis taking high-dose aspirin [152], and ranitidine reduces aspirin-induced bleeding in healthy volunteers [153]. Cimetidine reduces the fall in gastric mucosal potential difference in healthy volunteers given aspirin [154]. Healthy males given long-term aspirin therapy obtained significant protection against gastric and duodenal mucosal damage when ranitidine was co-administered [155].

In a double-blind, randomized study, patients received NSAIDs for rheumatoid arthritis or osteoarthritis and who had a normal upper gastrointestinal endoscopy were given either ranitidine 150 mg twice a day or a placebo together with the NSAID [156]. After 4 weeks, the incidence of new gastric erosions in the patients receiving ranitidine was not significantly different from that in patients on placebo. This suggests that the H$_2$-receptor antagonists are ineffective in preventing the early gastric mucosal damage attributable to NSAIDs. They may, however, protect against duodenal damage. In a randomized, double-blind study, patients receiving one of four commonly prescribed NSAIDs were given either ranitidine 150 mg twice a day or placebo with their NSAID [166]. All patients had a normal upper gastrointestinal endoscopy and had been off treatment with NSAIDs for 1 week before the start of the study. After 8 weeks, 1.5% of patients in the ranitidine group had developed duodenal ulceration compared with 8% in the placebo group, a statistically significant difference. The incidence of gastric ulceration was 6% in each group after 8 weeks.

The experience with H$_2$-receptor antagonists in the prevention of NSAID-related upper gastrointestinal ulceration is in marked contrast to that with synthetic prostaglandins. In a prospective study of patients taking NSAIDs for osteoarthritis [157], misoprostol, a synthetic derivative of prostaglandin E$_1$, significantly reduced the incidence of gastric ulceration during 3 months of treatment. Direct comparisons with the H$_2$-receptor antagonists will be awaited with interest.

Generally, NSAIDs should be discontinued if at all possible in patients found to have peptic ulceration. If this is not possible, the ulcer can be satisfactorily treated with an H$_2$-receptor antagonist although treatment may have to be continued for longer than usual.

The H$_2$-receptor antagonists protect the gastric mucosa against the damaging effect of aspirin, presumably by raising intragastric pH and so increasing the degree of ionization of aspirin and reducing its absorption by the gastric mucosa [158]. There is no evidence that they prevent new gastric damage due to non-aspirin NSAIDs, but they might give some protection to the duodenum although the incidence of damage here is low in any case [147].

IX. MAINTENANCE TREATMENT OF PEPTIC ULCERATION WITH H_2-RECEPTOR ANTAGONISTS

Duodenal ulceration is a chronic relapsing condition, and although the H_2-receptor antagonists are highly effective in alleviating pain and effecting ulcer healing, ulcers relapse once treatment is discontinued. Following withdrawal of H_2-receptor antagonists after treatment of duodenal ulceration, up to 80% of patients will relapse within 1 year [159]. Continuing treatment with an H_2-receptor antagonist beyond the point of ulcer healing does not influence the subsequent rate of relapse once treatment is eventually stopped [159].

The high relapse rates following withdrawal of treatment with H_2-receptor antagonists have encouraged the use of long-term maintenance treatment. Both cimetidine and ranitidine reduce the rate of symptomatic and asymptomatic ulcer relapse if they are prescribed as continuous maintenance treatment for patients with duodenal ulcer [160]. Standard maintenance doses are cimetidine 400 mg at bedtime, ranitidine 150 mg at bedtime, and famotidine 20 mg at bedtime. In two large-scale comparative trials, relapse rates were lower in patients on ranitidine than in those on cimetidine [161,162]. In these trials, the annual relapse rates for patients on ranitidine were 16% and 23%, respectively, compared with 43% and 37%, respectively, for patients on cimetidine.

Routine maintenance treatment is probably not necessary for every patient with duodenal ulceration, although this has recently been debated in terms of efficacy and cost [163,164]. Although maintenance treatment definitely reduces the total number of relapses, it has not been possible to demonstrate a significant reduction in ulcer complications [165,163]. Most patients with duodenal ulceration are adequately managed on intermittent courses of H_2-receptor antagonists given from symptomatic relapses [167,168]. Approximately two-thirds of patients can be managed in this way, although the remainder—including the elderly, those with other chronic disorders, those with a previous ulcer complication, and probably those on NSAIDs—should be given maintenance treatment.

Most of the therapeutic gain of maintenance treatment is lost if patients smoke cigarettes. In a placebo-controlled study of maintenance treatment with cimetidine in duodenal ulcer [169], the relapse rate for nonsmokers receiving placebo was not significantly different from that of smokers receiving cimetidine.

Gastric ulceration is also a relapsing disease. After healing of gastric ulcers, one-third of patients relapsed within 9 months [170]. The rate of relapse was not different whether the ulcers had healed on placebo, antacid, or cimetidine. Since gastric ulcers tend to occur in an older age group than duodenal ulcers and are associated with greater morbidity, it has been argued that all patients with healed gastric ulcers should be offered lifelong maintenance treatment [171].

The whole area of maintenance treatment for peptic ulcer disease has recently been reviewed by the American College of Gastroenterology Committee on FDA-related matters [172].

REFERENCES

1. Popielski L. Beta-imidazolylathylamin und die organextrakte. Erst tiel beta-imidazolyl-athylamin als machtiger erreger der magendrusen. Pflugers Arch Ges Physiol 1920; 178:214–36.

2. Ash ASF, Schild HO. Receptors mediating some actions of histamine. Br J Pharmacol Chemother 1966; 27:427–39.

3. Black JW, Duncan WAM, Durant GJ, Ganellin CR, Parsons ME. Definition and antagonism of histamine H$_2$ receptors. Nature 1972; 236:385–90.

4. Durant GJ, Parsons ME, Ganellin CR. Potential histamine H$_2$-receptor antagonists: 3-Methylhistamines. J Med Chem 1976; 19:923–8.

5. Hirschowitz BI. An update on histamine receptors and the gastrointestinal tract. Dig Dis Sci 1985; 30:998–1004.

6. Wolfe MM, Soll AH. The physiology of gastric acid secretion. N Engl J Med 1988; 319:1707–15.

7. Brimblecombe RW, Parsons ME. Histamine. In: Bloom SR, Ponk JM, eds. Gut hormones. London: Churchill Livingstone, 1981: 171–5.

8. Carter DC, Forrest JAH, Werner M, Heading RC, Park J, Shearman DJC. Effect of histamine H$_2$ receptor blockade on vagally-induced gastric secretion in man. Br Med J 1974; 3:554–6.

9. Thjodleifsson B, Wormsley KG. Effects of metiamide on the human stomach. Clin Sci 1975; 49:445–58.

10. Forrest JAH, Shearman DJC, Spencer R, Celestin LR. Neutropenia associated with metiamide. Lancet 1975; i:392–3.

11. Burland WL, Hunt RH, Mills JG, Milton-Thompson GJ. Drugs of the decade 1970–1979: cimetidine. Br J Pharmacother 1979:24–40.

12. Anon. Too many H$_2$-antagonists [editorial]. Lancet 1988; i:28–9.

13. Taylor DC, Cresswell PP, Bartlett DC. The metabolism and elimination of cimetidine, a histamine H$_2$-receptor antagonist, in the rat, dog and man. Drug Metab Disposition 1978; 6:21–30.

14. Somogyi A, Gugler R. Clinical pharmacokinetics of cimetidine. Clin Pharmacokinet 1983; 9:463–95.

15. Jones DB, Howden CW, Burget DW, Kerr GD, Hunt RH. Acid suppression in duodenal ulcer: a meta-analysis to define optimal dosing with antisecretory drugs. Gut 1987; 28:1120–7.

16. Kapur B, Mills JG, Glenny H, Bowland WL, Lunt M, Bardham KD. Evaluation of large single nighttime doses of cimetidine using continuous 24-hour ambulatory gastric pH monitoring. Gut 1985; 26:A559.

17. Howden CW, Jones DB, Peace KD, Burget DW, Hunt RH. The treatment of gastric

ulcer with antisecretory drugs: relationship of pharmacological effect to healing rates. Dig Dis Sci 1988; 33:619–24.

18. Gledhill T, Howard OM, Buck M, Paul A, Hunt RH. Single nocturnal dose of an H_2-receptor antagonist for the treatment of duodenal ulcer. Gut 1983; 24:904–8.

19. Galbraith RA, Michnovicz JJ. The effects of cimetidine on the oxidative metabolism of estradiol. N Engl J Med 1989; 321:269–74.

20. Van Thiel DH, Gavaler JS, Smith WI, Paul G. Hypothalamic-pituitary-gonadal dysfunction in men using cimetidine. N Engl J Med 1979; 300:1012–5.

21. Wang C, Lai CL, Lam KC, Yeung KK. Effect of cimetidine in gonadal function in man. Br J Clin Pharmacol 1982; 13:791–4.

22. Daubresse JC, Meunier JC, Ligny G. Plasma prolactin and cimetidine. Lancet 1978; i:99.

23. Morton R, Das A, Jacobs J, Fox N. Rates of adverse reactions to cimetidine and ranitidine. Am J Gastroenterol 1988; 83:1036. Abstract.

24. Richter JM, Colditz GA, Huse DM, Delea TE, Oster G. Cimetidine and adverse reactions: a meta-analysis of randomized clinical trials of short-term therapy. Am J Med 1989; 87:278–84.

25. Parkin JW, Ackroyd EB, Glickman S, Hobsley M, Lorpaz W. Release of histamine by H_2-receptor antagonists. Lancet 1982; ii:938–9.

26. Serlin MJ, Sibeon RR, Mossman S, et al. Cimetidine: interaction with oral anticoagulants in man. Lancet 1979; ii:317–9.

27. Hetzel DJ, Bochner F, Hallpike JF, Shearman DJC, Hann CS. Cimetidine interaction with phenytoin. Br Med J 1981; 282:1512.

28. Wood L, Grice J, Petroff V, McGuffie C, Roberts RK. Effect of cimetidine on the disposition of theophylline. Aust NZ J Med 1980; 10:586.

29. Somogyi A, Muirhead M. Pharmacokinetic interactions of cimetidine 1987. Clin Pharmacokinet 1987; 12:321–66.

30. Brogden RN, Carmine AA, Heel RC, Speight TM, Avery GS. Ranitidine: a review of its pharmacology and therapeutic uses in peptic ulcer disease and other allied diseases. Drugs 1982; 24:267–303.

31. Grant SM, Langtry HD, Brogden RN. Ranitidine. An updated review of its pharmacodynamic properties and therapeutic uses in peptic ulcer disease and other allied diseases. Drugs 1989; 37:801–70.

32. McNeil JJ, Mihaly GW, Anderson A, Marshall AW, Smallwood RA, Louis WJ. Pharmacokinetics of the H_2-receptor antagonist ranitidine in man. Br J Clin Pharmacol 1981; 12:411–5.

33. Chau NP, Zech PY, Pozet N, Hadj-Aissa A. Ranitidine kinetics in normal subjects. Clin Pharmacol Ther 1982; 31:770–4.

34. Zech PY, Chau NP, Pozet N, Labeeuw M, Hadj-Aissa A. Ranitidine kinetics in chronic renal impairment. Clin Pharmacol Ther 1983; 34:667–72.

35. Smith IL, Ziemniak JA, Bernhard H, Eshelman FN, Martin LE, Schentag JJ. Ranitidine disposition and systemic availability in hepatic cirrhosis. Clin Pharmacol Ther 1984; 35:487–94.

36. Howden CW, Tsai HH, Reid JL. Twenty-four-hour intragastric acidity in duodenal ulcer patients during dosing with placebo and 150 mg ranitidine twice or four times daily. Aliment Pharmacol Ther 1989; 3:253–8.

37. Lanzon-Miller S, Pounder RE, Chronos NAF, Hamilton M, Ball S, Raymond F. Can

high dose oral ranitidine eliminate intragastric acid, and what does it do to plasma gastrin? Gastroenterology 1987; 92:1491. Abstract.

38. Merki H, Witzel L, Harre K, Scheurle E, Neumann J, Rohmel J. Single dose treatment with H$_2$ receptor antagonists. Is bedtime administration too late? Gut 1987; 28:451–4.

39. Howden CW, Hunt RH. The relationship between suppression of acidity and gastric ulcer healing rates. Aliment Pharmacol Therap 1990; 4:25–33.

40. Savarino V, Giusti M, Mansi C, Marugo M, Delitala G, Celle G. Ranitidine and testosterone secretion in man. Br J Clin Pharmacol 1983; 15:578–9.

41. Wang C, Wong KL, Lam KC, Lai CL. Ranitidine does not affect gonadal function in man. Br J Clin Pharmacol 1983; 16:430–2.

42. Delitala G, Devilla L, Pende A, Canessa A. Effects of the H$_2$ receptor antagonist ranitidine on anterior pituitary hormone secretion in man. Eur J Clin Pharmacol 1982; 22:207–11.

43. Folsch UR, Wichmann GCh, Torossian A. Effect of 6-hourly intermittent intravenous boluses of oxmetidine and ranitidine on gastric acidity and serum prolactin. Eur J Clin Pharmacol 1987; 33:267–71.

44. Viana L. Probable case of impotence due to ranitidine. Lancet 1983; ii:635–6.

45. Epstein CM. Ranitidine and confusion. Lancet 1984; i:1071.

46. Silverstone PH. Ranitidine and confusion. Lancet 1984; i:1071.

47. Lauritsen K, Havelund T, Rask-Madsen J, Fenger C. Ranitidine and hepatotoxicity. Lancet 1984; ii:1471.

48. Lima MAS. Hepatitis associated with ranitidine. Ann Intern Med 1984; 101:207–8.

49. Black M, Scott WE, Kanter R. Possible ranitidine hepatotoxicity. Ann Intern Med 1984; 101:208–9.

50. Mitchard M, Harris A, Mullinger BM. Ranitidine drug interactions—a literature review. Pharmacol Ther 1987; 32:293–325.

51. Smith SR, Kendall MJ. Ranitidine versus cimetidine. A comparison of their potential to cause clinically important drug interactions. Clin Pharmacokinet 1988; 15:44–56.

52. Smith JL. Clinical pharmacology of famotidine. Digestion 1985; 32(Suppl 1):15–23.

53. Emde C, Bauerfeind P, Koelz HR, et al. Optimising the antisecretory effect of famotidine: early evening meal together with the drug is best. Gastroenterology 1987; 92: A1382. Abstract.

54. Somerville KW, Kitchingman GA, Langman MJS. Effect of famotidine on oxidative drug metabolism. Eur J Clin Pharmacol 1986; 30:279–81.

55. Humphries TJ. Famotidine: a notable lack of drug interactions. Scand J Gastroenterol 1987; 22(Suppl 134):55–60.

56. Callaghan JT, Bergstrom RF, Rubin A, et al. A pharmacokinetic profile of nizatidine in man. Scand J Gastroenterol 1987; 22(Suppl 136):9–17.

57. Dammann HG, Gottlieb WR, Walter TA, Muller P, Simon B, Keohane PP. The 24-hour acid suppression profile of nizatidine. Scand J Gastroenterol 1987; 22(Suppl 136):56–60.

58. Duroux P, Bauerfeind P, Emde C, et al. Optimising the effect of nizatidine on gastric pH: early evening meal together with the drug is best. Gut 1987; 28:A1339. Abstract.

59. Simon B, Cremer M, Dammann HG, et al. 300 mg nizatidine at night versus 300 mg ranitidine at night in patients with duodenal ulcer: a multicentre trial in Europe. Scand J Gastroenterol 1987; 22(Suppl 136):61–70.

60. Naccaratto R, Cremer M, Dammann HG, et al. Nizatidine versus ranitidine in gastric

ulcer disease: a European multicentre trial. Scand J Gastroenterol 1987; 22 (Suppl 136):71–8.

61. Van Thiel DH, Gavaler JS, Heyl A, Susen B. An evaluation of the anti-androgen effects associated with H_2 antagonist therapy. Scand J Gastroenterol 1987; 22(Suppl 136):24–8.

62. Klotz U. Lack of effect of nizatidine on drug metabolism. Scand J Gastroenterol 1987; 22(Suppl 136):18–23.

63. Collins JD, Pidgen AW. Pharmacokinetics of roxatidine in healthy volunteers. Drugs 1988; 35(Suppl 3):41–7.

64. Lassman HB, Ho I, Puri SK, Sabo R, Scheffler MR. The pharmacodynamics and pharmacokinetics of multiple doses of the new H_2-receptor antagonist, roxatidine acetate, in healthy men. Drugs 1988; 35(Suppl 3):53–64.

65. Dammann HG, De Looze SM, Bender W, Labs R. Clinical characteristics of roxatidine acetate: a review. Scand J Gastroenterol 1988; 23(Suppl 146):121–34.

66. Huttemann W. A comparison of roxatidine acetate and ranitidine in duodenal ulcer healing. Drugs 1988; 35(Suppl 3):90–5.

67. Hentschel E, Schutze K, et al. A comparison of roxatidine acetate 150 mg once daily and 75 mg twice daily in duodenal ulcer healing. Drugs 1988; 35(Suppl 3):96–101.

68. Judmaier G. A comparison of roxatidine acetate and ranitidine in gastric ulcer healing. Drugs 1988; 35(Suppl 3):120–6.

69. Rosch W. A comparison of roxatidine acetate 150 mg once daily and 75 mg twice daily in gastric ulcer healing. Drugs 1988; 35(Suppl 3):127–33.

70. Collins JD. Therapeutic approach in patients with concomitant disease/drug–drug interactions (roxatidine acetate). Scand J Gastroenterol 1988; 23(Suppl 146):89–99.

71. Meyrick-Thomas J, Misiewicz G. Histamine H_2-receptor antagonists in the short- and long-term treatment of duodenal ulcer. Clin Gastroenterol 1984; 13:501–41.

72. Chiverton SG, Hunt RH. Medical regimens in short- and long-term ulcer management. Baillere's Clin Gastroenterol 1988; 2(3):655–76.

73. Pounder RE, Williams JG, Hunt RH, Vincent SH, Milton-Thompson GJ, Misiewicz JJ. The effects of oral cimetidine on food-stimulated gastric acid secretion and 24-hour intragastric acidity. In: Cimetidine. Proceedings of the second international symposium on histamine H_2-receptor antagonists. Oxford: Excerpta Medica, 1977:189–206.

74. Johnston DA, Wormsley KG. The effect of food on ranitidine-induced inhibition of nocturnal gastric secretion. Aliment Pharmacol Ther 1988; 2:507–11.

75. Kempf M, Daufmann D, Walt RP, et al. TV snacks are bad for H_2 receptor blockade. Gastroenterology 1988; 94:A222. Abstract.

76. Merki H, Witzel L, Huttemann W, et al. Early evening ranitidine administration promotes faster duodenal ulcer healing. Am J Gastroenterol 1988; 83:362–4.

77. Rampal P, Alberola B, Pappo M. Ranitidine 300 mg od in acute duodenal ulcer: administration after dinner or at bedtime? A French multicenter comparative trial. Gastroenterology 1988; 94:A367. Abstract.

78. Grossman MI, Kirsner JB, Gillespie IE. Basal and histalog-stimulated gastric secretion in control subjects and in patients with peptic ulcer or gastric cancer. Gastroenterology 1963; 45:14–26.

79. Dent J. Medical treatment of gastroesophageal reflux disease. In: Starling JR, ed. Reflux esophagitis and the Angelchik prosthesis. New York: Elsevier, 1987:26–40.

80. Tytgat GNJ, Nio CY. Medical therapy of reflux esophagitis. Bailliere's Clin Gastroenterol 1987; 1:791–808.
81. Tytgat GNJ. Assessment of the efficacy of cimetidine and other drugs in oesophageal reflux disease. In: Baron JH, ed. Cimetidine in the 80s. Edinburgh: Churchill Livingstone, 1981:153–66.
82. Kimmig JM. Cimetidine and ranitidine in the treatment of reflux esophagitis. Gastroenterology 1984; 22:373–8.
83. Hunt RH, Howden CW, Jones DB, et al. The correlation between acid suppression and peptic ulcer healing. Scand J Gastroenterol 1986; 21(Suppl 125):22–9.
84. Bader JP, Stanescu L. Problems with patient compliance in peptic ulcer therapy. In: Hunt RH, ed. Advances in acid peptic disorders. J Clin Gastroenterol 1989; 11(Suppl 1):S25–8.
85. Gledhill T, Buck M, Hunt RH. Effect of no treatment, cimetidine 1 g/day, cimetidine 2 g/day and cimetidine combined with atropine on nocturnal acid secretion in cimetidine non-responders. Gut 1984; 25:1211–6.
86. Hunt RH. Non-responders to cimetidine treatment. In: Baron JH, ed. Cimetidine in the 80's. Edinburgh: Churchill Livingston, 1981: 331–41.
87. Bardhan KD. Non-responders to cimetidine treatment. In: Baron JH, ed. Cimetidine in the 80's. Edinburgh: Churchill Livingston, 1981:42–57.
88. Gledhill T, Buck M, Hunt RH. Cimetidine or vagotomy? Comparison of the effects of proximal gastric vagotomy, cimetidine or placebo on nocturnal intragastric acidity and acid secretion in patients with cimetidine-resistant duodenal ulcers. Br J Surg 1983; 70:704–6.
89. Bardhan KD. Refractory duodenal ulcer. Gut 1984; 25:711–7.
90. Anon. Cimetidine resistant duodenal ulcers [editorial]. Lancet 1985; i:23–4.
91. Piper DW. The refractory ulcer. World J Surg 1987; 11:268–73.
92. Pounder RE. What is an intractable duodenal ulcer and how should it be managed? Aliment Pharmacol Ther 1987; 1:439–46.
93. Walt RP, Danashmend TK. Resistant duodenal ulcers: when, why and, what not to do? Post Grad Med J 1988; 64:369–72.
94. Chiverton SG, Hunt RH. Smoking and peptic ulcer disease. In: Hunt RH, ed. Advances in acid peptic disorders. J Clin Gastroenterol 1989; 11(1):S29–33.
95. Domschke W, Lam SK, Pounder RE, Anderson D. H$_2$-Blocker resistant duodenal ulceration. Gastroenterol Int 1989; 2:85–91.
96. Rademaker JW, Hunt RH. Refractory duodenal ulcer. In: Benjamin SB, Collen MJ, eds. Pharmacology of peptic ulcer disease. 1991 (in press).
97. Freston JW. H$_2$-Receptor antagonists and duodenal ulcer recurrence: analysis of efficacy and commentary on safety, costs and patient selection. Am J Gastroenterol 1987; 82:1242–9.
98. Boyd EJS, Penston JG, Johnston KA, Wormsley KG. Does maintenance therapy keep duodenal ulcers healed? Lancet 1988; ii:134–7.
99. Hunt RH. Acid suppression and ulcer healing: dichotomy, degree, and dilemma. Am J Gastroenterol 1988; 83:964–6.
100. Collen MJ, Stanczak VJ, Ciarleglio CA. Refractory duodenal ulcers (non healing duodenal ulcers with standard doses of antisecretory medication). Dig Dis Sci 1989; 34:233–7.

101. Quatrini M, Basilico G, Bianchi PA. Treatment of cimetidine resistant chronic duodenal ulcers with ranitidine or cimetidine. Gut 1984; 25:1113–7.

102. Lam SK, Lee NW, Koo J, Hui WM, Fok K, Ng M. Randomized crossover trial of tripotassium dicitrato bismuthate versus high dose cimetidine for duodenal ulcers resistant to standard doses of cimetidine. Gut 1984; 25:703–6.

103. Bianchi-Porro G, Parente F, Lazzaroni M. Tripotassium dicitrato bismuthate versus two different dosages of cimetidine in the treatment of resistant duodenal ulcers. Gut 1987; 28:907–11.

104. Lam SK. Heterogeneous nature of hyperacidity in duodenal ulcer. In: Kreuning J, Samloff IM, Rotter JI, Eriksson AW, eds. Pepsinogens in man: clinical and genetic advances. Progress in clin biol res 173. New York: Liss, 1985:255–71.

105. Collen MJ. Idiopathic gastric acid hypersecretory states. Gastroenterology 1989; 96: A93.

106. Chiverton SG, Hunt RH. Initial therapy and relapse of duodenal ulcer: possible acid secretory mechanisms. Gastroenterology 1989; 96:632–9.

107. Aadland E, Berstad A, Semb LS. Effect of cimetidine on pentagastrin stimulated acid secretion in healthy man. Scand J Gastroenterol 1977; 12:501–6.

108. Aadland E, Berstad A. Parietal and chief cell sensitivity to histamine and pentagastrin stimulation before and after ranitidine treatment in healthy subjects. Scand J Gastroenterol 1986; 21:119–22.

109. Prichard PJ, Jones DB, Yeomans ND, et al. The effectiveness of ranitidine in reducing gastric acid secretion decreases with continued therapy. Br J Clin Pharmacol 1986; 22:663–8.

110. Marks IN, Young GO. Acid secretory response and parietal cell sensitivity in patients with duodenal ulcer before and after healing with sucralfate or ranitidine. S Afr Med J 1988; 73:660.

111. Jones DB, Howden CW, Burget DW, Kerr GD, Hunt RH. Acid suppression in duodenal ulcer: a meta-analysis to define optimal dosing with antisecretory drugs. Gut 1987; 28:1120–7.

112. Smith JLT, Gavey CJ, Nwokolo CU, Pounder RE. Tolerance during eight days H_2-blockade: placebo controlled studies of 24 hour acidity and gastrin. Gut 1989; 30: 1487.

113. Nwokolo CU, Gavey CJ, Smith JLT, et al. Tolerance during 29 days of conventional dosing with cimetidine, nizatidine, famotidine or ranitidine. Gut 1989; 30:1487.

114. Nwokolo CU, Smith JLT, Sawyer VA, et al. Intravenous pentagastrin can overcome H_2-blockade in man: a possible mechanism for tolerance. Gut 1989; 30:1487.

115. Nwokolo CU, Smith JLT, Pounder RE. Rebound intragastric acidity following dosing with cimetidine, nizatidine and famotidine. Gastroenterology 1989; 96:369.

116. Wilder-Smith CH, Ernst T, Gennoni M, et al. Acute tolerance to H_2-receptor antagonists. Gut 1989; 30:1489.

117. Lanzon-Miller S, Pounder RE, Hamilton MR, et al. Twenty-four hour intragastric acidity and plasma gastrin concentration before and during treatment with either ranitidine or omeprazole. Aliment Pharmacol Ther 1987; 1:239–51.

118. Pounder RE. Drug induced changes in plasma gastrin concentration. In: Hunt RH, ed. Peptic ulcer. North Am Clin Gastroenterol 1990; 19:141–53.

119. Richardson CT. Effect of H_2-receptor antagonists on gastric acid secretion and serum gastrin concentration: a review. Gastroenterology 1978; 74:366–70.

120. Hunt RH, Melvin MA, Mills JG. Gastric function after treatment with cimetidine. In: Torsoli A, Luccheli PE, Brimblecombe RW, eds. H$_2$-Antagonists. H$_2$-receptor antagonists in peptic ulcer disease and progress in histamine research. Amsterdam: Excerpta Medica, 1980:119–30.

121. Fullarton AM, McLaughlin G, MacDonald A, et al. Rebound nocturnal hypersecretion after four weeks treatment with an H$_2$-receptor antagonist. Gut 1989; 30:449–54.

122. Bardhan KD, Thompson M, Bose K, et al. Combined anti-muscarinic and H$_2$-receptor blockade in the healing of refractory duodenal ulcer. A double blind study. Gut 1987; 28:1505–9.

123. Pickard WR, MacKay C. Early results of surgery in patients considered cimetidine failures. Br J Surg 1984; 71:67–8.

124. Hansen JH, Knigge U. Failure of proximal gastric vagotomy for duodenal ulcer resistant to cimetidine. Lancet 1984; ii:84–6.

125. Primrose JN, Axon ATR, Johnston D. Highly selective vagotomy and duodenal ulcers that fail to respond to H$_2$-receptor antagonists. Br Med J 1988; 296:1031–5.

126. Anderson D, Amdrup E, Hanberg Sorenesk F. Parietal cell vagotomy in patients resistant to cimetidine. 1990; in press.

127. Chiverton SG, Burget DW, Hunt RH. Smoking and peptic ulcer—a meta-analysis. Gastroenterology 1988; 94:A69. Abstract.

128. Peura DA, Johnson LF. Cimetidine for prevention and treatment of gastroduodenal mucosal lesions in patients in an intensive care unit. Ann Intern Med 1985; 103:173–7.

129. Hastings PR, Skillman JJ, Bushnell LS, et al. Antacid titration in the prevention of acute gastrointestinal bleeding: a controlled randomized trial in 100 critically ill patients. N Engl J Med 1978; 298:1041–5.

130. Wilcox CM, Spenney JG. Stress ulcer prophylaxis in medial patients: who, what and how much? Am J Gastroenterol 1988; 83:1199–211.

131. Priebe JH, Skillman JJ, Bushnell LS, Long PC, Silen W. Antacid versus cimetidine in preventing acute gastrointestinal bleeding: a randomized trial in 75 critically ill patients. N Engl J Med 1980; 302:426–30.

132. MacDougall BRD, Bailey AJ, Williams R. H$_2$ Antagonists and antacids in the prevention of acute gastrointestinal haemorrhage in fulminant hepatic failure. Lancet 1977; i:617–8.

133. MacDougall BRD, Williams R. H$_2$-Receptor antagonist in the prevention of acute upper gastrointestinal haemorrhage in fulminant hepatic failure. Gastroenterology 1978; 74:464–5.

134. Merki HS, Ernst T, Zeyen B, et al. Individualized intragastric pH control using a computerized feedback infusion pump (PIP). Gastroenterology 1989; 96:A341. Abstract.

135. Tryba M, Zerounou F, Wruk G. Stress bleeding and pneumonia in patients under postoperative intensive care receiving ranitidine or pirenzepine. Dtsch Med Wochenschr 1988; 113:930–6.

136. Van Saene HKF, Stoutenbeck CP, Miranda DR, Zandstra DF. A novel approach to infection control in the intensive care unit. Acta Anaesthesiol Belg 1983; 3:193–208.

137. Craven DE, Kunches LM, Kilinsky V, et al. Risk factors for pneumonia and fatality in patients receiving continuous mechanical ventilation. Am Rev Resp Dis 1986; 133:792–6.

138. Driks MR, Craven DE, Celli BR, et al. Nosocomial pneumonia in intubated given sucralfate as compared with antacids or histamine type 2 blocker. N Engl J Med 1987; 317:1376–82.

139. Langman MJS. Upper gastrointestinal bleeding: the trials of trials. Gut 1985; 26:217–20.

140. Collins R, Langman M. Treatment with histamine H_2 antagonists in acute upper gastrointestinal haemorrhage. Implications of randomized trials. N Engl J Med 1985; 313:660–6.

141. Langman MJS. H_2 Antagonists in the treatment of upper gastrointestinal bleeding. Scand J Gastroenterol 1988; 23(Suppl 146):185–90.

142. Walt RP, Male PJ, Rawlings J, Hunt RH, Milton-Thompson GJ, Misiewicz JJ. Comparison of the effects of ranitidine, cimetidine and placebo on the 24 hour intragastric acidity and nocturnal acid secretion in patients with duodenal ulcer. Gut 1981; 22:49–54.

143. Green FW, Kaplan MM, Curtis LE, et al. Effect of acid and pepsin on blood coagulation and platelet aggregation: a possible contributor to prolonged gastroduodenal mucosal haemorrhage. Gastroenterology 1978; 74:38–43.

144. Walt RP, Gomes MdeFA, Wood EC, Logan LH, Pounder RE. Effect of daily oral omeprazole on 24 hour intragastric acidity. Br Med J 1983; 287:12–4.

145. Peterson WL. Pharmacotherapy of bleeding peptic ulcer—is it time to give up the search? Gastroenterology 1989; 97:796–7.

146. Langman MJS. Ulcer and ulcer complications from non-steroidal anti-inflammatory drugs: what is the risk? Aliment Pharmacol Therap 1988; 2S:27–31.

147. McCarthy DM. Nonsteroidal anti-inflammatory drug-induced ulcers: management by traditional therapies. Gastroenterology 1989; 96:662–74.

148. Croker JR, Cotton PB, Boyle AC, Kinsella P. Cimetidine for peptic ulcer in patients with arthritis. Ann Rheum Dis 1980; 39:275–8.

149. LoIudice TA, Saleem T, Lang JA. Cimetidine in the treatment of gastric ulcer induced by steroidal and nonsteroidal anti-inflammatory agents. Am J Gastroenterol 1981; 75:104–10.

150. Davies J, Collins AJ, Dixon AStJ. The influence of cimetidine on peptic ulcer in patients with arthritis taking anti-inflammatory drugs. Br J Rheumatol 1986; 25:54–8.

151. Manniche C, Malchow-Moller A, Andersen JR, et al. Randomised study of the influence of non-steroidal anti-inflammatory drugs on the treatment of peptic ulcer in patients with rheumatic disease. Gut 1987; 28:226–9.

152. Welch RW, Bentch L, Harris SC. Reduction of aspirin-induced gastrointestinal bleeding with cimetidine. Gastroenterology 1978; 74:459–63.

153. Hawkey CJ, Somerville KW, Marshall S. Human gastric mucosal protection by ranitidine. Gastroenterology 1986; 90:1454. Abstract.

154. MacKerecher PA, Ivey KJ, Baskin WN, Krause WJ. Protective effect of cimetidine on aspirin-induced gastric mucosal damage. Arch Intern Med 1977; 87:676–9.

155. Berkowitz JM, Rogenes PR, Sharp JT, Warner CW. Ranitidine protects against gastroduodenal mucosal damage associated with chronic aspirin therapy. Arch Intern Med 1987; 147:2137–9.

156. Bianchi-Porro G, Caruso I. Why are non-steroidal anti-inflammatory drugs important in peptic ulceration? Aliment Pharmacol Ther 1987; 1:540–7S.

157. Graham DY, Agrawal NM, Roth SH. Prevention of NSAID-induced gastric ulcer with misoprostol: multicentre, double-blind, placebo-controlled trial. Lancet 1988; ii: 1277–80.

158. Howden CW. Review: interactions between H$_2$-antagonists and non-steroidal anti-inflammatory drugs. Aliment Pharmacol Ther 1988; 2:93–100.

159. Bardhan KD, Cole DS, Hawkins BW, Franks CR. Does treatment with cimetidine extended beyond initial healing of duodenal ulcer reduce the subsequent relapse rate? Br Med J 1982; 284:621–3.

160. Van Deventer GM, Elashoff JD, Reedy TJ, Schneidman D, Walsh JH. A randomized study of maintenance therapy with ranitidine to prevent the recurrence of duodenal ulcer. N Engl J Med 1989; 320:1113–9.

161. Silvis SE. Final report on the United States multicenter trial comparing ranitidine to cimetidine as maintenance therapy following healing of duodenal ulcer. J Clin Gastroenterol 1985; 7:482–7.

162. Gough KR, Korman MG, Bardhan KD, et al. Ranitidine and cimetidine in prevention of duodenal ulcer relapse. A double-blind, randomised, multicentre comparative trial. Lancet 1984; ii:659–62.

163. Howden CW. Maintenance treatment with H$_2$ receptor antagonists in patients with peptic ulcer disease: rarely justified in terms of cost or patient benefit. Br Med J 1988; 297:1393–4.

164. Wormsley KG. Maintenance treatment with H$_2$-receptor antagonists in patients with peptic ulcer disease: reduces morbidity in a significant minority of patients. Br Med J 1988; 297:1392–4.

165. Wade AG, Rowley-Jones D. Long term management of duodenal ulcer in general practice: how best to use cimetidine? Br Med J 1988; 296:971–4.

166. Ehsanullah RSB, Page MC, Tildesley G, Wood JR. Prevention of gastroduodenal damage induced by nonstandard anti-inflammatory drugs trial of rantidine. Br Med J 1988; 297:1017–21.

167. Bardhan KD. Intermittent treatment of duodenal ulcer with cimetidine. Br Med J 1980; 281:20–2.

168. Bardhan KD. Intermittent treatment of duodenal ulcer for long term medical management. Postgrad Med J 1988; 64(Suppl 1):40–6.

169. Sontag S, Graham DY, Belsito A, et al. Cimetidine, cigarette smoking, and recurrence of duodenal ulcer. N Engl J Med 1984; 311:689–93.

170. Wolosin JD, Gertler SL, Peterson WL, Sanderfeld MA, Isenberg JI. Gastric ulcer recurrence: follow-up of a double-blind, placebo-controlled trial. J Clin Gastroenterol 1989; 11:12–6.

171. Miller TA. Gastric ulcer management: is long-term maintenance therapy necessary? Gastroenterology 1989; 97:803–4.

172. Sontag S. Current status of maintenance therapy in peptic ulcer disease. Am J Gastroenterol 1988; 83:607–17.

173. Howden CW, Jones DB, Hunt RH. Nocturnal doses of H$_2$-receptor antagonists for duodenal ulcer. Lancet 1985; i:647–8.

174. Morton DM. Pharmacology and toxicology of nizatidine. Scand J Gastroenterol 1987; 22(Suppl 136):1–8.

10

Therapy with Omeprazole, an Acid Pump Inhibitor

ANDERS WALAN

AB Hässle, Mölndal, Sweden

I. INTRODUCTION

The presence of acid is a prerequisite for the development of duodenal ulcer, gastric ulcer, and reflux esophagitis. Traditional therapies for acid-related diseases therefore include antacids, receptor antagonists, and surgery aimed at reducing acid secretion.

The parietal cell in the oxyntic part of the stomach is the source of the hydrochloric acid of the gastric secretion. There are three types of stimulatory receptors on the basolateral membrane of the parietal cell (Fig. 1). They react to stimulation by histamine, gastrin, and acetylcholine, respectively. Stimulation of the histamine receptor leads to activation of an adenylate cyclase system within the parietal cell. Stimulation of both the gastrin receptor and the muscarinic acetylcholine receptor is followed by an increase in cytosolic free calcium concentration. Subsequent steps in the process leading to acid secretion involve the stimulation of protein kinases, which phosphorylate regulatory proteins. Ultimately the regulation of acid secretion is achieved by changing the activity of a unique enzyme, an H^+/K^+-ATPase (the acid pump or proton pump) that uses the energy derived from splitting ATP to transport protons from the cytosol out of the cell into the lumen of the canaliculi in exchange for potassium (K^+) ions [1,2]. Separate channels account for the secretion of KCl from the cytosol to the lumen in the intracellular canaliculi. These processes are very energy-dependent, as the movement of the hydrogen ions occurs against a concentration gradient of several million (from pH 7.4 to pH 0.8) and the movement of the potassium ions occurs against a concentration gradient that is about tenfold.

217

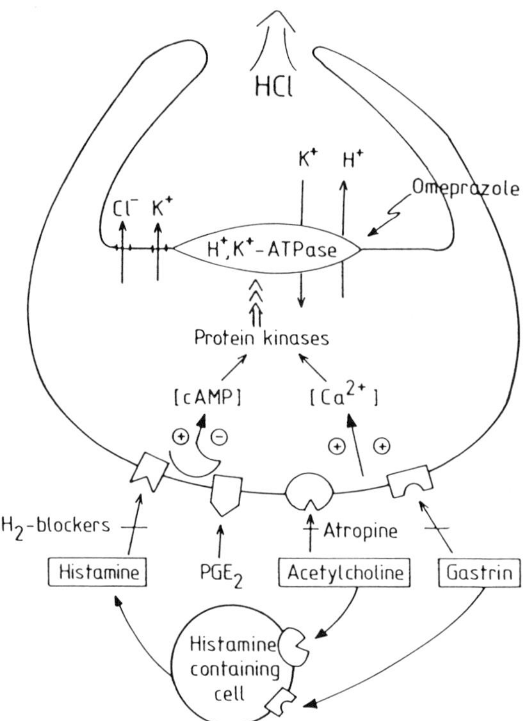

FIGURE 1 The mechanisms for stimulation and inhibition of hydrochloric acid secretion in the parietal cell.

Omeprazole is a substituted benzimidazole and is a weak base ($pK_a = 4.0$). After absorption in the small intestine, omeprazole will therefore be charged and trapped within the acid compartments of the parietal cell ($pH < 1.0$). Protonation of omeprazole causes a molecular rearrangement that transforms it from an inactive to an active form, a sulfenamide that then reacts with two cysteine SH groups on the luminal face of the H^+/K^+-ATPase [3] (Fig. 2). This covalent complex between the enzyme and the activated drug inhibits the enzyme so that no transport of protons can occur. Following inhibition of the acid pumps by omeprazole, normal resynthesis of the H^+/K^+-ATPase restores about one-third of the acid secretory capacity within 24 hr after each dose [4]. The duration of the inhibition is partly dependent on the life span of the enzyme, which has a half-life of 30–48 hr.

II. EFFECT OF OMEPRAZOLE ON ACID SECRETION

Omeprazole degrades rapidly in an acid environment. A formulation with enteric-coated granules in a gelatin capsule has therefore been developed to enable it to pass

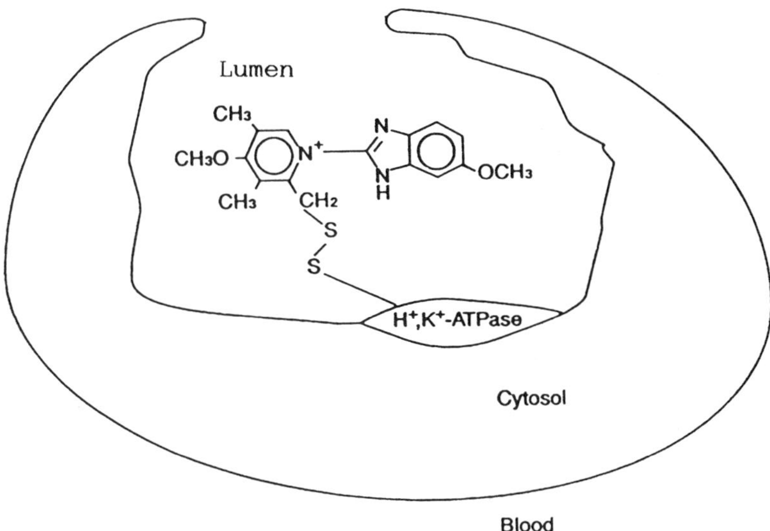

FIGURE 2   The structure of the final enzyme–inhibitor complex.

through the stomach. Omeprazole is then absorbed in the small intestine and transported to the parietal cell, where it is transformed to the active metabolite. This explains why there is no correlation between the actual concentration of omeprazole at a given moment and the degree of inhibition of acid secretion. There is, however, a correlation between the degree of acid inhibition and the area under the plasma concentration–time curve of omeprazole.

Omeprazole has a very long duration of action. When a single oral dose of 40 mg of omeprazole was given as a suspension with bicarbonate, pentagastrin-stimulated acid secretion was diminished by 90% during the second hour after administration and by 17% 72 hr after administration [4]. The bioavailability of a single oral dose of omeprazole in a capsule with enteric-coated granules is about 35%; this increases with repeated doses to about 60% [5]. The long duration of action and the increasing bioavailability with repeated doses explain why the effect of omeprazole on acid secretion increases during the first 3–4 days of treatment. After that time, during continuous treatment, the effect on gastric acid secretion and intragastric acidity is stable. With repeated daily dosing with omeprazole 20 mg, basal acid output is reduced by about 90% at 24 hr after the last dose, at which time pentagastrin-stimulated secretion is decreased by about 70% [6]. Intragastric acidity measured over 24 hr has often been used to express the effect of regimens used for treatment of peptic ulcer disease. Omeprazole causes a dose-dependent decrease of intragastric acidity. After repeated doses of 20 mg daily, the mean decrease in 24-hr intragastric acidity is about 80% [7]. Thus, treatment with omeprazole once daily does not induce achlorhydria. Systemically available omeprazole is rapidly eliminated with a plasma clearance of 400–600 mL/min and a $t^{1/2}$ of 0.5 hr [8]. Elimination occurs exclusively by biotransformation. Metabolites are eliminated by urinary excretion (80%) and biliary excretion (20%).

Pharmacokinetic parameters have also been investigated in elderly individuals, in patients with renal insufficiency, and in patients with hepatic impairment. In the elderly, the bioavailability is slightly higher and the plasma clearance slightly lower than in young healthy individuals or in duodenal ulcer patients. Except for a somewhat increased bioavailability, pharmacokinetic parameters in patients with renal impairment did not differ from those in duodenal ulcer patients. In patients with hepatic dysfunction, oral omeprazole was completely bioavailable and plasma $t^{1/2}$ was 2–3 hr. As the duration of effect of omeprazole is mainly regulated by resynthesis of new enzyme, this difference in pharmacokinetic profile will not lead to any change in dose recommendation in patients with decreased hepatic function.

III. EFFECT OF OMEPRAZOLE ON SECRETION OF INTRINSIC FACTOR AND PEPSIN

Intrinsic factor is also secreted from the parietal cell in humans. As omeprazole in the parietal cell acts only at the H^+/K^+-ATPase, that is, at the final site for acid production, treatment with omeprazole does not influence the secretion of intrinsic factor [9]. The secretion of pepsin is partly dependent on the flow through the gastric glands. Intravenous administration of omeprazole therefore caused a clear but short-lasting (a few hours) decrease in pepsin secretion. No changes in pentagastrin-stimulated pepsin output was seen 24 hr after seven daily doses of 40 mg of omeprazole [9].

In toxicological studies with omeprazole, some rats treated continuously with moderate to high doses of omeprazole developed carcinoids in the oxyntic part of the stomach. These carcinoids were found to consist of ECL cells. The development of an increase in ECL cells has been found to be correlated to an increase in serum gastrin concentration. Similar carcinoids have been observed in rats after administration of H_2 antagonists such as loxtidine and ranitidine and also in rats in whom a partial fundectomy had been performed. Thus the development of carcinoids was not caused by the drug itself but by the increase in gastrin consequent to lifelong increases in serum gastrin concentration.

Investigations of the gastric mucosa for detection of possible proliferation of endocrine cells have also been performed in patients who were treated with omeprazole for prolonged periods, some of them for many years. No carcinoids or marked proliferation of gastric endocrine cells were observed [10].

Omeprazole has not been found to have any effect in the gastrointestinal tract or in other organ systems other than those that can be ascribed to a decrease in acid secretion.

IV. EFFECT OF OMEPRAZOLE ON ACID-RELATED DISEASES

A. Duodenal Ulcer

1. Healing

A series of dose-finding studies in patients with active duodenal ulcer disease showed that with a daily dose of omeprazole of at least 20 mg, very high healing rates could be observed after treatment for 4 weeks [11].

The results from many studies have now been reported in which omeprazole in doses between 20 and 40 mg once daily were compared with cimetidine in doses varying between 400 mg and 600 mg twice daily or with ranitidine 150 mg twice daily or 300 mg at night (Table 1).

In these studies healing was assessed at 2 weeks and, in patients not healed at this time, also at 4 weeks and in three studies up to 8 weeks. The healing rates at 2 weeks in all but one of these comparisons were higher in patients randomized to treatment with omeprazole (range 58–86%) than with cimetidine (range 33–49%) or ranitidine (range 45–65%).

Also, at 4 weeks the healing rates were higher with omeprazole (range 84–100%) than with cimetidine (range 61–85%) in all but one of the comparisons. In one study the healing rates at 4 weeks with omeprazole and cimetidine were equal (85%).

In the comparisons between omeprazole and ranitidine, the healing rates at 4 weeks with omeprazole varied between 92 and 100% and with ranitidine between 82 and 93%. Higher healing rates were seen with omeprazole in all but one of the comparisons.

Figures 3 and 4 show the percentage difference in healing rates at 2 and 4 weeks and the confidence limits of this difference in the studies in patients with duodenal ulcer in which omeprazole was compared with ranitidine or cimetidine. The majority of the patients who were not healed after treatment for 4 weeks with omeprazole were smokers. Continued treatment for a further 2- or 4-week period resulted in healing in almost all patients receiving omeprazole, whereas 4–5% were still unhealed in patients randomized to H_2-receptor antagonists.

In some studies the influence of prognostic factors on healing rates has been investigated.

Ulcer Size.   Both with omeprazole and with H_2-receptor antagonists, ulcer size has a strong influence on healing rate; large ulcers take longer to heal than smaller ones. Overall, with omeprazole, 52% of large ulcers (larger than 10 mm in diameter) were healed within 2 weeks compared with 35% with H_2-receptor antagonists. The healing rate at 4 weeks in patients with large ulcers randomized to omeprazole was 80% compared to 68% of patients with large ulcers randomized to H_2-receptor antagonists.

Smoking.   It is a well-known fact that ulcer healing is slower in smokers than in nonsmokers. With omeprazole, the healing rates at 2 weeks were lower in smokers than in nonsmokers (67% versus 84%) but higher than in smokers treated with H_2-

Table 1 Duodenal Ulcer: Double-Blind Comparisons of Omeprazole with the H_2-Receptor Antagonists Ranitidine and Cimetidine

				Ulcer healing[b] (%)	
Reference	Drug[a]	n	Dose (mg)	2 wk	4 wk
Hui et al. [23]	Ome	83	10	77	95
	Ome	87	20	86	96
	Ran	84	150 bid	63†	93
Archambault et al. [24]	Ome	85	20	58	84
	Cim	84	600 bid	46	80
Bader et al. [25]	Ome	144	20	65	90
	Cim	154	400 bid	44†	79*
Crowe et al. [26]	Ome	98	20	62	85
	Cim	91	800 hs	33†	61†
Classen et al. [27]	Ome	168	20	72	95
	Ran	166	150 bid	60*	91
Mulder et al. [28]	Ome	91	20	63	91
	Ran	90	150 mg × 2	65	96
McFarland et al. [29]	Ome	125	20	79	91
	Ran	122	150 mg × 2	61†	80†
Chelvam et al. [30]	Ome	114	20	75	97
	Ran	115	300 hs	46‡	83‡
Marks et al. [31]	Ome	81	20	78	97
	Ran	79	300 hs	45†	82†
Bardhan et al. [32]	Ome	34	20	83	97
	Ome	36	40	83	100
	Ran	35	150 bid	53†	82†
Dahlgren et al. [33]	Ome	78	30	66	97
	Cim	73	400 bid	45*	84*
Hallberg et al. [34]	Ome	71	30	71	92
	Ran	72	150 bid	55	87
Lauritsen et al. [14]	Ome	67	30	72	92
	Cim	65	200 tds + 400 hs	46†	74†
Gustavsson et al. [35]	Ome	45	40	76	98
	Cim	43	400 bid	40‡	71†
Hetzel et al. [36]	Ome	48	40	82	100
	Cim	49	400 bid	49*	80*

[a]Ome = omeprazole; Ran = ranitidine; Cim = cimetidine.
[b]Significance: *p < .05; †p < .01; ‡p < .001.

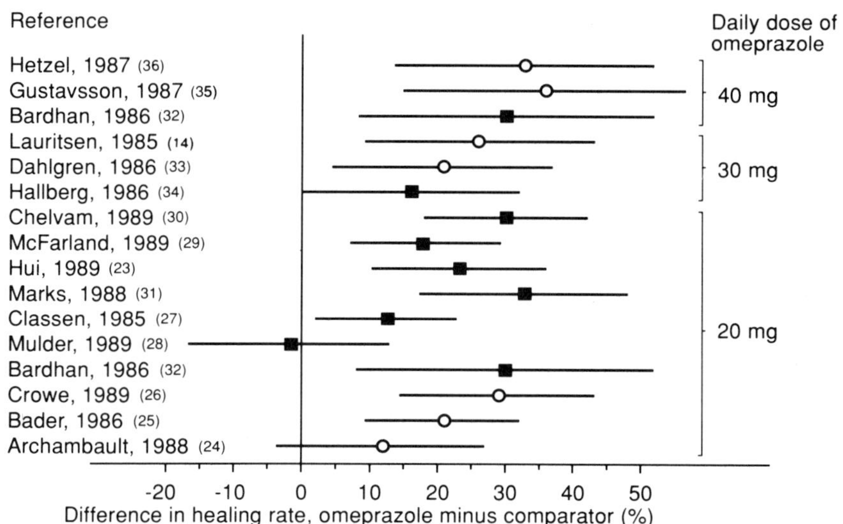

FIGURE 3 Difference in healing rate in duodenal ulcers at 2 weeks (95% confidence limits) between omeprazole and the H_2-receptor antagonists cimetidine (O) and ranitidine (■).

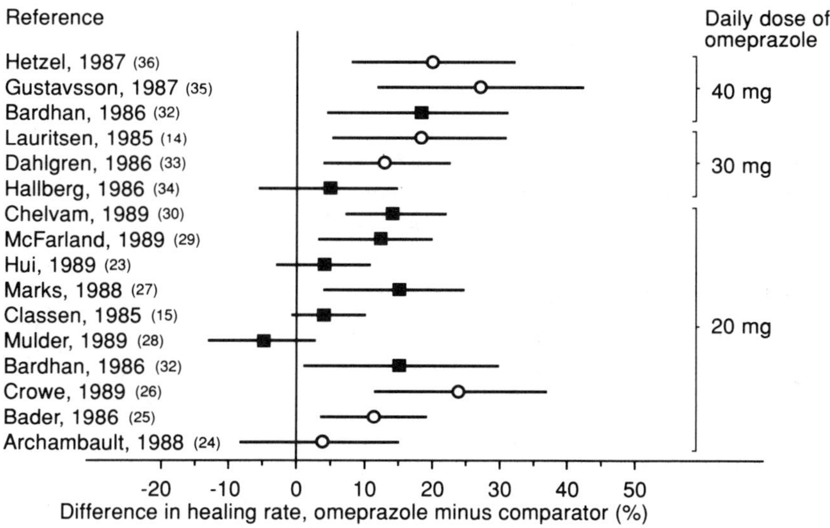

FIGURE 4 Difference in healing rate in duodenal ulcers at 4 weeks (95% confidence limits) between omeprazole and the H_2-receptor antagonists cimetidine (O) and ranitidine (■).

receptor antagonists and even higher than for nonsmokers receiving H_2-receptor antagonists.

Age. There has been a trend toward slightly faster healing in patients older than 65 years, probably reflecting a slightly higher bioavailability and lower elimination rate of omeprazole in elderly patients.

Gender and Alcohol Consumption. These factors have not been found to influence healing rates in patients treated with omeprazole.

2. Pain Relief

Since the institution of treatment with omeprazole or H_2-receptor antagonists, the degree of pain and frequency of attacks with pain have decreased rapidly, most often during the first 2 weeks. In several studies comparing omeprazole and H_2-receptor antagonists, the time to complete pain relief was investigated. The frequency of patients experiencing complete pain relief at 2 weeks was found to be 71% with omeprazole and 59% with ranitidine ($p < .001$). Both drugs gave equal relief of nocturnal pain [11].

3. Resistant Ulcers

A resistant ulcer has been defined as an ulcer that has not healed with treatment for at least 8 weeks at recommended doses. The effect of omeprazole 40 mg daily has been compared to continued or increased doses of H_2-receptor antagonists.

In one study by Bardhan et al. [12], patients were randomized to continued treatment with the same dose of H_2-receptor antagonists (cimetidine or ranitidine) or to omeprazole 40 mg daily. At endoscopy after 4 weeks, 39% of patients on ranitidine or cimetidine had healed compared to 87% of patients on omeprazole ($p < .001$), and at 8 weeks the healing rates were 60% and 98%, respectively ($p < .001$). Symptom relief was also faster and more pronounced in the omeprazole group.

Bardhan and colleagues also performed a study with omeprazole in so-called ultrarefractory ulcers [13], ulcers that had not healed after treatment for at least 12 weeks with increased doses of H_2-receptor antagonists. After treatment with omeprazole 40 mg daily for 1 month, 85% of the patients were healed, compared to 54% of patients with continued treatment with cimetidine either 2 or 3 g daily. The corresponding figures at 8 weeks were 92% and 67% ($p < .05$).

4. Relapse Rate after Discontinuation of Treatment

The relapse rate after healing of a duodenal ulcer was investigated in some trials. Ideally, all patients randomized to treatment should be followed independently of whether or not healing was achieved within the scheduled observation period. This was not, however, the case in these trials; only patients who were healed within 4–8 weeks were included in the follow-up. It has been the experience from many studies that patients who are slow or difficult to heal have a greater recurrence rate off treatment. Omeprazole healed more patients than H_2-receptor antagonists; almost all patients on omeprazole healed and would therefore also have a greater tendency to relapse. In the follow-up studies reported so far, only patients who healed during initial treatment were followed. Despite this fact, there was not any tendency for an increased recurrence rate during the first 6 months off treatment in patients healed with omeprazole compared to patients healed on ranitidine or cimetidine [14].

B. Gastric Ulcer

There have been several studies in which omeprazole in the clinically recommended doses was compared with ranitidine and cimetidine in patients with gastric ulcers. In the first of these studies, Classen et al. [15] compared omeprazole 20 mg daily with ranitidine 150 mg twice daily. High healing rates were observed in this study. At 4 weeks 81% and 80% healed with omeprazole and ranitidine, respectively. The healing rates at 8 weeks were 89% and 85% with omeprazole and ranitidine, respectively. In this study, patients with ulcers smaller than 5 mm in diameter were included. The study did not disclose any significant difference between the results of the two treatment regimens.

In a study by Bate et al. [16], omeprazole 20 mg daily was compared with cimetidine 400 mg twice daily. The healing rate at 4 weeks was 73% with omeprazole and 55% ($p < .05$) with cimetidine. After 8 weeks, 81% and 60% ($p < .01$) of patients randomized to omeprazole and cimetidine, respectively, were healed.

In a study by Barbara et al. [17], patients were randomized to treatment with omeprazole 20 mg every morning or 150 mg twice daily. In this study, endoscopies were performed after 2 weeks. The observed healing rates of 35%, 74%, and 96% with omeprazole and 9%, 53%, and 85% with ranitidine at 2, 4, and 8 weeks, respectively, were significantly different each time.

The largest study of gastric ulcers was an international multicenter study of 602 patients randomized to omeprazole 20 mg, omeprazole 40 mg, or ranitidine 150 mg twice daily [18]. At 4 weeks, 69% of the patients in the omeprazole 20 mg group were healed compared to 80% in the omeprazole 40 mg group and 59% in the ranitidine group. At 8 weeks, the corresponding figures were 89%, 96%, and 85%, respectively. After adjustment for an imbalance at entry in terms of ulcer size, both omeprazole groups produced significantly higher healing rates than the ranitidine group at 4 weeks, and the omeprazole 40 mg group had a significantly higher healing rate than the ranitidine group at 8 weeks. Ulcer symptoms were relieved faster on omeprazole.

This study also included a subgroup of patients with prepyloric ulcers. Such ulcers have often been found to be more resistant to treatment. Omeprazole 20 or 40 mg daily also showed a faster healing rate than treatment with ranitidine in patients with prepyloric ulcers.

In another subgroup of patients on continuous treatment with nonsteroidal anti-inflammatory drugs (NSAIDs), the healing rates with omeprazole 20 mg and 40 mg twice daily were 61% and 81%, respectively, at 4 weeks compared with 32% with ranitidine. At 8 weeks the healing rates were 82%, 95%, and 53% with omeprazole 20 or 40 mg twice daily and ranitidine 150 mg twice daily, respectively.

Patients were also followed during the first half-year period off treatment. During this period there was no increase in the recurrence rate in patients treated earlier with omeprazole compared with patients treated earlier with ranitidine.

C.   Reflux Esophagitis

The causes for the development of reflux esophagitis are several, including anatomical defects or changes and motor disorders resulting in a decreased tonus in the lower esophageal sphincter and/or decreased emptying from the lower esophagus and perhaps also decreased resistance in the esophageal mucosa. Independent of the individually most important factor, the result will be an increased exposure of the esophageal mucosa to gastrointestinal contents, which most often are very acidic. The esophageal mucosa is not equipped to withstand long-time exposure to high concentrations of acid and pepsin. Clinical evidence has also shown that the duration of exposure to high acidity is most crucial for the continuation of an inflammation, erosion, or ulcer. Treatment regimens that can reduce this time have also been found to result in increased healing of esophageal erosions or ulcers.

Omeprazole has been found to drastically decrease the duration of exposure to an acid milieu in the esophagus. In one investigation of patients with reflux esophagitis, the period with pH $<$ 4 over 24 hr was reduced from 11.2% without treatment to 3.1% with omeprazole 20 mg daily and to 0.7% with omeprazole 40 mg daily [19].

The influence of omeprazole on the healing of reflux esophagitis has also been investigated in several studies. In the first study in 64 patients with erosive or ulcerative esophagitis, patients were randomized to treatment with omeprazole 20 or 40 mg or placebo [20]. The healing rates after 4 weeks were 6% with placebo and 81% with omeprazole (code 20/40 mg not broken). The study was continued but now comparing only omeprazole 20 and 40 mg in a total of 164 patients. The healing rates after 4 weeks were 70% and 82% with omeprazole 20 and 40 mg, respectively, and after 8 weeks 79% and 85%. In parallel with a fast healing rate, a fast disappearance of symptoms was also observed. Since these initial studies were conducted, a large number of controlled studies comparing omeprazole in doses between 20 and 60 mg daily with cimetidine 1600 mg daily or ranitidine 300–600 mg daily have been published (Table 2). In all of these studies, the healing rates at 4, 8, and 12 weeks were higher with omeprazole, and in parallel the disappearance rate of heartburn was also faster than with the comparison therapy.

V.   LONG-TERM TREATMENT WITH OMEPRAZOLE

Omeprazole has also been used for long-term management of patients who did not respond to high-dose (450–600 mg) ranitidine. After treatment with omeprazole 40 mg daily until healing, these patients were offered long-term maintenance therapy

Table 2 Healing of Patients with Erosive or Ulcerative Reflux Esophagitis in Double-Blind Comparisons of Omeprazole with the H_2-Receptor Antagonists Ranitidine and Cimetidine

Reference	Drug[a]	n	Dose (mg)	Ulcer healing (%)		
				4 wk	8 wk	12 wk
Bate et al. [37]	Ome	137	20	56	71	
	Cim	133	1600	26[b]	35[b]	
Blum et al. [38]	Ome	79	20	77		
	Ran	83	300	55[b]		
Dehn et al. [39]	Ome	36	40	57	71	
	Cim	31	1600	29[b]	31[b]	
Havelund et al. [40]	Ome	80	40	74	86	90
	Ran	81	300	37[b]	54[b]	60[b]
Klinkenberg-Knol et al. [41]	Ome	25	60	76	88	
	Ran	26	300	27[b]	38[b]	
Lundell et al. [42]	Ome	51	40	63	86	90
	Ran	47	600	17[b]	38[b]	47[b]
Sandmark et al. [43]	Ome	73	20	67	85	
	Ran	77	300	31[b]	50[b]	
Vantrappen et al. [44]	Ome	26	40	85	96	
	Ran	25	300	40[b]	52[b]	
Zeitoun et al. [45]	Ome	76	20	81	95	
	Ran	80	300	45[b]	65[b]	

[a]Ome = omeprazole; Cim = cimetidine; Ran = ranitidine.
[b]Significance: $p < .01$

with the same dose for 5 years [21]. Fifty-nine of these patients had been treated for between 1 and 4 years. During maintenance therapy, no relapses occurred and no changes in the morphology of the gastric mucosa were observed.

Similar experience was reported for patients with reflux esophagitis resistant to H_2-receptor antagonists [22].

Inhibition of the acid secretion at the final site for acid production, the H^+/K^+-ATPase in the parietal cell, has thus been observed to induce unprecedented high healing rates in duodenal ulcer, gastric ulcer, and reflux esophagitis with concomitant reduction in symptoms of peptic ulcer or reflux esophagitis.

REFERENCES

1. Ganser AL, Forte JG. K^+-Stimulated ATPase in purified microsomes of bullfrog oxyntic cells. Biochim Biophys Acta 1973; 307:169–80.
2. Saccomani G, Helander HF, Crago S, Chang HH, Sachs G. Characterization of gastric

mucosal membranes. X. Immunological studies of gastric ($H^+ + K^+$)-ATPase. J Cell Biol 1979; 83:271–83.

3. Lindberg P, Nordberg P, Alminger T, Brändström A, Wallmark B. The mechanism of action of the gastric acid secretion inhibitor omeprazole. J Med Chem 1986; 29:1327–9.

4. Lind T, Cederberg C, Ekenved G, Haglund U, Olbe L. Effect of omeprazole—a gastric proton pump inhibitor—on pentagastrin stimulated acid secretion in man. Gut 1983; 24:270–6.

5. Andrén K, Andersson T, Cederberg C, Skånberg I, Regårdh CG. Omeprazole pharmacokinetics during repeated oral administration. Annual Pharmaceutical Congress, Stockholm, Sweden 1985; 112. Abstract 32.

6. Müller P, Seitz HK, Simon B, Dammann HG, Feurle G, Huefner M, Lichtwald K, Schmidt-Gayk H. Vierwöchige Omeprazol-Gabe: Einfluss auf Säureverhalten und basale Hormonspeigel. Z Gastroenterol 1984; 22:236–40.

7. Naesdal J, Bodemar G, Walan A, Effect of omeprazole, a substituted benzimidazole, on 24-h intragastric acidity in patients with peptic ulcer disease. Scand J Gastroenterol 1984; 19:916–22.

8. Regårdh CG, Gabrielsson M, Hoffman KJ, Löfberg I, Skånberg I. Pharmacokinetics and metabolism of omeprazole in animals and man—an overview. Scand J Gastroenterol 1985; 20(Suppl 108):79–94.

9. Kittang E, Aadland E, Schjønsby H. Effect of omeprazole on the secretion of intrinsic factor, gastric acid and pepsin in man. Gut 1985; 26:594–8.

10. Solcia E, Rindi G. Qualitative studies of gastric endocrine cells in patients treated long-term with omeprazole. International Symposium on omeprazole. Monaco, 11–12 November 1988:25.

11. Walan A. Omeprazole. Baillieres Clin Gastroenterol 1988; 2:629–40.

12. Bardhan KD, Naesdal J, Bianchi Porro G, et al. Omeprazole in the treatment of refractory peptic ulcer. Gastroenterology 1988; 94:A22.

13. Bardhan KD, Dhande D, Hinchliffe RFC, et al. Omeprazole in the treatment of ultrarefractory duodenal ulcer. Gastroenterology 1988; 94:A22.

14. Lauritsen K, Rune SJ, Bytzer P, et al. Effect of omeprazole and cimetidine on duodenal ulcer. A double-blind comparative trial. N Engl J Med 1985; 312:958–61.

15. Classen M, Dammann HG, Domschke W, Hengels KJ, Hütteman W, Londong W, Rehner M, Simon B, Witzel L, Berger J. Abheilungsraten nach Omeprazol- und Ranitidin-Behandlung des Ulcus ventriculi. Ergebnisse einer deutschen Multizenterstudie. Dtsch Med Wochenschr 1985; 110:628–33.

16. Bate CM, Bradby GVH, Wilkinson SP, et al. Omeprazole provides faster ulcer healing and symptom relief than cimetidine in the treatment of gastric ulcer. Gut 1988; 29:A1440–1.

17. Barbara L, Saggioro A, Olsson J, Cisternino M, Franceschi M. Omeprazole 20 mg om and ranitidine 150 mg bid in the healing of benign gastric ulcers—an Italian multicentre study. Gut 1987; 28:A1341.

18. Walan A, Bader JP, Classen M, Lamers CBHW, Piper DW, Rutgersson K, Eriksson S. Effect of omeprazole and ranitidine on ulcer healing and relapse rates in patients with benign gastric ulcer. N Engl J Med 1989; 320:69–75.

19. Pasqual JC, Hémery P, Bruley S, Galmiche JP. Comparison of the effects of two doses omeprazole on 24-hour esophageal pH in gastroesophageal reflux disease. Gastroenterology 1987; 92:1567.

20. Hetzel DJ, Dent J, Reed W, et al. Healing of peptic esophagitis with omeprazole: a dose-response study. Gastroenterology 1987; 92:1434.

21. Brunner G, Creutzfeldt W, Harke U, Lamberts R. Therapy with omeprazole in patients with peptic ulcerations resistant to extended high-dose ranitidine treatment. Digestion 1988; 39:80–90.

22. Klinkenberg-Knol EC, Jansen JBMJ, de Bruyne JW, et al. Long-term efficacy and safety of omeprazole on healing and prevention of resistant reflux esophagitis. Gastroenterology 1988; 94:A230.

23. Hui WM, Lam SK, Lau WY, et al. Omeprazole and ranitidine in duodenal ulcer healing and subsequent relapse: a randomized double-blind study with weekly endoscopic assessment. J Gastroenterol Hepatol 1989; 4(Suppl 2):35–43.

24. Archambault AP, Pare P, Bailey RJ, et al. Omeprazole (20 mg daily) versus cimetidine (1200 mg daily) in duodenal ulcer healing and pain relief. Gastroenterology 1988; 94:1130–4.

25. Bader JP. Etude de l'effet de l'omeprazole sur la cicatrisation des ulceres duodenaux: comparaison avec la cimetidine. Gastroenterol Clin Biol 1986; 10:190A.

26. Crowe JP, Wilkinson SP, Bate CM, et al. Symptom relief and duodenal ulcer healing with omeprazole or cimetidine. Aliment Pharmacol Ther 1989; 3:83–91.

27. Classen M, Dammann HG, Domschke W, Hengels KJ, Hüttemann W, Londong W, Rehner M, Simon B, Witzel L, Berger J. Kurzzeit-Therapie des Ulcus duodeni mit Omeprazol und Ranitidin. Ergebnisse einer deutschen Multizenter-Studie. Dtsch Med Wochenschr 1985; 110:210–5.

28. Mulder CJJ, Tijtgat GNJ, Cluysenaer OJJ, Nicolai JJ, Meyer WW, Hazenberg BP, Vogten AJM, Gerrits C, Stuifbergen WHNN. Omeprazole (20 mg o.m.) versus ranitidine (150 mg b.d.) in duodenal ulcer healing and pain relief. Aliment Pharmacol 1989; 3:445–51.

29. McFarland RJ, Bateson MC, Green JRB, O'Donoghue DP, Dronfield MW, Keeling PWN, Peers EM, Richardson PDI. Omeprazole provides faster symptom relief and heals a greater proportion of duodenal ulcers than ranitidine. Gut 1989; 30:A725.

30. Chelvam P, Goh KL, Leong YP, Leela MP, Yin TP, Ahmad H, Jalleh R, Wong NW, Lee HB, Mahendran T. Omeprazole compared with ranitidine once daily in the treatment of duodenal ulcer. J Gastroenterol Hepatol 1989; 4(Suppl 2):53–61.

31. Marks IN, Winter TA, Lucke W, Wright JP, Newton KA, O'Keefe SF, Marotta F. Omeprazole and ranitidine in duodenal ulcer healing. S Afr Med J. 1988; 74(Suppl):54–6.

32. Bardhan KD, Bianchi Porro G, Bose K, Daly M, Hinchliffe RFC, Jonsson E. Lazzaroni M, Naesdal J, Rikner L, Walan A. A comparison of two different doses of omeprazole versus ranitidine in treatment of duodenal ulcers. J Clin Gastroenterol 1986; 8:408–13.

33. Dahlgren S, Hradsky M, Norryd C, et al. The effect of omeprazole and cimetidine on ulcer healing in treatment of duodenal ulcer patient. A Swedish multicentre study. Dig Dis Sci 1986; 31(Suppl):44S.

34. Hallberg D, Backman L, Hellström M, et al. The effect of omeprazole and ranitidine on ulcer healing in treatment of duodenal ulcer patients. A Swedish multicentre study. Dig Dis Sci 1986; 31(Suppl):280S.

35. Gustavsson S, Nyrén O, Adami H-O, et al. Omeprazole heals duodenal and prepyloric

ulcers faster than cimetidine—a single-centre trial. Gastroenterology 1987; 92:1420. Abstract.

36.   Hetzel DJ, Korman MG, Hansky J, et al. A double blind multicentre comparison of omeprazole and cimetidine in the treatment of duodenal ulcer. Aust NZ J Med 1986; 16(Suppl 3):595. Abstract.

37.   Bate CM, Keeling PWN, O'Morain CA, et al. Omeprazole heals reflux oesophagitis in a greater proportion of patients than cimetidine, assessed endoscopically, histologically, and symptomatically. Hepatogastroenterology 1989; 36:279.

38.   Blum AL, Wienbeck M, Schiessel R, Carlsson R. Omeprazole is superior to ranitidine in the treatment of reflux esophagitis. Hepatogastroenterology 1989; 36:279.

39.   Dehn TCB, Shepherd HA, Colin-Jones D, Kettlevell MGW. Double blind comparative study of omeprazole (40 mg od) vs cimetidine (400 mg qds) in the treatment of erosive reflux oesophagitis. Gut 1988; 29:A1440.

40.   Havelund T, Laursen LS, Skoubo-Kristensen E, et al. Omeprazole and ranitidine in treatment of reflux oesophagitis: double blind comparative trial. Br Med J 1988; 296:89–92.

41.   Klinkenberg-Knol EC, Jansen JMBJ, Festen HPM, Meuwissen SGM, Lamers CBHW. Double-blind multicentre comparison of omeprazole and ranitidine in the treatment of reflux oesophagitis. Lancet 1987; i:349–51.

42.   Lundell L, Westin IH, Sandmark S, et al. Omeprazole or high dose ranitidine in the treatment of patients with reflux esophagitis not responding to standard doses of H_2-receptor antagonists. Gastroenterology 1989; 96:A310.

43.   Sandmark S, Carlsson R, Fausa O, Lundell L. Omeprazole or ranitidine in the treatment of reflux esophagitis. Scand J Gastroenterol 1988; 23:625–32.

44.   Vantrappen G, Rutgeerts L, Schurmans P, Coenegrachts J-L. Omeprazole (40 mg) is superior to ranitidine in short-term treatment of ulcerative reflux esophagitis. Dig Dis Sci 1988; 33:523–9.

45.   Zeitoun P, Rampal P, Barbier P, Isal J-P, Eriksson S, Carlsson R. Oméprazole (20 mg/j) comparé à ranitidine (150 mg 2 fois/j) dans le traitement de l'oesophagite par reflux. Résultats d'un essai multicentrique franco-belge, randomisé en double insu. Gastroenterol Clin Biol 1989; 13:457–62.

11

Prostaglandins as Regulators of Gastric Secretion and Gastrointestinal Mucosal Integrity

ANDRÉ ROBERT

The Upjohn Company, Kalamazoo, Michigan

I. INTRODUCTION

In the late 1960s there were two reasons for investigating the effect of prostaglandins (PGs) on the digestive system: (a) Several PGs had been identified in relatively large amounts in the gastrointestinal mucosa, and (b) they were believed to act mostly locally, that is, at their site of production, because of their rapid degradation in the body. Although these observations did not preclude activity by the systemic route, it was likely that if endogenous PGs affected gastrointestinal functions, they might do it primarily in the tissues where they were produced. The corollary was that by inhibiting synthesis of endogenous PGs with appropriate drugs, one would induce a tissue depletion of PG. This should result in alterations of gastrointestinal functions that would be opposite to changes obtained by administration of PGs.

We will review the major lines of experimentation in which these two approaches were explored, namely, the effect of administration of prostaglandins and the effect of inhibitors of PG synthesis on the gastrointestinal tract. The parameters studied include gastric secretion and gastrointestinal mucosal integrity.

II. GASTRIC SECRETION

Gastric acid secretion was studied in several species after administration of exogenous prostaglandins as well as after treatment with inhibitors of PG synthesis, particularly indomethacin.

A. Effect of Exogenous Prostaglandins

Several prostaglandins of the E type were administered to dogs whose gastric secretion was stimulated by various secretagogues (histamine, pentagastrin, food, and cholinergic stimuli such as carbachol, 2-deoxy-D-glucose, and vagal nerve stimulation). Initial studies were performed in animals. In all cases, the stimulation of acid secretion was markedly inhibited, in a dose-dependent manner [1–3]. In the case of natural PGs [PGE$_1$, PGE$_2$, PGA$_1$, prostacyclin (PGI$_2$)], the antisecretory effect occurred only after parenteral (intravenous or subcutaneous) administration. Certain methyl analogues (16,16-dimethyl PGE$_2$, 15S,15-methyl PGE$_2$, arbaprostil, misoprostol, enprostil, rioprostol) inhibited acid secretion after oral administration also [3–5]. Only when high doses of PGE$_2$ were orally administered was there a reduction in acid secretion [3].

Whereas the antisecretory effect of the natural PGs was short-lived (1–2 hr), the duration of action of most methyl analogues was much longer (6–10 hr). Most of these prostaglandins tended to elicit loose stools at doses approaching the antisecretory dose. However, a stable analogue of PGI$_2$ (U-68,215) was devoid of such a side effect; it inhibited acid secretion, but even at very high doses it did not induce diarrhea [6].

Several PGs of the E type also tended to stimulate uterine contractions. However, in some of these the dose ratio of the antisecretory over uterotonic activity was large. In the case of arbaprostil, doses that inhibited acid secretion by more than 90% did not induce significant uterine contractions, even in pregnant women whose uterine muscle is particularly sensitive [7]. U-68,215, a stable analogue of prostacyclin, was devoid of uterine contractile activity in pregnant monkeys at any dose [6].

The antisecretory effect of several prostaglandins was confirmed in humans [8–15]. This was the case after stimulation with either histamine, histalog, tetragastrin, pentagastrin, or food. Natural PGs, given parenterally, inhibited acid secretion, whereas several methyl analogues inhibited acid secretion even after oral administration. PGE$_2$ given orally at high doses (1.1 mg per subject) also inhibited meal-induced acid secretion.

Prostaglandins inhibit acid secretion by preventing histamine-induced formation of cAMP within parietal cells. This was shown in studies using isolated parietal cells in which acid secretion was measured by the uptake of aminopyrine [16,17]. Receptors for PGE$_2$ have also been identified on parietal cells. These receptors mediate the inhibition of acid secretion [18].

B. Effect of Inhibitors of PG Synthesis

The finding that natural prostaglandins inhibit gastric acid secretion suggested that these same substances produced endogenously by the stomach might exert a similar effect. If this were the case, endogenous PGs might be among the factors regulating gastric acid secretion. To test this possibility, inhibitors of PG synthesis were used. This was made possible by Vane's discovery [19] that most nonsteroidal anti-inflammatory drugs, such as indomethacin, are potent inhibitors of PG cyclooxygenase, the enzyme responsible for the transformation of arachidonic acid into endoperoxides, which in turn are transformed into PGs and thromboxanes. Administration of indomethacin depletes within minutes the body stores of PGs by blocking their synthesis [20,21]. When indomethacin was administered to various animal species, it stimulated gastric acid secretion. This was the case in rats [22–24], dogs [25], hamsters [26], and humans [27,28].

These results support the hypothesis that prostaglandins may regulate gastric acid secretion. The two facts favoring this hypothesis are that exogenously administered prostaglandins inhibit gastric acid secretion, whereas depletion of tissue levels of PGs by indomethacin stimulates it.

III. GASTROINTESTINAL MUCOSAL INTEGRITY

The antisecretory effect of prostaglandins suggest that these compounds might be useful for the treatment of peptic ulcer, because most drugs used for this disease act either by inhibiting acid secretion or by neutralizing acid already formed by the stomach.

A.   Anti-Ulcer Effect of Prostaglandins in Animal Models

Several experimental models of gastric and duodenal ulcers were used to determine whether antisecretory PGs would also prevent ulcer formation. Natural prostaglandins (PGE_1, PGE_2) as well as synthetic methyl analogues (15-methyl PGE_2 and 16,16-dimethyl PGE_2) all prevented formation of ulcers produced in rats by either corticoids (steroid-induced ulcers) [2,3], pylorus ligation (Shay ulcers), [2,3,26], stress (restraint, exertion) [29,30], or administration of nonsteroidal anti-inflammatory compounds (aspirin, indomethacin) [31–36].

Similar results were obtained in animal models of duodenal ulcers. This was the case for ulcers produced in rats by administration of cysteamine [37], proprionitrile [38], mepirizole [39,40], mefenamic acid [41], and gastric secretagogues (histamine, pentagastrin, carbachol) [3]. In all cases, the doses preventing ulcer formation also inhibited acid secretion.

These results indicated that PGs were indeed anti-ulcer, presumably because of their gastric antisecretory activity.

B.   Effect of Prostaglandins on Peptic Ulcer in Humans

Clinical trials confirmed the potential for certain PGs to heal duodenal ulcers. In one such study involving 173 patients, arbaprostil given orally at 100 μg four times a day healed 37% of patients in 2 weeks (versus 12% in placebo-treated), and 67% in 4 weeks (versus 39% in placebo-treated) [42]. Similar studies were obtained with misoprostol [43,44] and enprostil [45]. It was concluded that PGs of the E type are anti-ulcer as well as antisecretory and that their therapeutic efficacy is similar to that of cimetidine.

C. Cytoprotective Effect of Prostaglandins

The studies just cited established a close correlation between the antisecretory and anti-ulcer activity of PGs. The former appeared to be the cause of the latter. Additional studies, however, suggested that the anti-ulcer activity of prostaglandins was not due exclusively to inhibition of acid secretion. It was found that gastric lesions produced in rats by NSAIDs could be prevented by doses of PGs much below their antisecretory ED_{50}, and, moreover, certain prostaglandins such as $PGF_{2\beta}$, which are not antisecretory at any dose, could still prevent these lesions. This anti-ulcer effect of PGs, which was independent of inhibition of acid secretion, was called *cytoprotection* [34]. Since, however, gastric lesions caused by the NSAIDs could also be prevented by antisecretory drugs, such as histamine H_2 antagonists and anticholinergic agents, it was necessary to develop an experimental model of gastric damage that would not respond to inhibitors of acid secretion. Using such a model, PGs could be tested to determine whether they still could prevent gastric damage.

1. Models of Gastric Cytoprotection

Various necrotizing agents were administered intragastrically to fasted rats. These included absolute ethanol, 0.6 M HCl, 0.2 M NaOH, a hypertonic solution (25% sodium chloride), and 80 mM acidified taurocholate. These agents, given orally, produced extensive necrosis of the gastric mucosa almost instantaneously. When various types of prostaglandins were administered, orally or subcutaneously, prior to administration of these necrotizing agents, protection of the mucosa was observed [46,47]. The massive necrosis and hemorrhagic areas did not develop. The only damage that persisted was spotty exfoliation of the surface epithelium, a structure consisting of a single layer of epithelial cells that covers the mucosa [48]. The protective effect was almost immediate when the PGs were given orally, whereas the full effect required a few minutes after subcutaneous administration, presumably because of the time required for the PG to reach the stomach from the site of injection. Prostaglandins of the A, B, D, E, F_α, F_β, and I type were all cytoprotective, although their potency varied. The duration of protection lasted several hours. The longest acting PG tested was U-68,215, a prostacyclin analogue, whose activity lasted 8–10 hr [6].

2. Mechanisms of Cytoprotection

Although the mechanism by which prostaglandins exert cytoprotection has not been elucidated, several hypotheses have been tested.

Role of Mucus–Bicarbonate Barrier. Several prostaglandins of the E type stimulate secretion of gastric mucus and of bicarbonate by the gastric and duodenal mucosa [49–56]. Much of the bicarbonate is trapped into the mucus gel adherent to the mucosal surface. This alkaline unstirred layer creates a pH gradient between the lumen and the apical side of the gastric mucosal cells. The pH of gastric juice can fall as low as 1.5 while the pH of the interface between the surface epithelial cells and the mucus layer is maintained at 7 [56,57]. Only when the luminal pH falls below 1.3 does the pH of the mucosal surface decrease to below 7. This property of the unstirred layer to prevent the penetration of acid can obviously help maintain gastric mucosal integrity by avoiding contact of the cells with hydrogen ions. Since PGs increase both the bicarbonate content and the thickness of the mucus gel layer, they may protect the mucosa against acid-induced damage by this mechanism.

Gastric Mucosal Barrier.   The gastric mucosal barrier conceptualized by Theorell and studied extensively by Davenport is a phenomenon by which acid secreted into the gastric lumen does not back-diffuse into the mucosa. It was calculated that no more than 1% does back-diffuse under normal conditions. When, however, the gastric mucosa is exposed to irritants such as acetic acid, ethanol, bile salts, or lysolecithin, this barrier is broken, and hydrogen ions freely diffuse from the lumen into the mucosa. This induces the release of several mediators, including histamine, with consequent vasodilation, increased vascular permeability, edema, and histological damage to glandular cells. As hydrogen ions penetrate the mucosa, other cations, particularly sodium and potassium, move in the opposite direction from the blood to the gastric lumen [58,59]. As a result of this ionic equilibration, the electrical potential difference between the lumen and the blood falls precipitously. Administration of PGs of the E type reduces the ionic fluxes [60]. Therefore, one of the mechanisms of cytoprotection may involve the maintenance of the gastric mucosal barrier.

Gastric Mucosal Blood Flow.   Gastric mucosal blood flow, measured by the trapping of weak bases such as aminopyrine or aniline, by direct observation of the microvessels of the gastric submucosa through microscopic cinematography, or by the hydrogen gas clearance technique, was extensively studied after administration of irritants and necrotizing agents into the gastric lumen, as well as after administration of prostaglandin. The following findings were made:

1. Intragastric administration of ethanol slows the gastric microcirculation, leading to complete stasis within 1 min [61,62].
2. Gastric mucosal blood flow measured with the hydrogen gas clearance technique was also reduced (by 25%) by ethanol.
3. Unexpectedly, administration of 16,16-dimethyl PGE_2 to intact animals (without any damaging agent) reduced gastric mucosal blood flow by 20–25% [62].
4. A PG given prior to administration of ethanol prevented the slowing of the microcirculation, prevented the stasis, and, as observed in histological studies, also prevented formation of the necrohemorrhagic lesions [61].

It was concluded that although cytoprotective PGs by themselves do not increase gastric mucosal blood flow above the basal level, they prevent the decrease in blood flow elicited by necrotizing agents. This property may play a major role in protecting the gastric mucosa.

Vascular Permeability.   Absolute ethanol, in addition to producing vascular stasis, increases vascular permeability of the gastric mucosa to large molecules. This was shown by studies in rats using Evans blue intravenously. $PGF_{2\beta}$ reduced the extravasation of the dye [63]. This effect suggested that one of the primary targets of cytoprotection is the maintenance of vascular integrity. The capillary damage produced within 1 min of oral administration of absolute ethanol, as shown by light and electron microscopy, was prevented by $PGF_{2\beta}$ and by cysteamine. The vascular protection increased with the depth of the mucosa [64].

Surface-Active Phospholipids.   The surface of the gastric mucosa is hydrophobic. It was postulated that this hydrophobicity may contribute to the maintenance of mucosal integrity by preventing the entry of damaging agents into the mucosa. The hydrophobicity was ascribed to several phospholipids present on the surface of the mucosa and apparently secreted with mucus [65,66]. Several PGs markedly increased the amount of these gastric phospholipids. It was concluded that cytoprotection by PGs might be mediated by the formation of these hydrophobic phospholipids.

Sulfhydryl Agents.   Sulfhydryl compounds (e.g., cysteamine, penicillamine) markedly reduced gastric mucosal damage produced by absolute ethanol in rats [63,67]. It was suggested that endogenous sulfhydryl agents such as glutathione may mediate PG-induced cytoprotection [67]. Such a mechanism is uncertain in view of studies showing that agents that deplete the mucosal content of glutathione (diethyl maleate and buthionine sulfoximine) are cytoprotective, whereas *N*-acetyl cysteine, which raises the mucosal content of glutathione, aggravates ethanol-induced lesions [68,69].

Penetration of Necrotizing Agents.   One possible mechanism of cytoprotection by PGs is that these substances could prevent the entry of damaging agents into the mucosa. An earlier study had shown that 16,16-dimethyl PGE_2 did not prevent the entry of aspirin into the gastric mucosa after oral administration, although the PG inhibited the ulcerogenic effect of aspirin [70]. To further test this possibility, [^{14}C]-ethanol was administered orally to rats, and its progression through the gastric mucosa and eventually to the blood was measured as a function of time. At first, radioactive ethanol was very concentrated in the gastric juice (since it had been administered intragastrically); then the radioactivity proceeded through the mucosa and eventually reached the blood. This confirmed that ethanol had entered the gastric tissue. The penetration of ethanol was accompanied by extensive necrosis of the mucosa. When 16,16-dimethyl PGE_2 was administered at a cytoprotective dose prior to ethanol, no necrosis was observed in the gastric tissue. Nevertheless, the degree and rate of penetration of [^{14}C]-ethanol into the gastric mucosa was the same as in nonprotected animals that did not receive the PG [71]. It was concluded that prostaglandins are cytoprotective in spite of the fact that they do not prevent the penetration of ethanol into the gastric mucosa. A further conclusion was that in animals pretreated with PGs, gastric cells located deep in the mucosa are impregnated with ethanol; however, these cells become resistant to the damaging effect of the agent when a PG has been administered. This study helped to localize the site of action of cytoprotection, namely, that PGs appear to "strengthen" the resistance of the mucosal cells themselves to damage. Whether this resistance is located at the cell membrane has not been determined.

In Vitro Cytoprotection.   Support for the hypothesis that PGs may protect by a direct action on the cells was provided by experiments in which either dispersed gastric cells or isolated gastric glands were exposed to damaging agents such as aspirin, indomethacin, taurocholate, or ethanol. The indices of damage consisted of measuring the release of preloaded ^{51}chromium or of a cytosolic enzyme (lactic dehydrogenase), of determining trypan blue exclusion, and of electron microscopic changes.

These studies showed that whereas all these indices of damage were present when the injurious agents were applied to the cells, they were much less severe when the medium contained a PG [72–74]. It was concluded that cytoprotection by PGs can be observed in vitro, that is, with the exclusion of blood flow and nerves. These findings strongly suggest that cytoprotection is exerted at the cellular level.

3.   Duodenal Cytoprotection

Several animal models have been developed showing that prostaglandins can cyto-protect the stomach and the small and large intestines against a variety of noxious agents [75]. In the case of duodenal ulcers, however, cytoprotection could not be demonstrated in humans; a dose that healed such ulcers also reduced gastric acid secretion. In animal models of duodenal ulcers whose mechanism involves gastric hypersecretion, again doses of PG that prevented such ulcers were also antisecretory. This was the case particularly of duodenal ulcers produced in rats by administration of secretogogues (histamine, carbachol, pentagastrin) [3,76], of cysteamine [37], and of mepirizole [39,40]. However, other models were developed that are not associated with hypersecretion; in such models, PGs prevented the ulcers at doses that did not affect acid secretion. Three such models are reviewed.

Duodenal Ulcers Produced by Indomethacin Plus Bile Duct Ligation.   A single dose of indomethacin (10 mg/kg orally) given to rats following ligation of the bile duct produced within 12 hr one or two duodenal ulcers located within 1 cm of the pylorus [77]. These ulcers become more severe with time, and about 50% perforate after 3 days. Neither bile duct ligation nor indomethacin alone is ulcerogenic. Administration of a PG of the E type (PGE_2 or 16,16-dimethyl PGE_2) prevented formation of the ulcers, and this occurred at doses that are not antisecretory [77]. The pathogenesis of such ulcers is not clear, but it does not involve acid hypersecretion; actually, acid secretion tends to decrease. However, some gastric acid is necessary,

since antisecretory agents (methscopolamine bromide, cimetidine) can prevent formation of the ulcers. A plausible hypothesis is that the depletion of cytoprotective PGs
(caused by indomethacin) combined with a reduction in bicarbonate secretion by the
duodenum may render the duodenal mucosa particularly sensitive to acid. Exogenous
administration of a PG replaces the missing compound and also stimulates bicarbonate secretion by the duodenum [78,79].

Duodenal Ulcers Produced by Indomethacin Plus Histamine.   Fasted rats
given indomethacin, 5 mg/kg, followed by histamine, 40 μg/kg three times at 2.5-
hr intervals, develop duodenal ulcers in 24 hr. Treatment with dimethyl PGE_2, 10–
30 μg intraduodenally, markedly reduced the severity of the ulcers [80]. These doses
did not inhibit gastric acid secretion.

**Duodenal Ulcers Produced by Indomethacin and a Low Dose of Cyste-
amine.**   A single oral administration of indomethacin (10 mg/kg) combined with
subcutaneous injections of 100 mg/kg of cysteamine twice a day for 2 days produced
in rats one or two duodenal ulcers in the first centimeter of the duodenal bulb [80].
Neither indomethacin nor cysteamine was ulcerogenic at that dose. As in the case of
duodenal ulcers produced by indomethacin plus bile duct ligation, the duodenal
ulcers produced by indomethacin plus cysteamine may be due to a combination of
factors: a depletion of cytoprotective PG in the duodenal mucosa, a decrease of
duodenal secretion of bicarbonate, and the presence of acid in the duodenal lumen.
Low doses of PGs of the E type, doses much below the antisecretory range, prevented
the formation of these ulcers [81].

In these three models of duodenal ulcers, the common denominator appears to be a
depletion of the PG content of the duodenum induced by indomethacin. Under such
conditions, the duodenal mucosa becomes sensitive to agents that otherwise are not
ulcerogenic. In the case of cysteamine and histamine, it is likely that the hypersecretion of acid caused by these secretagogues can damage the mucosa only in the absence
of endogenous cytoprotective PGs. In the case of ulcers produced by indomethacin
plus bile duct ligation, the mechanism is unclear but may still involve relative
hyperacidity. Although gastric acid is not increased under those conditions, there is
acid flowing over the duodenum, and the inhibition of bicarbonate secretion caused
by indomethacin [78,79] reduces the buffering of acid.

4.   Adaptive Cytoprotection

The facts that exogenous prostaglandins are cytoprotective and that agents that
deplete the stomach of PG (aspirin, indomethacin) cause gastric erosions suggested
that natural PGs may play an important role in maintaining gastric mucosal integrity. If so, a stimulation of PG formation would be expected to protect the stomach
against damage produced by necrotizing agents. The following studies confirmed
that hypothesis.

Oral administration of a variety of mild irritants (20% ethanol, 0.3 M HCl,
0.075 M NaOH, 4% NaCl, 10 mM taurocholate) was found to prevent necrosis and
hemorrhages in the gastric mucosa caused by necrotizing agents (absolute ethanol,

0.6 M HCl, 0.2 M NaOH, 25% NaCl, 80 mM acidified taurocholate) [82,83]. The protection was abolished by prior treatment with indomethacin, an inhibitor of PG synthesis. Actual measurement of mucosal PG showed that mild irritants indeed markedly increased the formation of PGs [83]. It was concluded that mild irritants are cytoprotective mainly by stimulating the endogenous release of prostaglandins by the stomach.

It appears that one of the reasons the stomach maintains its structural integrity in spite of the constant presence of irritants (foods, spices, acid, gastrotoxic drugs) in its lumen is the continued synthesis of prostaglandins that serve as cytoprotective agents. These very irritants stimulate PG formation.

REFERENCES

1. Robert A, Nezamis JE, Phillips JP. Inhibition of gastric secretion by prostaglandins. Am J Dig Dis 1967; 12:1073–6.
2. Robert A, Nezamis JE, Phillips JP. Effect of prostaglandin E_1 on gastric secretion and ulcer formation in the rat. Gastroenterology 1968; 55:481–7.
3. Robert A, Schultz JR, Nezamis JE, Lancaster C. Gastric antisecretory and antiulcer properties of PGE_2, 15-methyl PGE_2, and 16,16-dimethyl PGE_2. Intravenous, oral and intrajejunal administration. Gastroenterology 1976; 70:359–70.
4. Tsai BS, Kessler LK, Collins P, Kramer S, Bauer RF. Antisecretory activity of misoprostol, its racemates, stereoisomers and metabolites in isolated parietal cells. Prostaglandins 1987; 33:30–9.
5. Roskowski AP, Garay GL, Baker S, Schuler M, Carter H. Gastric antisecretory and antiulcer properties of enprostil, ($\pm$)-11α,15α-dihydroxy-16-phenoxy-17,18,19,20-tetranor-9-oxoprosta-4,5,13(t) acid methyl ester. J Pharmacol Exp Ther 1986; 239:382–9.
6. Robert A, Aristoff PA, Wendling MG, Kimball FA, Miller WL Jr, Gorman RR. Cytoprotective and antisecretory properties of a non-diarrheogenic and nonuterotonic prostacyclin analog. Prostaglandins 1985; 30:619–49.
7. Euler AR, Leodolter S, Huber J, Lookabaugh J, Burns M, Phan T, Wood D, Bogaerts H. Arbaprostil (15R-15-methyl PGE_2) effects on intrauterine pressure in the nonpregnant and pregnant human female. A report of four clinical trials. Prostaglandins, Leuk Ess Fatty Acids 1989; 38:91–98.
8. Wilson DE, Phillips C, Levine RA. Inhibition of gastric secretion in man by prostaglandin A_1. Gastroenterology 1971; 61:201–6.
9. Classen M, Koch H, Deyhle P, Weidenhiller S, Demling L. Wirkung von prostaglandin E_1 auf die basale magensekretion des menschen. Klin Wochenschr 1970; 48:876–8.
10. Classen M, Koch H, Bickhardt J, Topf G, Demling L. The effect of prostaglandin E_1 on the pentagrastrin-stimulated gastric secretion in man. Digestion 1971; 4:333–44.
11. Carter DC, Karim SMM, Bhana D, Ganesan PA. Inhibition of human gastric secretion by prostaglandins. Br J Surg 1973; 60:828–31.
12. Konturek SJ, Kwiecien N, Swiereczek J, Oleksy J, Sito E, Robert A. Comparison of methylated prostaglandin E_2 analogues given orally in the inhibition of gastric responses to pentagastrin and peptone meal in man. Gastroenterology 1976; 70:683–7.

13. Robert A, Nylander B, Andersson S. Marked inhibition of gastric secretion by two prostaglandin analogs given orally to man. Life Sci 1974; 14:533–8.

14. Savarino V, Scalabrini P, Mela GS, Timoteo ED, Percario G, Magnolia MR, Celle G. Evaluation of antisecretory activity of misoprostol in duodenal ulcer patients using long-term intragastric pH monitoring. Dig Dis Sci 1988; 33:293–7.

15. Deakin M, Ramage J, Paul A, Gray SP, Billings J, Williams JG. Effect of enprostil, a synthetic prostaglandin E_2, on 24 hour intragastric acidity, nocturnal acid and pepsin secretion. Gut 1986; 27:1054–7.

16. Soll AH. Specific inhibition by prostaglandins E_2 and I_2 of histamine-stimulated (^{14}C)aminopyrine accumulation and cyclic adenosine monophosphate generation by isolated canine parietal cells. J Clin Invest 1980; 65:1222–9.

17. Soll AH, Chen MC, Amirian DA, Toomey M, Alvarez R. Prostanoid inhibition of canine parietal cells. Am J Med 1986; 81:5–11.

18. Seidler U, Beinborn M, Sewing K-F. Inhibition of acid formation in rabbit parietal cells by prostaglandins is mediated by the prostaglandin E_2 receptor. Gastroenterology 1989; 96:314–20.

19. Vane JR. Inhibition of prostaglandin synthesis as a mechanism of action for aspirin-like drugs. Nature (New Biol) 1971; 231:232–5.

20. Fitzpatrick FA, Wynalda MA. In vivo suppression of prostaglandin biosynthesis by nonsteroidal anti-inflammatory agents. Prostaglandins 1976; 12:1037–51.

21. Whittle BJR, Higgs GA, Eakins KE, Moncada S, Vane JR. Selective inhibition of prostaglandin production in inflammatory exudates and gastric mucosa. Nature 1980; 284:271–3.

22. Arai I, Hirose H, Usuki C, Muramatsu M, Aihara H. Synergism of indomethacin and cold-stress in gastric acid output, ulceration and gastric motility, and the effects of anti-ulcer agents in rats. Jpn J Pharmacol 1985; 39:278P.

23. Alino SF, Marti-Bonmati E, Torregrosa A, Callaghan R, Morcillo E, Garcia D. Prosta-glandin synthesis inhibition reverses the antisecretory activity of somatostatin in anaes-thetized rats. Hormones Metab Res 1985; 17:123–6.

24. Main IHM, Whittle BJR. Investigation of the vasodilator and antisecretory role of prostaglandins in the rat gastric mucosa by use of nonsteroidal anti-inflammatory drugs. J Pharmacol 1975; 53:217–24.

25. Gerkens JF, Shad DG, Flexner C, Nies AS, Dates JA, Data JL. Effect of indomethacin and aspirin on gastric blood flow and acid secretion. J Pharmacol Exp Ther 1977; 203:646–52.

26. Kolbasa KP, Lancaster C, Olafsson AS, Gilbertson SK, Robert A. Indomethacin-induced gastric antral ulcers in hamsters. Gastroenterology 1988; 95:932–44.

27. Feldman M, Colturi TJ. Effect of indomethacin on gastric acid and bicarbonate secretion in humans. Gastroenterology 1984; 87:1339–43.

28. Levine RA, Schwartzel EH. Effect of indomethacin on basal and histamine stimulated human gastric acid secretion. Gut 1984; 25:718–22.

29. Lee YH, Cheng WD, Bianchi RG, Mollison K, Hansen J. Effects of oral administration of PGE_2 on gastric secretion and experimental peptic ulcerations. Prostaglandins 1973; 3:29–45.

30. Dajani EZ, Driskill DR, Bianchi RG, Collins PW. Comparative gastric antisecretory

and antiulcer effects of prostaglandin E_1 and its methyl ester in animals. Prostaglandins 1975; 10:205–15.

31. Kawarada Y, Lambek J, Matsumoto T. Pathophysiology of stress ulcer and its prevention. II. Prostaglandin E_1 and microcirculatory responses in stress ulcer. Am J Surg 1975; 129:217–22.

32. Carmichael HA, Nelson LM, Russell RI. Cimetidine and prostaglandin: evidence for different modes of action on the rat gastric mucosa. Gastroenterology 1978; 74:1229–32.

33. Guth PH, Aures D, Paulsen G. Topical aspirin plus HCl gastric lesions in the rat. Cytoprotective effect of prostaglandin, cimetidine and probanthine. Gastroenterology 1979; 76:88–93.

34. Robert A. Antisecretory, antiulcer, cytoprotective and diarrheogenic properties of prostaglandins. Adv Prostaglandin Thromboxane Res 1975; 1:507–20.

35. Whittle BJR. Relationship between the prevention of rat gastric erosions and the inhibition of acid secretion by prostaglandins. Eur J Pharmacol 1976; 40:233–9.

36. Whittle BJR. Mechanisms underlying gastric mucosal damage induced by indomethacin and bile-salts, and the actions of prostaglandins. Br J Pharmacol 1977; 60:455–60.

37. Robert A, Nezamis JE, Lancaster C, Badalamenti JN. Cysteamine-induced duodenal ulcers: A new model to test antiulcer agents. Digestion 1975; 11:199–214.

38. Robert A, Nezamis JE, Lancaster C. Duodenal ulcers produced in rats by propionitrile: factors inhibiting and aggravating such ulcers. Toxicol Appl Pharmacol 1975; 31:201–7.

39. Takeuchi K, Ohtsuki H, Okabe S. Mechanisms of protective activity of 16,16-dimethyl PGE_2 and acetazolamide on gastric and duodenal lesions in rats. Dig Dis Sci 1986; 31:406–11.

40. Robert A, Tabata K, Joffe SN, Jacobson ED. Prostaglandin deficiency by itself is not the cause of mepirizole-induced duodenal ulcers in rats. Dig Dis Sci 1987; 32:997–1003.

41. Elliott G, Whited BA, Purmalis A, Davis JP, Field SO, Lancaster C, Robert A. Effect of 16,16-dimethyl PGE_2 on renal papillary necrosis and gastrointestinal ulcerations (gastric, duodenal, intestinal) produced in rats by mefenamic acid. Life Sci 1986; 39:423–32.

42. Vantrappen G, Janssens J, Popiela T, Kulig J, Tytgat GNJ, Huibregtse K, Lambert R, Pauchard JP, Robert A. Effect of 15(R)-15-methyl prostaglandin E_2 (arbaprostil) on the healing of duodenal ulcer. Gastroenterology 1982; 83:357–63.

43. Aenishaenslin W, Baerlocher C, Bernoulli R, Egger G, Eisner M, Fumagalli I. Misoprostol and cimetidine in the treatment of duodenal ulcer. A Swiss multicenter double blind study. Schweiz Med Wochenschr 1985; 115:1225–31.

44. Fich A, Goldin E, Zimmerman J, Ligumsky M, Rachmilewitz D. Comparison of misoprostol and cimetidine in the treatment of duodenal ulcer. Isr J Med Sci 1985; 21:102–6.

45. Winters L. Comparison of enprostil and cimetidine in active duodenal ulcer diseases. Summary of pooled European studies. Am J Med 1986; 81:69–74.

46. Robert A, Nezamis JE, Lancaster C, Hanchar AJ. Cytoprotection by prostaglandins in rats: prevention of gastric necrosis produced by alcohol, HCl, NaOH, hypertonic NaCl, and thermal injury. Gastroenterology 1979; 77:433–43.

47. Robert A. Cytoprotection by prostaglandins. Gastroenterology 1979; 77:761–7.

48. Lacy ER, Ito S. Microscopic analysis of ethanol damage to rat gastric mucosa after treatment with a prostaglandin. Gastroenterology 1982; 83:619–25.

49. Bolton JP, Cohen MM. Stimulation of nonparietal cell secretion in canine Heidenhain pouches by 16,16-dimethyl prostaglandin E_2. Digestion 1978; 17:291–9.

50. Kauffman GL Jr, Reeve JJ Jr, Grossman MI. Gastric bicarbonate secretion: effect of topical and intravenous 16,16-dimethyl prostaglandin E_2. Am J Physiol 1980; 239: G44–8.

51. Miller TA, Watkins LA, Henagen JM. 16,16-Dimethyl PGE_2 stimulates bicarbonate secretion in the canine stomach. Surg Forum 1980; 31:126–9.

52. Flemström G. Duodenal mucosal alkaline secretion in the rat: role of endogenous prostaglandin in stimulation by BW755C. In: Allen A, Flemström G, Garner A, Silen W, Turnberg LA. Mechanisms of mucosal protection in the upper gastrointestinal tract. New York: Raven, 1984:147–52.

53. Flemström G, Garner A, Nylander O, Hurst BD, Heylings JR. Surface epithelial HCO_3^- transport by mammalian duodenum in vivo. Am J Physiol 1982; 243:G348–58.

54. Flemström G, Heylings JR, Garner A. Gastric and duodenal HCO_3^- transport in vitro: effects of hormones and local transmitters. Am J Physiol 1982; 242:G100–10.

55. Bickel M, Kauffman GL. Gastric mucus gel thickness: effect of distention, 16,16-dimethyl prostaglandin E_2, and carbenoxolone. Gastroenterology 1981; 80:770–5.

56. Turnberg LA, Ross IN, Bahari HMM. pH gradient across gastric mucus. In: Allen A, Flemström G, Garner A, Silen W, Turnberg LA. Mechanisms of mucosal protection in the upper gastrointestinal tract. New York: Raven, 1984:223–6.

57. Rees WDW, Turnberg LA. Mechanisms of gastric mucosal protection: a role for the "mucus–bicarbonate" barrier. Clin Sci 1982; 62:343–8.

58. Davenport HW. Damage to the gastric mucosa: effects of salicylates and stimulation. Gastroenterology 1965; 49:189–96.

59. Davenport HW. Destruction of the gastric mucosal barrier by detergents and urea. Gastroenterology 1968; 54:175–81.

60. Tepperman BL, Miller TA, Johnson LR. Effect of 16,16-dimethyl prostaglandin E_2 on ethanol-induced damage to canine oxyntic mucosa. Gastroenterology 1978; 75:1061–5.

61. Guth PH, Paulsen G, Nagata H. Histologic and microcirculatory changes in alcohol-induced gastric lesions in the rat: effect of prostaglandin cytoprotection. Gastroenterology 1984; 87:1083–90.

62. Leung FW, Robert A, Guth PH. Gastric mucosal blood flow in rats after administration of 16,16-dimethyl prostaglandin E_2 at a cytoprotective dose. Gastroenterology 1985; 88:1948–53.

63. Szabo S, Trier JS, Brown A, Schmoor J. Early vascular injury and increased vascular permeability in gastric mucosal injury caused by ethanol in the rat. Gastroenterology 1985; 88:228–36.

64. Trier JS, Szabo S, Allan CH. Ethanol-induced damage to mucosal capillaries of rat stomach. Ultrastructural features and effects of prostaglandin $F_{2\beta}$ and cysteamine. Gastroenterology 1987; 82:13–22.

65. Lichtenberger LM, Graziani LA, Dial EJ, Butler BD, Hills BA. Role of surface-active phospholipids in gastric cytoprotection. Science 1983; 219:1327–9.

66. Lichtenberger LM, Richards JE, Hills BA. Effect of 16,16-dimethyl prostaglandin E_2 on

the surface hydrophobicity of aspirin-treated canine gastric mucosa. Gastroenterology 1985; 88:308–14.

67. Szabo S, Trier JS, Frankel PW. Sulfhydryl compounds may mediate gastric cytoprotection. Science 1981; 214:200–2.

68. Robert A, Eberle D, Kaplowitz N. Role of glutathione in gastric mucosal cytoprotection. Am J Physiol 1984; 247:G296–304.

69. Lu SC, Kuylenkamp J, Robert A, Kaplowitz N. Role of glutathione status in protection against ethanol-induced gastric lesions. Pharmacology 1989; 38:57–60.

70. Guth PH, Paulsen G. Prostaglandin cytoprotection does not involve interference with aspirin absorption. Proc Soc Exp Biol Med 1979; 162:128–30.

71. Robert A, Lancaster C, Davis JP, Field SO, Wickrema Sinha AJ, Thornburgh BA. Cytoprotection by prostaglandin occurs in spite of penetration of absolute ethanol into the gastric mucosa. Gastroenterology 1985; 88:328–33.

72. Terano A, Mach T, Stachura J, Tarnawski A, Ivey KJ. Effect of 16,16-dimethyl prostaglandin E_2 on aspirin-induced damage to rat gastric epithelial cells in tissue culture. Gut 1984; 25:19–25.

73. Terano A, Ota S, Mach T, Hiraishi H, Stachura J. Prostaglandin protects against taurocholate-induced damage to rat gastric mucosal cell culture. Gastroenterology 1987; 92:669–77.

74. Tarnawski A, Brzozowski T, Sarfeh J, Krause WJ, Ulrich TR, Gergely H, Hollander D. Prostaglandin protection of human isolated gastric glands against indomethacin and ethanol injury. J Clin Invest 1988; 81:1081–9.

75. Robert A. Effects of prostaglandins on the stomach and the intestine. Prostaglandins 1974; 6:523–32.

76. Robert A, Stowe DF, Nezamis JE. Prevention of duodenal ulcers by administration of prostaglandin E_2 (PGE_2). Scand J Gastroenterol 1971; 6:303–5.

77. Robert A, Nezamis JE, Lancaster C. Duodenal ulcers produced by nonsteroidal anti-inflammatory compounds plus bile duct ligation. Fed Proc 1975; 34:442.

78. Isenberg JI, Smedfors B, Johansson C. Effect of graded doses of intraluminal H^+, prostaglandin E_2 and inhibition of endogenous prostaglandin synthesis on proximal duodenal bicarbonate secretion in unanesthetized rat. Gastroenterology 1985; 88:303–7.

79. Takeuchi K, Furukawa O, Tanaka H, Okabe S. Determination of acid-neutralizing capacity in rat duodenum. Dig Dis Sci 1986; 31:631–7.

80. Takeuchi K, Furukawa O, Tanaka H, Okabe S. A new model of duodenal ulcers induced in rats by indomethacin plus histamine. Gastroenterology 1986; 90:636–45.

81. Gilbertson-Beadling, S, Olafsson AS, Lancaster C, Robert A. Duodenal ulcers produced by indomethacin and low dose of cysteamine. Gastroenterology 1989; 96:171.

82. Chaudhury TK, Robert A. Prevention by mild irritants of gastric necrosis produced in rats by sodium taurocholate. Dig Dis Sci 1980; 25:830–6.

83. Robert A, Nezamis JE, Lancaster C, Davis JP, Field SO, Hanchar AJ. Mild irritants prevent gastric necrosis through "adaptive cytoprotection" mediated by prostaglandins. Am J Physiol 1983; 83:G113–21.

12

Prostaglandin Therapy

DONALD E. WILSON

State University of New York Health
Science Center, Brooklyn, New York

I. INTRODUCTION

Prostaglandins (PGs) are cyclic fatty acids that are synthesized upon demand from dietary fatty acids stored in most mammalian cells. For humans of the western hemisphere, arachidonic acid (AA) is the major dietary substrate for "eicosanoid" synthesis, resulting in the synthesis of PG_2 series and leukotriene-4 series compounds (Fig. 1). These ubiquitous compounds bring about a variety of biological responses and in many instances act as modifiers of cellular action. Because of their rapid metabolism, prostaglandins do not circulate and thus do not act as hormones in the true sense. Vogt [1] isolated "Darmstoff," a material capable of stimulating smooth muscle and later found to be a mixture of PGE_1 and $PGF_{1\alpha}$. In 1961 there was only one published article on prostaglandins. Now thousands of related reports are published annually. Over the past two decades, the physiological and pharmacological effects of prostaglandins on the gastrointestinal tract have been delineated in great detail. Because prostaglandins both inhibit gastric acid secretion and strengthen the integrity of the gastroduodenal mucosa, they have the potential to affect both the aggressive and defensive factors involved in the pathogenesis of peptic ulcer disease. As such, these compounds may present a unique approach to peptic ulcer therapy.

II. GASTRIC ANTISECRETORY EFFECTS

A. Naturally Occurring Prostaglandins

The antisecretory effects of prostaglandins were first described by Robert et al. [2]. Their studies reported that prostaglandins E_1, E_2, and A_1 reduced basal and stimu-

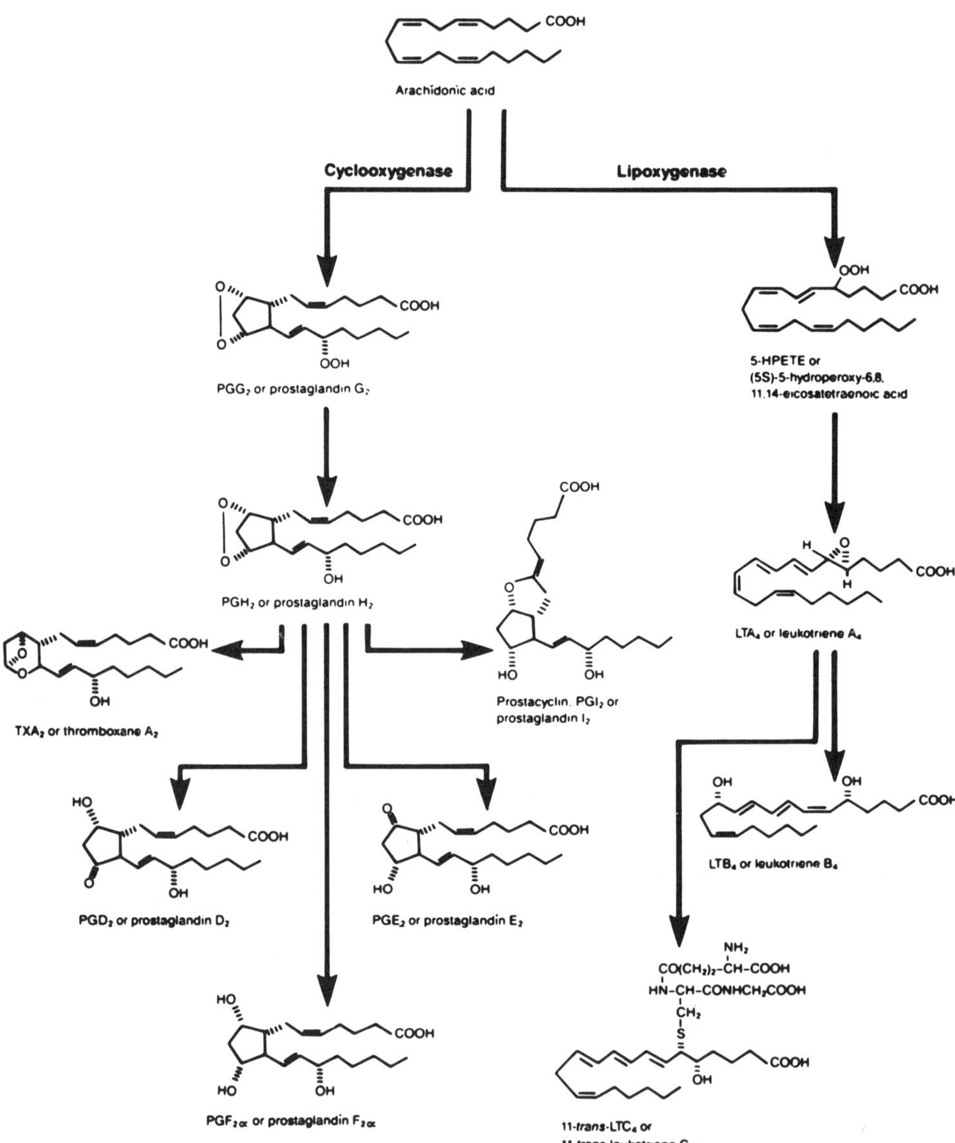

FIGURE 1 Biosynthesis of prostaglandins and other eicosanoids. Arachidonic acid cascade.

lated gastric acid secretion in the dog but that $PGF_{2\alpha}$ was essentially ineffective. Over the next several years, a number of reports confirmed the gastric antisecretory actions of naturally occurring prostaglandins in the rat and in dogs [3–5]. When administered to dogs by constant intravenous infusion, PGE_1 at a dose of 2 μg/kg per min inhibits histamine-stimulated acid secretion by more than 90%. The discovery that naturally occurring prostaglandins given in microgram amounts were capable of causing marked inhibition of acid secretion in animals led quite naturally to speculation that these compounds might be effective antisecretory agents in humans.

The mechanism of the PG antisecretory effect has not been precisely delineated. However, it is knwon that prostaglandins act directly on the parietal cell, where PG receptors have been described [6]. Whether PG-receptor activation inhibits histamine stimulation of adenylate cyclase, directly inhibits adenylate cyclase, or acts at other sites in the cellular pathway of activation of acid secretion is not yet clear (Fig. 2). Studies continue to delineate the exact site(s) in the acid secretory cascade where PGs exert their effect.

Wilson et al. [7] administered prostaglandin A_1 intravenously to healthy male volunteers at dosages of 0.5 and 1.25 μg/kg per min and observed a significant reduction in gastric juice volume and acid output. Maximal inhibition of volume and acid were approximately 40%. As previously observed in the dog [4], it was noted that the antisecretory effect was short-lived, disappearing within 15 min after discontinuance of the infusion. The infusion was well tolerated, with the only complaint being the passage of a more liquid than usual bowel movement 3–6 hr post-study in several subjects. Classen et al. [8] observed a similar antisecretory effect for PGE_1 given to humans but also observed the development of significant hypotension in several subjects during the infusion. The possible therapeutic use of natural prostaglandins as antisecretory compounds was seriously hampered by their rapid conversion to inactive metabolites in most tissues, particularly the lungs, liver, and gut [9–11]. With a circulatory half-life of several minutes, the antisecretory effect of parenteral prostaglandins was short-lived, with a constant infusion being required for prolonged effect. Orally administered prostaglandins were similarly metabolized and, moreover, were generally ineffective antisecretory agents except at dosages that caused significant diarrhea [12]. In 1970 prostaglandins were considered "interesting" antisecretory agents without much therapeutic benefit.

B.   Synthetic Prostaglandin Analogues

In the early 1970s, synthetic analogues of prostaglandins A, B, E, and F were developed. These compounds resisted rapid metabolism by the tissue enzymes, primarily PG 15-OH-dehydrogenase and 13,14-reductase. Not only were these synthetic analogues more resistant to degradation by tissues, but they were also more potent antisecretory agents than their naturally occurring counterparts. Several investigators [13–15] reported that 15-methyl and 16,16-dimethyl analogues of PGE_2

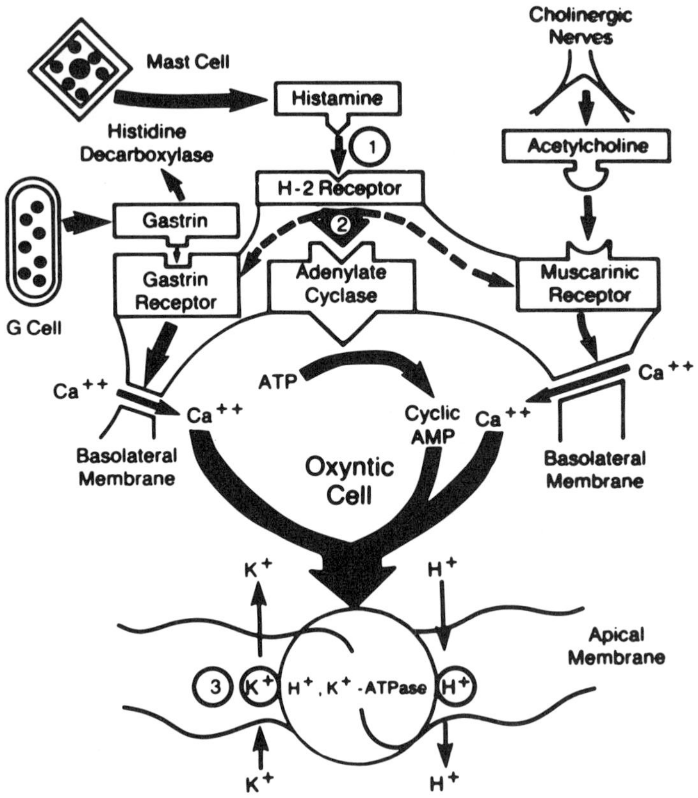

FIGURE 2 Currently proposed pathways of activation of parietal cell acid secretion. Prostaglandins may act primarily at receptor sites on the cell membrane or also at the basolateral membrane of other intracellular sites.

were effective inhibitors of basal and stimulated acid secretion in animals at dosages as little as one-twentieth of that required to achieve a smaller degree of acid inhibition with natural PGE_2. Additionally, these analogues were effective when administered orally. As observed with the natural PGs, the E and A compounds inhibited secretion but the F compounds did not.

Numerous antisecretory studies have been performed in humans using methylated analogues of PGE_1 or PGE_2 [16–21]. These reports indicate that the short-term administration of PGE_2 and PGE_1 analogues significantly reduces acid secretion for several hours following drug administration. A single 127-μg dose of 16,16-dimethyl PGE_2 inhibits basal acid secretion by more than 90% and histamine or pentagastrin-stimulated secretion by approximately 80% over a 3-hr period following drug administration. Misoprostol, a PGE_1 analogue, at a single dose of 400 μg inhibits pentagastrin-stimulated acid secretion in humans by 32% over a 3-hr period [21]. Additional PGE analogues such as arboprostil [15(R), 15-methyl PGE_2], rioprostil (16-methyl, 16-OH PGE_1), and trimoprostil [11(R), 16, 16-trimethyl PGE_2] have similar efficacy in varying dosages.

Prostaglandin analogues are effective inhibitors of histamine-, pentagastrin-, meal-, and caffeine-stimulated acid secretion as well as overnight secretion. For example, misoprostol 200 µg inhibits overnight secretion by approximately 60% [22], and enprostil, a PGE_2 analogue, given at night at a dose of 70 µg, reduces 24-hr intragastric acidity by one-third [23]. Although prostaglandin analogues are up to 1000 times as potent as H_2-receptor antagonists on a molar basis, they are generally similar to the H_2-receptor antagonists with respect to their maximal antisecretory effect. However, the duration of antisecretory action observed with prostaglandin analogues is generally less than that of the newer H_2-receptor antagonists. Thus, prostaglandins are moderate inhibitors of acid secretion.

III. MUCOSAL PROTECTIVE EFFECTS

Robert et al. [24] were the first to report that PGE_2 could prevent ulcer formation in the rat. The term "cytoprotection" was coined by Robert and Jacobson and may be paraphrased as "the ability of a compound to prevent or limit mucosal damage caused by a variety of diverse insulting agents, without affecting gastric acid secretion." In additional studies, Robert and his colleagues [14,25] observed that nonantisecretory prostaglandins (e.g., $PGF_{2\beta}$), as well as antisecretory PGs (e.g., PGE_1, PGE_2), when administered at less than antisecretory concentrations, prevented experimental gastric mucosal damage in animals if given prior to administering the insulting agent and noted further that prostaglandins protected against damage caused by diverse noxious agents such as acidified bile acids, ethanol, stress, and boiling water. These findings indicated efficacy for prostaglandins in preventing damage in both acid-dependent and acid-independent experimental models (Table 1).

Table 1 Lesion-Causing Agents from Which Prostaglandins Can Protect the Mucosa

Ethanol
Aspirin
Bile acids
Nonsteroidal anti-inflammatory drugs (NSAIDs)
Stress
Hypertonic/hypotonic solutions
Caustic solutions (lye)
Boiling water

We now know that protecting agents do not prevent damage to all cells in a tissue and that protection may be partial or limited to certain zonal regions of a tissue. Thus the term "mucosal protection" is somewhat more accurate than "cytoprotection."

A discussion of the mechanisms of mucosal protection as well as a review of the experimental data in animals is contained in Chapter 11. In order to appropriately review the anti-ulcer actions of prostaglandins in humans, a few concepts will be restated here.

Although the precise components of mucosal protection have not been fully defined and the exact mechanisms of action of prostaglandins are still being studied, there are certain clinically measurable factors that are thought to play a role in enhancing mucosal integrity (Table 2). The concept of the gastric mucosal barrier is discussed in detail in Chapter 1. For our purposes it is important to stress that the constant secretion of mucus glycoprotein and bicarbonate into the mucus gel (unstirred) layer on cell surfaces aids in providing a protective zone against the back-diffusion of acid and pepsin into mucosal cells. While it is clear that these two factors alone do not entirely explain the gradient observed between gastric intracellular and intraluminal H^+ concentration, the importance of this layer has been documented in several experimental studies by several groups of investigators [26–28]. The mucus gel layer is also important in maintaining the "hydrophobicity" of cells, a function dependent upon surface-active phospholipids. However, Robert et al. [29] did not find a correlation between the thickness of the mucus gel layer and protection of the gastric mucosa against irritants. It is also known that maintenance of the integrity of the gastric mucosal barrier and of mucus and bicarbonate secretion is dependent upon an intact blood supply to the mucosa (gastric mucosal blood flow). The interruption of normal vascular integrity will adversely affect mucosal function.

In general, the exogenous administration or endogenous stimulation of prostaglandins strengthens the gastric mucosal barrier and positively affects the protective factors listed above (Table 3). Conversely, in most instances, inhibition of PG synthesis has a negative effect on the mucosal integrity.

Table 2 Mucosal Resistance Factors

Mucosal barrier
    Adherent mucus gel layer
    Mucus synthesis/secretion
    Mucus viscosity
    Bicarbonate secretion
    Surface phospholipids
    Blood flow/vascular integrity
    Membrane stabilization
Mucosal regenerative capacity
    Cell turnover (DNA/RNA)

Table 3   Effects of Exogenous Prostaglandin
Administration

Prevent/reduce damage by barrier breakers
Increase thickness of mucus layer
Increase mucus secretion
Increase bicarbonate secretion
Maintain/increase mucosal blood flow
Stabilize tissue lysozymes/vascular endothelium
Improve mucosal regenerative capacity

A.   Protective Effects in Humans

Early in the course of our antisecretory studies, we noticed that subjects who had
received a prostaglandin had a more mucoid gastric juice than those receiving vehicle
or placebo. Several prostaglandin analogues stimulate the intragastric secretion of
mucus in humans [21,30]. Measurements of components of mucus glycoprotein
indicate that PG analogues increase both mucus concentration and output in the basal
state and total mucus output during secretory stimulation. Animal studies by Tao and
Wilson [31] showed that the mucogenic effect of prostaglandins is not restricted to
stimulation of secretion, which may lead to subsequent depletion of mucus stores, but
is also related to the stimulation of mucus synthesis. The exogenous administration of
16,16-dimethyl PGE_2 also increases mucus viscosity, significantly retarding mucus
penetration by H^+ and pepsin [32]. It is also interesting to note that a report by
Younan et al. [33] found that patients with gastric ulcers, and to a lesser extent those
with duodenal ulcers, produce a gastric mucus containing more lower molecular
weight glycoprotein, thereby indicating a weaker mucus structure.

As reported in animals, exogenous PGs stimulate gastroduodenal bicarbonate
secretion in humans [34]. The physiological increase in duodenal bicarbonate secretion seen in response to acid perfusion of the duodenum is markedly reduced by prior
inhibition of endogenous PG synthesis, indicating a role for prostaglandins in mediating this response. Isenberg et al. [35] reported that patients with peptic ulcer
disease secrete less duodenal bicarbonate than do non-ulcer subjects in response to acid
perfusion of the duodenum.

In studies measuring changes in intragastric electrical potential difference (EPD)
during the administration of acidified bile salts to humans, pretreatment with
misoprostol, a PGE_1 analogue, restored the EPD to normal more rapidly than did
placebo [36]. Similar observations have been made in animals.

Ethanol is a direct-acting gastroduodenal mucosal irritant. Prostaglandin analogues markedly reduce the deleterious effects of ethanol on the gastric mucosa in
humans [37]. Agrawal et al. [38] found misoprostol to be significantly superior to
cimetidine in reducing ethanol-induced damage. Although cimetidine also reduced

gastric damage, compared to placebo, misoprostol was far superior to cimetidine ($p <$ .001), essentially totally preventing damage.

IV. TREATMENT OF PEPTIC ULCER DISEASE

Because prostaglandins both inhibit acid secretion and possess cytoprotective properties, there is the potential that these compounds may be superior to standard therapy for peptic ulcer disease. The PG analogues developed to date, however, have achieved healing rates similar to those observed for other available drugs for treating "routine" gastric and duodenal ulcer disease. Rybicka and Gibinski [39] were the first to report a controlled study indicating that methylated analogues of PGE_2 significantly improved the healing of gastroduodenal ulcers. A large number of prostaglandin analogues are in various stages of development and approval as anti-ulcer therapy throughout the world (Table 4). Misoprostol (a PGE_1 analogue) and enprostil (a PGE_2 analogue) have undergone extensive clinical trials and are already available in many countries for the treatment of peptic ulcer disease, although neither drug has been approved in the United States for this indication. Ornoprostil (Alloca), a PGE_1 analogue, is available in Japan for treating gastric ulcers.

A. Duodenal Ulcers

A multicenter trial [40] reported that arbaprostil improved duodenal ulcer healing in a randomized clinical trial, with 67% versus 39% healing at 4 weeks for arbaprostil

Table 4 Status of Prostaglandin Analogues

Drug	Company	Stage
Arbaprostil	Upjohn/Chugai	Filed (Japan)
Enisoprost	Searle	Phase II
Enprostil	Syntex	Launched (Mex,Fr)
FCE-20700	Erbamont	Phase I
GR-63799	Glaxo	Preclinical
Mexiprostil	Merrell Dow	Phase II
Misoprostol	Searle	Launched[a]
Nileprost	Schering AG	Phase II
Nocloprost	Schering AG	Phase II
Ornoprostil	Upjohn/Ono	Launched (Japan)
Rosaprostol	IBI	Launched (Italy)
Trimoprostil	Roche	Filed (Japan)

[a]Approved in United States for prevention of NSAID gastric ulcers.
Source: From SCRIP No. 1395, March 1989.

and placebo, respectively. In a recent study, when arbaprostil was given at a "cyto-protective" dose (10 μg four times daily), no improvement in ulcer healing was noted [41].

Several international clinical trials, involving nearly 1800 patients, have shown misoprostol to be effective in promoting healing of duodenal ulcer [42–45]. In dosages of 100 and 200 μg four times daily or 400 μg twice daily, misoprostol significantly improved ulcer healing compared to placebo. Healing rates at 4 weeks ranged from 65% to 80%. Misoprostol 50 μg four times a day, a minimally antisecretory dose, was not superior to placebo. In comparison studies, misoprostol achieved healing rates similar to those of cimetidine [45]. Misoprostol 200 μg four times daily relieved pain more effectively than placebo but was less effective than cimetidine.

Fewer patients have been reported in enprostil trials. The healing rates are similar to those reported for misoprostol; however, enprostil is administered only on a twice-daily schedule [46–48]. Enprostil was significantly superior to placebo, with 4-week healing rates of 67–78% being reported for both 35 μg and 70μg twice daily. In trials comparing enprostil to H_2-receptor antagonists, Winters et al. [49] reported similar healing at 4 weeks, 75% versus 77% for enprostil 35 μg twice daily and cimetidine 400 mg twice daily, respectively, whereas Lauritsen et al. [50] found that the same dose of enprostil was significantly less effective than ranitidine 150 mg twice daily, with healing rates of 74% and 89%, respectively. Similarly, in a 6-week trial, enprostil (82% healing) was less effective than ranitidine (97% healing) [51]. In general, enprostil was superior to placebo in relieving pain but less effective than the H_2-receptor antagonists.

In a single reported study, trimoprostil 750 μg four times a day was less effective than cimetidine 200 mg three times a day, with 58% versus 89% healing at 4 weeks ($p < .05$) [52]. Rioprostil is a long-acting antisecretory prostaglandin analogue that can be administered once daily [53]. In a preliminary study, rioprostil given at a dose of 600 μg at night achieved a healing rate similar to cimetidine, 85% versus 90% at 4 weeks for rioprostil and cimetidine, respectively [54].

B. Gastric Ulcer

Considering the possible "dual approach" to treatment offered by prostaglandins, it was anticipated that they would prove to be superior to conventional therapy in gastric ulcer disease, a disorder in which a diminution in mucosal integrity is considered to play an important pathogenetic role. However, such superiority has not yet been clearly demonstrated, and prostaglandins appear to be similar to conventional therapy in that they are less effective in healing gastric ulcers than they are for duodenal ulcers and they are not superior to other proven treatment. However, there are some data to suggest that prostaglandins may be more effective than conventional therapy in healing gastric ulcers in certain high-risk groups (see below).

Results from over 1300 patients have been reported from clinical trials using misoprostol. Misoprostol 25 μg four times daily (a nonantisecretory dose) was not superior to placebo, but 100 μg four times daily resulted in 62% healing compared to 45% for placebo ($p < .05$) at 8 weeks in a U.S. study [55]. Rachmilewitz [56] found that misoprostol 200 μg four times daily and cimetidine 300 mg four times daily had similar healing rates, 54% and 61%, respectively, with both being superior to misoprostol 50 μg four times daily. Cimetidine, however, was superior in relieving pain. Shield [57], in a similar comparative study, reported similar results with 60% and 63% healing for misoprostol and cimetidine, respectively.

Relatively few (less than 300) patients have been reported in enprostil studies. Treatment with enprostil 35 μg twice daily resulted in significantly better healing than with placebo, 82% versus 50%, respectively, while enprostil 70 μg was numerically superior (70%) only at 6 weeks [58]. A comparison to ranitidine at 6 weeks resulted in similar healing efficacy, 80% and 84% for enprostil and ranitidine, respectively [59]. A group of investigators [60] compared rioprostil 100 μg twice daily to ranitidine 150 mg twice daily in treating prepyloric gastric ulcers. At the end of 8 weeks, ulcer healing was 60% and 90% for rioprostil and ranitidine, respectively ($p < .01$).

V. NONSTEROIDAL ANTI-INFLAMMATORY DRUGS AND GASTRODUODENAL DAMAGE

Nonsteroidal anti-inflammatory drug (NSAIDs) in general exert their beneficial effects primarily by reducing tissue levels of prostaglandins, by inhibiting the cyclo-oxygenase enzyme. A side effect common to all NSAIDs that do so is the reduction of the gastroduodenal protective PGs, such as PGE_2, $PGF_{2\alpha}$, and PGI_2 (prostacyclin). Gastrointestinal symptoms and gastroduodenal damage are common side effects of long-term NSAID therapy [61]. There is consensus that inhibition of mucosal prostaglandins correlates with mucosal damage in the stomach, although there is less concordance on duodenal ulceration [62,63]. Theoretically, inhibition of cyclo-oxygenase would increase arachidonic acid conversion to lipoxygenase metabolites (e.g., leukotrienes). There are preliminary data linking leukotrienes to experimental gastric injury [64]. There are both epidemiological and direct studies linking NSAID use to increased gastroduodenal complications in humans, including not only increased symptomatology and gastrointestinal bleeding, but also discrete lesions, including erosions and ulcers [65]. Somerville et al. [66] observed a three- to fourfold increase in number of NSAID users in patients entering hospital for gastrointestinal ulcer bleeding. Armstrong and Blower [67] found that 60% of patients entering hospital for ulcer complications were taking NSAIDs whereas only 10% of hospital patients with non-ulcer problems consumed NSAIDs. In several well-controlled endoscopic studies, gastroduodenal ulcers have been reported to occur in 15–22% of patients taking NSAIDs such as aspirin, tolmetin, ibuprofen, naproxene, or piroxicam for a 1-month period.

Yik et al. [68] reported that PGE_2 tablets prevented acute aspirin-induced blood loss in humans. In other short-term studies, enprostil was found to reduce antral and duodenal damage caused by aspirin [69,70]. Silverstein and coworkers [71,72] reported several studies showing that misoprostol protected the stomach against acute damage by aspirin. Lanza [73] found a similar protective effect for misoprostol in preventing or markedly reducing the gastroduodenal damage associated with 1 week of tolmetin 500 mg four times daily in humans.

There have been several studies comparing the efficacy of prostaglandins to H_2-receptor antagonists or sucralfate in preventing gastroduodenal damage. Lanza et al. [74] compared misoprostol to cimetidine in preventing gastroduodenal damage caused by tolmetin 400 mg four times daily for 6 days. While cimetidine significantly reduced gastric damage compared to placebo, misoprostol was superior to cimetidine in preventing gastric damage ($p < .001$). Overall duodenal damage was much less severe than that observed in the stomach, and misoprostol and cimetidine were equally effective in preventing such damage ($p < .001$, compared to placebo). Roth et al. [75] found only a placebo effect for cimetidine in preventing the progression of NSAID-induced gastric lesions. Lanza et al. [76] reported 100% successful prophylaxis for misoprostol against aspirin-induced (650 mg four times daily for 7 days) gastric damage, as compared to 20% for sucralfate ($p < .0001$) and 0% for placebo. Duodenal damage occurred only 60% of the time in this study, with both misoprostol and sucralfate significantly preventing this damage 100% of the time.

Recent studies by a group of investigators (Roth et al. [77]) indicated that 22% of patients with rheumatoid arthritis, taking their usual dosages of aspirin, developed a gastric ulcer after 1 month. When this group of patients were treated with either placebo or misoprostol 200 μg four times daily for 2 months while continuing aspirin therapy, approximately 30% and 65%, respectively ($p < .05$), experienced healing of their ulcers. Graham et al. [78] reported that misoprostol 100 or 200 μg four times daily was 94% and 99% effective, respectively, in preventing gastric ulceration associated with 3 months of NSAID therapy, compared to 78% efficacy for placebo ($p < .001$). Based in large part upon this and similar studies, misoprostol (Cytotec) has been approved for use in the United States to prevent NSAID-induced gastric ulcers.

VI. SMOKING AND PEPTIC ULCER DISEASE

Numerous studies have shown that cigarette smoking not only retards acute ulcer healing but also increases ulcer recurrence. While the association of smoking with ulcers appears stronger for gastric ulcers than for duodenal ulcers, there is strong evidence linking smoking to duodenal disease. Korman et al. [79] reported that duodenal ulcer patients on cimetidine therapy who smoked more than 29 cigarettes daily had a 40% healing rate at 4 weeks compared to an 89% healing rate for patients who smoked fewer than 10 cigarettes daily. The 12-month accumulated recurrence rate was also significantly less for nonsmokers compared to smokers. In a provocative study, patients whose duodenal ulcers healed on cimetidine were followed for 1 year to determine cumulative ulcer recurrences. Nonsmoking patients on placebo actually had a slightly lower recurrence rate (21%) at 1 year than smoking patients who received maintenance cimetidine (34%) [80]. One group of investigators [81] has reported that duodenal ulcers of both smoking and nonsmoking patients receiving misoprostol heal at the same rate, suggesting that prostaglandins may overcome the deleterious effect of cigarette smoking on ulcer healing. However, some other studies have not confirmed this finding.

There are experimental data on humans indicating that cigarette smoking reduces prostaglandin synthesis or output in the stomach and duodenum. Quimby et al. [82] found that smoking four cigarettes acutely reduced PGE_2 and 6-keto $PGF_{1\alpha}$ (stable metabolite of PGI_2) in the gastric fundic mucosa. McCready et al. [83] reported that three cigarettes reduced gastric luminal PGE_2. Moreover, while inhibiting prostaglandin synthesis, cigarette smoke stimulates platelet thromboxane A_2 production [84]. There are several reports in the literature indicating that this potent vasoconstrictor enhances the damaging effects of noxious agents on the gastric mucosa.

VII. PROSTAGLANDINS AND ULCER PATHOGENESIS

Hinsdale et al. [85] reported that patients with duodenal ulcers secreted less PGE in their gastric juice than did normal control subjects, noting that PGE secretion was diminished relative to gastric acid secretion. In the early 1980s, several groups of investigators confirmed this earlier report. However, the documentation of a prostaglandin deficiency in peptic ulcer disease remains controversial. Some investigators have found diminished synthesis and/or secretion of prostanoids only in the stomach of patients with duodenal ulcers [86]; others have also found a reduction in duodenal prostaglandin production [87]. Konturek et al. [63] found decreased prostanoid synthesis in gastric ulcers but not in duodenal ulcers. Ahlquist et al. [88] failed to find an absolute deficiency of PG synthesis but did note a decrease in PG output relative to the duodenal acid load.

Methodological difficulties in terms of both reproducible measurements of prostaglandins and the selection of patients in varying stages of ulcer disease make firm conclusions difficult. However, it does appear that many patients with peptic ulcer disease demonstrate an absolute or relative defect in prostaglandin synthesis and/or secretion.

VIII. RESISTANT ULCERS

In a multicenter study, 4 weeks of misoprostol 200 µg four times daily was compared to placebo healing of duodenal ulcers that had failed to heal on 4 or 8 weeks of therapy with H_2-receptor antagonist therapy [89]. Healing rates of 37% vs. 22% ($p = .02$) in patients who had received 4 weeks of H_2-receptor antagonist therapy was 42% vs.

20% ($p = .01$) in patients who had received 8 weeks of H_2-receptor antagonist therapy were observed for the misoprostol and placebo groups, respectively. Another group of investigators [90] added ornoprostil 10 μg twice daily to the ongoing treatment of resistant gastric ulcers and observed complete healing in 36% of patients after 8 weeks, with an additional 10% of patients showing substantial healing. In Japan, more than 90% of patients with ulcer disease are treated with more than one drug, with the average number being 3.2 concurrent drugs. Definitive studies comparing prostaglandin therapy alone to the continuation of original treatment or to other standard therapy have not yet been performed.

IX. SUMMARY

For two decades, the development of prostaglandins as a more effective therapy for peptic ulcer disease has been anticipated. These expectations have not yet been fully realized. Nearly a dozen PG analogues have been approved for use or are in various stages of development in a variety of countries throughout the world. Second-generation analogues are already being studied.

Naturally occurring prostaglandins play a unique role in normal gastroduodenal mucosal protection. There are data to indicate that prostaglandins may, in fact, provide more effective anti-ulcer therapy in certain unique high-risk groups (e.g., cigarette smokers and patients chronically taking NSAIDs) in whom the risk factors themselves may exert their deleterious effects by inhibiting endogenous mucosal prostaglandin synthesis. Certainly no other therapy to date appears to be as effective as prostaglandins in preventing NSAID-induced gastric ulceration. Prostaglandins may also be effective therapy for "resistant ulcers" and for gastric ulcers in the elderly; however, not enough data are currently available to warrant such conclusions.

In all probability, now that a prostaglandin analogue has been approved in the United States to prevent NSAID-associated gastric ulcers, an expansion of appropriate research will soon bring to realization the full potential of these "interesting" compounds.

REFERENCES

1. Vogt W. Uber die stoffiche grundlage der darmbewegungen und des vasqusriezes am darm. Arch Exp Pharmakol 1949; 206:1–11.
2. Robert A, Nezamis JE, Phillips JP. Inhibition of gastric secretion by prostaglandins. Am J Dig Dis 1967; 12:1073–6.
3. Ramwell PW, Shaw JE. Prostaglandin inhibition of gastric secretion. J Physiol 1968; 195:34–36P.
4. Wilson DE, Levine RA. Decreased canine gastric mucosal blood flow induced by prostaglandin E_1: a mechanism for its inhibitory effect on gastric secretion. Gastroenterology 1969; 56:1268–73.

5.   Main IHM. Effects of prostaglandin E_2 (PGE_2) on the output of histamine and acid in rat gastric secretion induced by pentagastrin or histamine. Br J Pharmacol 1969; 36:214–5P.

6.   Tsai BS, Kessler LK, Schoenhard, Collins PW, Bauer RF. Demonstration of specific E-type prostaglandin receptors using enriched preparations of canine parietal cells and [^{3}H] misoprostol free acid. Am J Med 1987; 83(Suppl 1A):9–14.

7.   Wilson DE, Phillips C, Levine RA. Inhibition of gastric secretion in man by prostaglandin A_1. Gastroenterology 1970; 61:201–6.

8.   Classen M, Koch H, Deyhle P, Weidenhiller S, Demling L. Wirkung von prostaglandin E_1 auf die basale magensekretin des menchen. Klin Wochenschr 1970; 48:876–8.

9.   Larsson C, Anggard E. Distribution of prostaglandin metabolizing enzymes in tissues of the swine. Acta Pharmacol Toxicol 1970; 28(Suppl 1):61.

10.   Ferreira SH, Vane JR. Prostaglandins: their disappearance from and release into the circulation. Nature 1967; 216:868–73.

11.   Dawson W, Jessup SJ, McDonald-Gibson W, Ramwell PW, Shaw J. Prostaglandin uptake and metabolism by the perfused rat liver. Br J Pharmacol 1970; 39:585–98.

12.   Horten EW, Main IHM, Thompson CJ, Wright PM. Effects of orally administered prostaglandin E_1 on gastric secretion and gastrointestinal motility in man. Gut 1968; 9:655–8.

13.   Robert A, Magerlein BJ. 15-Methyl PGE_2 and 16,16,-dimethyl PGE_2: potent inhibitors of gastric secretion. Adv Biosci 1973; 9:247–53.

14.   Robert A. Antisecretory, antiulcer, cytoprotective and diarrheogenic properties of prostaglandins. In: Samuelsson B, Paoletti R, eds. Advances in prostaglandin and thromboxane research, Vol. 2. 1976:507–20.

15.   Dajani EZ, Driskill DR, Bianchi RG, Collins PW, Pappo R. SC-29333: a potent inhibitor of canine gastric secretion. Dig Dis Sci 1976; 21:1049–57.

16.   Karim SMM, Carter DC, Bhana D, Ganesan PA. Effect of orally administered prostaglandin E_2 and its 15-methyl analogues on gastric secretion. Br Med J 1973; 1:143–6.

17.   Robert A, Nylander B, Anderson S. Marked inhibition of gastric secretion by two prostaglandin analogues given orally to man. Life Sci 1974; 14:533–8.

18.   Wilson DE, Winnan G, Quetermus J, Tao P. Effects of an orally administered prostaglandin analogue (16,16-dimethyl prostaglandin E_2) on human gastric secretion. Gastroenterology 1975; 69:607–11.

19.   Konturek SJ, Kwiecien N, Swierczek J, Olesky J, Sito E, Robert A. Comparison of methylated prostaglandin E_2 analogues given orally in the inhibition of gastric responses to pentagastrin and peptone meals in man. Gastroenterology 1976; 70:683–7.

20.   Wilson DE, Quertermus J, Raiser M, Curran J, Robert A. Inhibition of stimulated gastric secretion by an orally administered prostaglandin capsule: a study in normal men. Ann Intern Med 1976; 84:688–91.

21.   Wilson DE, Quadros E, Rajapaksa T, Adams A, Noar M. Effects of misoprostol on gastric acid and mucus secretion in man. Dig Dis Sci 1986; 31(Suppl):126–9S.

22.   Wilson DE. Antisecretory and mucosal protective actions of misoprostol: potential role in the treatment of peptic ulcer disease. Am J Med 1987; 83(Suppl 1A):2–8.

23.   Deakin M, Ramage J, Paul A, Gray SP, Billings J, Williams JG. Effect of enprostil, a synthetic prostaglandin E_2 on 24 hour intragastric acidity, nocturnal acid and pepsin secretion. Gut 1986; 27:1054–7.

24.   Robert A, Nezamis JE, Phillips JP. Effect of prostaglandin E_2 on gastric secretion and ulcer formation in the rat. Gastroenterology 1968; 55:481–7.

25. Robert A, Nezamis JE, Lancaster E, Hanchar AJ. Cytoprotection by prostaglandins in rats. Prevention of gastric necrosis produced by alcohol, HCl, NaOH, hypertonic NaCl and thermal injury. Gastroenterology 1979; 77:433–43.

26. Bahari HMM, Ross IN, Turnberg LA. Demonstration of a pH gradient across the mucus layer on the surface of human gastric mucosa in vitro. Gut 1982; 23:513–6.

27. McQueen S, Allen A, Garner A. Measurement of gastric and duodenal mucus gel thickness. In: Allen A, Flemstrom G, Garner A, Silen W, Turnberg LA, eds. Mechanisms of mucosal protection in the upper gastrointestinal tract. New York: Raven, 1984:215–21.

28. Takeuchi K, Magee D, Critchlow J, Matthews J, Silen W. Studies of the pH gradient and thickness of frog gastric mucus gel. Gastroenterology 1983; 84:331–40.

29. Robert A, Bottcher W, Golanska E, Kauffman GL. Lack of correlation between mucus gel thickness and gastric cytoprotection in rats. Gastroenterology 1984; 86:670–4.

30. Kaymakcalan H, Ramsamooj E, Wilson DE. The effect of a novel prostaglandin (PG)E$_1$ analogue (CL 115,574) on gastric acid and mucus secretion in man. Prostaglandins 1984; 28:5–12.

31. Tao P, Wilson DE. Effects of prostaglandin E$_2$, 16,16-dimethyl prostaglandin E$_2$ and a prostaglandin endoperoxide analogue (U-46619) on gastric secretory volume, [H]$^+$ and mucus synthesis and secretion in the rat. Prostaglandins 1984; 28:353–66.

32. Sarosiek J, Murty VLN, Nadziejko C, Slomiany A, Slomiany BL. Prostaglandin effect on the physical properties of gastric mucus glycoprotein and its susceptibility to pepsin. Prostaglandins 1986; 32:635–46.

33. Younan F, Pearson J, Allen A, Venables C. Changes in the structure of the mucous gel on the mucosal surface of the stomach in association with peptic ulcer disease. Gastroenterology 1982; 82:827–31.

34. Isenberg JI, Hogan DL, Selling JA, Koss MA. Duodenal bicarbonate secretion in humans: role of prostaglandins. Dig Dis Sci 1986; 31(Suppl):130S. Abstract.

35. Isenberg JI, Selling JA, Hogan DL, Koss MA. Impaired proximal duodenal mucosal bicarbonate secretion in patients with duodenal ulcer. N Engl J Med 1987; 316:374–8.

36. Fimmel CJ, Muller-Lissner SA, Blum AL. Bile salt-induced acute gastric damage in man: time course and effect of misoprostol, a PGE$_1$ analogue. Scand J Gastroenterol 1984; 19(Suppl 92):184–8.

37. Tarnowski A, Stachiura S, Ivey JJ, Mach T, Klimczyk B, Bogdal J. Protection by prostaglandin against ethanol induced gastric mucosal damage in man. An endoscopic and histological assessment. Gastroenterology 1981; 80:1300.

38. Agrawal NM, Godiwala T, Arimura A, Dajani EZ. Comparative cytoprotective effects against alcohol: misoprostol versus cimetidine. Dig Dis Sci 1986; 31(Suppl):142S. Abstract.

39. Rybicka J, Gibinski K. Methyl-prostaglandin E$_2$ analogues for healing of gastroduodenal ulcers. Scand J Gastroenterol 1978; 13:155–9.

40. Vantrappen G, Janssens J, Popiela T, Kulig J, Tytgat GNJ, Huibregtse K, Lambert R, Pauchard JP, Robert A. Effect of 15(R),15-methyl prostaglandin E$_2$ (arboprostil) on the healing of duodenal ulcer. A double-blind multicenter study. Gastroenterology 1982; 83:357–63.

41. Euler AR, Tytgat G, Berenguer J, Brunner H, Wood DR, Lookabaugh JL, Phan TD. Failure of a cytoprotective dose of arbaprostil to heal acute duodenal ulcers. Gastroenterology 1987; 92:604–7.

42. Sontag S, Mazure PA, Pontes JF, Beker SG, Dajani EZ. Misoprostol in the treatment of duodenal ulcer: a multicenter double-blinded placebo-controlled study. Dig Dis Sci 1985; 30(Suppl):159–63S.

43. Bright-Asare P, Sontag S, Gould RJ, Brand DL, Roufsil WM, and coinvestigators. Efficacy of misoprostol (twice daily dosage) in acute healing of duodenal ulcer: a multicenter double-blind controlled trial. Dig Dis Sci 1986; 31(Suppl):63–7S.

44. Brand DL, Roufail WM, Thomson ABR, Tapper EJ. Misoprostol, a synthetic PGE_1 analog in the treatment of duodenal ulcers: a multicenter double-blind study. Dig Dis Sci 1985; 30(Suppl):147—58S.

45. Nicholson PA. A multicenter international controlled comparison of two dosage regimens of misoprostol and cimetidine in the treatment of duodenal ulcers in out-patients. Dig Dis Sci 1985; 30(Suppl):171–7S.

46. Archambault AP, Halvorsen L, Lee SP, Maclaurin BP, Navert H, Sevelius H, Sutherland LR, Thompson RPH, Thomson ABR. Efficacy and safety of enprostil, a synthetic prostaglandin and placebo in patients with duodenal ulcer. Am J Gastroenterol 1984; 79:828.

47. Thomson ABR, Navert H, Halvorsen L, Maxton D, Archambault A, Sutherland L, Lee SP, Sevelius H. Treatment of duodenal ulcer with enprostil, a synthetic prostaglandin E_2 analogue. Am J Med 1986; 81(Suppl 2A):59–63.

48. Bright-Asare P, Krejs GJ, Santangelo WC, Brand DL, Brugge WR, Van Zuiden PEA, Tesler MA, Giannikopoulos I, Whiten JT, Bynum L. Treatment of duodenal ulcer with enprostil, a prostaglandin E_2 analogue. Am J Med 1986; 81(Suppl 2A):64–8.

49. Winters L, Willcox R, Ligny G, Barbier P, Deltenre M, Evreux M, Frexinos J, Michel H, Vicari F, Andrieu J, Guerre J, Carling L, Unge P, Hagg S, Cronstedt J, Alstrom C, Northfield T, Reed P, Salmon P, oare A, Cockel R, Schiller K, Trewby P, Edwards M, Mountford R, Dawson J, Elias E, Qureshi M, Miller JP. Comparison of enprostil and cimetidine in active duodenal ulcer disease. Summary of pooled European studies. Am J Med 1986; 81(Suppl 2A):69–74.

50. Lauritsen K, Laursen SK, Havelund T, Bytzer P, Svendsen LB, Madsen-Rask J. Enprostil and ranitidine in duodenal ulcer healing: a double-blind comparative trial. Br J Med 1986; 292:864–6.

51. Bardhan KD, Bose K, Hinchliffe RFC, Whittaker L, Morris P, Massey H, Thomson M. Enprostil (E) versus ranitidine in duodenal ulcer. Gut 1986; 26:A1149.

52. Bardhan KD, Whittaker L, Hinchcliffe RG, Cleur RN, Bose K. Trimoprostil vs cimetidine in duodenal ulcer. Gut 1984; 25:A580.

53. Shriver DA, Rosenthale ME, Kluender HC, Schut RN, McQuire JL, Hong E. Pharmacology of rioprostil, a new gastric cytoprotective/antisecretory agent. Arzneim Firsch/Drug Res 1985; 35:839–43.

54. Dammann HG, Walter TA, Muller P, Simon B. Nighttime rioprostil versus ranitidine in duodenal ulcer healing. Lancet 1986; i:335–6.

55. Agrawal NM, Saffouri B, Kruss DM, Callison DA, Dajani EZ. Healing of benign gastric ulcer: a placebo-controlled comparison of two dosage regimens of misoprostol, a synthetic analogue of prostaglandin E_1. Dig Dis Sci 1985; 30(Suppl):164–70S.

56. Rachmilewitz D, Chapman JW, Nicholson PA, on behalf of an international study group. A multicenter international controlled comparison of two dosage regimens of misoprostol with cimetidine in treatment of gastric ulcer in outpatients. Dig Dis Sci 1986; 31(Suppl):75–80S.

57. Shield MJ. Interim results of a multicenter international comparison of misoprostol and cimetidine in the treatment of out-patients with benign gastric ulcers. Dig Dis Sci 1985; 30(Suppl):178–84S.

58. Navert H, Thomson ABR, Archambault A, Halvorsen L, Lee F, Sutherland L, Sidorov J, Qureshi M, Miller JP. Treatment of gastric ulcer with enprostil. Am J Med 1986; 81(Suppl 2A):75–9.

59. Dammann HG, Huttemann W, Kalek HD, Rohner HG, Simon B. Comparative clinical trial of enprostil and ranitidine in treatment of gastric ulcer. Am J Med 1986; 81(Suppl 2A):80–4.

60. Lauritsen K, Staerk L, Havelund T, Bronnum-Schou J, Madsen-Rask J. Rioprostil and ranitidine in the treatment of prepyloric gastric ulcer. Scand J Gastroenterol 1989; 24:368–72.

61. Larkai EN, Smith JL, Lidsky MD, Graham DY. Gastroduodenal mucosa and dyspeptic symptoms in arthritic patients during chronic non-steroidal anti-inflammatory drug use. Am J Gastroenterol 1987; 82:1153–8.

62. Whittle BJR. Prostaglandin-cyclo-oxygenase inhibition and its relationship to gastric damage. In: Harmon JW, ed. Basic mechanisms of gastrointestinal mucosal cell injury and protection. Baltimore: William & Wilkins, 1981: 197–210.

63. Konturek SJ, Kwiecien N, Obtulowicz W, Olesky J, Sito E, Kopp B. Prostaglandins in peptic ulcer disease: effect of nonsteroidal antiinflammatory compounds (NOSAC). Scand J Gastroenterol 1984; 19(Suppl 92):250–4.

64. Quadros E, Wilson DE. Nordihydroguaiaretic acid (NDGA) prevents ethanol-induced gastric mucosal damage: role of arachidonic acid lipoxygenase pathway metabolites. Gastroenterology 1987; 92:1584.

65. Fries JF, Miller SR, Spitz PW, Williams CA, Hubert HB, Block DA. Toward an epidemiology of gastropathy associated with nonsteroidal anti-inflammatory drug use. Gastroenterology 1989; 96:647–55.

66. Somerville K, Faulkner G, Langman M. Non-steroidal anti-inflammatory drugs and bleeding peptic ulcer. Br J Clin Pract 1987; (May, Suppl):64–7.

67. Armstrong CP, Blower AL. Non-steroidal anti-inflammatory drugs and life threatening complications of peptic ulceration. Gut 1987; 28:527–32.

68. Yik KY, Dreidger AA, Watson WC. Prostaglandin E_2 tablets prevent aspirin-induced blood loss in man. Dig Dis Sci 1982; 27:972–974.

69. Cohen MM, McCredy DR, Clark L, Sevelius H. Protection against aspirin-induced antral and duodenal damage with enprostil. A double-blind endoscopic study. Gastroenterology 1985; 88:382–6.

70. Stiel D, Ellard KT, Hills LJ, Brooks PM. Protective effect of enprostil against aspirin-induced gastroduodenal mucosal injury in man. Am J Med 1986; 81(Suppl 2A):54–8.

71. Silverstein FE, Kimmey MB, Saunders DR, Levine DS. Gastric protection by misoprostol against 1300 mg of aspirin: an endoscopic study. Dig Dis Sci 1986; 31(Suppl): 137–41S.

72. Silverstein FE, Kimmey MB, Saunders DR, Surawicz CM, Willson RA, Silverman BA. Gastric protection by misoprostol against 1300 mg of aspirin: an endoscopic dose-response study. Am J Med 1987; 83(Suppl 1A):32–6.

73. Lanza FL. A double-blind study of prophylactic effect of misoprostol on lesions of gastric and duodenal mucosa induced by oral administration of tolmetin in healthy subjects. Dig Dis Sci 1986; 31(Suppl):131–6S.

74. Lanza FL, Aspinall RL, Swabb EA, Davis RE, Rack MF, Rubin A. A double-blind placebo-controlled endoscopic comparison of the cytoprotective effects of misoprostol and cimetidine on tolmetin-induced gastric mucosal injury. Gastroenterology 1987; 92:1491. Abstract.

75. Roth SH, Bennett RE, Mitchell CS, Charles S, Ruby J. Cimetidine therapy in non-steroidal anti-inflammatory drug gastropathy. Arch Intern Med 1987; 147:1798–1801.

76. Lanza FL, Peace K, Gustitus L, Rack MF, Dickson B. A blinded endoscopic comparative study of misoprostol versus sucralfate and placebo in the prevention of aspirin-induced gastric and duodenal ulceration. Am J Gastroenterol 1988; 83:143–6.

77. Roth S, Agrawal NM, Mahowald M, Montoya H, Robbins R, Miller S, Nutting S, Woods E, Crager M, Swabb E. Misoprostol heals gastroduodenal injury patients with rheumatoid arthritis receiving aspirin. Arch Intern Med 1989; 149:775–9.

78. Graham DY, Agrawal NM, Roth SH. Prevention of NSAID-induced gastric ulcer with misoprostol: multicentre, double-blind, placebo-controlled trial. Lancet 1988; ii:1277–80.

79. Korman MG, Hansky J, Eaves ER, Schmidt GT. Influence of cigarette smoking on healing and relapse in duodenal ulcer disease. Gastroenterology 1983; 85:871–4.

80. Sontag S, Graham DY, Belisto A, Weiss J, Farley A, Grunt R, Cohen N, Kinnear D, Davis W, Archambault A, Achord J, Thayer W, Gillies R, Sidorov J, Sabesin SM, Dyck W, Fleshler B, Cleator I, Wengerm J, Opekun A. Cimetidine, cigarette smoking and recurrence of duodenal ulcer. N Engl J Med 1984; 311:689–93.

81. Lam SK, Lau WY, Choi TK, Lai CL, Lok ASF, Hui WM, Ng MMT, Choi SKY. Prostaglandin E_1 (misoprostol) overcomes the adverse effect of chronic cigarette smoking on duodenal ulcer healing. Dig Dis Sci 1986; 31(Suppl):68–74S.

82. Quimby G, Bonnice CA, Burstein SH, Eastwood GL. Active smoking depresses prostaglandin synthesis in human gastric mucosa. Ann Intern Med 1986; 104:616–9.

83. McCready DR, Clark L, Cohen MM. Cigarette smoking reduces human gastric luminal prostaglandin E_2. Gut 1985; 26:1192–6.

84. Lubawy WC, Culpepper BT, Valentovic MA. Alterations in prostacyclin and thromboxane formation by chronic cigarette smoke exposure: temporal relationships and whole smoke vs. gas phase. J Appl Toxicol 1986; 6:77–80.

85. Hinsdale J, Engel JJ, Wilson DE. Prostaglandin E in peptic ulcer disease. Prostaglandins 1974; 6:495–500.

86. Sharon P, Cohen F, Zifroni A, Karmeli F, Ligumsky M, Rachmilewitz D. Prostanoid synthesis by cultured gastric and duodenal mucosa: possible role in the pathogenesis of duodenal ulcer. Scand J Gastroenterol 1983; 18:1045–9.

87. Hillier K, Smith CL, Jewell R, Arthur MJP, Ross G. Duodenal mucosa synthesis of prostaglandins in duodenal ulcer disease. Gut 1985; 26:237–40.

88. Ahlquist DA, Dozois RR, Zinmesiter AR, Malagelada JR. Duodenal prostaglandin synthesis and acid load in health and in duodenal ulcer disease. Gastroenterology 1983; 85:522–8.

89. Newman RD, Gitlin N, Lacayo EJ, Safdi AV, Ramsey EJ, Engel SL, Rubin A, Nissen CH, Swabb EA. Misoprostol in the treatment of duodenal ulcer refractory to H_2-blocker therapy. Am J Med 1987; 83(Suppl 2A):27–31.

90. Sasagawa C, Kimura A, Ogoshi K, Saito M, Niwa M, Tomizawa M, Sekine T, Shinohara T, Souma T, Sekine A, Murayama H, Watanabe Y, Oda K, Tomidokoro T, Toeda K, Tosaka T, Kawamura T. Gendai Iryo 1986; 18(Suppl):404.

13

Sucralfate: Efficacy and Basis for Therapy

I. N. MARKS

Gastrointestinal Clinic, Groote Schuur Hospital, and
University of Cape Town, Cape Town, South Africa

I.   INTRODUCTION

The past decade has seen profound changes in the management of peptic ulcer disease. Conventional antacid regimens have been seriously challenged by a bewildering array of newer ulcer-healing agents. The perception of the problem has also changed. Relapse rates and maintenance therapy have become virtual buzzwords, and controversies abound. These include the choice of treatment for short-term ulcer healing, the question as to whether relapse rates are higher following healing with some drugs than with others, the advisability and choice of maintenance therapy, and safety aspects. In addition, the management of reflux esophagitis and stress ulcer prophylaxis have added new dimensions to the therapeutic controversy.

Tentative advances have been made in our understanding of the ulcer diathesis, but, in general, the cause of ulcer disease remains elusive. Most current therapeutic options can be relied upon to heal the ulcer, but they do little to cure the disease. Perhaps the most vexing issue, therefore, is the choice of the most appropriate first-line treatment in peptic ulcer disease—a potent acid-inhibitory drug, a mucosal protective agent, or, indeed, antacids.

This review will focus on the current status of sucralfate, the most widely used mucosal protective agent.

II.   MODE OF ACTION

Sucralfate, a basic aluminum salt of sucrose octasulfate, is a unique, locally active ulcer-healing agent. It is essentially protective in character and involves two distinct mechanisms of action.

A. Ulcer-Coating Effect

Sucralfate becomes a viscous substance when exposed to gastric acid. This forms an adherent and protective chemical complex with proteins at the ulcer site that acts as an effective barrier against the deleterious actions of acid, pepsin, and bile salts. In addition, sucralfate absorbs pepsin [1] and bile salts [2], and its basic aluminum moieties may serve to buffer hydrogen ions somewhat [3].

The selective binding of sucralfate to proteins at the ulcer site has been demonstrated in both experimental animals and humans. Significant binding of ^{14}C-sucralfate at the ulcer site was still present after 6 hr in the rat [4,5], and gastric ulcer patients given sucralfate 1.5 g 12–16 hr before gastric resection showed, on an average, six to seven times as much sucralfate per square centimeter in the ulcer area as in the healthy mucosa of the same patient [6]. A biopsy study in duodenal ulcer patients given sucralfate 1 g, 3–12 hr previously showed similar evidence of selective binding to the ulcer site [7].

B. Mucosa-Protective Effects

Apart from the formation of a protective barrier on ulcerated surfaces, there is evidence that sucralfate acts on the gastric and duodenal mucosa in a more general and complex fashion. The latter may explain the finding of Danesh et al. [8] that sucralfate protection against mucosal injury induced by aspirin and bile acids in the rat may occur in a near-neutral pH milieu. It would appear that sucralfate protects the stomach against injury by prostaglandin-dependent and prostaglandin-independent mechanisms [9]. Sucralfate stimulates prostaglandin E_2 luminal release and mucus output in the rat [10], and in vitro studies suggest that it improves the barrier property of pig mucus by increasing viscosity and reducing the permeability to hydrogen ions [11]. Mucosal bicarbonate secretion is increased in the isolated amphibian mucosal model [12], and, remarkably, ethanol-induced microvascular damage can be prevented by large doses of sucralfate given subcutaneously in the rat [13]. There is some evidence that sucralfate binding to epidermal growth factor facilitates delivery of the latter to the ulcer base [14]. This carrier role of sucralfate may be relevant to ulcer healing.

Sucralfate prevents gastric mucosal damage caused by ethanol, taurocholic acid, and aspirin, and it is thought that endogenous prostaglandins may mediate, at least in part, in this protective action. The protective effect of sucralfate against aspirin-induced gastric damage, however, cannot be entirely attributed to mucosal prostaglandins, because the latter are suppressed under these conditions [15]. By the same token, the drug has been shown to stimulate mucus output even in the presence of aspirin [16]. These findings suggest that sucralfate protection against aspirin damage is probably unrelated to mucosal prostaglandins, and the same may pertain to other experimental models. One can but speculate as to whether the luminal release of prostaglandins in the rat is not perhaps linked to disruption and exfoliation of surface epithelial cells following administration of large doses of sucralfate of the order of 500 mg per kilogram body weight [10]. Studies on the effect of sucralfate on mucosal prostaglandins in humans have been equally controversial [15,17].

Studies have been carried out to determine whether the mucosa-protective effect of sucralfate might perhaps be attributable to any of its individual components. The sulfate radical has been shown to be the most important in protection against acute gastric and esophageal damage [18,19]. Sucralfate, however, was at least twice as active as its individual components, suggesting an additive or potentiating interaction among them [18].

III.   CLINICAL EVALUATION

A.   Short-Term Ulcer Healing

1.   Efficacy in Ulcer Healing

Sucralfate given in a dose of 4 g/day (1 g three times daily 30 min before meals and 1 g at night) has been shown to be significantly better than placebo and as effective as cimetidine (0.8–1.2 g/day) or ranitidine (150 mg twice daily) in healing both duodenal and gastric ulcers [20,21] (Figs. 1–3). Healing rates after 4 weeks of sucralfate therapy range from 60 to 92% in duodenal ulcer patients and from 47 to 62% in gastric ulcer patients. Gastric ulcer healing rates after 8 weeks of therapy are of the order of 75–83% [20,22,23].

2.   Smoking and Duodenal Ulcer Healing

Data derived from six duodenal ulcer healing studies [21,24] suggest that smoking has no adverse effect on healing in sucralfate-treated patients. The healing rate among

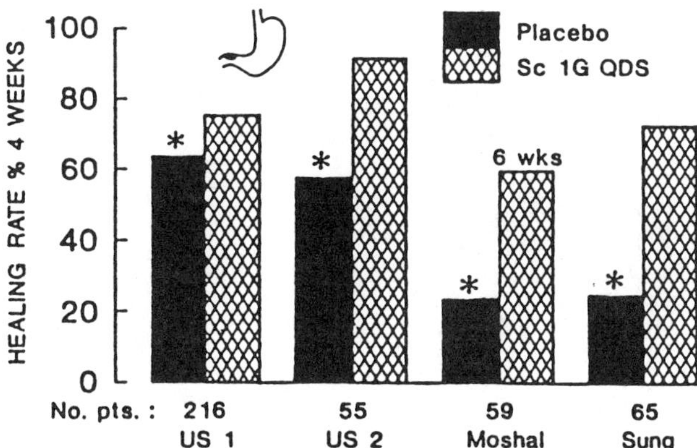

FIGURE 1   Short-term duodenal ulcer healing rates at 4 weeks with sucralfate (Sc) and placebo. (From Marks [21].)

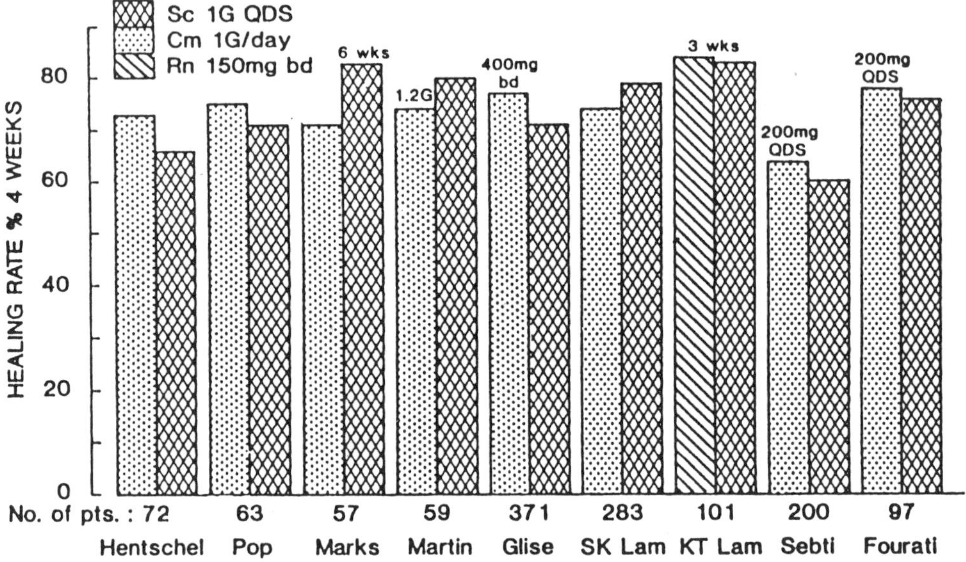

FIGURE 2   Short-term duodenal ulcer healing rates at 4 weeks with sucralfate (Sc), cimetidine (Cm), and ranitidine (Rn). (From Marks [21].)

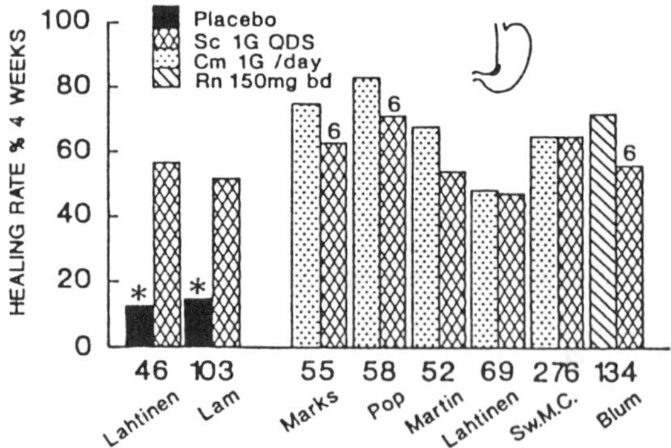

FIGURE 3   Short-term gastric ulcer healing rates at 4 weeks with sucralfate (Sc), cimetidine (Cm), ranitidine (Rn), and placebo. (From Marks [21].)

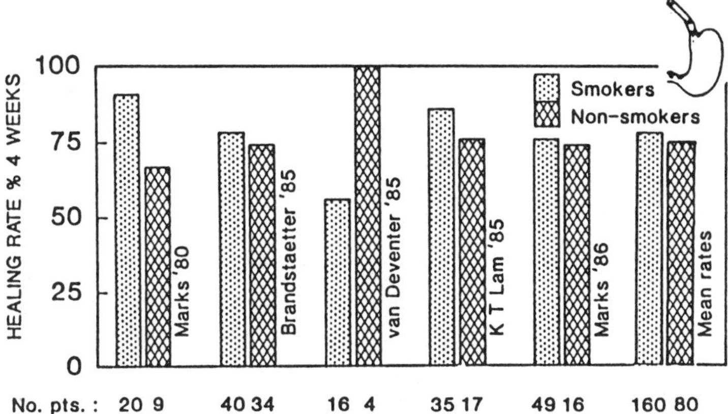

FIGURE 4   Smoking does not influence duodenal ulcer healing in sucralfate-treated patients. (From Marks [21].)

198 smokers and 173 nonsmokers culled from these studies was 79% and 77%, respectively (Fig. 4).

3.   Newer Dosage Regimen

Single-blind studies have shown that sucralfate given in a dose of 2 g twice daily (on waking and before bed) is as effective as the conventional dose of 1 g four times daily [25,26]. These findings have been confirmed in a double-blind study [27].

4.   Newer Preparations

Sucralfate is available in tablet form (1 g), in a granular form (1-g sachet), and in a palatable suspension. The suspension contains 1 g of sucralfate per 5 mL in some countries, and 1 g/10 mL in others. The suspension is the preferred formulation in the treatment of reflux esophagitis, in the intensive care setting, and in patients who experience difficulty in swallowing the 1-g tablet.

B.   Maintenance Treatment

1.   Duodenal Ulcers

The efficacy of sucralfate in maintenance therapy has been amply confirmed in a number of placebo- and cimetidine-controlled studies. Figure 5 shows the results of available 12-month maintenance studies. Sucralfate was significantly better than placebo and at least as effective as cimetidine or ranitidine. The dose of sucralfate in these studies was of the order of 2–2.5 g/day and in all but one of them the drug was given in divided doses.

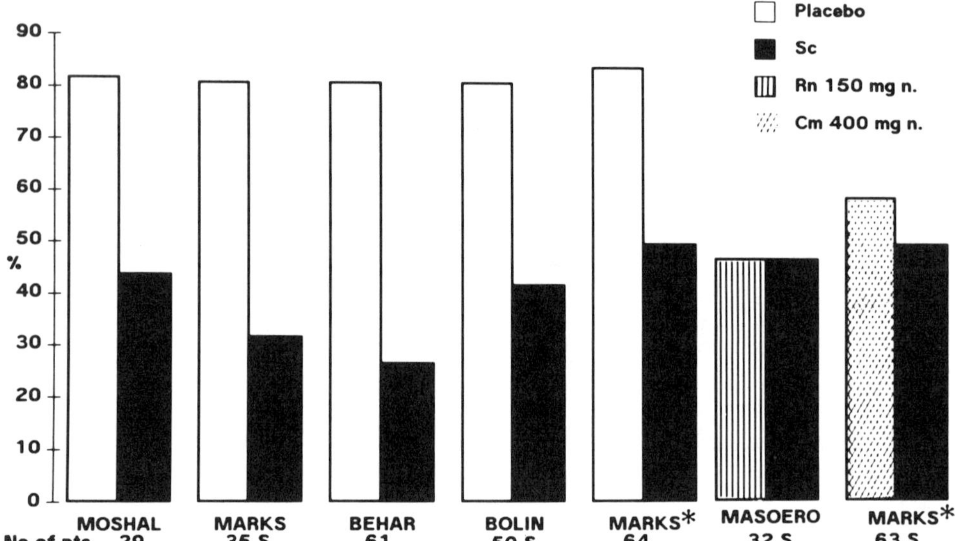

FIGURE 5 Duodenal ulcer relapse rates on maintenance treatment with sucralfate 1 g twice daily (Sc), ranitidine 150 mg at night (Rn), cimetidine 400 mg at night (Cm), and placebo at 1 year. * = sucralfate 2 g at night; S = single-blind study. (From Marks et al. [34].)

2. Gastric Ulcers

Figure 6 shows the results of available placebo- and cimetidine-controlled 6-month maintenance studies. An early study by Classen et al. [28] failed to show a significant advantage of sucralfate 1 g twice a day over placebo, but subsequent studies showed that sucralfate 1 g in the morning and 2 g at night [29] or, indeed, sucralfate 2 g at night [30] were clearly efficacious. Cimetidine-controlled studies have shown the drug to be at least as effective as cimetidine [31,32].

The superiority of sucralfate 2 g/day over placebo in the maintenance treatment of gastric ulcer has recently been confirmed in a 12-month maintenance study. Relapses occurred in 20 of 49 (41%) sucralfate-treated and in 32 of 42 (76%) placebo-treated patients [33].

3. Newer Maintenance Schedules

Gastric and duodenal ulcer maintenance studies have shown that a single daily dose of sucralfate 2 g at night offers meaningful protection against ulcer recurrence [30,34].

C. Reflux Esophagitis

Sucralfate given in a dose of 1 g four times daily is as effective as cimetidine 400 mg four times daily [35] or ranitidine 150 mg twice daily [36] in the management of

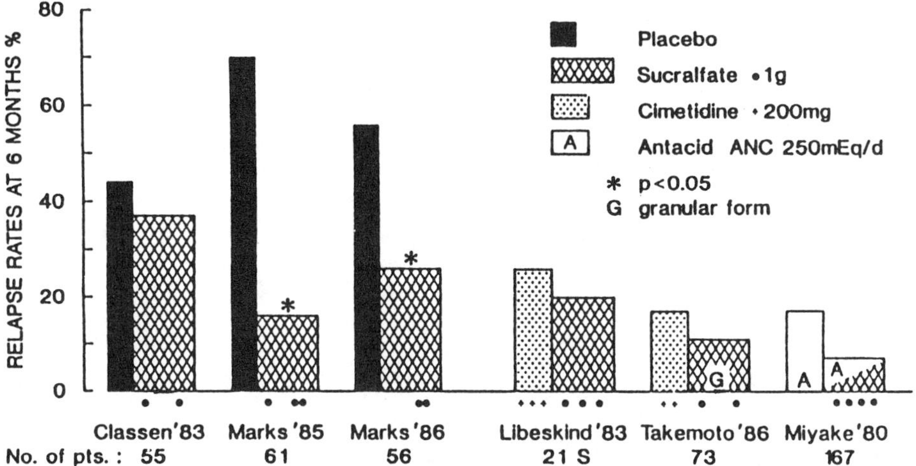

FIGURE 6 Gastric ulcer relapse rates with maintenance treatment with sucralfate, placebo, cimetidine, or antacids. ANC = acid-neutralizing capacity; S = single-blind study. (From Marks [21].)

reflux esophagitis. The drug has been shown to be significantly better than placebo after 12 weeks of treatment [37], but a more recent placebo-controlled study failed to show an unequivocal advantage of sucralfate over placebo after 8 weeks of therapy [38]. Available evidence suggests that a 12-week course of treatment is warranted or, alternatively, that a larger dose of sucralfate (6 g/day) be considered.

D. Stress Ulcer Prophylaxis

Sucralfate given in a dose of 1 g every 6 hr is as effective as antacids or H_2-receptor blockers in stress ulcer prophylaxis [39,40], but recent evidence suggests that a larger dose of sucralfate may be more effective than an H_2-receptor blocker. Laggner et al. [41] treated 85 patients in the intensive care setting with either sucralfate 6 g daily or ranitidine 300–600 mg daily. Bleeding occurred more commonly in the ranitidine-treated patients ($p < .05$), and the latter showed, in addition, a higher incidence of positive bacterial cultures in blood ($p < .05$) and bronchial secretions ($p < .01$). These findings were in keeping with the observations of Driks et al. [42] and Tryba [43] regarding a significantly greater incidence of nosocomial pneumonia in patients treated with antacids or an H_2-receptor blocker than in those treated with sucralfate. An increased gastric pH predisposes to bacterial overgrowth in the stomach, retrograde colonization of the pharynx, and an increased liability to nosocomial pneumonia. The use of a prophylactic agent against stress ulcer bleeding that preserves the natural gastric acid barrier against bacterial overgrowth may thus be preferable to antacids and H_2-receptor blockers [44]. It should be noted that untreated patients in the intensive care setting not infrequently show an increased gastric pH. Despite this, sucralfate remains the drug of choice in stress ulcer prophylaxis.

IV. RELAPSE RATES AFTER SUCRALFATE THERAPY

Recurrence rates after initial duodenal ulcer healing appear to have shown a marked increase over those reported in earlier studies. Reasons for this include the intensity of follow-up, the availability of duodenoscopy, and, paradoxically, the remarkable efficacy of the newer ulcer-healing agents in short-term healing. A larger proportion of deeply penetrating ulcers—with their profound liability to relapse—are now being healed. The increase in the use of endoscopy has led to the earlier and more frequent finding of ulcer relapse, and asymptomatic recurrences detected during routine follow-up examination now account for up to 25% of relapses in many controlled studies. The reported increase also raises the question as to whether the potent acid-inhibitory agents do not, in themselves, invite a higher relapse rate [45].

A. Relapse Rates After Short-Term Treatment

It is generally accepted that duodenal ulcers recur within a year in 75–90% of patients treated initially with an H_2-receptor blocker, and the same is almost certainly true with regard to omeprazole. Relapse rates following initial treatment with colloidal bismuth agents are appreciably, and often significantly, lower than those following

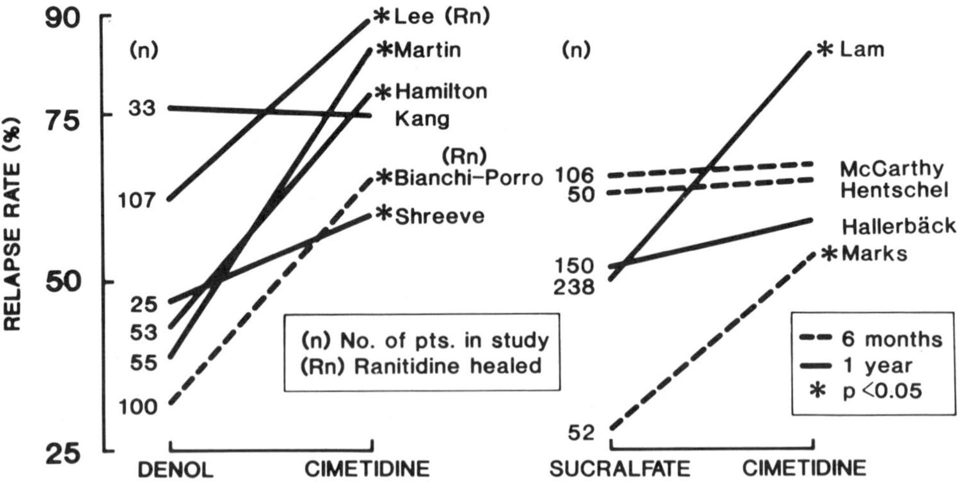

FIGURE 7 Comparative relapse rates following duodenal ulcer healing by an H_2-receptor antagonist or a mucosa-protective agent. (From Marks [102].)

initial treatment with an H_2-receptor blocker, and a similar advantage has been reported in some studies in patients healed initially with sucralfate [46] (Fig. 7).

An early study [47] showed that sucralfate-healed ulcers have a longer duration of remission than those following short-term treatment with cimetidine. Relapse rates in the sucralfate-healed group were appreciably lower at 3 and 6 months, but the rates were comparable after a year. Three subsequent studies [48–50] showed only a marginal advantage of sucralfate over cimetidine. A comprehensive study of 238 patients by Lam et al. [24], however, shows that the remission period following sucralfate healing was double that of cimetidine, suggesting that sucralfate may indeed have an advantage over cimetidine in terms of ulcer relapse.

B.   Relapse Rates after Maintenance Therapy

1.   Gastric Ulcer Disease

An early study suggested that gastric ulcer relapse rates after 6 months of maintenance treatment with sucralfate were lower than those following treatment with antacids [51]. Takemoto et al. [32] more recently showed lower relapse rates in gastric ulcer patients after maintenance treatment with sucralfate than in those treated with cimetidine.

2.   Duodenal Ulcer Disease

Takemoto et al. [32], in the same study, were unable to confirm this advantage of maintenance sucralfate over cimetidine in duodenal ulcer patients. Tovey et al. [52], however, noted a lower relapse rate after maintenance treatment with sucralfate than with cimetidine, in keeping with the earlier observations of Libeskind [31].

3.   Initial Treatment and Relapse on Maintenance Therapy

There is, in addition, some slender evidence concerning the possible advantage of sucralfate healing on subsequent duodenal ulcer relapse in the maintenance setting. Patients healed initially on H_2-receptor blockers alone fared less well than those healed initially on sucralfate with or without an H_2-receptor blocker or antacids in a maintenance study comparing sucralfate, cimetidine, and placebo [34]. Blum and Bethge [33] were unable to confirm this observation in patients following treatment for gastric ulcer.

C.   Parietal Cell Sensitivity

The reason for the trend toward lower relapse rates after ulcer healing with mucosa-protective, as opposed to acid-inhibitory, agents is not clear. The antimicrobial action of the colloidal bismuth agents against *Helicobacter* (*Campylobacter*) *pylori* may have some relevance [53,54], and the possibility that these agents may continue to exert an effect once treatment is withdrawn cannot be excluded. Gavey et al. [55] recently confirmed the observation that bismuth accumulates in the body during short-term treatment with a colloidal bismuth agent [56]. These possible mechanisms cannot be invoked in the case of sucralfate. Lower relapse rates following healing with sucralfate and, presumably, the colloidal bismuth agents may be reconciled with increased parietal cell sensitivity (PCS) after treatment with an H_2-receptor blocker [57–59]. The notion of increased PCS in patients with an active duodenal ulcer is not a new one, but it is only in recent years that its relevance in early relapse has become apparent.

1. Definitions

The terms parietal cell responsiveness and parietal cell sensitivity define the sensitivity of the parietal cells in terms of the response to a low-dose stimulus. They are, at best, rather arbitrary. The stimuli may differ, the low dose employed by different workers is not necessarily the same, and the response may or may not be corrected for basal secretion. (See Table 1.) Parietal cell responsiveness may be measured, simply, as the response to a minimal or submaximal stimulus expressed in milliequivalents per hour, whereas PCS is derived from dose–response curves or the ratio of a low-dose or submaximal response to the maximum acid output (MAO) expressed as a percentage. Transformation of the dose–response data may allow calculation of the ED_{50}, the dose required for producing 50% of the MAO. This provides yet another measure of PCS or parietal cell responsiveness.

2. PCS and Duodenal Ulcer Healing

There is good evidence to show that PCS is increased in patients with an active duodenal ulcer [60–63]. There is a lot less to indicate whether this increased PCS falls

Table 1   Measurement of Parietal Cell Responsiveness

   I.   Response to minimal or submaximal stimulus (mEq/hr)
-   A. Antral distention
-   B. Low dose: pentagastrin, tetragastrin, histamine, and impromidine
-   C. Simulated test meal/chewing gum
-   D. Nocturnal acid secretion
-   E. Basal acid secretion

  II. Parietal cell sensitivity (PCS)
-   A. Dose–response curves: pentagastrin, tetragastrin, histamine, and impromidine
  -     1. Ratio of low or submaximal responses to MAO (%)
  -     2. ED_{50}—dose required for 50% MAO
-   B. Other submaximal response MAO ratios (%)
  -     1. Antral distention vs. MAO
  -     2. Chewing gum response vs. MAO
  -     3. Nocturnal acid secretion vs. MAO
  -     4. Basal acid secretion vs. MAO

---

with ulcer healing. Antral distention studies by Celestin [64] and Bergegardh and Olbe [65] suggested that this increased PCS diminishes on ulcer healing, and Achord [66] found both basal and peak acid outputs to be higher in patients with an active duodenal ulcer than in others with a healed duodenal ulcer. The concept of a reduction in parietal cell responsiveness and PCS on duodenal ulcer healing received strong support from a recent study in 20 patients with active duodenal ulceration [67]. Ten patients were randomly assigned to treatment with ranitidine 300 mg at night, and the other ten were put on a regimen of sucralfate 2 g twice daily for 6 weeks. The acid-secretory response to low- and high-dose infusions of the secretory stimulants penta-gastrin or histamine acid phosphate was determined before treatment and 60–84 hr after treatment had been withdrawn and endoscopic healing confirmed. PCS was calculated as the ratio of low-dose to high-dose acid output expressed as a percentage. The acid-secretory responses and PCS in the entire group showed a significant fall on ulcer healing (Fig. 8). The reduction in PCS, however, was significant only in the sucralfate-treated subgroup and not in the ranitidine-treated subgroup (Fig. 9). These differences can be reconciled with the findings in a number of recent studies examining the effect of short- or long-term treatment with an H_2-receptor blocker in control and duodenal ulcer subjects.

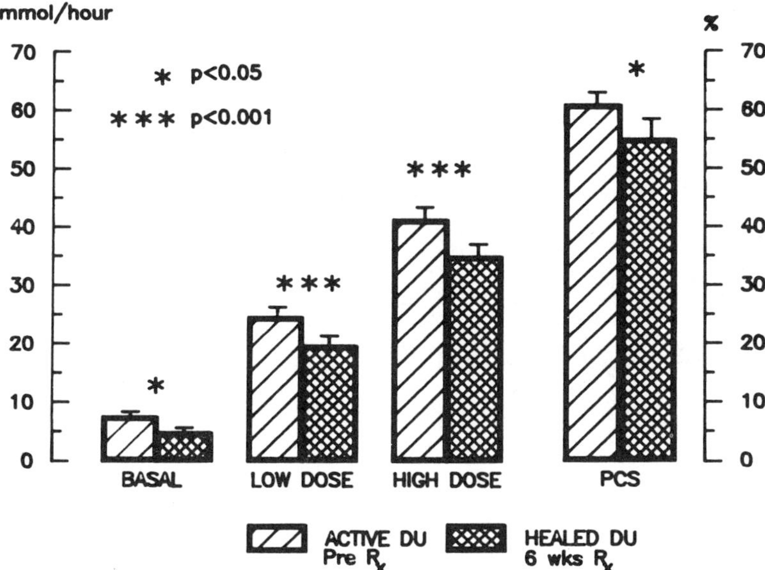

FIGURE 8 Acid secretory responses (mean ± SEM) before and after duodenal ulcer healing in 20 patients treated with ranitidine ($n = 10$) or sucralfate ($n = 10$). (From Marks et al. [67].)

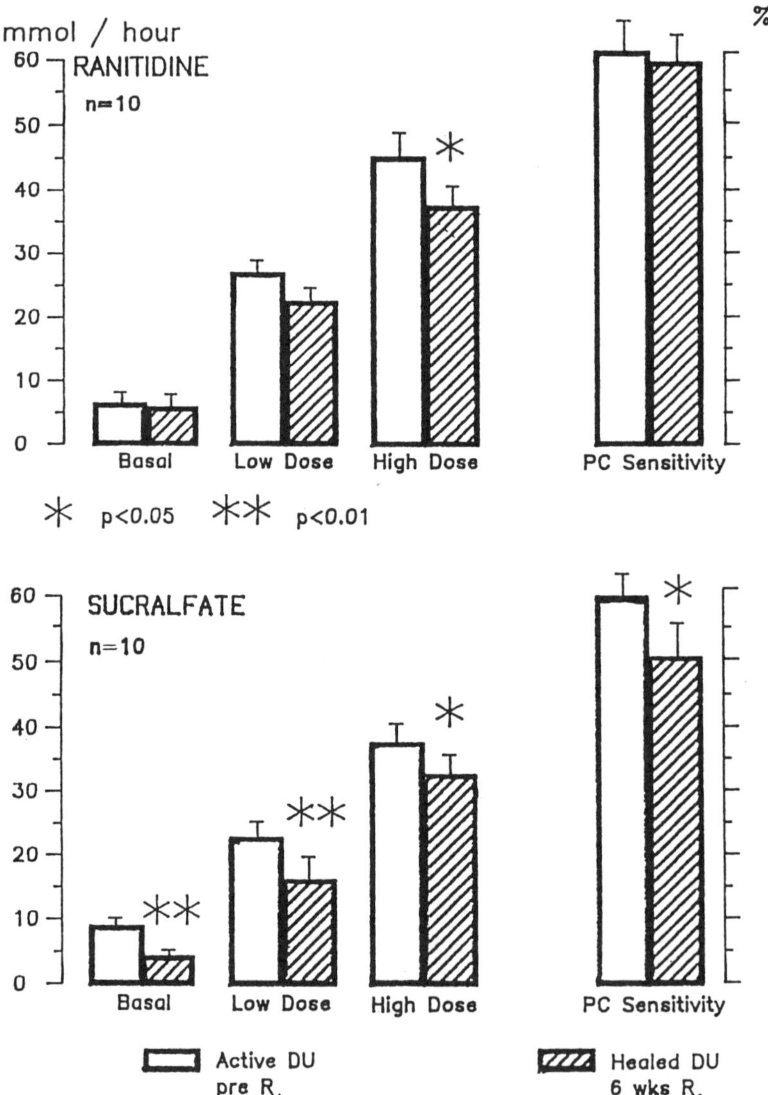

FIGURE 9   Acid secretory responses (mean ± SEM) before and after duodenal ulcer healing with ranitidine or sucralfate. The scale for PCS corresponds to that for acid output. (From Marks et al. [67].)

3.   Influence of H_2-Receptor Blockers on PCS

Aadland and Berstad [68] and Frislid et al. [57] reported a transient increase in PCS in control subjects following 4 weeks of treatment with cimetidine 1 g/day and ranitidine 150 mg twice a day, respectively. Jones et al. [58] showed increased responses to graded doses of impromidine following 3 months of maintenance treatment with ranitidine 150 mg at night in a small group of duodenal ulcer patients in remission, and Fullarton et al. [59] noted a significant increase in nocturnal acid secretion in a similar group of patients treated with nizatidine 300 mg at night for 1 month. Aadland and Berstad [69], however, found no consistent change in PCS following duodenal ulcer healing in a group of 10 patients treated with cimetidine 1 g/day for 6–8 weeks. This, in retrospect, is hardly surprising, because any increase in PCS attributable to treatment with an H_2-receptor blocker may well have been tempered by the fall in PCS on ulcer healing. It is of interest that Walsh et al. [70] found increased acid secretory responses following 4 weeks of treatment with omeprazole in a mixed group of 46 duodenal ulcer patients, in which only 14 of the ulcers were inactive.

The finding of increased acid-secretory responses following treatment with an acid-inhibitory agent is not unique to humans. The Inselspital group reported increased parietal cell responsiveness in the rat following prolonged treatment with metiamide [71] or omeprazole [72], and Coruzzi and Bertaccini [73] demonstrated a transient increase in PCS in the conscious cat after prolonged treatment with ranitidine.

4.   Predictive Value of PCS on Ulcer Relapse

The clinical relevance of an increased PCS on ulcer healing has been studied by two independent groups of workers. The methodologies differed somewhat, but the conclusions were the same.

Marks and Young [74] followed up a group of 21 patients with an active duodenal ulcer that healed after treatment with either ranitidine 300 mg at night or sucralfate 2 g twice daily for 6 weeks, and this study has since been extended to 32 patients [75]. Endoscopy and acid-secretory studies were performed before and after active treatment and repeated after a further 4 weeks of treatment with token antacids. An early relapse was noted in 13 (41%) of the 32 patients. The majority of patients in the early-relapse group showed persistent elevation of the low-dose acid output (LD_{AO}) and PCS after initial ulcer healing, whereas the patients who did not develop an early relapse showed a significant fall in LD_{AO} and PCS on ulcer healing (Fig. 10). An increase in the LD_{AO} and PCS on ulcer healing was thus of value in predicting an early relapse within the next 4 weeks. Another interesting aspect of the study was the difference in the relapse rates in the two treatment groups. Ten of 15 ranitidine-healed patients had an early relapse compared to only 3 of 17 sucralfate-healed patients. These differences could also be reconciled with differences in the fall in LD_{AO} and PCS with ulcer healing.

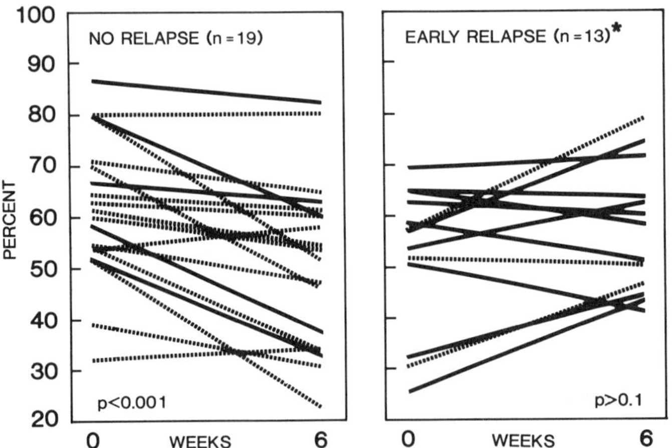

FIGURE 10 Parietal cell sensitivity before and after duodenal ulcer healing in patients in whom a subsequent early relapse was, or was not, found. Solid lines, ranitidine treatment; dotted lines, sucralfate treatment; * = relapse 4–6 weeks later. (After Young et al. [75].)

Yanaka and Muto [76] carried out a tetragastrin dose–response study in each of 65 patients within a week of documented duodenal ulcer healing. The patients had been treated with antacids with or without a short course of cimetidine. Routine endoscopies were done at 3-month intervals, and a repeat dose–response study was carried out in some patients. The patients were divided into three groups based on the 2-year endoscopic follow-up study. The early-recurrence group consisted of 16 patients with recurrence occurring within 3 months of documented healing, and the late-recurrence group included 25 whose ulcers recurred after 3 months. The remaining 24 had no recurrence during the 2-year follow-up period. Patients in the early-recurrence group showed a significant increase in PCS following ulcer healing (Fig. 11), and studies in a few patients in the late-recurrence group suggested that PCS increases within 3 months of recurrence. They concluded that increased PCS correlates strongly with duodenal ulcer recurrence.

The high incidence of early relapses following duodenal ulcer healing in the Cape Town study may be construed as being at variance with the generally accepted relapse rate of 75–90% after 1 year. The recurrence rate of 67% in patients off active treatment for a mere 4 weeks after ranitidine healing, while surprisingly high, should be compared with the 22% rate found by Boyd et al. [77] in patients 1 month after starting *maintenance ranitidine* following duodenal ulcer healing with ranitidine. The relapse rate on maintenance ranitidine in their study was 28% at 2 months and 48% at 1 year. The majority of endoscopic relapses, it would seem, develop within the first few months after ulcer healing.

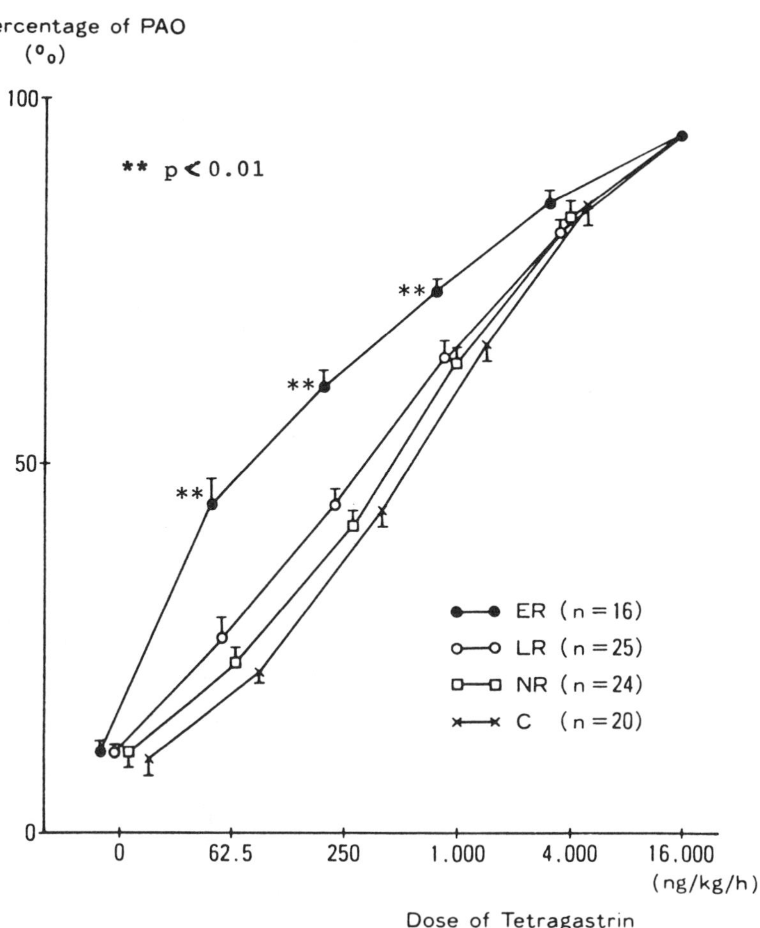

FIGURE 11 Acid-secretory responses expressed in percent of peak acid output (PAO) to graded doses of tetragastrin in early relapse (ER), late relapse (LR), no relapse (NR), and control (C) groups. Mean ± SEM. **$p < .01$. (After Yanaka and Muto [76].)

It should be noted that the 18% early-relapse rate (3 of 17 patients) in the sucralfate-healed group compares favorably with the 25% (16 of 65 patients) found by Yanaka and Muto [76] within 3 months of healing in their essentially antacid-treated group of patients. The Cape Town data suggest that the advantage of sucralfate over H_2-receptor blockers in terms of ulcer relapse applies particularly to the first month or two following ulcer healing.

The available data do not answer the question as to the cause of the raised PCS in patients with, or at risk of, duodenal ulcer. There is some evidence that prolonged treatment with an H_2-receptor blocker may result in "up-regulation" of both H_2 and gastrin receptors, with increased responsiveness to physiological stimuli once treatment is withdrawn [78]. This, it may be argued, might invite an early relapse in patients following ulcer healing with an H_2-receptor blocker. Although this attractive hypothesis may help explain the large number of early relapses in the ranitidine-treated patients in the Cape Town study, it cannot be reconciled with relapses in antacid- or sucralfate-healed patients. Attention has recently been refocused on the time-honored "duodenal brake" concept of acid-secretory control [79]. One can but speculate as to whether the loss of the "duodenal brake" mechanism by duodenal ulcer or, indeed, gross duodenitis may be a contributory factor in increased parietal cell responsiveness.

V. SAFETY ASPECTS

A. Clinical

Sucralfate is particularly well tolerated. Constipation, which occurs in about 2% of patients, was encountered more frequently in a few studies. Nausea and mild headaches were rarely troublesome.

B. Biochemical and Metabolic

Concern has been expressed in some quarters about the aluminum content of the drug, possible phosphate and vitamin B_{12} binding, and drug–drug interaction. They appear unwarranted.

1. Aluminum

The total aluminum load in patients on full-dose sucralfate therapy (4 g/day) is of the order of 800 mg/day. This is somewhat less than the aluminum load in patients on a low-dose regimen with a potent antacid tablet [80,81] and appreciably lower than that in patients on full-dose treatment with a variety of antacid gels. Sucralfate is only minimally absorbed [84], and the small amount of aluminum that is absorbed poses no hazard in patients with normal renal function. A transient increase in blood and urinary levels of aluminum has been shown in normal volunteers on full-dose sucralfate, but these levels returned to normal within a week of stopping treatment. The urinary levels are comparable to those found following an aluminum-containing antacid with a similar aluminum content [82]. The finding of normal bone aluminum levels in patients given full-dose sucralfate for 2 months opposes the theoretical possibility of aluminum deposition in the tissues [83]. It is of interest that no elevation in serum aluminum levels was noted in patients with normal renal function on maintenance sucralfate, 2 g/day [85].

2.   Phosphate and Vitamin B_{12} Binding

No alteration in serum phosphate levels have been reported in patients on maintenance sucralfate [29,30,34,85] or, indeed, after 6–12 weeks of full-dose therapy [86]. Sucralfate given in a larger dose of 6 g/day was considered a possible phosphate binder in patients with advanced renal failure. As with aluminum hydroxide-containing antacids given in this setting, however, phosphate binding was associated with raised aluminum levels [87]. Because of this, sucralfate and other aluminum-containing preparations should be used with caution in patients with reduced renal function. Yolk-bound ^{57}Co vitamin B_{12} studies have shown sucralfate to have no consistent effect on vitamin B_{12} absorption [88].

3.   Drug Interactions

Because sucralfate has no effect on gastric acidity and is only minimally absorbed, it is unlikely that the absorption, metabolism, or elimination of other drugs will be affected to any great extent [89]. However, pharmacological studies show a reduction in the bioavailability of phenytoin in the dog [90] and in humans [91]. There is a single case report suggesting a possible drug reaction with warfarin [92], but a subsequent study in patients on long-term warfarin therapy showed that sucralfate did not significantly change prothrombin time, partial thromboplastin time, or plasma warfarin concentrations [93].

For the rest, drug interactions between sucralfate and non-ulcer healing agents are either trivial or nonexistent. Studies in dogs have shown that sucralfate does not affect the absorption of quinidine, propanolol, aminophylline, tetracycline, or digoxin [90]. Studies in healthy subjects have shown that sucralfate has no effect on the bioavailability of aspirin [94], ibuprofen [95], or prednisone [96], and only a slight effect on digoxin kinetics [97].

Concomitant administration of sucralfate may reduce the bioavailability of the H_2-receptor blockers. Maconochie et al. [98], in a single-dose study in 12 normal volunteers, showed a 29% reduction in the bioavailability of ranitidine 150 mg given together with sucralfate 2 g. Mullersman et al. [99], on the other hand, noted no significant effect in a similar study using sucralfate 1 g. Sucralfate has been shown to reduce the bioavailability of cimetidine by 18% in the dog [100,101]. Staggering the dosing of the two drugs by 2 hr restored the bioavailability of cimetidine [101], and it is probable that the same pertains to ranitidine, phenytoin, and digoxin in humans.

VI.   CONCLUSION

The choice of first-line treatment in the management of peptic ulceration, reflux esophagitis, and stress ulcer prophylaxis is one of the more compelling issues in gastroenterology. Current favorites comprise the H_2-receptor blockers, sucralfate, and, perhaps, a potent antacid regimen.

This review draws attention to the efficacy and safety of sucralfate in the treatment of these conditions. Available data suggest that it is at least as effective as cimetidine in the short- and long-term treatment of peptic ulcer, and limited ranitidine-controlled studies indicate that this applies also to the other available H_2-receptor blockers. Evidence has also been presented to show that the new liquid formulation of sucralfate is of value in reflux esophagitis and that sucralfate is perhaps the drug of choice in stress ulcer prophylaxis.

This review also highlights the developing concept of the predictive value of increased PCS in early relapse. It is now appreciated that PCS tends to rise following prolonged treatment with a potent acid-inhibitory agent; that the increased PCS in patients with an active duodenal ulcer tends to fall with ulcer healing; that this fall is more marked in sucralfate-treated than in ranitidine-treated patients; and that increased PCS following healing predisposes to early relapse. Lower early-relapse rates following healing with sucralfate compared to an H_2-receptor blocker can now be reconciled with increased parietal cell sensitivity after treatment with an H_2-receptor blocker.

I wish to acknowledge support received from The Medical Research Council of South Africa.

REFERENCES

1. Bighley LD, Giesing D. Mechanism of action studies of sucralfate. In: Caspary WF, ed. Duodenal ulcer–gastric ulcer. Munich: Urban & Schwarzenberg, 1981:3–12.

2. Bruusgaard A, Elsborg L, Reinicke V. Bile acid "binding" properties of sucralfate. In: Caspary WF, ed. Duodenal ulcer–gastric ulcer. Munich: Urban & Schwarzenberg, 1981: 28–31.

3. Samloff IM. Inhibition of peptic aggression by sucralfate: the view from the ulcer crater. Scand J Gastroenterol 1983; 18(Suppl 83):7–11.

4. Nagashima R, Hinohara Y, Hirano T. Selective binding of sucralfate to ulcer lesion in experiments on rats with duodenal ulcer receiving ^{14}C-labelled sucralfate. Arzneim Forsch/Drug Res 1980; 30:88–91.

5. Steiner K, Garbe A. Specific binding of ^{14}C-sucralfate to acetic acid-induced gastric and duodenal ulcers of the rat. In: Caspary WF, ed. Duodenal ulcer–gastric ulcer. Munich: Urban & Schwarzenberg, 1981:19–21.

6. Nakazawa S, Nagashima R, Samloff IM. Selective binding of sucralfate to gastric ulcer in man. Dig Dis Sci 1981; 26:297–300.

7. Sasaki H, Hinohara Y, Tsunoda Y, Hagashima R. Binding of sucralfate to duodenal ulcer in man. Scand J Gastroenterol 1983; 18(Suppl 83):13–4.

8. Danesh BJZ, Duncan A, Russell RI. Is an acid pH required for the protective effect of sucralfate against mucosal injury? Am J Med 1987; 83(Suppl 3B):11–3.

9. Hollander D, Tarnawski A. Are antacids cytoprotective? Gut 1989; 30:145–7.

10. Tarnawski A, Hollander D, Krause WJ, Zipser RD, Staschura J, Gergely H. Does sucralfate affect the normal gastric mucosa? Histological, ultrastructural and functional assessment in the rat. Gastroenterology 1986; 90:893–905.

11. Slomiany BL, Laszewicz W, Slomiany A. Effect of sucralfate on the viscosity of gastric mucus and the permeability to hydrogen ion. Digestion 1986; 33:146–51.

12. Crampton JR, Gibbons LC, Rees WDW. Effect of certain ulcer-healing agents on amphibian gastroduodenal bicarbonate secretion. Scand J Gastroenterol 1986; 21(Suppl 125):113–6.

13. Szabo S. Discussion. Scand J Gastroenterol 1986; 21(Suppl 125):118.

14. Nexo E, Poulsen SS. Does epidermal growth factor play a role in the action of sucralfate? Scand J Gastroenterol 1987; 22(Suppl 127):45–9.

15. Konturek SJ, Kwicien N, Obtulowicz W, Kopp B, Olesky J. Double-blind controlled study on the effect of sucralfate on gastric prostaglandin formation and microbleeding in normal and aspirin-treated man. Gut 1986; 27:1450–6.

16. Shea-Donohue T, Steel L, Montcalm E, Dubois A. Gastric protection by sucralfate: role of mucus and prostaglandins. Gastroenterology 1985; 88:1583.

17. Roost R, Wright JP, Young GO, et al. The effect of aspirin and anti-ulcer drugs on gastric mucosal prostaglandin E. S Afr Med J 1986; 70:594–7.

18. Szabo S, Brown A. Prevention of ethanol-induced vascular injury and gastric mucosal lesions by sucralfate and its components: possible role of endogenous sulfhydryls. Proc Soc Exp Biol Med 1987; 185:493–7.

19. Orlando RC, Turjman NA, Tobey NA, Schreiner VJ, Powell DW. Mucosal protection by sucralfate and its components in acid-exposed rabbit esophagus. Gastroenterology 1987; 93:352–61.

20. Marks IN. Clinical summary of the 2nd International Sucralfate Symposium. Scand J Gastroenterol 1983; 18(Suppl 83):75–7.

21. Marks IN. Sucralfate: worldwide experience in recurrence therapy. J Clin Gastroenterol 1987; 9(Suppl 1):18–22.

22. Lam SK, Lau WY, Lai CL, et al. Efficacy of sucralfate in corpus, prepyloric and duodenal ulcer-associated gastric ulcers. A double-blind placebo controlled study. Am J Med 1985; 79(2c):24–31.

23. Herrerfas JM, Sego J, Castillo P. Comparison of sucralfate and ranitidine in short-term treatment of gastric ulcer. Dig Dis Sci 1986; 31(Suppl Oct):497S.

24. Lam SK, Hui WM, Lau WY, et al. Sucralfate overcomes adverse effect of cigarette smoking on duodenal ulcer healing and prolongs subsequent remission. Gastroenterology 1987; 93:1193–1201.

25. Brandstaetter G, Kratochvil P. Comparison of two sucralfate dosages (2 g twice a day versus 1 g four times a day) in duodenal ulcer healing. Am J Med 1985; 79(2c):36–8.

26. Coste T, Rautureau J, Beaugrand M, et al. Comparison of two sucralfate dosages presented in tablet form in duodenal ulcer healing. Am J Med 1987; 83(3B):86–90.

27. Marks IN, Wright JP, Gilinsky NH, et al. A comparison of sucralfate dosage schedules in duodenal ulcer healing. J Clin Gastroenterol 1986; 8:419–23.

28. Classen M, Bethge H, Brunner G, et al. Effect of sucralfate on peptic ulcer recurrence: a controlled, double-blind multicentre study. Scand J Gastroenterol 1983; 18(Suppl 83):61–8.

29. Marks IN, Wright JP, Girdwood AH, Gilinsky NH, Lucke W. Maintenance therapy with sucralfate reduces rate of gastric ulcer recurrence. Am J Med 1985; 79(2C):32–5.

30. Marks IN, Girdwood AH, Wright JP, et al. Nocturnal regimen of sucralfate in maintenance treatment of gastric ulcer. Am J Med 1987; 83(2B):95–8.

31. Libeskind M. Maintenance treatment of patients with healed peptic ulcer with sucralfate, placebo and cimetidine. Scand J Gastroenterol 1983; 18(Suppl 83):69–70.

32. Takemoto T, Kimura K, Okita K, et al. Efficacy of sucralfate in the prevention of recurrence of peptic ulcer—double-blind multicentre study with cimetidine. Scand J Gastroenterol 1987; 22(Suppl 140):49–60.

33. Blum AL, Bethge H. Sucralfate in the treatment and prevention of gastric ulcer. Gastroenterology 1988; 94:A39.

34. Marks IN, Girdwood AH, Newton KA, O'Keefe SJD, Marotta F, Lucke W. Maintenance sucralfate 2 g nocte reduces the relapse rate in duodenal ulcer disease—a one-year follow-up study. Am J Med 1989; 86(Suppl 6A):136–40.

35. Tytgat GNJ. Clinical efficacy of sucralfate in reflux oesophagitis. Comparison with cimetidine. Am J Med 1987; 83(Suppl 3B):38–42.

36. Simon B, Mueller P. Comparison of the effect of sucralfate & ranitidine in reflux oesophagitis. Am J Med 1987; 83(Suppl 3B):43–7.

37. Weiss W, Brunner H, Buttner GR, et al. Therapie der refluxoesophagitis mit sucralfat. Dtsch Med Wochenschr 1983; 108:1706–11.

38. Williams RM, Orlando RC, Bozymski EM, et al. Multicentre trial of sucralfate suspension for the treatment of reflux oesophagitis. Am J Med 1987; 83(Suppl 3B):61–6.

39. Borrero E, Bank S, Margolis I, Schulman WD, Chardavoyne R. Comparison of antacid and sucralfate in prevention of gastrointestinal bleeding in patients who are critically ill. Am J Med 1985; 79(Suppl 2c):62–4.

40. Tryba M, Zevounou F, Torok M, Zeuz M. Prevention of acute stress bleeding with sucralfate, antacids or cimetidine. Am J Med 1985; 79(Suppl 2c):55–61.

41. Laggner AN, Lenz K, Grainger W, et al. Stress ulcer prophylaxis in a general intensive care unit: sucralfate versus ranitidine. Anaesthetist 1988; 37:704–10.

42. Driks MR, Craven DE, Celli BR, et al. Nosocomial pneumonia in intubated patients given sucralfate as compared with antacids or histamine type 2 blockers. N Engl J Med 1987; 317:1376–82.

43. Tryba M. Risk of acute stress bleeding and nosocomial pneumonia in ventilated intensive care unit patients: sucralfate vs antacids. Am J Med 1987; 83(Suppl 3B):117–24.

44. Malan JF, Michell WL. Prophylaxis for gastrointestinal bleeding in the critically ill. S Afr J Contin Med Educ 1988; 6:53–7.

45. Marks IN. A sceptical view of medical treatment. In: Truelove SC, Willoughby CP, eds. Topics in gastroenterology, Vol. 7. Oxford: Blackwell, 1979:111–29.

46. Marks IN. Site-protective agents. Baillieres Clin Gastroenterol 1988; 2:609–20.

47. Marks IN, Wright JP, Lucke W, Girdwood AH. Relapse rates after initial ulcer healing with sucralfate and cimetidine. Scand J Gastroenterol 1982; 17:429–32.

48. Hentschel F, Schutze K, Dufek W. Rezidive des ulcers duodeni nach therapie mit sucralfat oder cimetidin. Wien Klin Wochenschr 1984; 96(4):153–6.

49. McCarthy PG, Norton L, Kronborg I, et al. Duodenal ulcer relapse following cimetidine healing: failure of modification by short-term sucralfate treatment. Gastroenterology 1986; 90:1541.

50. Hallerback B, Solhaug J-H, Carling L, et al. Recurrent ulcer after treatment with cimetidine or sucralfate. Scand J Gastroenterol 1987; 22:791–7.

51. Miyake T, Ariyoshi J, Suzaki T, Oishi M, Sakai M, Ueda S. Endoscopic evaluation of the

effect of sucralfate therapy and other clinical parameters on the recurrence rate of gastric ulcers. Dig Dis Sci 1980; 25:1–7.

52. Tovey FI, Husband EM, Yui YC, et al. Differences in mucosal appearances and in relapse rates in duodenal ulceration treated with sucralfate or cimetidine. Am J Med 1989; 86(Suppl 6A):141–4.

53. Lambert JR, Hansky J, Davidson A, Pinkard K, Stockman K. *Campylobacter*-like organisms (CLO)—in vivo and in vitro susceptibility to antimicrobial and antiulcer therapy. Gastroenterology 1985; 88:1462.

54. Marshall J, Armstrong JA, Francis J, Nokes NT, Wee SH. Antimicrobial action of bismuth in relation to *Campylobacter pyloridis* colonisation and gastritis. Digestion 1987; (Suppl 2):16–30.

55. Gavey CJ, Szeto ML, Nwokolo CU, Sercombe J, Pounder RE. Bismuth accumulation in the body during treatment with tripotassium dicitrato bismuthate. Aliment Pharmacol Ther 1989; 3:21–8.

56. Hamilton I, Worsley BW, O'Connor HJ, Axon ATR. Effects of tripotassium dicitrato bismuthate tablets or cimetidine in the treatment of duodenal ulcer. Gut 1983; 24: 1148–51.

57. Frislid K, Aadland E, Berstad A. Augmented postprandial gastric secretion due to exposure to ranitidine in healthy subjects. Scand J Gastroenterol 1986; 21:119–22.

58. Jones DB, Howden CW, Burget DW, Silletti C, Hunt RH. Alteration of H_2-receptor sensitivity in duodenal ulcer patients after maintenance treatment with an H_2-receptor antagonist. Gut 1988; 29:890–3.

59. Fullarton GM, McLaughlan G, Macdonald A, Crean GP, McColl KEL. Rebound nocturnal hypersecretion after 4 weeks H_2-antagonist therapy. Gut 1989; 30:449–54.

60. Roland M. Gastric secretory response to graded doses of pentagastrin alone or in combination with carbacholine in unoperated duodenal ulcer patients. Scand J Gastroenterol 1975; 10:603–8.

61. Isenberg JI, Grossman MI, Maxwell V, Walsh JH. Increased sensitivity to stimulation of acid secretion by pentagastrin in duodenal ulcer. J Clin Invest 1975; 55:330–7.

62. Halter F, Bangerter U, Hacki WH, et al. Sensitivity of the parietal cell to pentagastrin in health and duodenal ulcer disease. A reappraisal. Scand J Gastroenterol 1982; 17:539–44.

63. Lam SK, Koo J. Gastrin sensitivity in duodenal ulcer. Gut 1985; 26:485–90.

64. Celestin LR. Antral activity and symptom periodicity in duodenal ulceration. Gut 1967; 8:318–24.

65. Bergegardh S, Olbe L. Gastric acid response to antrum distension in man. Scand J Gastroenterol 1975; 10:171–6.

66. Achord JL. Gastric pepsin and acid secretion in patients with acute and healed duodenal ulcer. Gastroenterology 1981; 81:15–8.

67. Marks IN, Young GO, Tigler-Wybrandi NA, Bridger S, Newton KA. Acid secretory response and parietal cell sensitivity in patients with duodenal ulcer before and after healing with sucralfate or ranitidine. Am J Med 1989; 86(Suppl 6A):145–7.

68. Aadland E, Berstad A. Parietal and chief cell sensitivity to histamine and pentagastrin stimulation before and after cimetidine treatment in healthy subjects. Scand J Gastroenterol 1979; 14:933–8.

69. Aadland E, Berstad A. Parietal and chief cell sensitivity to pentagastrin stimulation before and after cimetidine treatment for duodenal ulcer. Scand J Gastroenterol 1979; 14:111–4.

70. Walsh JH, Sytnik B, Maxwell V, et al. Reversibility of plasma gastrin changes induced by omeprazole or ranitidine in man. Am J Gastroenterol 1988; 83:1042. Abstract.

71. Halter F, Witzel L, Haecki WH, Olah AJ, Hietz P, Varga L. Gastric secretion, the parietal cell and gastrin response to histamine H_2-receptor antagonists in the rat. In: Creutzfeld W, ed. Cimetidine. (Proc. International Symposium on Histamine H_2-receptor antagonists. 1977.) Amsterdam: Excerpta Medica, 1978:108–13.

72. Inauen W, Eigenmann F, Koelz HR, Halter F. Omeprazole reduces trophic effects on parietal cells by endogenous gastrin and treatment with atropine. Gastroenterology 1986; 90:1471.

73. Coruzzi G, Bertaccini G. Increased parietal cell sensitivity after chronic treatment with ranitidine in the conscious cat. Agents Actions 1989; 28:215–17.

74. Marks IN, Young GO. Changes in acid secretory response and parietal cell sensitivity on healing predict early relapse in patients with duodenal ulcer. Am J Gastroenterol 1988; 83:1075. Abstract.

75. Young GO, Marks IN, Tigler-Wybrandi NA, Bridger SA, Newton KA. Changes in acid secretory response and parietal cell sensitivity on healing predict early relapse in patients with duodenal ulcer. S Afr Med J 1989; 75(Suppl 3 June):2.

76. Yanaka A, Muto H. Increased parietal cell responsiveness to tetragastrin in patients with recurrent duodenal ulcer. Dig Dis Sci 1988; 33:1459–65.

77. Boyd EJS, Penston JG, Johnston DA, Wormsley KG. Does maintenance therapy keep duodenal ulcers healed? Lancet 1988; i:1324–7.

78. Bertaccini G. Increased parietal cell sensitivity. S Afr Med J 1988; 74(Suppl to 2 July):14.

79. Parekh D, Lawson HH, van der Walt LA, et al. Omeprazole-induced hypergastrinaemia in the dog and primate; the role of duodenal mechanisms. S Afr Med J 1988; 73:659–60.

80. Weberg R, Berstad A, Aaseth J, Falch JA. Mineral-metabolic side effects of low-dose antacids. Scand J Gastroenterol 1985; 20:741–6.

81. Weberg R, Aubert E, Dahlberg O, et al. Low-dose antacids or cimetidine for duodenal ulcer? Gastroenterology 1988; 95:1465–9.

82. Haram E-M, Weberg R, Berstad A. Urinary excretion of aluminum after ingestion of sucralfate and an aluminum-containing antacid in man. Scand J Gastroenterol 1987; 22:615–8.

83. Bannwarth B, Gaucher A, Burnel D, Netter PJ. Long-term sucralfate therapy. J Rheumatol 1986; 13(6):1187(L).

84. Kinoshita H, Kumaki K, Nakano H, et al. Plasma aluminum levels of patients on long-term sucralfate. Res Commun Chem Pathol Pharmacol 1982; 35:515–8.

85. Bolin TD, Davis AE, Duncombe VM, Billington B. Role of maintenance sucralfate in prevention of duodenal ulcer recurrence. Am J Med 1987; 83(Suppl 3B):91–4.

86. Marks IN, Wright JP, Denyer M, Garisch JAM, Lucke W. Comparison of sucralfate with cimetidine in short-term treatment of chronic peptic ulcers. S Afr Med J 1980; 57:567–73.

87. Leung ACT, Henderson IS, Halls DJ, Dobbie JW. Aluminium hydroxide versus sucralfate as a phosphate binder in uraemia. Br Med J 1983; 286:1379–81.

88. Hanslip JI, Gidden D, Boyd EJS, Marks IN, Wormsley KG. The effect of mucosal protective and antisecretory drugs on assimilation of food-bound vitamin B_{12}. Gut 1987; 28(1C):1341–2. Abstract.

89. Chiverton SG, Hunt RN. Pharmacokinetics and pharmacodynamics of treatments for peptic ulcer disease in the elderly. Am J Gastroenterol 1988; 83:211–5.

90. Lacz JP, Groschang AG, Giesing DH, et al. The effect of sucralfate on drug absorption in dogs. Gastroenterology 1982; 82:1108. Abstract.

91. Smart HL, Somerville KW, Williams J, Richens A, Langman MJS. The effects of sucralfate upon phenytoin absorption in man. Brit J Clin Pharmacol 1985; 20:238–40.

92. Mungall D, Talbert RL, Phillips C, et al. Sucralfate and warfarin. Ann Intern Med 1983; 98:557. Letter.

93. Talbert RL, Dalmady-Israel C, Bussey HI, et al. Effect of sucralfate on plasma warfarin concentration in patients requiring chronic warfarin therapy. Drug Intell Clin Pharmacol 1985; 19:456–7.

94. Lau A, Chang CW, Schlesinger P. Evaluation of a potential drug interaction between sucralfate and aspirin. Drug Intell Clin Pharm 1985; 19:457. Abstract.

95. Pugh MC, Small RE, Garnett WR, et al. Effect of sucralfate on ibuprofen absorption in normal volunteers. Clin Pharm 1984; 3:630–3.

96. Gambertoglio JG, Romac DR, Yong C-L, Birnbaum J, Lizak P, Amend WJC. Lack of effect of sucralfate on prednisone bioavailability. Am J Gastroenterol 1987; 82:42–5.

97. Giesing DH, Lanman RC, Dimmitt DC, Runser DJ. Lack of effect of sucralfate on digoxin pharmacokinetics. Gastroenterology 1983; 85:1165. Abstract.

98. Maconochie JG, Thomas M, Michael MF, Jenner WR, Tanner RJN. Ranitidine sucralfate interaction. Clin Pharmacol Ther 1987; 41:205. Abstract P110-2.

99. Mullersman G, Gotz VP, Russell WL, Derendorf H. Lack of clinically significant in vitro and in vivo interactions between ranitidine and sucralfate. J Pharm Sci 1986; 75:995–8.

100. Ritschel WA, Banerjes PS, Koch HP, et al. Cimetidine-sucralfate drug interaction. Methods Find Exp Clin Pharmacol 1984; 6:261–3.

101. Lacz J, Drees D, Browne R. The effect of sucralfate on the absorption of cimetidine and other drugs in dogs. Am J Gastroenterol 1982; 77:689. Abstract.

102. Marks IN. The medical management of duodenal ulcer. S Afr J Contin Med Educ 1988; 6:29–36.

14

Colloidal Bismuth Subcitrate

G. Bianchi Porro **and** M. Lazzaroni

L. Sacco Hospital, Milan, Italy

I. INTRODUCTION

The first clinical application of bismuth salts in the treatment of diseases of the gastrointestinal tract dates back to the end of the 19th century. Compounds such as bismuth subnitrate, subgallate, and subcarbonate showed a certain degree of efficacy in reducing the severity of dyspeptic manifestations, vomiting, and bowel disorders.

Despite these promising results, reports of significant side effects, often due to uncontrolled use, and the development of more specific, more easily managed products mitigated against the use of bismuth compounds in clinical practice. More recently, however, the synthesis of a highly water-soluble compound, colloidal bismuth subcitrate (CBS), has been recognized as an important innovation in the treatment of peptic ulcer. In the light of current knowledge, this bismuth derivative, from the point of view of the etiopathogenesis of peptic ulcer, may be regarded, if not as a first-choice therapeutic agent, then at least as a valid alternative to traditional antisecretory compounds.

II. PHYSICOCHEMICAL CHARACTERISTICS

The chemical name for the active ingredient of DeNol is the double ammonium and potassium salt of bismuth citrate hydroxide, a colloidal complex. In the international literature it is cited briefly either as colloidal bismuth subcitrate (CBS) or as tripotassium dicitratobismuthate (TDB). Its quantitative composition is expressed by the formula $Bi_2(OH)_3(C_6H_5O)$. The CBS molecule has a peculiar chemical structure capable of forming complex salts. Its dimensions are such as to give rise to the formation of colloids in an aqueous environment.

Unlike the other bismuth salts, CBS is characterized by a high degree of water solubility. The pH of the colloidal solution tends to be basic, pH 9–10. The stability of the complex decreases with the pH. In an acid environment, the bismuth precipitates, probably owing to disruption of the bismuth–citrate bond, with the formation of various insoluble salts. The simplest of these is bismuth oxychloride (BiOCl); more complex structures contain COOH free radicals and groups containing Bi [1–5]. All these compounds have a particular affinity for organic molecules, amino acids, and proteins, with which they form stable compounds. This latter property, as we shall see, accounts for the clinical activity of colloidal bismuth.

III. PHARMACODYNAMICS

A. Prevention of Experimental Gastric Mucosal Lesions

Numerous in vivo experimental observations in animals have confirmed the efficacy of colloidal bismuth in the prevention of gastric mucosal lesions. In particular, the anti-ulcer activity of colloidal bismuth has been tested in rats with gastric lesions induced by using the Shay technique. The introduction of 8 mL of solution with differing CBS concentrations [1,6] and even with an acid pH [7] approximately 1 hr after pylorus ligation proved capable of significantly reducing the ulcer incidence, compared to other bismuth salts, by means of a mechanism that is certainly unrelated to acid secretion.

The ID_{50}, expressed as mg/kg of BiO, was 132, with a range of 107–161. The same efficacy was also observed after the administration of reserpine (1 mg/kg) [1]. Pretreatment with oral CBS brought a significant reduction in the ulcerogenic index with an ID_{50} of 169 mg/kg of BiO for the number of ulcers and 134 for ulcer size. Significant anti-ulcer activity has also been reported in the rat after the administration of histamine [6] and other gastric damaging drugs such as aspirin [6,8,9], phenylbutazone [6], cortisone [6], ethanol [10,11], and 0.2 N NaOH [10].

In ulcers induced by different mechanisms—for instance, by restraint stress with or without the administration of indomethacin [5,6,8]—it has been observed that colloidal bismuth, at doses ranging from 4 to 8 mg/kg, is capable of promoting more rapid healing of lesions, though this activity appears to be somewhat reduced by pretreatment with indomethacin, a potent inhibitor of prostaglandin synthesis [12].

Of great interest for the purposes of clarifying the mechanism of action of the drug were, among other things, the results obtained using an experimental model involving exposure of the mucosa to contact with acetic acid, a model that rules out any nonantisecretory activity of prostaglandins [12,13]. CBS (400 mg/kg per day for 9 days) produced 61% and 47% reductions in the mean sizes of duodenal and gastric ulcers, respectively, with complete healing after 2 weeks.

To the observations obtained with colloidal bismuth subcitrate solution we should also add the results emerging from more recent experiments with a different formulation, namely chewable or coated tablets [14]. In this formulation, colloidal bismuth has proved capable of significantly reducing the number and size of ulcers induced in the rat by contact of the gastric mucosa with acetic acid.

B.   Effects on Gastric and Duodenal Mucosal Ultrastructure

The first results of an investigation on the effects of CBS on mucosal ultrastructure were reported by Moshall et al. [15] in a group of duodenal ulcer patients treated for 6 weeks with cimetidine or CBS. In the CBS group, unlike patients healed on the antisecretory agent, biopsy samples taken from the edges of the ulcer scar showed a better restoration of mucosal integrity, with well-developed normal villi, thickening of the glycocalyx, and replacement of cells secreting acid mucins with other cells secreting neutral mucins.

The possibility that this effect may be secondary to the formation of complexes between bismuth and mucoproteins secreted from the ulcer was confirmed in a later study by the same group [16] and also by other investigators [17] by means of ultrastructural investigations that showed the presence of electron-dense corpuscular material adhering to the plasmalemma and glycocalyx 1 hr after administration of CBS.

This process, moreover, appears to be reversible. It has been observed that the bismuth concentration in the brush border and in the lysosomes of enterocytes is inversely proportional to the time elapsing after administration, with a 90% reduction after only 72 hr, probably as a result of systemic absorption and cellular exfoliation [18].

Further confirmation of the potential positive interference of colloidal bismuth in cell function is provided by data concerning the ability of the metal to inhibit intestinal alkaline phosphatase [19], and above all by the microscopic and ultrastructural demonstration of the way in which the drug protects the gastric mucosa against ethanol-induced lesions [20]. In an experiment with rats administered 1 mL of absolute ethanol, pretreatment by infusion of CBS (120 mg/kg) proved capable of drastically reducing the histological alterations of the gastric mucosa and of protecting both the foveolar mucosal and deep glandular cells.

Necrotic lesions were virtually absent in animals protected by colloidal bismuth, with complete restoration of normal mucosal integrity within 6 hr.

More controversial appears to be the action of colloidal bismuth on macrophages, which are known to play an important role in the healing process. In the study by Koo et al. [21], optical and electron microscopic analysis of chronic gastric ulcer sections in rats treated with CBS (120 mg/5 mL) showed significantly increased concentrations of macrophages containing abundant amounts of the metal. After 6 hr, the concentration was similar to that in controls.

This observation, however, was not confirmed by Soutar and Coghill [22]. Under similar experimental conditions, but using more refined and more suitable investigative methods—for example, the use of nonspecific esterases as markers of macrophages—no increase in macrophage concentration was observed even in response to repeated administration of CBS. What was observed, on the other hand, was a rapid phagocytosis of metal granules by macrophage precursor monocytes. The process of phagocytosis was accelerated and thus promoted by plasma proteins, allowing the formation of large CBS aggregates. The formation of these plasma protein–CBS aggregates is thought to constitute the microscopic substratum for the protective layer macroscopically observable on the ulcer crater after the administration of colloidal bismuth.

1. Reduction of Intragastric Acid-Peptic Activity

In vitro and in vivo studies both in animals and in humans have clearly shown not only that bismuth possesses no antacid activity [23], but also that it does not even interfere with acid secretion. The short- and long-term administration of CBS in rats and in dogs did not affect the hydrogen-ion concentration or secretory volume either in basal conditions [12,24] or after a test meal [24]. These findings were later confirmed in humans with respect to both basal and pentagastrin-stimulated acid output [23,25,26]. More controversial, however, is the effect of CBS on pepsin. The positive results obtained in elegant in vitro studies contrast with the conflicting in vivo findings in humans.

In vitro, CBS, unlike aluminum-based antacids or other bismuth salts, has shown an antipepsin activity related to environmental pH [27]. This activity was maximal at pH values theoretically allowing inhibition also of pepsin fraction 1, which is known to be the fraction most involved in the ulcerogenic mechanism. These results were confirmed by other experiments, which incubated colloidal bismuth at different concentrations with human gastric juices [28]. At predetermined pH values (pH 2), a dose-dependent reduction in pepsin was observed, and particularly in type 1 pepsin. The inhibition was 29% and 39% for CBS concentrations of 13.7 and 27 mmol/L, respectively. Although these concentrations are high and are very likely to be reached in vivo in humans, it is nevertheless reasonable to assume that they may be produced within the ulcer crater, where the drug is known to concentrate. The results obtained in vivo, as previously mentioned, are contradictory. In the rat, the distinct dose-dependent antipepsin activity observed by certain investigators [1,24] contrasts with the negative findings reported by Konturek and colleagues [12]. The same can be said of the results in humans. The negative findings of Flavell-Matts and Schwan [23] contrast with the results reported by Baron and colleagues [26], who claim to have demonstrated a marked reduction in pepsin output in basal conditions (16% and 13% in patients with duodenal and gastric ulcer, respectively) and after pentagastrin stimulation (42% and 36%, respectively).

Although, with our present knowledge, we are not in a position to rule out, with any degree of certainty, the existence of a mechanism of inhibition of the proenzyme pepsinogen, we may reasonably postulate that the antipepsin activity of CBS is produced via the formation, in an acid environment, of an insoluble complex capable of inactivating pepsin.

Relatively few data are available regarding the effects of colloidal bismuth on another factor potentially capable of damaging the gastric mucosa, namely, bile acids [29]. No activity has been observed at pH values of 4 or above. At pH 2, however, bismuth has been found capable of binding the conjugated bile salts predominant in bile by varying amounts. The maximum effect is observed with glychenodeoxycholate [29].

2. Cytoprotective Activity

As far as gastric mucus is concerned, bismuth has been found to be capable of interfering with the mucus by mechanisms that are complex and as yet by no means clearly defined but that can be summarized as follows:

1. Ability to reduce mucus permeability to hydrogen ions
2. Stimulation of greater mucus production
3. Interference with the composition of mucus

The first clear demonstration of an interaction between bismuth and gastric mucus glycoproteins was provided by Lee in 1982 [3]. The addition of colloidal bismuth to a glycoprotein solution prepared from human gastric juices produced a precipitate consisting of a glycoprotein–bismuth complex capable of reducing the migration of hydrogen ions to a significantly greater extent than the mucus barrier alone. This aspect was studied in greater depth and the findings substantiated by Tasman-Jones et al. [30], who showed that the CBS–mucin binding decreases with increasing pH and that, in any case, the formation of possible complexes does not affect the ion-exchange properties of gastric mucus.

In addition to this barrier effect, colloidal bismuth is also thought to stimulate mucus output and, even more important, to have an effect on the quality of mucus composition. In the rat, short-term administration of CBS causes an increase in the bound glycoprotein fraction and a reduction in the unbound fraction [24]. This effect, already observed in the case of carbenoxolone, is regarded as being an expression of the protective activity of the gastric mucosal barrier.

In humans, the quantitative changes in mucus after CBS treatment are controversial. Reports by certain investigators [31,32] suggest a positive effect of the drug and in this sense contrast with the findings of Baron et al. [26], who observed a significant reduction in pentagastrin-stimulated mucus production in patients with gastric or duodenal ulcers healed after treatment with DeNol.

Definitely accepted, on the other hand, is colloidal bismuth's ability to modify the quality of mucus composition with an increased stimulation of neutral acid mucins as compared to controls [31,32]. In particular, the protection index—the ratio of neutral to acid mucins—is increased even after withdrawal of the drug. This finding may be interpreted as one of the mechanisms underlying the ability of CBS to reduce the risk of relapse of the ulcer lesion.

An important role in the complex pharmacological action of colloidal bismuth is played by endogenous prostaglandins. In experimental conditions, CBS has been seen to be capable of inducing the endoluminal synthesis [9–11,13] and release of PGE_2 [10,13] to a dose- and time-dependent extent [11,33]. The increase in luminal concentration ranges from 70% with CBS doses of 30 mg/kg to 300% with doses of 480 mg/kg. The stimulating action sets in immediately. Maximum synthesis is thought to occur 15 min after administration, with subsequent reductions at 60, 120, and 240 min and normalization after 6 hr. Pretreatment with indomethacin proved capable of drastically reducing PGE synthesis without significantly interfering with the drug's protective effect on the gastric mucosa. These experimental findings were later confirmed in humans after both a single administration of CBS in volunteers [34] and a 3-week course of treatment in patients with gastric and duodenal ulcers [35]. It should be stressed, however, that in the latter study an increase in PGE_2 was observed in the duodenal cap and in the gastric antrum not only after the administration of colloidal bismuth, but also after aluminum hydroxide antacid.

Probably secondary to the synthesis of endogenous prostaglandins is the role of colloidal bismuth with regard to the secretion of gastric bicarbonates, which is definitely known to be involved in cytoprotection. In vitro, in isolated amphibian mucosa, it has been seen that application of bismuth subcitrate is capable of inducing production of bicarbonates to a dose-dependent extent [36]. This effect was later confirmed in vivo in humans in an elegant experiment [34], in the course of which it also proved possible to demonstrate that pretreatment with prostaglandin synthesis inhibitors completely inhibited the CBS-induced alkaline secretion.

The hypothetical role played by endogenous sulfhydryl radicals in DeNol-induced cytoprotection is still no more than speculative but is undoubtedly suggestive. It has been observed that the protective action of the drug against vascular damage induced by 85% ethanol is significantly increased by pretreatment with a sulfhydryl compound such as cysteamine [37].

3. Physical Protection

As mentioned in Section III.A, colloidal bismuth appears to form a protective coating, with elective stratification over the ulcer crater. Recent sophisticated investigations seem to confirm this. By means of particular histochemical staining techniques using brucine sulfate, the presence of an orange or reddish bismuth precipitate has clearly been demonstrated in the ulcer crater and, to a lesser extent, on the surrounding mucosa. Formation of the precipitate is achieved only with bismuth subcitrate and not with other bismuth salts [1,4,5,21,38].

Further investigations [3] have provided additional explanations regarding the mechanism whereby the protective layer forms both in vitro and in vivo in humans.

Using titration with 0.1 N HCl, it was observed in vitro that approximately 50% of the colloidal bismuth precipitates at pH values of 4.0 ± 0.1. In vivo, the optimum pH for precipitation is 3.5 ± 0.3. This difference may be due to the interference by proteins and glycoproteins with the gastric juice.

Bismuth precipitation in the stomach takes the form of crystals, which differ in structure according to the pH. At a pH of 1.5 only amorphous material is present, whereas at pH 2 complex crystalline forms of morular appearance are observed. At pH values of 3–5, the morphology varies from a diamond-shaped to a rhomboid or needle-shaped structure [17,39]. At the base of the ulcer in vivo, only the diamond-shaped form is observed. It has been demonstrated that the pH at the edge of the ulcer is certainly above 1.5 as a result of the protonization of free amino acids, and approaches the optimum values for precipitation of the drug.

These complex chemical interactions can be observed both in histological sections [3] and by endoscopy, even several hours after administration of the colloidal bismuth [40–42].

3. Antibacterial Activity

The hypothetical role of an infectious agent in the etiology of gastritis and peptic ulcer is deeply rooted in the history of medicine. From as early as 1883, a whole series of studies by numerous authors [43–49] reported the presence of spiral bacteria in stomachs from gastroresected patients or in autopsy findings. Scanty knowledge of the physiology of secretion and the inability to isolate the alleged etiological agent, however, made it impossible to formulate any single, acceptable, pathogenetic hypothesis. The first attempt in this direction was made by Warren [50] and Marshall [51], who succeeded in attributing a possible clinical significance to the presence in the gastric antral mucosa of a particular microorganism, which, after a certain amount of taxonomic uncertainty, was eventually named *Helicobacter pylori*.

In the wake of the initial observation came a veritable "explosion" of scientific publications aimed at demonstrating and emphasizing what was regarded as the probable decisive role of bacterial infection in the genesis of acute and chronic inflammatory processes of the gastric antral mucosa and perhaps also in peptic ulcer.

Helicobacter pylori is a spiral gram-negative organism with morphological characteristics that permit easy development even in a particular environment such as the gastric mucosa. It can move rapidly even in a viscous medium such as gastric mucus, with preferential localization in those areas having a congenial, slightly alkaline pH in the gastric foveolae in the vicinity of the intercellular junctions [52,53]. In these sites, the microorganism, which exhibits high urease [54] and proteolytic [55] activity, is capable of damaging the gastric mucosal barrier with hydrogen-ion back-diffusion and hypochlorhydria. In addition to this, the bacterium is able to penetrate into cells, causing alterations of the membrane profiles, depletion of the mucus-secreting microvilli, disruption of the cellular junctions, and secondary infiltration of activated polymorphs [56] (Fig. 1).

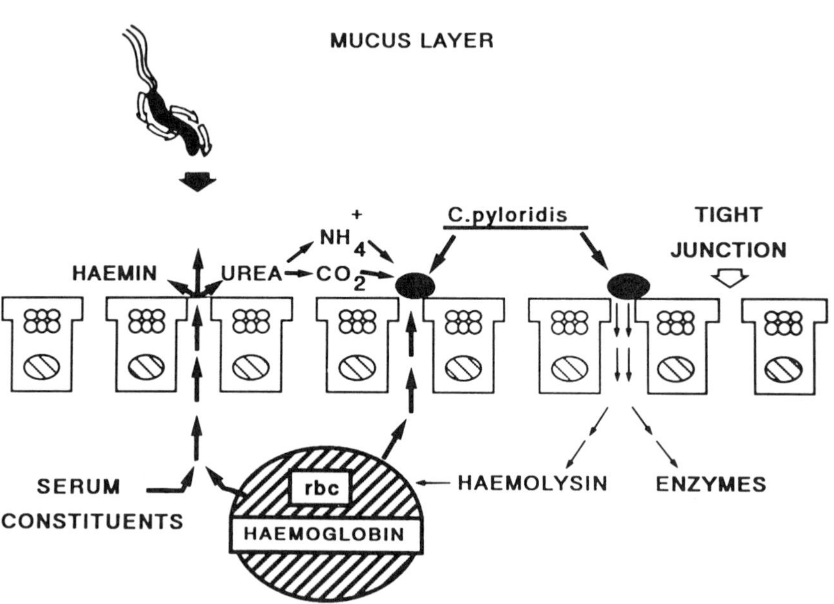

FIGURE 1 Diagrammatic representation of possible events in colonisation of the gastric mucosa by *H. pylori*. rbc = red blood cell. (From Hazell et al. [53].)

Despite its irregular distribution, *H. pylori* shows an elective tropism for the gastric mucosa, particularly in the antrum [57]. In the duodenal cap, the preferential site is in areas of gastric metaplasis [58] and possibly, though at minimal concentrations, in the mucosa surrounding the ulcer [59]. In contrast, it does not colonize areas of intestinal metaplasia of the gastric antrum and is not present in intestinal mucosa.

The epidemiological evidence currently available has confirmed, with rare exceptions, a significant prevalence of *H. pylori* infection (roughly 85%) in type B gastritis, particularly in the active form [60–68]. To this we must add clear experimental demonstrations in humans of an effective causative role of the bacterium [69,70]. On the other hand, the relationship between *Helicobacter* and peptic ulcer is still a matter of controversy [71,72]. Despite a profusion of speculative, yet suggestive, hypotheses [73], the actual information available is essentially of the indirect type, extrapolated from clinical trials conducted for the purposes of verifying the usefulness of drugs active against the organism in short-term therapy and in the prophylaxis of ulcer relapse [74]. To this end, colloidal bismuth subcitrate plays a particular role. It is the only compound usable in ulcer therapy that shows a significant degree of bactericidal activity against *H. pylori* both in vitro and in vivo. In vitro, the minimum inhibitory concentration (MIC) ranges from 4 to 32 μg/mL, which is significantly lower than that of cimetidine: 400–600 mg/L [75–77]. This activity, unlike that of other antibiotics such as erythromycin, spiramycin, and profloxacin [78,79], is maintained virtually unaltered also in vivo.

In patients with duodenal ulcer, CBS, when used as monotherapy, and even more when used in combination with other bactericidal compounds (amoxicillin, metronidazole, tinidazole), not only confirms its well-known ulcer-healing action, but also shows simultaneous bactericidal activity with resolution of antral gastritis in a mean 60% of patients, though the results reported by the various investigators [80–86] show a significant degree of variability (30–90%).

The action mechanisms are complex. Both a direct bactericidal effect, distinctly prevalent and already detectable in vitro, and an interference with the metabolic disorders induced by the microorganisms have been hypothesized. As regards the direct mechanism, electron microscopy of biopsy specimens from infected patients has shown the onset of irreversible alterations in the microorganism as early as 2 hr after administration of CBS [87,88]. In particular, evidence has been found of a loss of adherence to the gastric epithelium and the onset of parietal fragmentation and irreversible condensation of the cell contents, probably related to a deposition of bismuth aggregates on the surface and within the bacteria. The alterations of the epithelial profile and microvilli are no longer observable after 4 weeks of therapy, with restoration of the mucosa to normal, in complete agreement with the findings observed by Moshall et al. [15].

The indirect mechanisms are still speculative [88]. It has been postulated that CBS may inactivate the bacterial enzymes responsible for the metabolic damage or may interfere with mucolytic activity via the well-known action of glycoprotein chelation and by stimulation of production of endogenous prostaglandins, mucus, and parietal bicarbonates.

IV. PHARMACOKINETICS

Although colloidal bismuth has been proposed essentially as nonsystemic therapy for peptic ulcer, the studies currently available, which are still scanty and almost exclusively confined to short-term treatment, indicate a variable degree of absorption of the drug by the body in both animals and humans.

In experimental animals (dogs and rats), administration of CBS at doses ranging from 160 to 640 mg/kg (two to eight times the therapeutic dose in humans) for a period of 3–6 months did not induce any significant changes in serum and urinary bismuth levels, which varied from 5 to 14 μg/L depending upon the dose. The organs in which the highest concentrations were detected were the cecum and the kidneys [1].

Additional information in this connection was supplied by Stiel et al. [18] in an experiment conducted to evaluate the absorption and intracellular distribution of CBS in the gastrointestinal tracts of rats 24 hr after administration of the drug. Bismuth absorption by the gastric fundus and antrum was significantly less than that detected in the duodenum, jejunum, and small bowel.

Although the tissue concentration showed a progressive reduction, 10% of the bismuth absorbed was still detectable 72 hr after discontinuation of treatment, located mainly in the membrane border and in the cytosol of enterocytes. The same enterocyte accumulation phenomenon was also demonstrated in humans by Coghill et al. after endocytosis [17,39].

Data on plasma bismuth concentrations are available that were obtained after 4–6-week courses of therapy both with the liquid formulation and with chewable tablets. It has been calculated that at least 0.2% of the oral dose is absorbed in the course of routine treatment [89]. Overall, the maximum plasma bismuth values detected proved significantly lower than the warning threshold of 50 ng/mL [29,89–96].

An exception to these findings is reported by Nwokolo et al. [97], who found peak plasma bismuth concentrations above 50 ng/mL in 14 of 16 volunteers and above 100 ng/mL in 9 of the 16. Plasma bismuth values with the liquid formulation proved lower than those observed with tablets. The explanation is by no means simple. It may be assumed that there is poorer patient compliance among patients who are candidates for ingestion of a product with a disagreeable ammoniacal taste.

Only in one study have plasma bismuth concentrations been evaluated after long-term administration (up to 7 months) of colloidal bismuth 240 mg/day [96]. The values observed throughout the experiment, 40 ng/mL, were 75% lower than those documented in the course of short-term treatment.

Absorption is very rapid, the plasma peak being reached only 30 min after ingestion of two coated tablets. This presupposes a proximal absorption site. Although the information in this regard is still uncertain, the findings of Coghill et al. [17] of the presence of bismuth deposits in the esophageal epithelium, and in particular in the duodenum, suggest that the latter organ is the preferential absorption site, with a mechanism that remains unknown.

The finding that the plasma peak is reached earlier after morning administration than after evening administration suggests a transport mechanism liable to saturation. This suggestive hypothesis, however, requires further verification, as we cannot rule out the possible effect of the intragastric contents on the delayed onset of the evening plasma peak [97].

The data available on bismuth metabolism and half-life are scanty and have been extrapolated from observations in patients intoxicated with unidentified bismuth preparations [98]. The plasma half-life is believed to be approximately 5.2 days. More information is available regarding the modality and duration of urinary excretion. After CBS administration for a period of at least 4 weeks, urinary concentrations of the metal have been observed ranging from 17 to 710 μg/mL [89,90,92,94,99], with a relative increase of up to 350-fold compared to the pretreatment period [89].

The duration of elimination is also variable. The initial findings of Lee [3], who extrapolated a urinary elimination value of 2.6% per day, contrast with those of Pounder's group [89], who documented a urinary concentration four times the normal value as long as 3 months after discontinuation of the treatment. Prolonged urinary excretion even after normalization of plasma bismuth concentrations suggests an accumulation of the metal in the body with mechanisms and sites as yet by no means clearly defined. Bismuth is thought to accumulate preferentially in the kidney, spleen, liver, and bones.

In rats, evidence has been found that the metal crosses the blood–brain barrier and accumulates in the central nervous system [1, 100].

V. CLINICAL APPLICATIONS

A. Dosage Regimens

The dosage regimen originally proposed involved the administration of CBS in a liquid formulation at the dose of 5 mL (120 mg) diluted in 20 mL of water, to be taken four times daily, $\frac{1}{2}$ hr before each of the three main meals and 2 hr after dinner. The need to overcome two major drawbacks (the smell and unpleasant ammoniacal taste) capable of undermining patient compliance with the therapy led to the development of the 120-mg chewable tablet (which, however, caused brownish discoloration of the teeth and mucosa of the mouth) and eventually to the use of coated tablets.

Experience in controlled studies has shown that the three formulations possess virtually the same degree of healing activity [91, 92, 101–103] (Table 1). As far as the comparison between liquid and tablet formulations is concerned, healing rates range from 72 to 89% for the liquid form and from 69 to 89% for chewable tablets.

The proposed twice-daily administration regimen (two 120-mg tablets, morning and evening) is the logical conclusion of a progressive tendency toward simplification

Table 1 Therapeutic Efficacy of Various CBS Formulations in Peptic Ulcer Therapy

				Healing rates (%)		
Reference	Patients	Diagnosis	Weeks	Liquid	Chewable tablets	Coated tablets
Hamilton and Axon [92]	32	DU	4	85	75	—
Toussaint and Cremer [103]	33	GU	4	75	82	—
Kellow et al. [102]	26	DU	4	76	89	—
Lane et al. [101]	35	DU	8	89	89	—
Dekker et al. [91]	189	DU	4	—	72	76

DU = duodenal ulcer; GU = gastric ulcer.

of the therapeutic regimen to make it as acceptable as possible for the patient. In this connection, two single-blind studies are available.

In the study by Hollanders [104], the healing rates with the twice daily and four times daily regimens were 72% and 67%, respectively, at 4 weeks and 92% and 81% at 8 weeks. In the other study [105] also, no significant differences were found between the two regimens, though there was a numerical superiority in favor of the four times daily regimen (95%) as compared to twice daily (70%).

This finding was confirmed by Coghlan et al. [106], who observed a greater degree of activity with the four times daily regimen in inducing eradication of *H. pylori*. The eradication rates were 64% and 32%, respectively.

In the light of the results of these studies, the therapeutic regimen recommended consists in the administration of 480 mg daily in two or four doses, though, as we have seen, the most recent reports appear to testify in favor of the twice daily regimen.

B.   Short-Term Treatment of Duodenal Ulcer

The efficacy of colloidal bismuth in the short-term treatment of peptic ulcer has been documented in a broad range of clinical trials, the results of which have been gathered in six international symposia and in numerous comprehensive critical reviews [107–111].

The first clinical indications concerning the use of colloidal bismuth were provided by four pilot studies, which, although open to substantial criticism from the methodological point of view, demonstrated that the drug was capable of healing ulcers in 57–96% of cases [112–114] or of inducing a significant degree of improvement in 96% of patients [115]. These preliminary findings were later confirmed both in open studies [99,116,117] and controlled clinical trials versus placebo and, particularly, versus H_2 antagonists.

1.   Comparison with Placebo

The experience currently available comparing CBS versus placebo consists of 13 double-blind, controlled studies conducted with DeNol in the liquid formulation [90,118–129] and two studies with the chewable tablet formulation [130,131]. The scheduled duration of therapy was 4–6 weeks with endoscopic control examinations and X-ray control in only one case [126].

With the exception of the studies by Glover et al. [128] and Manousos [124], which were characterized by high placebo healing rates (60% and 42%, respectively), all of these trials showed significantly enhanced ulcer healing with the active drug. Healing rates ranged from 50 to 100% for colloidal bismuth and from 10 to 60% for placebo. The mean therapeutic gain with CBS was 43% with the liquid formulation and 52% with the tablets.

2.   Comparison with H_2-Receptor Antagonists

Exhaustive data are also available for comparisons between CBS and histamine H_2-receptor antagonists, particularly cimetidine. The controlled studies available compare CBS in the liquid formulation [132–140] (Table 2) or in the form of chewable tablets [25,141–148] (Table 3) with cimetidine at doses of 1.0 g/day or 400 mg morning and evening. With the exception of Baars et al.'s contribution [139], no significant differences were observed between the two drugs after 4, 6, or 8 weeks of treatment, although an overall analysis of the data appears to show a slight tendency in favor of CBS.

With the coated tablet formulation, the 4-week healing rates ranged from 57 to 84% for colloidal bismuth and from 38 to 72% for cimetidine, with a mean therapeutic gain of 21% in favor of the former. At week 6, this difference was drastically reduced to no more than 6%.

In the case of the liquid formulation, the 4-week healing rates ranged from 60 to 100% and were essentially similar to the cimetidine healing rates (54–89%). At week 8, peak healing rates were 95% for bismuth and 96% for cimetidine. The mean therapeutic gains for CBS over cimetidine at 4 and 8 weeks were 3% and 5%, respectively.

In two studies, CBS was compared with a dosage regimen consisting in the administration of cimetidine 400 mg twice daily [137, 147]. The 4-week healing rates were similar, but at week 8, CBS showed a slight 8% and 12% therapeutic gain over cimetidine.

The experience comparing CBS versus ranitidine 150 mg morning and evening is

Table 2 Controlled Trials Comparing CBS Liquid versus Cimetidine in Duodenal Ulcer Therapy

| | Healing rates (%) | | | |
| | 4 weeks | | 8 weeks | |
Reference	CBS	C	CBS	C
Paccini and Espejo [132]	63	69	—	—
Martin et al. [133]	66	60	89	85
Ward et al. [134]	74	83	84	89
Badial Aceves et al. [135]	60	64	—	—
Kang and Piper [136]	70	83	96	96
Lazzaroni et al. [137]	75	75	—	—
Shreeve et al. [138]	75	54	78	55
Baars et al. [139]	100	56	—	—
Gibinski et al. [140]	91	72	95	89
Mean therapeutic gain, CBS vs. cimetidine	3%		5%	

C = cimetidine.

Table 3 Controlled Trials Comparing CBS Tablets versus Cimetidine in Duodenal Ulcer Therapy

| | Healing rates (%) | | | | | |
| | 4 weeks | | 6 weeks | | 8 weeks | |
Reference	CBS	C	CBS	C	CBS	C
VanTrappen et al. [141]	67	57	86	86	—	—
Moshal et al. [142]	—	—	89	92	—	—
Anzures and Mugiuro [143]	75	33	—	—	—	—
Harley and Alp [144]	82	58	93	81	—	—
Hamilton et al. [25]	—	—	80	85	—	—
Oosthoek et al. [145]	57	38	—	—	—	—
Bianchi Porro et al. [146]	—	—	79	75	—	—
Bianchi Porro et al. [147]	84	72	—	—	100	88
Hamilton et al. [148]	—	—	81	74	—	—
Mean therapeutic gain, CBS vs. cimetidine	21%		6%		—	

C = cimetidine.

much more limited [149–151] (Table 4). The clinical efficacy of the two drugs was found to be practically identical after both 4 and 8 weeks of therapy, with mean therapeutic gains of 3% and 1%, respectively, in favor of colloidal bismuth. Alongside the healing efficacy, colloidal bismuth shows a comparable analgesic activity. In all studies, a rapid, significant reduction in antacid consumption was observed, similar to that found for H_2 antagonists.

3. Comparison with Other Drugs

Colloidal bismuth has been compared with another drug possessing a mainly cytoprotective action, namely sucralfate at the dosage of 4 g/day. In this connection, a contribution has been made by Chinese investigators [152]. In this study, the healing efficacy of colloidal bismuth was found to be significantly superior to that of the comparator drug, with healing rates of 25% versus 4% at 4 weeks and 72% versus 36% at 8 weeks. A difference of the same order in favor of CBS was also found with regard to analgesic efficacy, with 88% versus 59% reductions in symptomatic patients on CBS and sucralfate, respectively.

These data are interesting but require further confirmation in larger patient samples, particularly in the light of the undoubtedly modest sucralfate healing rates observed in this study.

Table 4 Controlled Trials Comparing CBS Tablets versus Ranitidine in Duodenal Ulcer Therapy

| | Healing rates (%) | | | |
| | 4 weeks | | 8 weeks | |
Reference	CBS	R	CBS	R
Bianchi Porro et al. [149]	84	68	96	92
Lee et al. [150]	90	81	97	97
Ward et al. [151]	76	87	91	94
Mean therapeutic gain, CBS vs. ranitidine	3%		1%	

R = ranitidine.

4. Use of Colloidal Bismuth in Patients with Duodenal Ulcers Resistant to Antisecretory Drugs

Colloidal bismuth would appear to play a particular role in "resistant" duodenal ulcers, which are defined as ulcer lesions that fail to heal or show at least a 25% reduction in diameter after a course of therapy, ranging from 6 to 12 weeks, with cimetidine 1.0–1.2 g/day or ranitidine 300 mg/day. The reasons for this have yet to be defined, though impairment of the defensive capability of the gastric and duodenal mucosa is thought to play an important role regardless of acid-pepsin secretory output.

The results obtained with colloidal bismuth in the two studies currently available are undoubtedly interesting and appear to confirm this hypothesis. The study by Lam et al. [153] was conducted using a crossover design, the percentage of nonresponders healed with colloidal bismuth (85%) proved to be significantly superior to that observed after a further course of high doses of cimetidine (400 mg, four times daily) (<40%). These findings were confirmed in a larger study by Bianchi Porro et al. [154] conducted in a group of 52 subjects with duodenal ulcers unhealed after 8 weeks of treatment with cimetidine 1.2 g/day or ranitidine 300 mg/day. Patients were allocated at random to treatment with (a) CBS 120 mg four times daily, (b) cimetidine 1.2 g/day, or (c) cimetidine 2.0 g/day for 4–8 weeks. After 4 weeks, healing rates were 82% (14/17), 39% (7/18), and 44% (7/16) for CBS, cimetidine 1.2 g/day, and cimetidine 2.0 g/day, respectively. At week 8, the respective healing rates were 94%, 65%, and 75%.

C.   Short-Term Treatment of Gastric Ulcer

The first data regarding the efficacy of CBS in the short-term therapy of gastric ulcer were provided by pilot studies conducted by Weiss and Kallmeyer in 1967 [113], by Sobotka [114], and by Cruickshank and Wright [115] in limited patient populations using radiological [113,114] or purely clinical [115] evaluation criteria.

Since Lanza's first endoscopic investigation [41], subsequent open studies over 4 and 8 weeks have demonstrated the efficacy of DeNol, with healing rates ranging from 55 to 92% after 4 weeks and from 83 to 87% after 8 weeks [16,117,155].

The results of these studies have been further confirmed and added to in numerous placebo-controlled studies, which have shown significantly higher healing rates and analgesic efficacy for CBS [94,123,126–129,157–160]. Healing rates range from 61 to 100% for the active drug and from 18 to 43% for placebo, with a mean therapeutic gain of 44% in favor of CBS.

As for comparisons with H_2 antagonists, the data currently available are limited almost entirely to comparisons versus cimetidine administered according to the classic regimen of 200 mg at mealtimes and 400 mg at bedtime for periods of 4, 6, or 8 weeks [94,139,140,157,160–164]. No significant difference has been observed between CBS (in the liquid or tablet formulation) and the comparator H_2-receptor antagonist. Four-week healing rates range from 57 to 81% for CBS and from 43 to 79% for cimetidine, with a marked 15% mean therapeutic gain in favor of CBS. There is practically no difference in healing rates at 6 weeks, but a 10% gain in favor of CBS is observed at 8 weeks. In view of the scanty data available from studies beyond 4 weeks, further confirmation in larger patient samples is required.

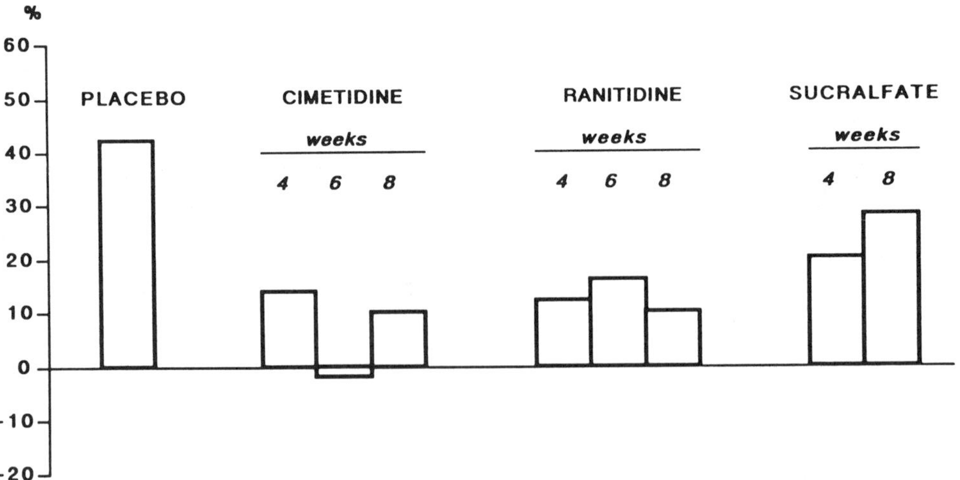

FIGURE 2   Mean therapeutic gain of colloidal bismuth subcitrate over placebo, H_2 blockers, and sucralfate in gastric ulcer.

To date the results of only two studies are available for comparison with ranitidine. In a study by Parente et al. [165], the efficacy of bismuth tablets was compared to that of ranitidine 300 mg/day for a maximum period of 2 months. The healing rates obtained were 70% and 63% for CBS and ranitidine, respectively, at week 4, and 88% and 79% at week 8. Identical analgesic activity was observed, as evaluated on the basis of antacid consumption. Similar results were obtained in another study [166] comparing CBS 240 mg morning and evening with ranitidine 150 mg morning and evening. After 6 weeks of therapy, the respective healing rates were 89% and 74%. The superior therapeutic efficacy of CBS is also confirmed in comparison with sucralfate [152,167,168], pirenzepine [167], vitamin A [167], antacids [169], and glycyrrhizinic acid [170].

As far as sucralfate in particular is concerned, the three studies available show healing rates ranging from 58 to 90% for CBS and from 17 to 63% for the comparator drug. Figure 2 illustrates the mean therapeutic gains for CBS as compared to placebo, H_2-receptor antagonists, and sucralfate.

D. Prophylaxis of Ulcer Relapse

The use of colloidal bismuth was not envisaged in the prophylaxis of ulcer relapse, but the results reported in the literature suggest that short-term treatment with CBS may positively affect the subsequent natural history of ulcer disease. Since the first report by Martin et al. [133], numerous controlled investigations over periods ranging from 3 to 12 months have shown that relapse rates after healing with DeNol are significantly lower than those observed after healing with cimetidine or ranitidine [86,95, 138,148–150] (Fig. 3). Relapse rates after 12 months ranged from 39 to 76% for CBS and from 60 to 100% for the H_2 antagonists. Only in one study [136] were equivalent relapse rates reported: 76% with CBS versus 75% with cimetidine.

On pooling the results of the individual trials eligible for meta-analysis, Dobrilla et al. [171] conclude that there is sufficient clinical evidence in favor of a long-term protective effect of De-Nol with a reduction of the relapse risk as compared to antisecretory agents of 26% at 6 months and 27% at 12 months. Further confirmation of these data is provided by Bianchi Porro et al. [146], who show that the relapse risk in duodenal ulcer patients healed with DeNol and followed up for 12 months is comparable to that observed in subjects healed with cimetidine and subsequently given prophylactic treatment with the same drug at doses of 400 mg at night.

To date, we have the results of only one study on the efficacy and tolerability of long-term prophylactic treatment with CBS [96]. The relapse rates after 6 months of treatment with colloidal bismuth 120 mg nightly were significantly lower than those observed with placebo, 39% versus 80%. These results, which are admittedly preliminary, are undoubtedly suggestive and deserve further study. The reasons for the long-term protective effect of colloidal bismuth are by no means clear. It is postulated that factors possibly contributing to this may be a longer-lasting therapeutic effect due to the slow elimination of body deposits of bismuth [25] and, even more

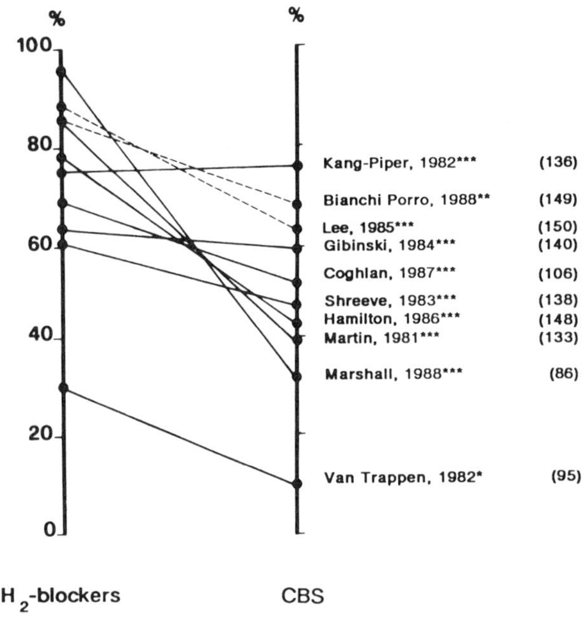

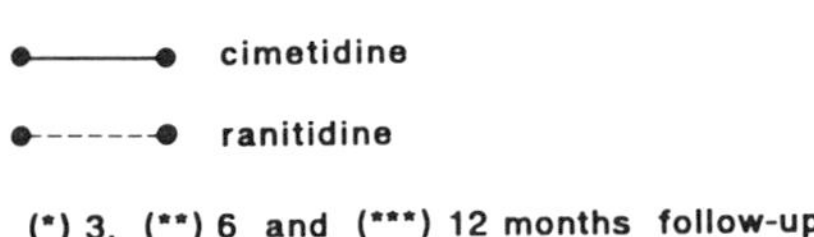

FIGURE 3 Summary of results of studies comparing ulcer relapse rates after healing with CBS, cimetidine, or ranitidine.

important, the bactericidal action of the drug on *H. pylori,* which appears to play a permissive role in the onset of gastric or duodenal ulcer [73].

The bactericidal action of CBS, which is undoubtedly enhanced by a combination with antibiotics (amoxicillin, nitroimidazoles), is associated with a significant reduction in inflammatory phenomena in the gastric and duodenal mucosa with restoration of mucinogenesis levels to normal (Fig. 4) and restoration of mucosal integrity [88], which is a sine qua non for reducing the risk of early relapse of ulcer disease [86, 172–

FIGURE 4 Gastritis scores (mean and SD) after treatment with cimetidine, CBS, or CBS plus antibiotic. CP = *Campylobacter pylori*; PMNs = polymorphonuclear leukocytes; MONOs = lymphocytes and plasma cells. (From Marshall et al. [88].)

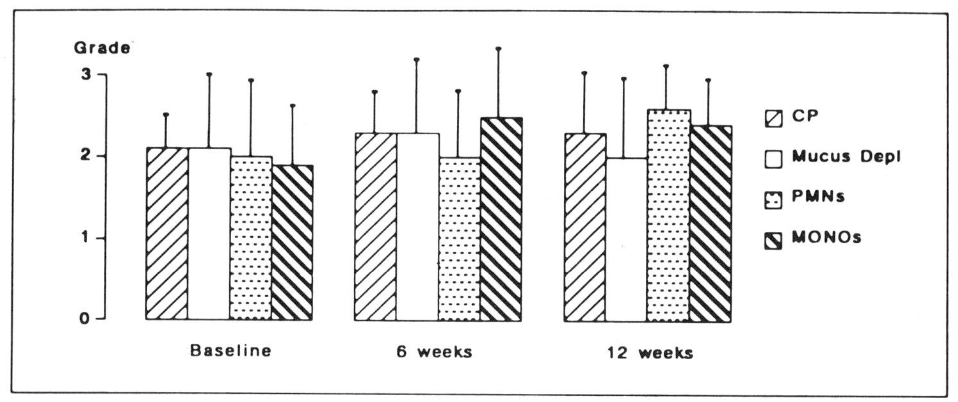
Grade
3
2
1
0
Baseline
6 weeks
12 weeks
CP
Mucus Depl
PMNs
MONOs

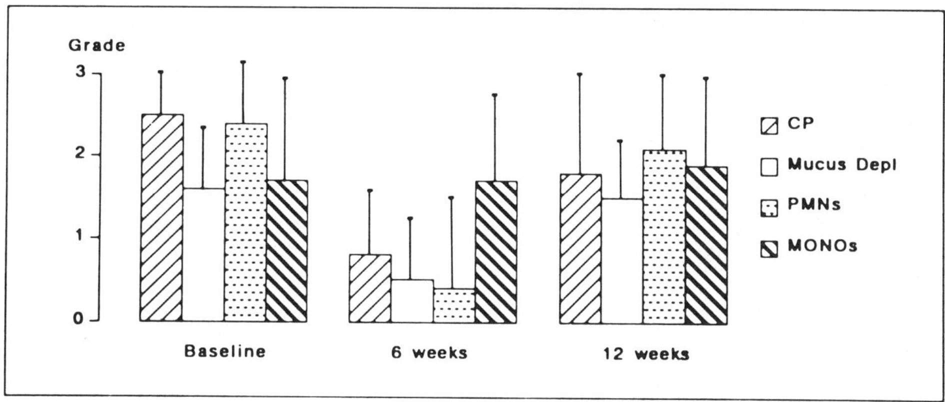
Grade
3
2
1
0
Baseline
6 weeks
12 weeks
CP
Mucus Depl
PMNs
MONOs

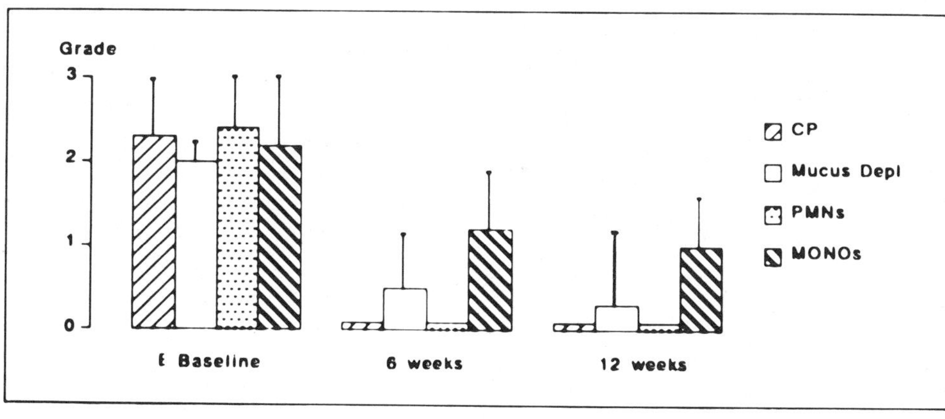
Grade
3
2
1
0
Baseline
6 weeks
12 weeks
CP
Mucus Depl
PMNs
MONOs

175]. Analysis of the data currently available has revealed that the relapse risk is significantly higher (72%) in patients with persistent antral infection than in negative control subjects (19%).

Paradigmatic results were obtained by Marshall et al. [86] in a sample of 100 duodenal ulcer patients with *H. pylori* infection and receiving acute treatment with cimetidine or CBS in combination with placebo or tinidazole and then subjected to clinical follow-up for 12 months. Persistence of *H. pylori* was detected in 100% of cases treated with cimetidine, in 95% of those treated with cimetidine plus tinidazole, in 73% of patients treated solely with CBS, and in 30% of cases treated with CBS plus tinidazole. The healing rates after eradication of the microorganism were significantly higher (92%) than in cases with persistent infection (61%). The percentages for remission at 12 months for the four treatment groups are shown in Figure 5. The relapse rate at 12 months in the HP-negative cases was significantly lower (21%) than in HP-positive controls (84%).

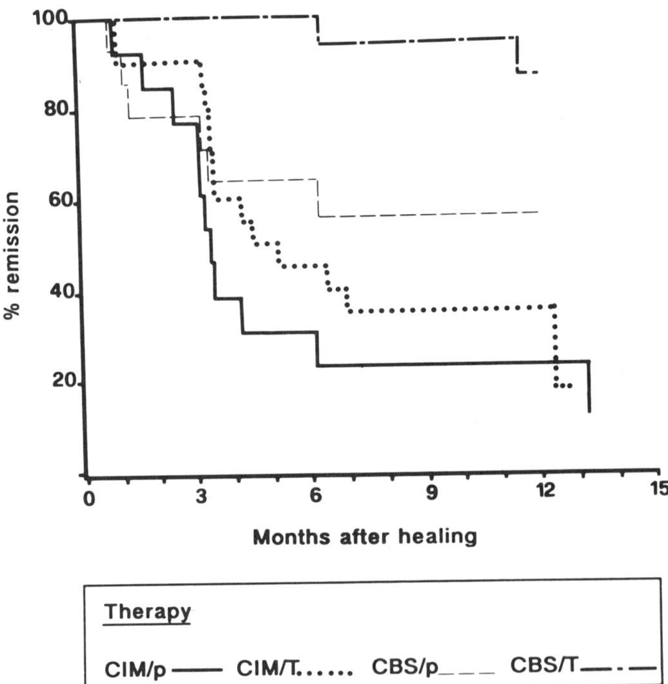

FIGURE 5 *Helicobacter pylori* and duodenal ulcer 12-month relapse rates after short-term treatment with cimetidine plus placebo (CIM/p), cimetidine plus tinidazole (CIM/T), CBS plus placebo (CBS/p), and CBS plus tinidazole (CBS/T). (From Marshall et al. [86].)

E.   Treatment of Non-Ulcer Dyspepsia and Antral Gastritis

The fact that a close etiopathogenetic relationship has been established between *H. pylori* infection and onset of acute and chronic inflammatory phenomena in the antral mucosa has opened up new prospects for an etiological, and not merely symptomatic, therapy for type B gastritis and the dyspeptic clinical manifestations associated with it.

Marshall et al. [88] and Rauws et al. [82] have provided sound evidence of the histological improvements in the gastric antral mucosa observed in approximately 50% of patients on short-term therapy with colloidal bismuth. In particular, an increase in mucinogenesis has been documented as well as a significant reduction in polymorphonuclear infiltrate, lymphocytes, and plasma cells in the lamina propria and also in the epithelium (Fig. 4). Combination with antibiotics (amoxicillin and/or nitroimidazoles) not only permits a more incisive antibacterial action in a significantly higher percentage of patients, even as high as 100%, but also, more important, reduces the risk of early relapse of infection.

Numerous controlled studies are available that document the efficacy of CBS in the treatment of antral gastritis [81,82,88,176–180]. The data on treatment on dyspepsia are more limited. Contributions by Lambert et al. [81], Borody et al. [176], and Rokkas et al. [180] have provided evidence of the specific efficacy of the drug in this context compared to placebo. In particular, the results of the study conducted by Rokkas et al. [180] in 52 patients with non-ulcer dyspepsia show that an 8-week course of treatment with CBS is capable of eradicating *H. pylori* in 83% of cases with a significant improvement in histological findings and in clinical manifestations compared to placebo.

In contrast with the findings in *Helicobacter*-positive patients, no therapeutic effect was detectable in *Helicobacter*-negative dyspeptic subjects even after DeNol, thus demonstrating the close link, at least in the study population examined, between *H. pylori* infection and clinical manifestations. These data, which are undoubtedly suggestive, require further confirmation, particularly in the light of the results obtained in a previous trial [78] in which no correlation was found between symptom improvement and *H. pylori* eradication in a sample of patients with non-ulcer dyspepsia treated with bismuth salicylate, erythromycin, or placebo.

It may be hypothesized that the beneficial effect of colloidal bismuth subcitrate on the functional state of gastric mucosa may be produced via a mechanism of action that is far more complex than simple antibacterial activity.

F.   Treatment of Reflux Esophagitis

The data available on reflux esophagitis are extremely limited, though the pharmacological properties of CBS suggest that it may be potentially useful, at least in the liquid formulation, in the treatment of peptic esophagitis. An indication of this was provided by the study conducted by Chaparala et al. [181], who demonstrated the efficacy of another bismuth compound (PeptoBismol) in preventing experimental lesions in the rabbit esophagus.

In humans, the only results we can refer to are those of a single study conducted by Borkent and Beker [182] in a group of 20 patients with grades 3 and 4 esophagitis that failed to respond to a 3-month treatment with H_2 antagonists. *Helicobacter pylori* was detected in the esophageal mucosa in nine of these patients. The patients were treated, according to a double-blind protocol, with cimetidine 800 mg nightly either alone or in combination with CBS 120 mg four times daily in the form of tablets dissolved in saline and administered topically via an esophageal tube left in situ for the entire duration of the therapy, which was scheduled to last for a maximum period of 3 weeks. Of the 10 patients treated with the drug combination, seven presented no endoscopic signs of esophagitis at the end of therapy, while grade 1 esophagitis was found in the other three. In contrast, in the cimetidine control group, six patients showed no change, three presented grade 2 esophagitis, and one presented grade 1 esophagitis. Nine patients with grade 2 or grade 3 esophagitis at the end of the course of the cimetidine treatment were then treated with the combination. After 3 weeks, six of these exhibited endoscopic healing.

These data suggest that CBS may have a precise role to play in the treatment of peptic esophagitis. However, more extensive investigation is needed in the light of the current potential offered by antisecretory proton-pump inhibitors in the treatment of resistant esophagitis.

VI.   TOLERABILITY AND SIDE EFFECTS

The large body of data currently available, acquired over the period since 1971 when the drug was first launched upon the market, shows that CBS is a well-tolerated compound [183]. The development of the coated tablet formulation has overcome both the problem of the characteristic unpleasant ammoniacal taste of the liquid formulation and that of the darkening of the teeth and mucosa of the mouth induced by chewable tablets. The darkening of the feces due to the formation of bismuth sulfate, on the other hand, is an inevitable consequence of ingestion of the metal and may occasionally cause differential diagnosis problems in relation to the passage of melenic feces.

Side effects, in the strict sense of the term, include dizziness, headache, bowel disorders (diarrhea or constipation), and skin rashes [25,96,181,184]. As far as the monitoring of blood chemistry variables is concerned, only rare cases of slight, temporary increases in ALT and AST values have been reported [132,184].

It should be stressed, however, that despite the excellent tolerability profile of CBS, bismuth compounds are potentially capable of causing a serious side effect, bismuth encephalopathy. The risk of onset of this severe clinical manifestation is closely related to the plasma levels of the metal. In a review of 310 reported cases of bismuth encephalopathy secondary to the uncontrolled administration of bismuth salts [185], only 22 occurred with plasma bismuth concentrations close to 100 μg/L (0.48 μmol), as against 194 with values ranging from 100 to 1000 μg/L, and 94 with values from 1000 to 2000 μg/L and above. On the basis of these findings, a normal range has been established with margins of absolute safety, namely anything up to 50 μg/L, while the danger zone lies between 50 and 100 μg/L, with a maximum acceptable value of 100 μg/L.

As mentioned, the mean variations in plasma bismuth concentrations detected in the course of controlled studies are very slight, not exceeding 7.0 μg/L, which is well within the safety limits [183]. To date, there has been an isolated report of a patient with neurotic symptoms after prolonged therapy with CBS [186] 600 mg four times daily for 2 months followed by 240 mg/day for two consecutive years. These neurological manifestations, which occurred during the last 2 months of therapy, gradually regressed over a 10–12-month period after discontinuation of the drug.

Food for thought, however, is provided by the results of a recent trial in a group of 16 healthy volunteers [97]. After three administrations of CBS in the form of coated tablets, peak bismuth concentrations exceeding 50 μg/L for 10–265 min were detected in 14 cases. Values exceeding 100 μg/L for 10–145 min were detected in nine cases. The overall 24-hour plasma bismuth values, however, showed no significant changes compared to basal values. This latter finding, although reassuring, does not entirely allay the misgivings prompted by the unusual variations in peak plasma concentrations, particularly in view of the fact that, in terms of time, the threshold value above which bismuth induces toxic effects on the CNS is not known. Further in-depth investigations are therefore necessary to clarify this important issue.

REFERENCES

1. Wiericks J, Hespe W, Jaitly HD, Koekkoek PH, Lang V. Pharmacological properties of colloidal bismuth subcitrate (CBS, DeNol). Scand J Gastroenterol 1982; 17(Suppl 80): 11–6.
2. Williams DR. Analytical and computer simulation studies of colloidal bismuth subcitrate system used as an ulcer treatment. Inorg Nucl Chem 1977; 39:711–4.
3. Lee SP. A potential mechanism of action of colloidal bismuth subcitrate: diffusion barrier to hydrochloric acid. Scand J Gastroenterol 1982; 17(Suppl 80):17–21.
4. Lavy V, Koekkoek PH, Jaitly HD. Anti-ulcer activity of colloidal bismuth subcitrate in Shay rats. Arch Int Pharmacodyn Ther 1976; 222:291–8.
5. Wilson TR. The pharmacology of TDB. Postgrad Med J 1975; Suppl 51:18–21.
6. Wilson TR. Effect of tri-potassium di-citrate bismuth (TDB) on healing of experimental gastric ulcers in rats. Postgrad Med J 1975; Suppl 51:22–5.
7. Bianchi RG, Dajani EZ, Casler JJ. Gastric anti-ulcer and anti-secretory effects of bismuth salts in the rat. Pharmacologist 1980; 22:168A.
8. Konturek SJ, Radecki T, Piastucki I, Drozdowicz D. Advances in the understanding of the mechanism of cytoprotective action by colloidal bismuth subcitrate. Scand J Gastroenterol 1986; 21(Suppl 122):6–10.

9. Konturek SJ, Radecki T, Piastucki I, Brzozowski T, Drozdovicz D. Gastrocytoprotection by CBS (DeNol) and sucralfate. The role of endogenous prostaglandins. Gut 1987; 28:201–5.

10. Malandrino S, Campagnoli G, Borsa M, Guidoboni R, Tonon GC. Prevention of gastric mucosal lesions in rats by tri-potassium dicitrato bismuthate. Arzneim Forsch 1984; 34:30–1.

11. Hall SWR, VanDeHoven WE. Gastric mucosal protection and prostaglandin E_2 generation in rats by colloidal bismuth subcitrate (DeNol). Arch Int Pharmacodyn 1986; 286:308–9.

12. Konturek SJ, Radecki T, Piastucki L, Drozdowicz D. Studies on the gastro-protective and ulcer healing effects of colloidal bismuth subcitrate. Digestion 1987; 37(Suppl 2):8–15.

13. Konturek SJ, Stachura J, Radecki T, Drozdowicz D, Brozozowski T. Cytoprotective and ulcer healing properties of prostaglandin E_2, colloidal bismuth and sucralfate in rats. Digestion 1987; 38:103–13.

14. Hall SWR, DeWijn SR. Bismuth from DeNol swallow tablets (ST) bind to acetic acid induced stomach ulcers in the rat. Abstract 766. XII International Congress of Gastroenterology, Lisboa, Portugal, 1984.

15. Moshall MG, Gregory MA, Pillay C, Spitaels JM. Does the duodenal cell ever return to normal? A comparison between treatment with cimetidine and DeNol. Scand J Gastroenterol 1979; Suppl 54:48–51.

16. Gregory MA, Moshall MG, Spitaels JM. The effect of tripotassium dicitrato bismuthate on the duodenal mucosa during ulceration. An ultrastructural study. S Afr Med J 1982; 62:52–5.

17. Coghill SB, Hopwood D, McPherson S, Hislop S. The ultrastructural localisation of colloidal tripotassium dicitrato bismuthate (DeNol) in the upper gastrointestinal tract of man and rodents following oral and instrumental administration. J Pathol 1983; 139:105–14.

18. Stiel D, Murray DG, Peters TJ. Uptake and sub-cellular localisation of bismuth in the gastrointestinal mucosa of rats after short-term administration of colloidal bismuth subcitrate. Gut 1985; 26:364–8.

19. Kamoda T, Sonoda M, Ikeda M, Hokari S, Sakagishi Y. Inhibition of alkaline phosphatase by bismuth. Clin Chim Acta 1981; 116:161–9.

20. Hall DWR, VanDenHoven WE. Light microscopic and ultrastructural evaluation of rat gastric mucosa protection by DeNol. Gut 1986; 27:A1236.

21. Koo J, Ho J, Lam SK, Wong J, Ong GB. Selective coating of gastric ulcer by TDB in the rat. Gastroenterology 1982; 82:864–70.

22. Soutar RL, Coghill SB. Interaction of tripotassium dicitrato bismuthate with macrophages in the rat and in vitro. Gastroenterology 1986; 91:84–93.

23. Flavell Matts SQ, Schwan CHJ. Initial evaluation of a new bismuth compound in the therapy of peptic ulcer with in vivo gastric analysis. Postgrad Med J 1965; 41:109–11.

24. Soldani G, del Tacca M, Barnardini C, Polloni A, Martinotti E, Malandrino S, Orsa M, Tonon GC. Gastric pharmacological activities of tripotassium dicitrato bismuthate in rats and in dogs. Pharmacol Res Commun 1985; 17:1017–26.

25. Hamilton I, Worsley BW, O'Connor HJ, Axon TR. Effects of tripotassium dicitrato bismuthate (TDB) tablets or cimetidine in the treatment of duodenal ulcer. Gut 1983; 24:1148–51.

26. Baron JH, Barr J, Batten J, Sidebotham R, Spencer J. Acid pepsin and mucus secretion in patients with gastric and duodenal ulcer before and after colloidal bismuth subcitrate (DeNol). Gut 1986; 27:486–90.

27. Hollander D, Morissey SM, Mehta J. Mucus secretion in gastric ulcer patients treated with tripotassium dicitrato bismuthate (DeNol). Br J Clin Pract 1983; 37:112–4.

28. Roberts NB, Taylor WH. Effect of tripotassium dicitrato bismuthate (DeNol) upon individual human pepsins. Clin Sci 1982; 63:65.

29. Stiel D, Peters TJ. Tripotassium dicitrato bismuthate (DeNol) binds conjugated bile acids in vitro. Possible mechanism in gastric ulcer healing. Proc Aust Soc Med Res 1983; 16:18A.

30. Tasman-Jones C, Maher C, Thomsen L, Lee SP, Vanderwee M. Mucosal defences and gastroduodenal disease. Digestion 1987; 37(Suppl 2):1–7.

31. Mekel R. Panel discussion. Present and future treatment of peptic ulcer and potential role of DeNol. Scand J Gastroenterol 1982; 17(Suppl 80):49–57.

32. Anon. Panel discussion: Present and future treatment of peptic ulcer and the potential role of DeNol. Scand J Gastroenterol 1982; 17(Suppl 80):49–57.

33. Hall DWR, VanDenHoven WE. Protective properties of colloidal bismuth subcitrate on gastric mucosa. Scand J Gastroenterol 1986; 21(Suppl 122):11–3.

34. Konturek SJ, Kwiecien N, Obtolowicz W, Hebzda Z, Oleski J. Effects of protective drugs on gastric alkaline secretion in man. Scand J Gastroenterol 1987; 22:1059–63.

35. Estela R, Feller A, Backhouse C, Castro R, Ugarte G. Efectos del subcitrato de bismuto coloidal e hidroxido de alumino sobre los niveles gastricos y duodenales de prostaglandina E_2. Rev Med Chile 1984; 112:975–81.

36. Crampton JR, Gibbons LC, Rees WDW. Effect of certain ulcer healing agents on amphibian gastroduodenal bicarbonate secretion. Scand J Gastroenterol 1986; 21(Suppl 125):113–6.

37. Malandrino S, Bestetti A, Campagnoli G, Guidoboni R, Tonon GC. Gastric cytoprotection in rats by tripotassium dicitrato bismuthate: role of mucosal sulphydryl compounds. XXII Congress of Italian Pharmacological Society 1984: 399A.

38. Goldenberg MM, Honcomp LH, Burrock SE, et al. Protective effect of PeptoBismol liquid on the gastric mucosa of rats Gastroenterology 1975; 69:636–40.

39. Coghill SB, Meehan SE, Milne G, Hopwood D. The localization of DeNol (tripotassium dicitrato bismuthate) in gastric ulcers and the normal upper G-I tract of man and rodents by light and electron microscopy. S Pathol 1983; 139:487.

40. Lam SK, Koo J, Cheng CH, et al. Treatment of corpus and prepyloric gastric ulcer with tripotassium dicitrate bismuthate (DeNol). Gastroenterology 1981; 80:1202A.

41. Lanza FL. An endoscopic evaluation of gastric ulcer treated with a mixture containing bismuth ammonium citrate. Curr Ther Res 1970; 12:779–88.

42. Weiss G, Kallmeyer K. Pilot trial of a colloidal bismuth preparation in the treatment of peptic ulcer. S Afr Med J 1968; 42:317–20.

43. Bizzozzero G. Ueber die schlauchfoermigen druden des magendarmkanals un die beziehungen epithels zu dem oberfachenepithel der schleimhaut. Arch Mikrobiol Anat 1883; 42:82–152.

44. Salomon H. Ueber das spirillium des saugetiermagens und sein verhalten zu der belegzellen. Zentralbl Bakteriol Mikrobiol Hyg 1896; 19:433–42.

45. Kreinitz W. Ueber das auftreren von spirochaeten verschiedener formin magenihalt bei carcinoma ventriculi. Dtsch Med Wochenschr 1906; 32:872.

46. Rosenow EC, Sanford C. The bacteriology of ulcer of the stomach and duodenum in man. J Infect Dis 1915; 17:219–26.

47. Appelmans R, Vassiliadis P. Etudes sur la flore microbienne des ulcères gastroduodenaux et des cancers gastriques. Rev Belge Sci Med 1932; 4:198–203.

48. Doenges JL. Spirochetes in the gastric glands of *Macacus rhesus* and human without definite history of related disease. Proc Soc Exp Med Biol 1938; 38:536–58.

49. Freedburg S, Barron LE. The presence of spirochetes in the human gastric mucosa. Am J Dig Dis 1940; 7:443–5.

50. Warren JR. Unidentified curved bacillus on gastric epithelium in active chronic gastritis. Lancet 1983; i:1273. Letter.

51. Marshall BJ. Unidentified curved bacillus on gastric epithelium in active chronic gastritis. Lancet 1983; i:1273–5. Letter.

52. Marshall BJ, Barrett LJ, Prakesh C, et al. Survival of *Campylobacter pyloridis* at acid pH. Gastroenterology 1987; 92:1517.

53. Hazell S, Lee A, Brady L, Hennessy W. *Campylobacter pyloridis* gastritis: association with intercellular spaces and adaptation to an environment of mucus as important factors in colonisation of the gastric epithelium. J Infect Dis 1986; 153:658–63.

54. Hazell S, Lee A. *Campylobacter pyloridis,* urease, hydrogen ion back diffusion and gastric ulcers. Lancet 1986; ii:15–7.

55. Slomiany BL, Bilsky J, Sarosiek M, et al. *Campylobacter pyloridis* degrades mucin and undermines gastric mucosa integrity. Biochem Biophys Res Commun 1987; 144:307–14.

56. Chen XG, Correa P, Offerhaus J, et al. Ultrastructure of the gastric mucosa harboring *Campylobacter*-like organisms. Am J Clin Pathol 1986; 86:575–82.

57. Thomas JM, Poynter D, Gooding C, et al. Gastric spiral bacteria. Lancet 1984; ii:100. Letter.

58. Philips AD, Hine KR, Holmes GKT, Woodings DF. Gastric spiral bacteria. Lancet 1984; ii:1000–1.

59. Hui WM, Lam SK, Chau PY, Ho J, Lui L, Lai CL, Lok ASF, Ng MMT. Persistence of *Campylobacter pyloridis* despite healing of duodenal ulcer and improvement of accompanying duodenitis and gastritis. Dig Dis Sci 1987; 32:1555–60.

60. Goodwin CS, Blincow E, Warren JR, et al. Evaluation of cultural techniques for isolating *Campylobacter pyloridis* from endoscopic biopsies of gastric mucosa. J Clin Pathol 1985; 138:1127–31.

61. Gilman RH, Leon-Barua RE, Kock J, et al. Rapid identification of pyloric *Campylobacter* in Peruvian with gastritis. Dig Dis Sci 1986; 31:1089–95.

62. McNulty CA, Watson DM. Spiral bacteria of gastric antrum. Lancet 1989; i:1068–9.

63. Rollason TP, Stone J, Rhodes JM. Spiral organisms in endoscopic biopsies of the human stomach. J Clin Pathol 1984; 37:23–6.

64. Price A, Levi J, Dolby JM, et al. *Campylobacter pyloridis* in peptic ulcer disease, microbiology, pathology and scanning electron microscopy. Gut 1985; 26:1183–8.

65. Buck GE, Gourley WK, Lee WK. Relation of *Campylobacter pyloridis* to gastritis and peptic ulcer. J Infect Dis 1986; 153:664–9.

66. Graham DY, Kein PD. *Campylobacter pyloridis* gastritis: the past, the present and speculations about the future. Am J Gastroenterol 1987; 82:283–6.

67. Blaser MJ. Gastric *Campylobacter*-like organisms, gastritis and peptic ulcer disease. Gastroenterology 1987; 93:371–83.

68. Dooley CP, Cohen H. The clinical significance of *Campylobacter pylori*. Ann Intern Med 1988; 108:70–9.

69. Marshall BJ, Armstrong JA, McGechie DB, Clancy RJ. Attempt to fulfill Kock's postulates for pylori *Campylobacter*. Med J Aust 1985; 142:436–9.

70. Morris A, Nicholson G. Ingestion of *Campylobacter pyloridis* causes gastritis and raised fasting pH. Am J Gastroenterol 1987; 82:297–301.

71. Bartlett JG. *Campylobacter pylori*: fact or fancy? Gastroenterology 1988; 94:228.

72. Stadler PH, Blum AL. *Campylobacter pylori* est-il responsable de la maladie ulcereuse? Gastroenterol Clin Biol 1989; 13:3–7.

73. Goodwin CS. Duodenal ulcer, *Campylobacter pylori* and the "leaking roof" concept. Lancet 1988; ii:1467–9.

74. Bianchi Porro G, Lazzaroni M. *Campylobacter pylori* and peptic ulcer therapy. Gastroenterol Clin Biol 1989; 13:107–11.

75. Goodwin CS, Blake P, Blincow E. The minimum inhibitory and bactericidal concentration of antibiotics and anti-ulcer agents against *Campylobacter pyloridis*. J Antimicrob Chemother 1986; 17:309–14.

76. Andreasen JJ, Andersen LP. In vitro susceptibility of *Campylobacter pyloridis* to sucralfate, bismuth and sixteen antibiotics. Acta Pathol Microbiol Immunol Scand 1987; Sect B; 95:147–9.

77. Hirschl AL, Stanek G, Rotter ML. *Campylobacter pyloridis*: frequency of occurrence, serology and susceptibility to antibiotics and ulcer drugs. The IV International Workshop on *Campylobacter pylori* Infection, Goteborg, June 16–18, 1987. Abstract 64.

78. McNulty CM, Gearty JC, Crump B, Davis M, Donovan I, Melikian V, Lister DM, Wise R. *Campylobacter pyloridis* and associated gastritis: investigator blind, placebo controlled trial of bismuth salicylate and erythromycin ethylsuccinate. Br Med J 1986; 293:645–9.

79. McNulty CM, Dent JC, Ford GA, Wilkenson SP. Antimicrobial concentrations in the gastric mucosa. The IV International Workshop on *Campylobacter pylori* Infection, Goteborg, June 16–18, 1987. Abstract 113.

80. Johnston BJ, Ali MH, Haines K, Reed PL. *Campylobacter*-like organisms in the duodenal mucosa and the effect of ulcer treatment on their presence. Gastroenterology 1985; 88:1463.

81. Lambert JR, Borromeo M, Korman MG, Ansky J, Eaves ER. Effect of colloidal bismuth (DeNol) on healing and subsequent relapse of duodenal ulcers. Role of *Campylobacter pyloridis*. Gastroenterology 1987; 92:1479.

82. Rauws EAJ, Langenberg W, Houthoff HJ, Zanen HC, Tytgat GNJ. *Campylobacter pyloridis* associated chronic active antral gastritis. A prospective study of its prevalence and the effects of antibacterial and anti-ulcer treatment. Gastroenterology 1988; 94:33–40.

83. Humphreys H, Bourke S, Dooley CW, McKenna D, Power B, Keane CT, Sweeney EC, O'Morain C. Effect of treatment on *Campylobacter pylori* in peptic disease; a randomised prospective trial. Gut 1988; 29:279–83.

84. Borsch G, Mai U, Opperkuch W. Oral triple therapy may effectively eradicate *Campylobacter pylori* in man. A pilot study. Gastroenterology 1988; 94:44.

85. Borody T, Cole P, Nooman S, Morgan A, Ossip G, Maysey J, Brandl S. Long-term *Campylobacter pylori* recurrence posteradication. Gastroenterology 1988; 94:43.

86.   Marshall BJ, Goodwin CS, Warren JR. Prospective double-blind trial of duodenal ulcer relapse after eradication of *Campylobacter pylori*. Lancet 1988; ii:1437–41.

87.   Armstrong JA, Wee SH, Goodwin CS, Wilson DH. Response of *Campylobacter pyloridis* to antibiotics, bismuth and an acid reducing agent in vitro—an ultrastructural study. J Med Microbiol 1987; 24:343–50.

88.   Marshall BJ, Armstrong JA, Francis GJ, Nokes NT, Wee SH. Antibacterial action of bismuth in relation to *Campylobacter pyloridis* colonization and gastritis. Digestion 1987; 37(Suppl 12):16–30.

89.   Gavey CJ, Szeto ML, Nwokolo CU, Sercombe J, Pounder RE. Bismuth accumulates in the body during treatment with tripotassium dicitrato bismuthate. Alimen Pharmacol Ther 1989; 3:21–8.

90.   Dekker W, Reisma K. Double-blind controlled trial with colloidal bismuth subcitrate in the treatment of symptomatic duodenal ulcers with special references to blood and urine bismuth levels. Ann Clin Res 1979; 11:94–7.

91.   Dekker W, dal Monte PR, Bianchi Porro G, Van Bentem N, Boekorst JC, et al. An international multi-clinic study comparing the therapeutic efficacy of colloidal bismuth subcitrate coated tablets with chewing tablets in the treatment of duodenal ulceration. Scand J Gastroenterol 1986; 21(Suppl 122):46–50.

92.   Hamilton I, Axon ATR. Controlled trial comparing DeNol tablets with DeNol liquid in the treatment of duodenal ulcer. Br Med J 1981; 282:362.

93.   Lee SP. Studies on the absorption and excretion of tripotassium dicitrato bismuthate in man. Res Commun Chem Pathol Pharmacol 1981; 34:359–64.

94.   Tytgat GNJ, VanBentem N, VanOffen G, Dekker W, Rutgeerts L, et al. Controlled trial comparing colloidal bismuth subcitrate tablets, cimetidine and placebo in the treatment of gastric ulceration. Scand J Gastroenterol 1982; 80:31–8.

95.   VanTrappen G, Schurrmans P, Rutgeerts L, Janssen J. A comparative study of colloidal bismuth subcitrate and cimetidine on the healing and recurrence of duodenal ulcer. Scand J Gastroenterol 1982; 17(Suppl 80):23–30.

96.   Bianchi Porro G, Lazzaroni M, Cortvriendt WRE. Maintenance therapy with colloidal bismuth subcitrate in duodenal ulcer disease. Digestion 1987; 37(Suppl 2):47–52.

97.   Nwokolo CU, Gavey CJ, Smith JTL, Pounder RE. The absorption of bismuth from oral doses of tripotassium dicitrato bismuthate. Aliment Pharmacol Ther 1989; 3:29–39.

98.   Allain P, Chaleil D, Emile J. L'elevation des concentrations de bismuth dans les tissue des malades intoxiques. Therapie 1980; 35:303–4.

99.   Tomecki R, Habior A, Medrzejewski W. Ocena kliniczna preparatu DeNol. Pol Tyf Lek 1984; XXXIX:1247–8.

100. Lee SP, Lim TH, Pybus J, Clarke C. Tissue distribution of orally administered bismuth in the rat. Clin Exp Pharm Physiol 1980; 7:319–24.

101. Lane M, Lee S, Tasman-Jones C, Nicholson G. Tripotassium dicitrato-bismuthate tablets vs. liquid in the treatment of duodenal ulcers. NZ Med J 1985; 98:191–2.

102. Kellow JW, Barr GD, Middleton WRJ, Piper DW. Comparison of colloidal bismuth subcitrate tablets and liquid in duodenal ulcer healing. J Clin Gastroenterol 1983; 5:417–20.

103. Toussaint J, Cremer M. A comparative trial of the DeNol chewing tablets and DeNol liquid in the treatment of gastric ulcers. Scand J Gastroenterol 1982; 17(Suppl 78):100.

104. Hollanders D. Twice daily tripotassium dicitrato bismuthate in the treatment of duodenal ulceration. Postgrad Med J 1986; 62:19–21.

105. Lazzaroni M, Parente F, Prada A, Bianchi Porro G. Colloidal bismuth subcitrate as coated tablets: four times versus twice daily dosage in duodenal ulcer. Scand J Gastroenterol 1986; 21(Suppl 122):51–3.

106. Coghlan G, Gilligan D, Humphreys H, McKenna D, Sweeney E, et al. Efficacy of different dosage regimes in duodenal ulcer healing and *Campylobacter pylori* eradication. Abstract presented at the Irish Society of Gastroenterology, Londonderry, June 5–6, 1987.

107. Brogden RN, Pinder RM, Phyllis R, Sawyer R, Speight TM, Avery GS. Tripotassium dicitrato bismuthate: a report of its pharmacological properties and therapeutic efficacy in peptic ulcer. Drugs 1976; 12:401–11.

108. Bianchi Porro G. Modern medical treatment of peptic ulcer. In: Axon TR, ed. Pathogenesis and the treatment of peptic ulcer disease. Amsterdam: Excerpta Medica, 1985:13–38.

109. Tytgat GNJ. Colloidal bismuth subcitrate in peptic ulcer—a review. Digestion 1987; 37(Suppl 2):31–41.

110. Wagstaff AJ, Benfield P, Monk J. Colloidal bismuth subcitrate. Review of its pharmacodynamic and pharmacokinetic properties and its therapeutic use in peptic ulcer disease. Drugs 1988; 36:132–57.

111. Barbara L, Corinaldesi R, Rea E, Paternico A, Stanghellini V. The role of colloidal bismuth subcitrate in the short-term treatment of duodenal ulcer. Scand J Gastroenterol 1986; 21(Suppl 122):30–4.

112. Paulus GE. A successful management of peptic ulcer patient in industry. Ind Med Surg 1966; 35:21–3.

113. Weiss G, Kallmeyer C. Pilot trial of colloidal bismuth preparation in the treatment of peptic ulcer. S Afr Med J 1969; 42:317–9.

114. Sobotka JJ. Peptic ulcer—simplified ambulatory therapy. Curr Ther Res 1970; 12:47–51.

115. Cruickshank GW, Wright T. A multi-centre pilot study of tripotassium dicitrato bismuthate (DeNol) in general practice. Curr Med Res Op 1973; 1:529–635.

116. Séchaud R. Un autre traitement des ulcères gastro-duodenaux. Schweiz Rundschaul Med 1980; 69:213–5.

117. Nogueire JR, Noyol J, Santoyo R, Esquivel RF. Results of treatment with bismuth subcitrate (Kurull) in patients with peptic ulcer. Compend Invest Clin Latinoamer 1982; 2(Suppl 1):66–70.

118. Salmon PR, Brown P, Williams R, Read E. Evaluation of colloidal bismuth (DeNol) in the treatment of duodenal ulcer employing endoscopic selection and follow-up. Gut 1974; 15:189–93.

119. Moshal MG. The treatment of duodenal ulcers with TDB: a duodenoscopic double-blind cross-over investigation. Postgrad Med J 1975; 51(Suppl 5):36–40.

120. Shreeve DR. A double-blind study of tripotassium dicitrate bismuth in duodenal ulcer. Postgrad Med J 1975; 51(Suppl 5):33–6.

121. Connon JJ. DeNol an effective drug in the therapy of duodenal ulceration. J Ir Med Assoc 1977; 70:206–7.

122. Coughlin GP, Kupa A, Alp M. The effect of tripotassium dictrato bismuth (DeNol) on the healing of chronic duodenal ulcers. Med J Aust 1977; 1:294–8.

123. Lee SP, Nicholson GI. Increased healing of gastric and duodenal ulcers in a controlled trial using tripotassium dicitrato bismuthate. Med J Aust 1977; 1:808–12.

124. Manousos O. Treatment of duodenal ulcer with tripotassium dicitrato bismuthate. Iat Chron 1977; 17:174.

125. Vissoulis C, Vissoulis G, Goldis G, Psimeros G. Endoscopic evaluation of TDB in the treatment of duodenal ulcer. Iat Chron 1977; 17:157–64.

126. Poulantzas J, Plyneropoulos S, Papsomoatious A. A double-blind evaluation of the effect of tripotassium dicitrato bismuthate in peptic ulcer. Br J Clin Pract 1978; 32:379–84.

127. Morales A, Antezana C, Roman I, Hurtado C. Effecto de un derivado del bismuto (DeNol) en la cicatrizacion de ulceras gastricas y duodenales. Rev Med Chile 1982; 110:959–63.

128. Glover SC, Cantlay JS, Weir J, Mowat NAG. Oral tripotassium dicitratobismuthate in gastric and duodenal ulceration. A double-blind controlled trial. Dig Dis Sci 1983; 28:13–7.

129. Tripathi BM, Misra NP, Dube S. A double-blind randomised study of tripotassium dicitrato bismuthate in the treatment of peptic ulcer. J Assoc Phys Indian 1984; 38:964–5.

130. Bank S, Marks IN, Novis IH, Barbezat GO. Colloidal bismuth tablets in the treatment of peptic ulceration. Gastroenterology 1979; 76:1093.

131. Wilson P, Alp MH. Colloidal bismuth subcitrate tablets and placebo in chronic duodenal ulceration: a double-blind randomised trial. Med J Aust 1982; 1:222–3.

132. Paccini G, Espejo H. Colloidal bismuth subcitrate and cimetidine in the treatment of peptic ulcers. Trib Med 1980; 16:30–6.

133. Martin DF, Hollanders D, May SJ, Ravenscroft MM, Tweedle DEF, Miller JP. Difference in relapse rates of duodenal ulcer after healing with cimetidine or tripotassium dicitrato bismuthate. Lancet 1981; i:7–10.

134. Ward M, Pollard EJ, Cowen A. Double-blind trial of cimetidine versus tripotassium dicitrato bismuthate in chronic duodenal ulceration. Med J Aust 1981; 1:363–4.

135. Badial Aceves F, Morales OP, Ramos RH, Saenz FV. Subcitrato de bismuto vs cimetidine en el tratamiento de la ulcero peptica. Compend Invest Clin Latinoam 1982; 2(Suppl 1):55–60.

136. Kang JY, Piper DW. Cimetidine and colloidal bismuth in treatment of chronic duodenal ulcer: comparison of initial healing and recurrence. Digestion 1982; 23:73–9.

137. Lazzaroni M, Petrillo M, DeNicola C, Bianchi Porro G. DeNol liquid and cimetidine twice daily in the treatment of duodenal ulcer. A preliminary study. Br J Clin Pract 1983; 37:379–81.

138. Shreeve DR, Klass HJ, Jones PE. Comparison of cimetidine and tripotassium dicitrato bismuthate in healing and relapse of duodenal ulcers. Digestion 1983; 28:96–101.

139. Baars H, Oekhorst JC, VanDommelen CKV, Van Leuween AA, et al. DeNol versus cimetidine (Tagamet). Een verglikend onderzoek bij de internisten praktijk. TGD/ JDR 1984; 9:187–90.

140. Gibinski K, Nowak A, Markicz et al. Dicytrynianobizmutan trojpotasowy w leczeniu wrzodu trawiennego i zapobieganiu nawrotowi wrzodu. Pol Tyg Lek 1984; 39:1547– 50.

141. VanTrappen G, Rutgeerts P, Brockaert L, Janssens J. Randomised open controlled trial of colloidal bismuth subcitrate tablets and cimetidine in the treatment of duodenal ulcer. Gut 1980; 21:329–33.

142. Moshal MG, Spitaels JM, Khan F. Tripotassium dicitrato bismuthate chewing tablets in the treatment of duodenal ulcers: a double-blind, double-dummy comparative study. S Afr Med J 1981; 60:420–3.

143. Anzures ME, Murguia D. Resultados preliminares del estudio dobie ciego en 30 pacientes con ulcera peptica tratados con subcitrato de bismuto, cimetidina o placebo. Comp Invest Clin Latinoam 1982; 2(Suppl 1):51–4.

144. Harley H, Alp MH. Treatment of chronic duodenal ulceration. Effectiveness of colloidal bismuth subcitrate tablets compared with cimetidine. Med J Aust 1983; ii:627–8.

145. Oosthoek D, Wille JJ, Naber FB, Khaap KC. DeNol versus Tagamet, een vergelijkend onderzoek bi peptisch ulcus. TGD/JDR 1983; 8:1553–9.

146. Bianchi Porro G, Lazzaroni M, Petrillo M, DeNicola C. Relapse rates in duodenal ulcer patients formerly treated with bismuth subcitrate or maintained with cimetidine. Lancet 1984; ii:698. Letter.

147. Bianchi Porro G, Petrillo M, DeNicola C, Lazzaroni M. A double-blind endoscopic study with DeNol tablets and cimetidine for duodenal ulcer. Scand J Gastroenterol 1984; 19:905–8.

148. Hamilton J, O'Connor HJ, Wood NC, Bradbury J, Axon ATR. Healing and recurrence of duodenal ulcer after treatment with tripotassium dicitrato bismuthate (TDR) tablets or cimetidine. Gut 1986; 27:106–10.

149. Bianchi Porro G, Lazzaroni M, Barbara L, Corinaldesi R, Dal Monte PR, D'Imperio N, Mazzacca G, D'Arienzo A, Cheli R, Bovero E. Tripotassium dicitrate bismuthate and ranitidine in duodenal ulcer healing and influence on recurrence. Scand J Gastroenterol 1988; 23:1232–6.

150. Lee FL, Samloff IM, Hardman M. Comparison of tripotassium dicitrato bismuthate tablets with ranitidine in healing and relapse of duodenal ulcers. Lancet 1985; i:1299–1305.

151. Ward M, Haliday C, Cowen AE. A comparison of colloidal bismuth subcitrate tablets and ranitidine in the treatment of chronic duodenal ulcers. Digestion 1986; 34:173–7.

152. Dang Z, Wang K, Tao J, Zhu L, Hu X. A clinical trial comparing colloidal bismuth subcitrate (DeNol liquid) with sucralfate in the treatment of peptic ulceration. Clin Trials J 1986; 23:235–41.

153. Lam SK, Lee NW, Koo J, Hui WM, Fok HK, et al. Randomised cross-over trial of tripotassium dicitrato bismuthate versus high dose cimetidine for duodenal ulcers resistant to standard dose of cimetidine. Gut 1984; 25:703–6.

154. Bianchi Porro G, Parente F, Lazzaroni M. Tripotassium dicitrato bismuthate (TDB) versus two different dosages of cimetidine in the treatment of resistant duodenal ulcers. Gut 1987; 28:907–11.

155. Park YT, Choi KW. An open endoscopic evaluation of the clinical effectiveness of tripotassium dicitrato bismuthate in peptic ulcer disease. Korean J Gastroenterol 1982; 14:63–7.

156. VanBentem N, Tytgat GNJ, Dekker W, DeBoer J. Bismutsubcitrate (DeNol), cimetidine en placebo een prospectief asekect onderzoek bij ulcus ventriculi. Ned T Geneesk 1982; 126:542.

157. Boyes BE, Woolf IL, Wilson RY, Cowley DJ, Dymock IW. Treatment of gastric ulceration with a bismuth preparation. Postgrad Med J 1975; 51(Suppl 5):29–32.

158. Lam SK, Koo J, Cheng CH, Ho J, Ong GB. Treatment of corpus and prepyloric gastric ulcers with tripotassium dicitrato bismuthate (DeNol). Gastroenterology 1981; 80: 1202.

159. Sutton DR. Gastric ulcer healing with tripotassium dicitrato bismuthate and subsequent relapse. Gut 1982; 23:621–4.

160. Tanner AR, Colishaw JL, Cowen AE, Ward M. Efficacy of cimetidine and tripotassium dicitrato bismuthate (DeNol) in chronic gastric ulceration. Med J Aust 1979; 1:1–2.

161. Austad WL, Hillamn LC, Luey K, Pomare EW, Scobie BA, et al. Gastric ulcer—a treatment comparison of colloidal bismuth with cimetidine and 30 months follow-up. Abstract. New Zealand Soc Gastroenterol meeting, Dunedin, 23–25 November, 1983.

162. Soltoft J, Iversen TO, Linde NC, Rahbek I, Jacobsen O. Kolloidal vismut subcitrat (DeNol) labletter versus cimetidin ved behandling af ulcus ventriculi. Ugeskr Laeg 1985; 147:1850–1.

163. Shou Po C, GuoZong P. Short-term treatment with colloidal bismuth subcitrate (DeNol) and cimetidine in Chinese patients with gastric ulcer. Clin Trials J 1986; 23:215–9.

164. Kisfalvi I. Comparative trial with DeNol, cimetidine and carbenoxolone in the healing of benign gastric ulceration. Non-systemic ulcer therapy with DeNol efficacy and tolerance. Proceedings of a symposium, IIIrd Congress of the Polish Gastroenterological Society, Lublin, June 1, 1985. Excerpta Medica, 1986:26–32.

165. Parente F, Lazzaroni M, Petrillo M, Bianchi Porro G. Colloidal bismuth subcitrate and ranitidine in the short-term treatment of benign gastric ulcer: an endoscopically controlled trial. Scand J Gastroenterol 1986; 21(Suppl 122):42–5.

166. Cipollini F, Altilia F. Comparison of tripotassium dicitrato bismuthate (TDB) with ranitidine in healing and relapse of gastric ulcer. Br J Clin Pract 1987; 41:707–9.

167. Patty I, Tarnok F, Simon L, Javor T, Deak G, Benedek SZ, Kenez P, Nagy L, Mozsik GY. A comparative dynamic study of the effectiveness of gastric cytoprotection by vitamin A, DeNol, sucralfate and ulcer healing by pirenzepine in patients with chronic gastric ulcer (multiclinical randomised study). Acta Physiol Hung 1984; 64:379–84.

168. Scuro LA, Cavallini G. Multi-centre study on the clinical efficacy of DeNol versus sucralfate in the treatment of gastric ulcer patients. Abstract presented at the 3rd International Congress of Ulcer Therapy, Lacco meno d'Ischia, Naples, June 26–28, 1986.

169. Patty L, Deak G, Mozsik GY, Nagy L, Tarnok F. A controlled clinical trial with DeNol (tripotassium dicitrato bismuthate) in patients with gastric ulcer. Int J Tissue React 1983; 4:397–401.

170. Scobie B. Successful bismuth (DeNol) therapy for gastric ulcer. NZ Med J 1976; 84:192–3.

171. Dobrilla G, Vallaperta P, Amplatz S. Influence of ulcer healing agents on ulcer relapse after discontinuation of acute treatment. Pooled estimate of controlled clinical trials. Gut 1988; 29:181–7.

172. Axon TR. *Campylobacter pyloridis*. What role in gastritis and peptic ulcer? Br Med J 1986; 293:772–3.

173. Miller JP, Faragher EB. Relapse of duodenal ulcer: does it matter which drug is used in initial treatment? Br Med J 1986; 293:1117–8.

174. Tytgat GNJ, Rauws E, Langenberg ML. The *Campylobacter pylori* story. Acta Endosc 1986; 16:141–4.

175. Coghlan JG, Gilligan D, Humphries H, McKenna D, Dooley C, et al. *Campylobacter pylori* and recurrence of duodenal ulcers. 12 months follow-up study. Lancet 1987; ii:1109–11.

176. Borody T, Hennessy W, Daskalopulos G, Garrick J, Hazell S. Double-blind trial of DeNol in non-ulcer dyspepsia associated with *Campylobacter pyloridis* gastritis. Gastroenterology 1987; 92:1394.

177. Humphries H, Bourke S, Dooley C, et al. Effect of treatment of *Campylobacter pylori* in peptic disease: a randomised prospective trial. Gut 1988; 29:279–83.

178. Malferthweiner P, Stanescu A, Bachako K, Vanek E, Bode G, Ditschimeit H. Bismuth subsalicylate treatment of chronic erosive gastritis associated with *Campylobacter pylori*. Dtsch Med Wochenschr 1988; 113:923–9.

179. Dooley CP, McKenna D, Humphreys H, Bourke S, Keane CT, Sweeney E, O'Morain C. Histological gastritis in duodenal ulcer: relationship to *Campylobacter pylori* and effect of ulcer therapy. Am J Gastroenterol 1988; 83:278–82.

180. Rokkas T, Pursey C, Uzoechina E, Dorrington L, Simmons N, Filipe MI, Sladen GE. Non-ulcer dyspepsia and short-term DeNol therapy: a placebo controlled trial with particular reference to the role of *Campylobacter pylori*. Gut 1988; 29:1386–91.

181. Chaparala LC, Manning RG, Hueskin JE, Harmon JW. PeptoBismol protects against experimental esophagitis. Gastroenterology 1987; 92:1342A.

182. Borkent MV, Beker JA. Treatment of ulcerative reflux esophagitis with colloidal bismuth subcitrate in combination with cimetidine. Gut 1988; 29:385–9.

183. Bader JP. The safety profile of DeNol. Digestion 1987; 37(Suppl 2):53–9.

184. Wu L, Liang Q, Chen C. Treatment of active peptic ulcers with tripotassium dicitrate bismuthate. Chin J Dig 1984; 4:86.

185. Martin-Bouyer G, Foulon B, Guerbois H, Barin C. Aspects epidemiologiques des encephalopathies apres administration de bismuth par voir orale. Therapie 1980; 35:307–13.

186. Weller MPI. Neuropsychiatric symptoms following bismuth intoxication. Postgrad Med J 1988; 64:308–10.

15

Therapy of Ulcers with Sulfhydryl and Nonsulfhydryl Antioxidants

GYULA MÓZSIK AND TIBOR JÁVOR

Medical University of Pécs, Pécs, Hungary

I. INTRODUCTION

Research on peptic ulcer disease has greatly increased in the last two decades [1–6].
The evaluation of aggressive factors has been the main trend, and currently the details
of possible mechanisms of mucosal defense are being emphasized [7,8]. The complex
pathology of ulcer disease suggests a multifactorial pharmacology, which was recently
summarized [9].

Szabó and Bynum [10] reviewed the mechanistic classification of anti-ulcer compounds based on known or suspected mechanism of action:

1. Antisecretory agents (e.g., decrease of HCl and pepsin secretion)
2. Prosecretory agents (e.g., increase of HCO_3^- and mucus)
3. Antioxidants (e.g., scavengers)
4. Oxidizing agents (e.g., mild irritants, metals)

Factors involved in gastric mucosal defense include (a) surface pH gradients (e.g.,
adherent mucus gel, bicarbonate secretion); (b) hydrophobic lining (e.g., adsorbed
phospholipids); (c) gastric mucosal barrier (e.g., apical cell membrane and tight
junction; (d) acid–base balance (e.g., intracellular pH regulator and mucosal blood
flow); (e) migration of cells (e.g., cellular restitution); (f) division of cells (cellular
turnover); and (g) endogenous modulators (e.g., prostaglandins, sulfhydryls, scavengers). These systems have been reviewed by Garner [11] and Wenzl et al. [12].

A.   Phenomenon of Gastric Cytoprotection

Gastric "cytoprotection" was discovered by Robert et al. [13], who described gastric mucosal protection by prostaglandins (PGs) as an action that differed from their inhibitory effects on the gastric H^+ secretion. This study opened a new avenue in ulcer research. Very low doses of PGs were able to prevent the gastric mucosal damage produced in rats by various chemicals. Further studies indicated that other compounds also showed this protective action (e.g., sulfhydryl and non-sulfhydryl antioxidants, vitamin A and other carotenoids, and drugs) (for details, see later) [14–22]. International research became focused on the importance of the gastric mucosa [7,8,19,23,24].

B.   Oxygen Free Radicals, Lipid Peroxidation, and Scavengers

Free radicals have been implicated in the pathogenesis of tissue damage caused by physical agents (e.g., radiation), chemicals (e.g., ethanol, NaOH, NaCl, nonsteroidal anti-inflammatory compounds, HCl), or ischemia and reperfusion [25]. Lipid peroxidation is considered one of the biochemically measurable processes by which free radicals cause membrane damage and cell and tissue injury [26,27]. Numerous compounds with and without the sulfhydryl (SH) moiety scavenge free radicals, decrease lipid peroxidation, and prevent cell and/or organ injury [25,28].

The existence of lipid peroxidation or oxygen free radicals is suggested by the fact that many chemically unrelated compounds (e.g., 96% ethanol, 0.2 N NaOH, 25% NaCl, 0.6 N HCl, acetic acid, nonsteroidal anti-inflammatory compounds, epinephrine, reserpine, digoxin) and many pathologically unrelated conditions (thermal injury, ischemia by blood loss, sepsis, burn, trauma) damage the gastric mucosa.

Because these agents and conditions result in damage to gastric mucosal cells, it has been suggested that direct measurements of membrane-located enzyme (e.g., membrane ATPase, adenylate cyclase) and ATP, ADP, AMP, and cAMP may lead to a better understanding of the development of mucosal damage and its prevention [29–36].

Since SH drugs and carotenoids are free radical scavengers, our attention has been focused on the possible role of free radicals and lipid peroxidation in the pathogenesis of acute gastric mucosal lesions and on their prevention [25,37–40].

II.   NONPROTEIN SULFHYDRYLS (NPSH) AND PROTEIN SULFHYDRYL (PSH)

Sulfhydryls (SH) represent one group of compounds that can influence gastrointestinal mucosal healing. This approach became especially plausible after the demonstration of relatively high levels of glutathione in the stomach and duodenum, which implicated SH groups in gastric [41] and duodenal [42] ulcer. These findings led to the hypothesis that endogenous SH might mediate the gastric mucosal protection offered by agents with different chemical structures and physicochemical properties. Based on the initial hypothesis concerning SH, as presented above, it was shown that drugs given intragastrically or subcutaneously 30 min before alcohol administration exerted a significant and dose-dependent protection against the hemorrhagic gastric lesion caused by 1 ml of absolute ethanol [41,43]. Sulfhydryl blockers such as iodoacetamide or N-ethylmaleide (NEM) injected subcutaneously 10 min after the protecting agents abolished gastric cytoprotection [41,43]. These SH blockers were equally effective in abolishing the protective actions of SH drugs such as BAL and cysteamine in the ethanol model. The intact adrenal cortex is necessary to obtain gastric cytoprotection by SH drugs, which are dependent on glucocorticoids [44] but not on mineralocorticoids. Gastric ulcers produced by indomethacin [23,45], phenylbutazolone, piroxicam, diclofenac [46,47], aspirin [48], and acidified ethanol [49,50] were also prevented by SH compounds in experimental animals.

Szabó et al. [41] demonstrated that the protection by SH drugs was associated with elevation of gastric mucosal levels of nonprotein sulfhydryls (NPSH). Diethylmaleate (DEM), which depletes gastric glutathione (GSH), aggravated stress ulcers [51] and phenylbutazolone-, piroxicam-, or diclofenac-induced gastric lesions [46]. More recently, in an attempt to evaluate more SH compounds for efficacy in preventing aspirin-induced hemorrhagic gastric erosions administered in parallel with aspirin, four compounds (N-acetylcysteine, methionine, sodium thiosulfate, and thiodipropionic acid) demonstrated a dose-related effect even in the coadministration regimen in rats [48]. These studies opened new therapeutic possibilities of giving the protective SH compounds together with aspirin-related drugs [28].

The biological effect of SH antagonists (NEM and iodoacetamide, which alkylate SH groups) also shows involvement of SH compounds in preserving the integrity of the gastric mucosa. The consumption of low doses of NEM and iodoacetamide in drinking water produces a diffuse and severe gastritis in rats [52] that is located in the glandular portion of the mucosa.

Szabó et al. [28] concluded that administration of SH groups prevents the acute erosive effect produced by several damaging agents, and that prolonged treatment with SH blockers results in diffuse inflammatory damage in the stomach [52].

In most of the biochemical studies, SH compounds are analyzed as NPSH and PSH. The majority (about 90%) of nonprotein sulfhydryls exist as GSH, and a small fraction of them are other naturally occurring SH compounds (cysteine, cysteamine). In PSH, cysteine and its oxidized dimer cystine are the components of major amino acids, but mixed disulfides can also be detected (e.g., interaction between protein cysteine and GSH or cysteamine from the NPSH fraction). The methods applied for determination of reduced GSH (reduced SH groups) are based on the colorimetric measurements of reduced SH groups by Ellman's reagent in the supernate of tissue homogenates after the precipitation of proteins by trichloroacetic acid [53]. A new high-performance liquid chromatographic (HPLC) technique opened the possibility of monitoring GSH and cysteine in the NPSH fraction and direct measurement of cysteine in the protein hydrolysates of gastric tissues [54,55]. These results indicated that the effect of agents that contain SH (e.g., cysteamine), deplete GSH (e.g., DEM), or bind SH [e.g., divalent metals such as $CuCl_2$, $Pb(NO_3)_2$, $ZnCl_2$] on endogenous NPSH fractions is variable, but all of these agents decreased the concentration of protein cysteine in the gastric mucosa [54,56]. N-Ethylmaleide, which antagonizes any form of gastric mucosal protection, increased free cysteine in the protein fraction. It has been concluded from these studies that these diverse protective agents have in common the blocking of protein SH groups by disulfide or mixed disulfide formation, as with cysteamine, oxidation with DEM, or binding by metals [28]. The endogenous SH groups are involved in the development of gastric mucosal damage produced by various necrotizing agents and its prevention by various compounds having altered chemical structures [28].

A. Sulfhydryl Compounds and the PG System in the Gastrointestinal Mucosa

Because PGs are also protective compounds in the gastric mucosa, studying the correlation between SH (NPSH and PSH)-induced gastric cytoprotection and the mucosal PG system was one of the aims of research done in this field. Endogenous PGs probably play an essential role in the development of SH group-induced gastric cytoprotection. The cytoprotective effect of $PGF_{2\beta}$ could be abolished by the SH alkylator NEM, suggesting an SH-sensitive process in gastroprotection by both PGs and SH compounds such as BAL and N-acetylcysteine [28]. The possible role of PGs in the gastric cytoprotection produced by SH compounds was suggested by experiments using indomethacin (an inhibitor of cyclooxygenase), which blocked the adaptive cytoprotection produced by 20% ethanol and interfered by only about 50% with the mucosal protection offered by BAL and cysteine [20,57]. Thus, SH drugs were able to offer substantial gastric cytoprotection even in the presence of indomethacin pretreatment. This conclusion indicated that the actions of SH groups are (at least in part) independent of the endogenous PGs of gastric mucosa.

The interaction (such as additive or potentiating) between the PG effect (PGE_2) and N-acetylcysteine is shown in the diminishing of indomethacin-induced gastric mucosal lesions [28]. Sulfhydryl groups scavenge free radicals and consequently prevent the membrane damage produced by various compounds via lipid peroxidation. All these results are in a good agreement with the results of biochemical measurements done with PSH and NPSH [28]. The early vascular injury of gastric mucosa can be regulated directly (via metabolites or chemicals) or indirectly (by the production of vasoactive compounds or others that modify them) by SH groups [28].

The following can be concluded from the results of observations reported by Szabó et al. [28]:

1. Compounds with SH groups in reduced form (e.g., N-acetylcysteine, cysteine) or various states of oxidation (e.g., cystine, methionine, sucralfate)

prevent the acute gastric hemorrhagic erosions produced by ethanol, non-steroidal anti-inflammatory compounds, or stress in animal experiments.

2. The action of these new groups of gastric mucosal agents is partly (about 50%) mediated by endogenous PGs, and this action is completely abolished by the SH alkylator NEM.

3. Sulfhydryl protein or cysteine levels (e.g., sulfoproteins) modulate the beneficial effect of SH groups.

4. The common mechanism of gastric cytoprotective agents seems to be vasoactive in the case of SH derivatives and PGs.

The potential role of sulfhydryl compounds was also reviewed by Strubelt [47].

III. NON-SULFHYDRYL ANTIOXIDANTS

Another main line of ulcer research was started in 1980, when Jávor et al. [17] demonstrated the mucosa-protective effect of vitamin A on the ethanol-induced gastric mucosal damage in rats. It was also demonstrated that the gastric mucosal protection by vitamin A and other carotenoids differed from the inhibition of gastric acid secretion [18]. It has been concluded that the gastric mucosal protection is consistent with "true gastric cytoprotection."

Vitamin A and other carotenoids are natural (but non-sulfhydryl) antioxidants that scavenge oxygen free radicals.

The phenomenon of gastric cytoprotection by vitamin A and several C_{40} plant carotenoids was demonstrated by Jávor et al. [18]. Our statement concerning the structure–activity relationship for gastric cytoprotection should be regarded as preliminary. However, some conclusions can be drawn from the data summarized in Table 1:

1. Gastric cytoprotection does not depend on vitamin A activity. For example, the vitamin A activity of β-carotene (β,β-carotene) is completely eliminated by modifications such as the introduction of a hydroxyl group at C-3(3′), substituting the E-end group for the β-end group. Although zeaxanthin (3,3′-dihydroxy-β,β-carotene) and lutein (3,3′-dihydroxy-β + carotene) are not precursors of vitamin A, they do exert a cytoprotective effect similar to that of vitamin A precursors β-carotene (β,β-carotene) and β-cryptoxanthine (3-hydroxy-β,β-carotene).

2. Gastric cytoprotection cannot be related exclusively to a conjugated polyene chain present in carotenoids, because, for example, acyclic lycopene (γ,γ-carotene) with an undecene chromophore, and cyclic capsorubin (3,3′-di-hydroxy-K,K-carotene-6,6′-dione) with a nonene-dione chromophore, are inactive. Furthermore, cytoprotective zeaxanthin and lutein have different chromophore systems.

3. Gastric cytoprotection by asymmetrical C_{40} carotenoids cannot be explained

Table 1 Correlation Between Gastric Cytoprotection, Vitamin A Effect, and Chemical Structures of Carotenoids

| | | | | Effect on gastric mucosa[a] | |
Compounds	Formula	Relative polarity	Vitamin A activity	Number	Severity
A. Vitamin A	R = a		Yes	+	+++
B. β-Carotene	X = Y = a	0.00	Yes	+++	+++
C. β-Cryptoxanthin	X = a, Y = b	1.00	Yes	++	++
D. Zeaxanthin	X = Y = b	2.00	No	++	++
E. Lutein	X = b, Y = c	1.89	No	+++	++
F. Capsorubin	X = Y = d	3.44	No	None	None
G. Capsanthin	X = b, Y = d	2.72	No	None	None
H. Capsanthol	X = b, Y = e	3.00	No	None	None
I. Lycopene	X = Y = f	0.00	No	None	None

[a]Effective dosage: +, 10 mg/kg; ++, 1–10 mg/kg; +++, 0.1–10 mg/kg.
Source: Based on results published by Jávor et al. [18].

by a splitting of the molecules at the central double bond, which would result in two C_{20} units with or without cytoprotective properties. According to such conversion, one might expect that capsanthin (3,3′-dihydroxy-β,K-carotene-6′-one) would be cytoprotective, as its molecule can be built up from an active (½ zeaxanthin) and an inactive (½ capsorubin) C_{20} unit. The lack of gastric cytoprotection by capsanthin argues against such a conversion. It should be noted that capsanthol, the reduction product of capsanthin, is also inactive.

A. Mechanisms of Action of Carotenoids

No inhibitory effects on gastric acid secretion were shown, either in animal experiments [18] or in human observations [58], by vitamin A and other carotenoids, but these agents prevented the gastric mucosal damage produced by 96% ethanol or 0.6 M HCl in rats or by indomethacin in healthy persons.

An acid-dependent (HCl model) and a non-acid-dependent (ethanol model) gastric ulcer model were used to evaluate the biochemical background of β-carotene-induced gastric cytoprotection [32,59]. The tissue levels of ATP, ADP, AMP, cAMP, lactate, adenylate pool (ATP + ADP + AMP), "energy charge" [(ATP + 0.5 ADP)/(ATP + ADP + AMP)], and ATP/ADP ratio were measured without and with administration of β-carotene in these models. The tissue levels of ATP, AMP, and cAMP decreased significantly, while the tissue level of ADP was unchanged in the ethanol model and increased in the HCl model. The biochemical changes could be dose-dependently reversed by the administration of β-carotene in the gastric mucosa (during the 1-hr experimental period). Gastric mucosal injury can be macroscopically detected at 1–5 min after the administration of necrotizing agents (ethanol, HCl), and about 50% of maximum damage is observed at 1 hr after giving ethanol or HCl [36,60,61]. An early (from 0 to 5 or maximally 15 min) and a late (from 15 to 60 min) period could be separated on the basis of the changes in gastric mucosal biochemistry when the measurements were carried out at 0, 1, 5, 15, 30, and 60 min after administration of necrotizing agents. The second (late) phase is associated with the repair function of the gastric mucosa [62–65]. The gastric mucosal damage prevention by PGI_2 appears in the first period, and that by β-carotene in the second period [65].

B. Correlation Between Prostaglandins and Carotenoids

$PGF_{2\alpha}$ and PGI_2 are able to prevent the gastric mucosal injury produced by ethanol or HCl in rats [64,66,67]. However, PGI_2 was able to increase the ATP–cAMP transformation in the first (early) phase after ethanol administration, in association with a decrease of ATP–ADP transformation in the gastric mucosa.

Gastric mucosal injury was produced by intragastric administration of ethanol or HCl, and the animals were killed at 0, 1, 5, 15, 30, and 60 min after administration of necrotizing agents. The animals were pretreated with various doses of PGI_2 (5 and 50 μg/kg administered intragastrically) or β-carotene (1 and 10 mg/kg ig). PGI_2 could inhibit the ethanol- or HCl-induced gastric mucosal damage in the early period, while mucosal protection was obtained by β-carotene in the second phase (Figs. 1 and 2).

The correlation between the gastric cytoprotective effect of PGI_2 and β-carotene was pharmacologically studied, and potentiation was proved by pharmacologic isobolic methods [68].

According to our biochemical studies, the gastric mucosal level of cAMP was dose-dependently increased by both PGI_2 and β-carotene, but the effects of these agents could be separated according to the time after administration of ethanol (Tables 2 and 3).

The β-carotene dose-dependently inhibited the development of indomethacin-induced gastric mucosal lesions in association with a dose-dependent increase of gastric mucosal cAMP [34]. It was recently demonstrated that β-carotene alone could not increase the tissue level of PGE_2 in intact and as well as indomethacin-treated rats [69]. It has been concluded that the β-carotene-induced gastric cytoprotection differs from that of the endogenous PGs but depends on the changes of membrane-bound ATP-dependent energy systems in the gastric mucosa.

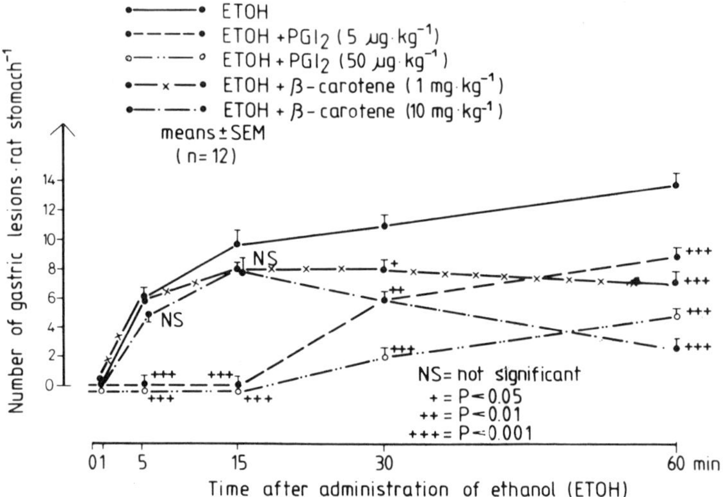

FIGURE 1   Effects of PGI_2 (given in doses of 5 and 50 μg/kg) and β-carotene (given in doses of 1 and 10 mg/kg) on the number of gastric mucosal lesions (ulcers) produced by intragastric administration of 96% (1 ml) ethanol. The PGI_2 and β-carotene was freshly dissolved and given intragastrically at 30 min prior to administration of ethanol, in 1 ml volume. The animals were killed at 0, 1, 5, 15, 30, and 60 min after administration of ethanol, and the number of gastric mucosal lesions (ulcers) was calculated. The results were expressed as means + SEM. *P* values were calculated by the unpaired Student's *t* test between the control (untreated) and treated groups at each time.

C.   Oxygen Free Radicals and Development of Gastric Mucosal Damage Without and With Carotenoids

The possible causative roles of oxygen free radicals were suggested in the development of gastric mucosal damage, because vitamin A and other carotenoids are natural antioxidants (e.g., scavengers).

Various parameters, such as the activities of catalase [70], glutathione peroxidase [53], and superoxide dismutase [71,72], were determined from the total homogenate of gastric mucosa of rats treated with 96% ethanol, 0.6 N HCl, acidified salicylate, and indomethacin. In addition, the tissue contents of reduced glutathione (as a major part of NPSH) [73] and malondialdehyde [74,75] were measured.

The results of 1-hr experiments with 96% ethanol and 0.6 N HCl without and with application of β-carotene (given in doses of 1 and 10 mg/kg intragastrically at 30 min prior to the administration of necrotizing agents) are summarized in Table 4. Surprisingly, the changes in these measured parameters showed some differences in the two experimental models without and with administration of β-carotene. Mean-

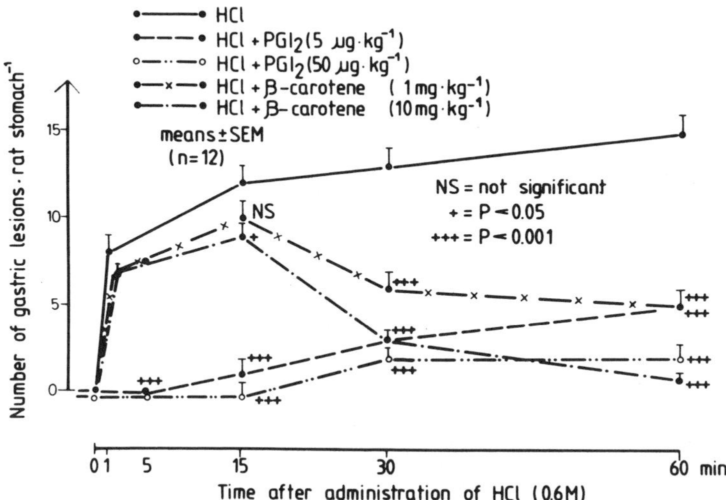

FIGURE 2 Effects of PGI₂ (given in doses of 5 and 50 μg/kg) and β-carotene (given in doses of 1 and 10 mg/kg) on the number of gastric mucosal lesions produced by intragastric administration of 0.6 M (1 ml) HCl. The PGI₂ and β-carotene were freshly dissolved and given intragastrically at 30 min prior to administration of HCl. The animals were killed at 0, 1, 5, 15, 30, and 60 min after administration of HCl. The results were expressed as means ± SEM. P values were calculated by the unpaired Student's t test between the control (untreated) and treated groups at each time.

while, the development of gastric mucosal damage and its prevention represented similar tendencies in the models [59]. These discrepancies could be explained in either of two ways: (a) No close correlation exists between the oxygen free radicals, mucosal damage, and its prevention, or (b) the time choice (1 hr) for examination is not optimal for the correct evaluation of these complex problems. Various arguments could be suggested for the existence of the second possibility:

1. The superoxide dismutase (SOD) activity in the gastric mucosa at first increased (at 2–3 hr); thereafter, its activity decreased at 4 hr in the pyloric-ligated plus aspirin-treated rats [76].
2. The results of experiments with ethanol or HCl indicated that the macroscopic appearance of gastric mucosal damage could be detected at 5 min (to about half the maximum extent of gastric mucosal damage obtained 1 hr after administration of necrotizing agents), whereas the oxygen free radicals changed later; so it seems that oxygen free radicals developed in consequence (and did not act as a cause) of gastric mucosal injury [36].

Table 2 Correlation Between the Gastric Cytoprotective Effect of PGI_2 and Changes in Gastric Mucosal Level of cAMP in Rats Treated with Ethanol (1 mL 96% ig)[a]

Treatments	Time after administration of ethanol (EtOH) (min)					
	0	1	5	15	30	60
	Number of gastric ulcers					
EtOH alone	0 ± 0	0 ± 0	5.8 ± 0.6	9.7 ± 1	11 ± 1	14 ± 1
EtOH + PGI_2 (5 μg/kg)	0 ± 0	0 ± 0	0 ± 0	0 ± 0	6 ± 1	9 ± 1
EtOH + PGI_2 (50 μg/kg)	0 ± 0	0 ± 0	0 ± 0	0 ± 0	2 ± 1	5 ± 0.5
	Gastric mucosal level of cAMP					
EtOH alone	3.3 ± 0.04	5.02 ± 0.01	4.6 ± 0.03	1.8 ± 0.03	1.8 ± 0.02	1.8 ± 0.02
EtOH + PGI_2 (5 μg/kg)	5.2 ± 0.1	7.00 ± 0.6	6.0 ± 0.5	2.0 ± 0.5	2.0 ± 0.05	2.2 ± 0.04
EtOH + PGI_2 (50 μg/kg)	7.2 ± 0.1	9.00 ± 0.4	7.0 ± 0.4	3.0 ± 0.4	2.9 ± 0.05	3.3 ± 0.05

[a]The PGI_2 was given intragastrically at 30 min prior to administration of ethanol. The number (sum per one rat stomach) and cAMP (pmol/mg mucosal protein) were expressed as means ± SEM ($n = 12$).

Table 3 Correlation Between the Gastric Cytoprotective Effect of β-carotene and Changes in Gastric Mucosal Level of cAMP in Rats Treated with 96% Ethanol (EtOH) ig[a]

	Time after administration of EtOH (min)					
Treatments	0	1	5	15	30	60
	Number of gastric ulcers					
EtOH alone	0 ± 0	0 ± 0	5.8 ± 0.6	9.7 ± 1	11 ± 1	14 ± 1
EtOH + β-carotene (1 mg/kg)	0 ± 0	0 ± 0	6.0 ± 0.6	8.0 ± 1	8 ± 1	7.4 ± 0.8
EtOH + β-carotene (10 mg/kg)	0 ± 0	0 ± 0	5.0 ± 1	8.0 ± 1	6 ± 0.5	2.8 ± 0.4
	Gastric mucosal level of cAMP					
EtOH alone	3.3 ± 0.04	5.02 ± 0.01	4.6 ± 0.03	1.8 ± 0.03	1.8 ± 0.02	1.8 ± 0.02
EtOH + β-carotene (1 mg/kg)	3.2 ± 0.04	3.0 ± 0.02	2.00 ± 0.01	3.0 ± 0.04	5.0 ± 0.01	6.0 ± 0.03
EtOH + β-carotene (10 mg/kg)	3.3 ± 0.02	3.5 ± 0.02	2.0 ± 0.02	3.2 ± 0.02	6.0 ± 0.02	8.0 ± 0.02

[a]β-Carotene was freshly dissolved in sunflower oil and given intragastrically at 30 min prior administration of EtOH. The number (sum per one rat stomach) and cAMP (pmol/mg mucosal protein) were expressed as means ± SEM ($n = 12$).

Table 4 Changes in the Oxygen Free Radicals of the Gastric Mucosa During the Development of Ethanol (96%)- and HCl (0.6 M)-Induced Gastric Mucosal Injury and Its Prevention Produced by β-Carotene Given in Doses of 1 and 10 mg/kg ig. 30 min prior to Administration of Necrotizing Agents[a]

Experimental parameters	Ethanol model			HCl model		
	A	B	C	A	B	C
Ulcer number	$100 \pm 7^{+++}$	$53 \pm 7^{+++}$	$20 \pm 3^{+++}$	$100 \pm 10^{+++}$	$33 \pm 7^{+++}$	$7 \pm 7^{+++}$
Ulcer severity	$100 \pm 7^{+++}$	$55 \pm 3^{+++}$	$18 \pm 2^{+++}$	$100 \pm 6^{+++}$	$60 \pm 2^{+++}$	$20 \pm 7^{+++}$
Catalase activity	90 ± 10^{NS}	$130 \pm 10^{++}$	$125 \pm 10^{+}$	$150 \pm 10^{+++}$	$90 \pm 10^{+++}$	$74 \pm 13^{+++}$
GSH px. activity	$600 \pm 8^{+++}$	$310 \pm 20^{+++}$	$115 \pm 10^{+++}$	$150 \pm 15^{++}$	$90 \pm 10^{+++}$	$60 \pm 6^{+++}$
Reduced GSH. content	80 ± 5^{NS}	98 ± 12^{NS}	$125 \pm 10^{+++}$	$150 \pm 15^{++}$	$90 \pm 10^{+++}$	$60 \pm 6^{+++}$
SOD activity	$150 \pm 10^{+++}$	$110 \pm 8^{++}$	$120 \pm 8^{++}$	$30 \pm 10^{+++}$	50 ± 8^{NS}	54 ± 11^{NS}
MDA content	$145 \pm 10^{+++}$	$80 \pm 10^{+++}$	$82 \pm 10^{+++}$	95 ± 10^{NS}	80 ± 8^{NS}	71 ± 5^{NS}

A, rats treated with ethanol (left) or HCl (right); B, rats treated with ethanol plus 1 mg/kg β-carotene (left) or HCl plus β-carotene (1 mg/kg) (right); C, rats treated with ethanol (left) or HCl (right) plus 10 mg/kg β-carotene.

P values (by unpaired Student's *t* test): A groups, untreated vs. ethanol or HCl-treated rats; B groups, A groups vs. B groups; C groups, A groups vs. C groups.

[a]Results are expressed as means ± SEM (in % values of control, untreated animals = 100%) (*n* = 12).

Source: Mózsik et al. [59].

3. When these observations were carried out at 0, 1, 5, 15, 30, and 60 min after intragastric administration of necrotizing agents, other tendencies were noted in their changes [60].

It was concluded that a correct time sequence analysis is needed between these parameters and the development of gastric mucosal damage and its prevention by natural antioxidants [61,64,67] (Table 4).

D. Time-Sequence Analysis of the Correlations Between the Oxygen Free Radicals, Gastric Mucosal Damage, and Its Prevention by β-Carotene

The biochemical parameters of oxygen free radicals were measured at 0, 1, 5, 15, 30, and 60 min after the administration of necrotizing agents (ethanol and HCl) [61]. The number and severity of gastric mucosal damage increased significantly from 5 min after administration of ethanol or HCl, whereas no close correlation was obtained between the tissue levels of endogenous antioxidants (catalase, glutathione peroxidase, SOD activity, tissue content, and reduced GSH and MDA) (Table 5). On the other hand, the changes in the tissue content of endogenous antioxidants differed significantly in ethanol- and HCl-induced gastric mucosal damage, while the macroscopic appearance showed similar tendencies in these models [67]. It has been concluded that the natural behavior of oxygen free radicals differs in these models; for example, their behavior depends, at least to some extent, on the nature of the necrotizing agents used [77]. It has also been concluded that the changes of oxygen free radicals in the gastric mucosa are probably the consequence of development of gastric mucosal damage (Table 5).

β-Carotene was given (in doses of 1 and 10 mg/kg intragastrically) at 30 min prior to administration of necrotizing agents, and the same parameters were measured. The number and severity of ethanol- and HCl-induced gastric mucosal lesions could be dose-dependently prevented by β-carotene, whereas no close correlation was obtained between the β-carotene-induced gastric cytoprotective effects and the changes in oxygen free radicals. Additionally, important changes were obtained in the oxygen free radicals at a later time (from 15 min after the administration of necrotizing agents) [40].

These results suggested that (a) dominant changes in the gastric mucosal free radicals can be obtained in the later phase, in connection with the development of β-carotene-induced gastric cytoprotection, and (b) the β-carotene-induced changes in the gastric mucosal free radicals are associated with an increased repair function in the gastric mucosa. When the PGI_2 was used as a protective agent (one of endogenous protective but nonantioxidant compounds), then these changes in the gastric mucosal oxygen free radicals were obtained primarily in the early phase (1–15 min) [39]. In light of these results, the etiological roles of oxygen free radicals can be better understood in the development of PGI_2-induced gastric cytoprotection than that by β-carotene.

Table 5 Time-Sequence Analysis of the Correlation Between Ethanol (96% ig)- and HCl (0.6 M)-induced Gastric Mucosal Damage and Oxygen Free Radicals in Rats

Experimental parameters	Time after administration of necrotizing agents (min)					
	0	1	5	15	30	60
Ethanol-induced gastric mucosal injury						
Ulcer number	0 ± 0	0 ± 0	42 ± 4	69 ± 7	79 ± 7	100 ± 7
Ulcer severity	0 ± 0	0 ± 0	54 ± 4	71 ± 6	77 ± 6	100 ± 6
Catalase activity	100 ± 16	161 ± 16	93 ± 7	91 ± 11	74 ± 11	86 ± 7
GSH px. activity	100 ± 9	150 ± 14	178 ± 9	144 ± 9	672 ± 39	563 ± 25
Reduced GSH content	100 ± 6	118 ± 7	124 ± 6	125 ± 7	153 ± 11	87 ± 5
SOD activity	100 ± 5	113 ± 5	117 ± 8	124 ± 8	136 ± 7	145 ± 5
MDA content	100 ± 10	102 ± 19	103 ± 15	96 ± 16	137 ± 15	182 ± 19
HCl-induced gastric mucosal injury						
Ulcer number	0 ± 0	53 ± 7	66 ± 6	80 ± 6	87 ± 6	100 ± 6
Ulcer severity	0 ± 0	50 ± 4	54 ± 4	70 ± 5	100 ± 4	100 ± 4
Catalase activity	100 ± 7	62 ± 9	118 ± 15	124 ± 9	152 ± 11	169 ± 15
GSH px. activity	100 ± 7	243 ± 13	148 ± 13	134 ± 10	151 ± 10	154 ± 10
Reduced GSH content	100 ± 6	242 ± 8	146 ± 10	141 ± 12	142 ± 8	153 ± 15
SOD activity	100 ± 6	148 ± 10	126 ± 10	167 ± 10	129 ± 8	34 ± 10
MDA content	100 ± 10	81 ± 6	99 ± 10	95 ± 7	93 ± 8	84 ± 9

[a]Results are expressed as means ± SEM (in % values of controls = 100%) ($n = 12$).

E. Gastric Mucosal Membrane-Bound ATP-Dependent Energy Systems, Oxygen Free Radicals, and Gastric Mucosal Damage and Its Prevention by PGI$_2$ and β-Carotene

The changes in gastric mucosal energy systems (ATP, ADP, AMP, cAMP, ATP/ADP, adenylate pool, "energy charge," lactate) were measured in ethanol [36] and HCl [32] models. The extent of ATP–ADP transformation was significantly increased in the early phase (from 0 to 15 min), while the ATP–cAMP transformation was inhibited during practically the entire experimental period. Thus an increased ATP–ADP transformation was associated with a decreased ATP–cAMP transformation. These correlations could be explained by different direct and indirect relationships between the routes of ATP breakdown and their regulation (modification) by neural, hormonal, and pharmacological influences [30,31,34–36]. The direction of ATP–ADP and ATP–cAMP transformations could be modified by prostacyclin, atropine, cimetidine [30,33], and β-carotene [32]. The ATP–cAMP transformation was increased by PGI$_2$ in the early phase. In contrast, the transformation was increased by β-carotene in the late phase in the ethanol (Tables 2 and 3) and HCl models [64].

The changes in gastric mucosal activity of SOD—one of the key enzymes that scavenges free radicals in the gastric mucosa after administration of damaging agents (e.g., 96% ethanol, 0.6 N HCl, 0.2 N NaOH, 25% NaCl) without and with protecting agents (e.g., vitamin A, β-carotene, PGI$_2$, atropine, and cimetidine)—showed important differences in these models [25,77]. The SOD activity was increased in the ethanol model but decreased in the other models (e.g., 0.6 N HCl, 0.2 N NaOH, 25% NaCl) [77]. Vitamin A, β-carotene [78], PGI$_2$, atropine, and cimetidine [79] decreased the gastric mucosal SOD activity in the ethanol model but increased it in the HCl model [38,39]. Interestingly, the effects of vitamin A and β-carotene were significantly greater than those produced by atropine, PGI$_2$, and cimetidine on the gastric mucosal SOD activity in the ethanol model, while vitamin A and β-carotene effects were significantly less than those obtained by PGI$_2$, atropine, and cimetidine in the HCl model [37]. The biochemical changes (e.g., ATP, ADP, AMP, cAMP, lactate, adenylate pool, "energy charge") showed similarities in the different models.

Based on these results, it has been concluded that:

1. No close correlation exists between the gastric mucosal energy state and production of natural antioxidant enzymes.
2. The gastric mucosal SOD activity was regulated by vitamin A and β-carotene differently than by PGI$_2$, atropine, and cimetidine.
3. The effects of externally applied non-sulfhydryl natural antioxidants can probably be summarized with the effects of endogenous natural antioxidant enzymes.
4. The changes in the gastric mucosal biochemistry seem to be more constant than changes in oxygen free radicals.

F.   Natural Non-Sulfhydryl Antioxidants
and Enhanced Gastric Mucosal Repair Function
in the Rat and Human

The increased repair function of the gastric mucosa was proved by β-carotene in rats treated with ethanol or HCl (Figs. 1 and 2) [65]. Von Ritter et al. [80] indicated that hemorrhagic shock-induced gastric mucosal damage could be prevented by application of SOD albumin during the reperfusion of baboons. These results indicated that (a) free radicals are independent of the blood perfusion of the stomach and (b) the natural antioxidants could promote the repair function in the gastric mucosa.

The increased healing rate of gastric ulcer by vitamin A treatment was proved in patients with chronic gastric ulcer at 2 weeks after the beginning of treatment [81,82]. The increased ulcer healing rate was calculated in comparison to results of various drugs (e.g., pirenzepine, sucralfate, and De-Nol), and this value was found to be 20% superior to that produced by other compounds ($p < .01$) [83,84]. These observations were made in randomized, multicenter, prospective studies in patients with chronic gastric ulcer.

It has been concluded that:

1.   Gastric cytoprotection by carotenoids exists in animals as well as in patients.
2.   Considering that the oxygen free radicals play only a secondary role in the development of gastric mucosal damage, the natural antioxidants (which act as scavengers) have an essential role in ulcer healing in patients.
3.   Vitamin A and β-carotene are natural non-sulfhydryl antioxidants that are closely connected to human nutrition ("nutritional gastric cytoprotection").
4.   A correlation can be suggested between the gastric cytoprotection phenomenon and cancer prevention by the natural non-sulfhydryl antioxidants [85].

IV.   FUTURE

The main results with sulfhydryl and non-sulfhydryl antioxidants were summarized from the point of peptic ulcer therapy. The results indicate a correlation between the gastric cytoprotection phenomenon and their preventive effects; however, the mechanisms of action of sulfhydryl and non-sulfhydryl antioxidants seem to be different. Sulfhydryls act partly via the endogenous PG system, whereas the effects of carotenoids are independent of PGs. Many arguments have proved that sulfhydryls and non-sulfhydryls act by different mechanisms. No close correlation was obtained between the development of gastric mucosal damage versus oxygen free radicals and oxygen free radicals versus membrane-bound ATP-dependent energy systems. The natural antioxidants are capable of promoting the repair function in acutely and chronically damaged gastric mucosa in rats and humans.

REFERENCES

1. Ivy AC, Grossmann MI, Bachrach WH. Peptic ulcer. Philadelphia: Blackiston, 1950.
2. Gheorghiu T, ed. Experimental ulcer: models, methods and clinical validity. Brussels: Gerhard Witzstrock, 1975.
3. Mózsik G, Jávor T, eds. Progress in peptic ulcer. Budapest: Akadémiai Kiadó, 1976.
4. Pfeiffer CJ, ed. Peptic ulcer. Philadelphia: Lippincott, 1971.
5. Szabó S, Pfeiffer CJ, eds. Ulcer disease: new aspects of pathogenesis and pharmacology. Boca Raton, Fla.: CRC Uniscience Press, 1989.
6. Umehara S, Ito H, eds. Advances in experimental ulcer. Proceedings of 4th International Conference on Experimental Ulcer, Tokyo, 1982.
7. Mózsik G, Hänninen O, Jávor T, eds. Gastrointestinal defense mechanisms. Advances in physiological sciences, 29. Oxford: Pergamon; Budapest: Akadémiai Kiadó, 1981.
8. Allen A, Flemström G, Garner A, Silen W, Turnberg LA, eds. Mechanisms of mucosal protection in the upper gastrointestinal tract. New York: Raven, 1984.
9. Szabó S, Trier JS, Brown A, LaRocque M. Protection against aspirin-induced hemorrhagic gastric erosions and mucosal vascular injury by co-administration of sulfhydryl drugs. Gastroenterology 1987; 88:1604.
10. Szabó S, Bynum TE. Alternatives to the acid-oriented approach to ulcer disease: does "cytoprotection" exist in man? Scand J Gastroenterol 1988; 23:1–6.
11. Garner A. Stimulants of duodenal alkaline secretion. In: Szabó S, Mózsik G, eds. New pharmacology of ulcer disease. New York: Elsevier, 1987:37–47.
12. Wenzl E, Feil W, Starlinger M, Schliessel R. Acid tolerance of rabbit duodenum: the role of alkaline secretion. In: Szabó S, Mózsik G, eds. New pharmacology of ulcer disease. New York: Elsevier, 1987:48–56.
13. Robert A, Nemazis JE, Lancaster C, Hanchar AJ. Cytoprotection by prostaglandins in rats. Gastroenterology 1979; 77:433–43.
14. Robert A. Cytoprotection by acetazolamide. Digestion 1985; 31:149.
15. Kusterer K, Pihan G, Szabó S. Role of lipid peroxidation in gastric mucosal lesions induced by HCl, NaOH, or ischemia. Am J Physiol 1987; 252:G811–6.
16. Konturek SJ, Brozowski T, Piastucki I, Radecki T, Dupuy D, Szabó S. Gastric mucosal protection by agents altering gastric mucosal sulfhydryls. Digestion 1987; 37:65–71.
17. Jávor T, Bata M, Kutor G, Lovász L, Mózes G, Tárnok F, Mózsik G. Gastric mucosal resistance to physical and chemical stress. In: Mózsik G, Hänninen O, Jávor T, eds. Gastrointestinal defense mechanisms. Advances in physiological sciences 29. Oxford: Pergamon, 1981:141–59.
18. Jávor T, Bata M, Lovász L, Morón F, Nagy L, Patty I, Szabolcs J, Tárnok F, Tóth G, Mózsik G. Gastric cytoprotective effects of vitamin A and other carotenoids. Int J Tiss Reac 1983; 5:289–96.
19. Mózsik G, Pár A, Bertelli A, eds. Recent advances in gastrointestinal cytoprotection. Budapest: Akadémiai Kiadó, 1984.
20. Robert A, Eberle D, Kaplowits N. Role of glutathione in gastric mucosal cytoprotection. Am J Physiol 1984; 247:G296–304.
21. Morón F, Barreras N, Achong M, Nagy L, Jávor T, Mózsik G. Cytoprotective effect of disodium cromoglycate (Intal) in gastric lesions induced by several necrotizing agents in rats. Digestion 1985; 31:172.

22. Morón F, Barreras N, Achong M, Jávor T, Nagy L, Mózsik G. Cytoprotective effect of disodium chromoglycate (Intal) on the gastric mucosal lesions induced by necrotizing agents in rats. In: Szabó S, Mózsik G, eds. New pharmacology of ulcer disease. New York: Elsevier, 1987:525–33.

23. Johansson C, Bergstrom S. Prostaglandins and protection of the gastroduodenal mucosa. Scand J Gastroenterol 1982; 17:21–46.

24. Mózsik G, Jávor T, Kitajima M, Pfeiffer CJ, Rainsford KD, Simon L, Szabó S, eds. Advances in gastrointestinal cytoprotection: topics 1987. Acta Physiol Hung 1989:111–391.

25. Mózsik G, Pihan G, Szabó S, Jávor T, Czeglédi B, Tigyi A, Tárnok F, Zsoldos T. Free radicals, nonsulfhydryl antioxidants, drugs, and vitamins in acute gastric mucosal injury and protection. In: Szabó S, Mózsik G, eds. New pharmacology of ulcer disease. New York: Elsevier, 1987:197–207.

26. Freemann BA, Crapo JD. Biology of disease: free radicals and tissue injury. Lab Invest 1982; 47:412–26.

27. Slater TF. Free radical mechanisms in tissue injury. London: Pion, 1972.

28. Szabó D, Pihan G, Dupuy D. The biochemical pharmacology of sulfhydryl compounds in gastric mucosal injury and protection. In: Szabó S, Mózsik G, eds. New pharmacology of ulcer disease. New York: Elsevier, 1987:424–36.

29. Mózsik G, Morón F, Jávor T. Cellular mechanisms of the development of gastric mucosal damage and of gastrocytoprotection induced by prostacyclin in rats. A pharmacological study. Prostaglandins, Leucotrienes Med 1982; 9:71–84.

30. Mózsik G, Morón F, Fiegler M, Jávor T, Nagy L, Patty I, Tárnok F. Interrelationships between membrane-bound ATP-dependent energy systems, gastric mucosal damage produced by NaOH, hypertonic NaCl, HCl, and alcohol, and prostacyclin-induced gastric cytoprotection in rats. Prostaglandins, Leukotrienes Med 1983; 12:423–36.

31. Mózsik G, Morón F, Fiegler M, Jávor T, Nagy L, Patty I, Tárnok F. Membrane-bound ATP-dependent energy systems and gastric cytoprotection by prostacyclin, atropine and cimetidine in the rat. Int J Tiss Reac 1983; 5:263–78.

32. Mózsik G, Bata M, Fiegler M, Jávor T, Nagy L, Patty I, Tóth G, Tárnok F. Interrelationships between the membrane-bound ATP-dependent energy systems of the gastric mucosa and the gastric cytoprotective effect of beta-carotene on the development of gastric mucosal damage produced by 0.6M HCl in rats. Acta Physiol Hung 1984; 64:301–7.

33. Mózsik G, Fiegler M, Jávor T, Morón F, Nagy L, Patty I, Tárnok F. In: Kecskeméti V, Gyires K, Kovács G, eds. Prostanoids. Proc 4th Congr Hung Pharmacol Soc. Oxford: Pergamon, Budapest: Akadémiai Kiadó, 1986:461–72.

34. Mózsik G, Fiegler M, Jávor T, Morón F, Nagy L, Patty I, Tárnok F. Correlations between the membrane-bound ATP-dependent energy systems and ulcer treatment in the rat and man. In: Szabó S, Mózsik G, eds. New pharmacology of ulcer disease. New York: Elsevier, 1987:11–36.

35. Mózsik G, Fiegler M, Morón M, Nagy L, Patty I, Tárnok F. Molecular biochemistry and pharmacology of peptic ulcer treatment. A review. Acta Med Hung 1987; 44:3–29.

36. Mózsik G, Jávor T. A biochemical and pharmacological approach to the genesis of ulcer disease. I. A model study of ethanol-induced injury to gastric mucosa in rats. Dig Dis Sci 1988; 33:92–105.

37. Mózsik G, Czeglédi B, Sütö G, Vincze Á, Zsoldos T. In: Matkovics B, Boda D, Kalász H, eds. Oxygen free radicals and tissue injury. Budapest: Akadémiai Kiadó, 1988:225–34.

38. Sütö G, Vincze Á, Zsoldos T, Mózsik G. In: Matkovics B, Boda D, Kalász H, eds. Oxygen free radicals and tissue injury. Budapest: Akadémiai Kiadó, 1988:357–64.

39. Vincze Á, Sütö G, Zsoldos T, Mózsik G. In: Matkovics B, Boda D, Kalász H, eds. Oxygen free radicals and tissue injury. Budapest: Akadémiai Kiadó, 1988:389–95.

40. Vincze Á, Garamszegi M, Jávor T, Sütö G, Tigyi A, Tóth G, Zsoldos T, Mózsik G. The free radical mechanisms in beta-carotene induced gastric cytoprotection in HCl model. Acta Physiol Hung 1989; 73:351–5.

41. Szabó S, Trier JS, Frankel PW. Sulfhydryl compounds may mediate gastric cytoprotection. Science 1981; 214:200–2.

42. Bailey KA, Szabó S. Effects of duodenal ulcerogens, cysteamine and propionitrile on tissue glutathione in rats. Fed Proc 1978; 37:302.

43. Szabó S. Role of sulfhydryls and early vascular lesions in gastric mucosal injury. Acta Physiol Hung 1984; 64:203–14.

44. Szabó S, Gallagher GT, Horner HC, Frankel PW, Underwood RH, Konturek SJ, Brozowski T, Trier JS. Gastroenterology 1983; 85:1384–90.

45. Bálint G, Varró V. On the cytoprotective action of sulfhydryl-containing substances. Acta Physiol Acad Sci Hung 1982; 60:139–42.

46. Strubelt O, Hoppenkamps R. Relations between gastric glutathione and the ulcerogenic action of non-steroidal anti-inflammatory drugs. Arch Int Pharmacodyn 1983; 262: 268–78.

47. Strubelt O. The role of sulfhydryls in the ulcerogenic action of nonsteroidal antirheumatics. In: Szabó S, Mózsik G, eds. New pharmacology of ulcer disease. New York: Elsevier, 1987:397–446.

48. Szabó S, Trier JS, Brown A, LaRocque M. Protection against aspirin-induced hemorrhagic gastric erosions and mucosal vascular injury by co-administration of sulfhydryl drugs. Gastroenterology 1985; 88:1604.

49. Ezer E. Orally administered aspirin prevents the severe gastric damage induced by acidified ethanol, and sulfhydryl blocker pretreatment counteracts this protective effect in the rat. Gastroenterology 1985; 88:1377.

50. Mizui T, Doteuchi M. Effect of polyamines on acidified ethanol-induced gastric lesions in rats. Jpn J Pharmacol 1983; 33:939–45.

51. Boyd SC, Sasame HA, Boyd MR. High concentrations of glutathione in glandular stomach: possible implications for carcinogenesis. Science 1979; 205:1010–2.

52. Szabó S, Trier JS, Brown A, Schnoor J. Sulfhydryl blockers induce severe inflammatory gastritis in the rat. Gastroenterology 1984; 86:1271.

53. Sedlak J, Lindsay R. Estimation of total, protein-bound, and nonprotein sulfhydryl groups in tissue with Ellman's reagent. Anal Biochem 1968; 25:192–205.

54. Dupuy D, Szabó S. Protection by metals against ethanol-induced gastric mucosal injury in the rat. Gastroenterology 1986; 91:966–74.

55. Raza A, Szabó S. Biochemical changes in endogenous sulfhydryls in gastric mucosal injury and protection: studies with diethylmaleate and N-ethylmaleimide. Dig Dis Sci 1985; 30:397.

56. Dupuy D, Szabó S. Protective effects of heavy metals on ethanol-induced gastric erosions. Fed Proc 1984; 43:946.

57. Szabó S, Maull EA, Movahedi S. Sulfhydryl drugs: a new type of gastric cytoprotective agent. Gastroenterology 1981; 80:1298.

58. Mózsik G, Morón F, Nagy L, Ruzsa C, Tárnok F, Jávor T. Evidence of the gastric cytoprotective effects of vitamin A, atropine and cimetidine on the development of gastric mucosal damage produced by administration of indomethacin in healthy subjects. Int J Tiss Reac 1986; 8:85–90.

59. Mózsik G, Garamszegi M, Jávor T, Sütö G, Vincze Á, Tóth G, Zsoldos T. In: Tsuchiya M, et al., eds. Free radicals and digestive diseases. Amsterdam: Elsevier, 1988:111–6.

60. Mózsik G, Fiegler M, Garamszegi M, Jávor T, Nagy L, Sütö G, Vincze Á. PGI_2 prevents the development of gastric mucosal damage, β-carotene stimulates the repair mechanisms in ethanol-induced gastric mucosal damage in rats. Dig Dis Sci 1988; 33:906.

61. Mózsik G, Fiegler M, Garamszegi M, Jávor T, Nagy L, Sütö G, Vincze Á, Tóth G, Zsoldos T. In: Hayaishi O, Niki E, Konolo M, Yoshikawa T, eds. Medical, biochemical and chemical aspects of free radicals. Amsterdam: Elsevier, 1989:1421–5.

62. Lacy ER, Ito S. Microscopic analysis of ethanol damage to rat gastric mucosa after treatment with a prostaglandin. Gastroenterology 1982; 83:619–25.

63. Lacy ER, Ito S. Rapid epithelial restitution of the rat gastric mucosa after ethanol injury. Lab Invest 1984; 51:573–83.

64. Mózsik G, Garamszegi M, Fiegler M, Jávor T, Nagy L, Sütö G, Vincze A. Biochemical backgrounds of the development of gastric mucosal damage produced by intragastric administration of ethanol or HCl in the rat. Dig Dis Sci 1988; 33:906.

65. Sütö G, Garamszegi M, Jávor T, Vincze Á, Mózsik G. Similarities and differences in the cytoprotection induced by PGI_2 and beta-carotene in experimental ulcer. Acta Physiol Hung 1989; 73:155–8.

66. Czeglédi B, Zsoldos T, Mózsik G. Effect of $PGF_{2\alpha}$ administered in cytoprotective and antisecretory doses on the ethanol- and HCl-induced gastric mucosal damage and gastric mucosal superoxide dismutase activity in rats. Acta Physiol Hung 1984; 64:331–7.

67. Mózsik G, Garamszegi M, Fiegler M, Nagy L, Sütö G, Vincze Á, Zsoldos T, Jávor T. In: Hayaishi O, Niki E, Konolo M, Yoshikawa T, eds. Medical, biochemical and chemical aspects of free radicals. New York: Elsevier, 1988; 1427–31.

68. Sütö G, Garamszegi M, Tóth G, Vincze Á, Jávor T, Mózsik G. Interaction between the PGI_2- and β-carotene-induced gastric cytoprotection. Quart Bull Hung Gastroenterol 1988; 6:102.

69. Vincze Á, Garamszegi M, Sütö G, Tóth G, Jávor T, Mózsik G. β-carotene-induced gastric cytoprotection differs from gastric mucosal PGE_2 in indomethacin-treated rats. Quart Bull Hung Gastroenterol 1988; 6:54.

70. Beers RF, Sizer JW. A spectrophotometric method for measuring the breakdown of hydrogen peroxide by catalase. J Biol Chem 1952; 195:133–40.

71. Misra HP, Fridovich I. The role of superoxide anion in the autoxidation of epinephrine and a simple assay for superoxide dismutase. J Biol Chem 1972; 247:3170–5.

72. Matkovics B, Novák R, Hank HD, Szabó L, Varga SI, Zalesna G. A comparative study of some more important experimental animal peroxide metabolism enzymes. Comp Biochem Physiol 1977; 56:31–4.

73. Ellmann GL. Tissue sulfhydryl groups. Arch Biochem Biophys 1959; 82:70–7.
74. Fong KL, McKay PB, Polyer JL. Evidence that peroxidation of lysosomal membranes is initiated by hydroxyl free radicals produced during flavin enzyme activity. J Biol Chem 1973; 248:7792–7.
75. Zsoldos T, Tigyi A, Monskó T, Puppi A. Lipid peroxidation in the membrane damaging effect of silica-containing dust on rat lungs. Exp Pathol 1983; 23:73–8.
76. Czeglédi B, Jávor T, Nagy L, Patty I, Tigyi A, Tárnok F, Zsoldos T, Mózsik G. The interrelationships between the lipid peroxidation, superoxide dismutase activity, development of gastric H^+ secretion and gastric mucosal damage produced by intragastric administration of aspirin in pylorus-ligated rats. Int J Tiss Reac 1986; 8:23–30.
77. Mózsik G, Jávor T, Zsoldos T, Tigyi A. The interrelationships between the development of ethanol-, HCl, NaOH, and NaCl-induced gastric mucosal damage and the gastric mucosal superoxide dismutase activity in the rat. Acta Physiol Hung 1984; 64:309–14.
78. Mózsik G, Jávor T, Tóth G, Zsoldos T, Tigyi A. Interrelationships between the gastric cytoprotective effects of vitamin A and beta-carotene and the gastric mucosal superoxide dismutase activity in rats. Acta Physiol Hung 1984; 64:315–8.
79. Zsoldos T, Czeglédi B, Tigyi A, Jávor T, Mózsik G. Interrelationships between the development of the gastric cytoprotective effects of prostacyclin, atropine, cimetidine and the gastric mucosal superoxide dismutase activity in rats. Acta Physiol Hung 1984; 64:325–30.
80. von Ritter C, Hinder RA, Oosthuizen MMJ, Svensson LG, Hunter SJS, Lambrecht H. Gastric mucosal lesions induced by hemorrhagic shock in baboons. Dig Dis Sci 1988; 33:857–64.
81. Patty I, Benedek S, Deák G, Jávor T, Kenéz P, Nagy L, Simon L, Tárnok F, Mózsik G. Controlled trial of vitamin A therapy in gastric ulcer. Lancet 1982; ii:876.
82. Patty I, Benedek S, Deák G, Jávor T, Kenéz P, Morón F, Nagy L, Simon L, Tárnok F, Mózsik G. Cytoprotective effect of vitamin A and its clinical importance in the treatment of patients with chronic gastric ulcer. Int J Tiss Reac 1983; 5:301–7.
83. Patty I, Tárnok F, Simon L, Jávor T, Deák G, Benedek S, Kenéz P, Nagy L, Mózsik G. A comparative dynamic study of the effectiveness of gastric cytoprotection by vitamin A, De-Nol, sucralfate and ulcer healing by pirenzepine in patients with chronic gastric ulcer (a multiclinical and randomized study). Acta Physiol Hung 1984; 64:379–84.
84. Mózsik G, Bertelli A, Deák G, Nagy L, Patty I, Simon L, Tárnok F, Jávor T. Some aspects of the critical evaluation of peptic ulcer therapy in patients. Int J Clin Pharmacol Res 1985; 5:447–55.
85. Mózsik G, Snodgrass W. In: Rozman K, Hänninen O, eds. Gastrointestinal toxicology. New York: Elsevier, 1986:436–63.

16

Endoscopic Therapy of Peptic Ulcer Disease

GUENTER J. KREJS

Karl Franzens University, Graz, Austria

I. INTRODUCTION

The introduction of fiberoptic endoscopy in gastroenterology during the last 20 years and its general availability have allowed accurate diagnosis of peptic ulcer disease, exact assessment of healing rates with drug treatment, and the possibility of therapeutic intervention in cases of ulcer bleeding. Although many of the endoscopic therapeutic approaches have a sound and promising rationale, in several instances controlled clinical trials have not supported the optimistic hopes of many investigators.

II. PEPTIC ULCER BLEEDING: NATURAL HISTORY

Bleeding from peptic ulcers has remained a major clinical problem and still is responsible for a considerable number of deaths. Mortality rates from peptic ulcer bleeding range from 2 to 15% in several large series, with 10% being frequently reported [1]. This high mortality is disturbing in the face of major accomplishments in resuscitation, intensive care, and surgery. It may, however, be due in part to the increasing age of the population, with many patients who bleed being above 60 years of age. One might speculate that the increased use of nonsteroidal anti-inflammatory agents may also play a role [2].

A major problem in selecting patients for therapeutic endoscopy is that in the majority of patients, bleeding from peptic ulcers ceases spontaneously. Only about 5–10% of patients continue to bleed. However, recurrence of bleeding during hospital admission occurs in about 25–30% of patients [3,4].

Endoscopic treatment has thus been aimed for use in patients who continue to bleed or are at high risk for rebleeding. The appropriate selection of patients for therapeutic endoscopy is thus of utmost importance. Recognized risk factors for continued or recurrent bleeding are based on both clinical and endoscopic findings. A clinical predictor is the amount of blood lost prior to admission, as evidenced by hypovolemia and/or a hemoglobin level of less than 10 g/dL [5]. Endoscopic risk factors include a spurting vessel, a fresh clot on the ulcer base, or a visible vessel [6,7]. The latter, however, has not been shown unequivocally to be a risk factor for recurrent bleeding [8,9]. Patients at low risk for rebleeding are those who have a clean ulcer base.

III.   THERAPEUTIC INTERVENTIONS

The decision for intervention is based on the above-mentioned considerations concerning risk for continued or recurrent bleeding and the likelihood of preventing such events by the use of a given technique. In addition, the risk associated with the endoscopic procedure must be taken into account. Most techniques carry a 1–2% chance of perforation or of induced bleeding [8,10].

A.   Electrocoagulation

Two types of electrocoagulation techniques are available: monopolar and bipolar. With monopolar coagulation the current flows from the tip of the probe through the tissue at the point of contact and through the body of the patient to a grounding plate [11]. With bipolar coagulation the electric circuit is completed between two separate points on the tip of the probe. (A multipolar probe has three pairs of electrodes on the tip.)

With monopolar electrocoagulation, several disadvantages are encountered, and these include difficulties in controlling current flow, corrosiveness of coagulation, and sticking of the probe to the coagulated area. For these reasons, although several controlled trials are available [12,13], most investigators do not recommend monopolar electrocoagulation.

With bipolar or multipolar electrocoagulation there is less tissue corrosion, since the temperature reached does not exceed 100°C. The probe allows compression of the vessel before or at the time of current delivery (coaptive coagulation). Multipolar coagulation has convincingly been shown to be effective in stopping peptic ulcer bleeding and is now one of the preferred methods [14,15].

B.   Laser

Laser light transmitted through a flexible quartz fiber inserted through the biopsy channel of an endoscope is another form of energy delivery for photocoagulation of tissue. Numerous studies in experimental models have shown efficacy [16,17]. Because of the low energy of the argon laser, its use [18,19] has practically been discontinued in favor of the higher-energy neodymium-YAG laser.

Two major studies with different results deserve closer analysis and discussion. A significant benefit of Nd:YAG laser treatment was shown by Swain and colleagues in England [20], while a group in Dallas failed to show any benefit [8]. One main difference between the two studies lies in the outcome of patients in the control groups. Since such differences are of great importance and determine the outcome of a study, they are shown in detail in Table 1.

The results of standard therapy in London were such that laser treatment easily provided a significant benefit. In Dallas, results with standard therapy "were so good" [8] that laser treatment was not able to add a significant benefit. These studies show that the same technique may yield completely different results in different patient settings. The mean age of the Dallas patients was 49 years, and that of the patients in London was 70 years. Thus, one might conclude that life in the U.S. leads to ulcer bleeding early (age 49) but carries a good prognosis (2% mortality), whereas the British life style leads to ulcer bleeding late (age 70) but carries a very bad prognosis (mortality 13%). The Dallas study [8], like the recent study by Wara [9], also questions the importance and predictive value of visible vessels, which may have been overemphasized in the past [7]. A comparison of the results with laser therapy in the two studies is shown in Table 2.

Further disadvantages of the laser are its high price and poor portability. It is also claimed that the Nd:YAG laser is more difficult to use than other devices. For all these reasons, lasers now receive low priority in recommendations for use in peptic ulcer bleeding (see NIH consensus statement, Section IV).

Table 1 Outcome of Patients in Control Groups of Nd:YAG Laser Studies in Bleeding Peptic Ulcers

	Swain et al. [20] (London)	Krejs et al. [8] (Dallas)
Number of patients	61	90
Rebleeding (%)	39	20
Rebleeding from ulcers with visible vessels (%)	55	19
Urgent surgery (%)	31	16
Mortality (%)	13	2

Table 2 Outcome of Nd:YAG Laser-Treated Patients

	Swain et al. [20] (London)	Krejs et al. [8] (Dallas)
Number of patients	62	86
Rebleeding (%)	8	17
Rebleeding from ulcers with visible vessels (%)	11	33
Urgent surgery (%)	8	14
Mortality (%)	2	1
Complications of laser	None	Started bleeding, 4 (2, surgery); perforation, 1

C. Heater Probe

With this device the application of heat and pressure (coaptive coagulation) allows sealing of arteries up to 2.5 mm in diameter [21]. Measurements by Swain et al. [22] of the size of arteries that bled in peptic ulcers necessitating surgical resection showed diameters up to 1.8 mm with a mean of 0.7 mm. Thus, the heater probe would appear to be a suitable tool for controlling even the most severe spurting bleeding [23]. In an ongoing trial funded by NIH (D. M. Jensen, personal communication), patients with active bleeding or a visible vessel are managed either medically or treated with the heater probe. Continued bleeding or recurrent bleeding was observed in 93% of the medical group but in only 19% of the patients treated with the heater probe. The need for urgent surgery was correspondingly reduced. More results are necessary [24,25] to fully judge the heater probe; however, it appears to be a safe and effective device and is now widely recommended for endoscopic use.

D. Injection Therapy

Injection therapy appears to be a promising technique, and several studies are now in progress. The technique is attractive because it can be readily practiced by any experienced endoscopist without expensive equipment. Injection is carried out with hypertonic saline and epinephrine [26], thrombin in saline [27], ethanol [28,29] or, more recently, fibrin tissue glues. It is my impression that injection therapy may become an important modality in the control of gastrointestinal bleeding from peptic ulcers. Results of controlled trials will become available in the near future.

IV.   NIH CONSENSUS STATEMENT 1989

In March 1989 a consensus conference was held at the National Institutes of Health in Bethesda, Maryland, to assess the merit of currently available methods of therapeutic endoscopy in peptic ulcer bleeding. Fourteen speakers (this author was one of them) provided the basis for 15 panelists to come up with the following statement, which is used as a summary for this chapter:

> In the United States, more than 100,000 patients a year bleed from peptic ulcers. Despite advances in diagnosis and treatment, the mortality rate from bleeding ulcers has averaged between 6 and 10 percent during the past 30 years.
>
> Bleeding from peptic ulcers stops spontaneously in 70 to 80 percent of patients. A major predictor of significant persistent or recurrent bleeding is the magnitude of blood loss before evaluation. Documented coagulopathy and the onset of the bleeding episode in a patient already hospitalized for a related or unrelated condition are predictive. The first and most important endoscopic predictor of persistent or recurrent bleeding is active bleeding at the time of endoscopy.
>
> Some pigmented protuberances within the ulcer crater imply a high risk of rebleeding even when not associated with bleeding during endoscopy. These are often referred to by endoscopists as "visible vessels" or "sentinel clots." The prognostic implications of the anatomic location of the ulcer crater are unclear. Patients at low risk for rebleeding are those whose ulcers have a clean ulcer base or a flat pigmented spot.
>
> The most effective techniques for treating ulcers are multipolar (also known as bipolar) electrocoagulation and the heater probe. These achieve immediate hemostasis and prevent rebleeding in actively bleeding patients. Further advantages are lack of need for an "en face" approach to the bleeding point, ability to control the depth of tissue injury, and portability and ease of use of the instruments.
>
> The Nd-YAG laser photocoagulation is effective but somewhat more difficult for endoscopists to learn and to use. Injection therapies (as with sodium chloride, epinephrine, and ethanol) appear promising for early control of bleeding, and further study of these is recommended. Other therapeutic endoscopic techniques reviewed by the panel are not recommended.
>
> Safety may be compromised by patient characteristics such as hemodynamic instability and illnesses, by the depth and location of the ulcer, and by excessive depth of penetration of energy or injectant during endoscopic therapy. Therapeutic endoscopy should be performed only by an endoscopist experienced and qualified in the specific therapeutic technique. In a patient in such hands, the rate of complications of endoscopic/hemostatic therapy is acceptably low considering the natural history of bleeding peptic ulcers. A surgeon should be involved from the outset in the team caring for patients with bleeding peptic ulcers.
>
> Therapeutic/hemostatic endoscopy should be directed at selected high-risk patients. These include bleeding patients with substantial blood loss manifested by hemodynamic instability, ongoing transfusion requirement, red hematemesis, or red stool. Also at high risk are patients older than 60 years, or who have associated diseases, or whose bleeding begins in the hospital, or who rebleed there.

These important issues should be given high priority for continuing scientific evaluation using multicenter, randomized controlled trials: (1) standardize use of terminology, (2) quantitate rebleeding risk associated with certain endoscopic features and with different host factors; (3) develop a composite system using clinical and endoscopic features to predict risk of persistent or recurrent bleeding, (4) define optimal treatment regimens, and (5) explore improved diagnostic and therapeutic technology with biomedical engineers. (NIH Consensus Conference [30].)

REFERENCES

1. Allan R, Dykes P. A study of the factors influencing mortality rates from gastrointestinal haemorrhage. Q J Med 1976; 45:533–50.
2. Armstrong CP, Blower AL. Non-steroidal antiinflammatory drugs and life threatening complications of peptic ulceration. Gut 1987; 28:527–32.
3. Peterson WL, Barnett CC, Smith HJ, Allen MH, Corbett DB. Routine early endoscopy in upper-gastrointestinal-tract bleeding. A randomized, controlled trial. N Engl J Med 1981; 304:925–9.
4. Avery Jones F. Hematemesis and melena: with reference to causation and to the factors influencing the mortality from bleeding peptic ulcers. Gastroenterology 1956; 30:166–90.
5. Bornman PC, Theodorou NA, Shuttleworth RD, Essel HP, Marks IN. Importance of hypovolaemic shock and endoscopic signs in predicting recurrent haemorrhage from peptic ulceration: a prospective evaluation. Br Med J 1985; 291:245–7.
6. Bown SG. Controlled studies of laser therapy for haemorrhage from peptic ulcers. Acta Endosc 1985; 15:1–12.
7. Griffiths WJ, Neumann DA, Welsh JD. The visible vessel as an indicator of uncontrolled or recurrent gastrointestinal hemorrhage. N Eng J Med 1979; 300:1411–3.
8. Krejs GJ, Little KH, Westergaard H, Hamilton JK, Spady DK, Polter DE. Laser photocoagulation for the treatment of acute peptic-ulcer bleeding. A randomized controlled clinical trial. N Engl J Med 1987; 316:1618–21.
9. Wara P. Endoscopic prediction of major rebleeding—a prospective study of stigmata or haemorrhage in bleeding ulcer. Gastroenterology 1985; 55:1209–14.
10. Rutgeerts P, Vantrappen G, Van Hootegem P, Broeckaert L, Janssens J, Coremans G, Geboes K. Neodymium-YAG laser photocoagulation versus multipolar electrocoagulation for the treatment of severely bleeding ulcers: a randomized comparison. Gastrointest Endosc 1987:199–202.
11. Papp JP. Electrocoagulation. In: Papp JP, ed. Endoscopic control of gastrointestinal hemorrhage. Boca Raton, Fla.: CRC, 1981:31–42.
12. Freitas D, Donato A, Monteiro JG. Controlled trial of liquid monopolar electrocoagulation in bleeding peptic ulcers. Am J Gastroenterol 1985; 80:853–7.
13. Moreto M, Zaballa M, Ibanez S, Setien F, Figa M. Efficacy of monopolar electrocoagulation in the treatment of bleeding gastric ulcer: a controlled trial. Endoscopy 1987; 19:54–6.
14. Laine L. Multipolar electrocoagulation in the treatment of active upper gastrointestinal hemorrhage: a prospective controlled trial. N Engl J Med 1987; 316:1613–7.

15. Laine L. Multipolar electrocoagulation in the treatment of ulcers with non-bleeding visible vessels: a prospective, controlled trial. Gastroenterology 1986; 1:464.

16. Silverstein FE, Protell RL, Gulacsik C, Auth DA, Dennis MB, Rubin CE. Argon versus neodymium-YAG laser photocoagulation of experimental canine ulcers. Gastroenterology 1979; 77:491–6.

17. Johnston JH, Jensen DM, Mautner W, Elashoff J. YAG laser treatment of experimental bleeding canine gastric ulcers. Gastroenterology 1981; 80:708–16.

18. Vallon AG, Cotton PB, Laurence BH, Armengol Miro JR, Salord Oses JC. Randomised trial of endoscopic argon laser photocoagulation in bleeding peptic ulcers. Gut 1981; 22:228–33.

19. Swain CP, Bown SG, Storey DW, Kirkham JS, Northfield TC, Salmon PR. Controlled trial of argon laser photocoagulation in bleeding peptic ulcers. Lancet 1981; ii:228–33.

20. Swain CP, Kirkham JS, Salmon PR, Bown SG, Northfield TC. Controlled trial of Nd-YAG laser photocoagulation in bleeding peptic ulcers. Lancet 1986; i:1113–7.

21. Johnston JH, Jensen DM, Auth D. Experimental comparison of endoscopic yttrium-aluminium-garnet laser, electrosurgery, and heater probe for canine gut arterial coagulation: the importance of vessel compression and avoidance of tissue erosion. Gastroenterology 1987; 92:1101–8.

22. Swain CP, Storey DW, Bown SG, Heath J, Mills TN, Salmon PR, Northfield TC, Kirkham JS, O'Sullivan JP. Nature of the bleeding vessel in recurrently bleeding gastric ulcers. Gastroenterology 1986; 90:595–608.

23. Johnston J, Sones J, Long B, Posey EL. Heater probe is superior to YAG laser in clinical endoscopic treatment of major bleeding from peptic ulcers. Gastrointest Endosc 1985; 31:175–80.

24. Matthewson D, Swain CP, Bland M, Kirkham JS, Bown SG, Northfield TC. Randomized comparison of Nd YAG laser, heater probe, and no endoscopic therapy for bleeding peptic ulcer. Gastroenterology 1987; 92:1522. Abstract.

25. Hirao M, Kobayashi T, Masuda K, Yamaguchi S, Noda K, Matsuura K, Naka H, Kawauchi H, Namiki M. Endoscopic local injection of hypertonic saline-epinephrine solution to arrest hemorrhage from the upper gastrointestinal tract. Gastrointest Endosc 1985; 31:313–7.

26. Fuchs KH, Wirtz HJ, Schaube H, Elfeldt R. Initial experience with thrombin as injection agent for bleeding gastroduodenal lesions. Endoscopy 1986; 18:146–8.

27. Sugawa C, Fujita Y, Ikeda T, Walt AG. Endoscopic hemostasis of bleeding of the upper gastrointestinal tract by local injection of 98% dehydrated ethanol. Surg Gynecol Obstet 1986; 162:159–63.

28. Asaki S, Nishimura T, Satoh A, Ohara S, Shibuya D, Ogitsu Y, Goto Y. Endoscopic hemostasis of gastrointestinal hemorrhage by local application of absolute ethanol: a clinical study. Tohoku J Exp Med 1983; 141:373–83.

29. Chen PC, Wu CS, Liaw YF. Hemostatic effect of endoscopic local injection with hypertonic saline-epinephrine solution and pure ethanol for digestive tract bleeding. Gastrointest Endosc 1986; 32:319–23.

30. NIH Consensus Conference on Therapeutic Endoscopy and Bleeding Ulcers, March 6–8, 1989. Bethesda, Md: National Institutes of Health, Office of Medical Applications of Research, 1989.

17

Surgical Treatment of Peptic Ulcer Disease: Past, Present, and Future

Michael P. Hocking and E. R Woodward

University of Florida College of Medicine and
Gainesville Veterans Administration Medical Center,
Gainesville, Florida

I. INTRODUCTION

As with the medical therapy of peptic ulcer disease (PUD), surgical treatment has evolved from empiricism to procedures based on sound scientific principles. As our medical colleagues have been able to refine and improve their therapy, based on an increasing understanding of the physiology and pathophysiology of gastric secretion, so too has surgical therapy advanced. What follows is a brief summary of the evolution of the surgical treatment of peptic ulcer disease, a review of the procedures currently available, and some conjecture on future trends in surgical therapy.

II. HISTORY

Little more than 100 years has passed since Billroth performed the first successful gastric resection in 1881 [1]. That same year, his associate Wolfler performed the first gastroenterostomy [2]. This procedure was technically simpler than gastric resection and eventually became quite popular in surgical circles. Whereas the first gastric operations were directed toward the therapy of gastric neoplasia, only a few years elapsed before the surgical indications were broadened to include the treatment of peptic ulcer disease. VonRydygier, in 1884, is credited with performing the first gastroenterostomy for a patient with an obstructing duodenal ulcer [3]. Doyen performed a similar procedure eight years later for an obstructing gastric ulcer [4].

351

A. Gastroenterostomy

The understanding of the pathophysiology of peptic ulcer disease (which was then considered a rare entity) was rudimentary prior to the turn of the 20th century. Because of its initial successes, gastroenterostomy was empirically used to treat obstructing and eventually nonobstructing peptic ulcers. The increasing use of gastroenterostomy paralleled the increasing incidence of duodenal ulcer disease after the turn of the century. The major advantage of gastroenterostomy was its low morbidity and mortality rates. Operative mortality rates in the 0.5–1% range were reported [5]. Somewhat surprisingly, the original duodenal ulcer healed in the vast majority of cases. This success was probably due to the partial diversion of acid away from the duodenum, along with neutralization of gastric contents secondary to intestinal reflux [6].

B. Partial Gastrectomy

Gastroenterostomy was less successful for the therapy of gastric ulcer, however. VonRydygier described the first partial gastrectomy with gastroduodenostomy for gastric ulcer in 1882, and Billroth performed the first gastrectomy with gastro-jejunostomy (Billroth II) for a gastric ulcer 2 years later [7,8]. Gastric resection soon became the favored technique for the surgical treatment of gastric ulcer. In 1906 Edkins published his description of the gastric phase of acid secretion [9] and surgeons, especially in Europe, began to advocate gastric resection for the surgical treatment of duodenal ulcer as well.

Because of the increased morbidity and mortality following gastric resection in that era, however, surgeons were slow to abandon gastroenterostomy. Nevertheless, by the late 1920s, surgeons, led by Lewisohn and Berg in the United States, Pribram in Europe, and others, began to appreciate the high incidence of marginal ulceration following gastroenterostomy [10–12]. This rate reached 34% or higher. Interestingly, these marginal ulcers often occurred late in the postoperative period, with marginal ulcers being reported to occur at a mean of 11.2 years postoperatively in a series reported from the Mayo Clinic [13]. The reason for this late occurrence of marginal ulcers is unknown. A high-lying gastroenterostomy can stimulate gastric acid secretion, presumably secondary to continual distention of the gastric antrum by alkaline secretion [14]. However, a dependent gastroenterostomy should have no such effect. Perhaps the jejunum is truly less resistant to the deleterious effects of continual exposure to an acid and peptic environment. Partial bypass of the duodenum, with its neural and humoral negative feedback to gastric acid secretion, may also play a role. Regardless, gastroenterostomy was slowly abandoned, and partial gastrectomy gradually accepted, by surgeons during the late 1930s and early 1940s.

C. Subtotal Gastrectomy

The trend in the late 1930s and 1940s was toward more radical subtotal gastrectomy, with the rationale being resection of more and more of the parietal cell region of the stomach. Eventually, two-thirds to three-fourths of the stomach was removed [8]. Although the results in terms of ulcer recurrence were quite satisfactory, with reported recurrence rates generally in the 5–10% range (and some even less than 5%), the procedure was associated with a relatively high incidence of postgastrectomy symptoms (10–20%), so that there was still room for improvement [8,15,16].

D.   Vagotomy

Following Pavlov's report of his experimental studies on the cephalic phase of acid secretion, published in London in 1910, various European surgeons had attempted clinical vagotomy. These included Exner, Bircher, Latarjet, and Schiassi, among others [17]. However, the vagotomies were not always complete, and the indications for surgery were often obscure. Although it was understood that vagotomy resulted in decreased gastric acid secretion, it was also proposed that vagal denervation would diminish gastric sensation as well as "relax" the stomach in patients with "hypermotility." Vagotomy was not generally adopted by the surgical community in that era.

In 1943, Dragstedt, who can be considered the father of the modern era of the surgical treatment of peptic ulcer disease, reintroduced vagotomy as the treatment for duodenal ulcer (Fig. 1) [18]. In animal investigations he documented the ability of truncal vagotomy to decrease acid secretion. He produced hypersecretion in a dog model by isolating the stomach surgically, with preservation of the vagal trunks [19]. This preparation causes gastric hypersecretion and results in experimental peptic ulcers. However, concomitant or subsequent vagotomy prevents the gastric hypersecretion, and peptic ulcers do not develop.

Dragstedt felt that the main pathophysiology of duodenal ulcer disease was basal acid hypersecretion, which is vagal in origin [20]. In contrast to other species, humans exhibit a relatively high basal acid secretion in the interdigestive period. This basal secretion reaches nearly 7–10% of maximal acid output and follows a circadian rhythm, with the highest output between 5 p.m. and 2 a.m. [21]. Thus maximal basal secretion usually occurs during sleep, when food cannot be ingested to buffer it. This basal secretion does not correlate with serum gastrin levels and is abolished by vagotomy [20,22]. Thus, truncal vagotomy, which abolishes the cephalic phase of gastric acid secretion and diminishes nocturnal acid production, seemed the perfect surgical treatment for duodenal ulcer disease.

Dragstedt emphasized the acid secretory changes that occurred postvagotomy. His first patient was a young man who was reluctant to undergo the accepted procedure of the time, namely, subtotal gastrectomy, because close relatives had undergone this procedure with subsequent severe postgastrectomy symptoms. Instead, the patient underwent transthoracic truncal vagotomy. Postoperatively, Dragstedt documented a dramatic fall in basal acid output. He also documented that clinical improvement was due to this decreased acid secretion, and not to decreased gastric sensation, as installation of 0.1 N HCl in the early postoperative period reproduced the patient's preoperative symptoms.

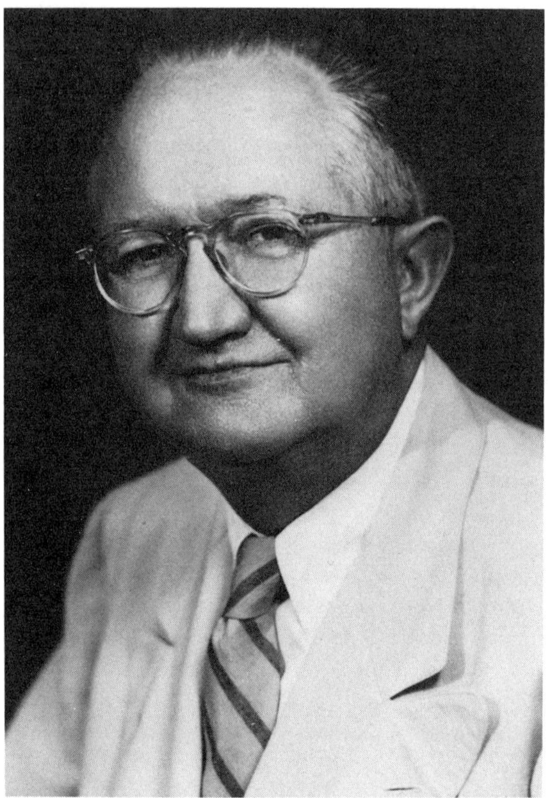

FIGURE 1   Lester R. Dragstedt, father of the modern era of the surgical treatment of peptic ulcer disease.

Nevertheless, surgeons, being generally a conservative lot, were reluctant to accept the new procedure. Although the complications of extensive subtotal gastrectomy were well known, the procedure had been effective in terms of curing the ulcer diathesis. Some of the initial reluctance was related to the complication of gastric stasis, which was observed in nearly a third of patients following truncal vagotomy alone [23]. The initial vagotomies were performed transthoracically. The change to a transabdominal approach and the addition of gastroenterostomy (V&GE) and, later, pyloroplasty (V&P), led to effective prevention of this complication.

E.   Vagotomy and Antrectomy

In the early 1950s, several surgeons combined vagotomy with partial gastrectomy [24,25]. Animal experiments in the 1940s had demonstrated conclusively that a powerful hormone was liberated by the gastric antrum in response to food and distention, confirming Edkins' report of 1906 [26]. With the concomitant ablation of both the cephalic and gastric phases of acid secretion, the probability of surgical cure was now even higher than it had been with high subtotal gastrectomy.

F.   Selective Vagotomy

Both vagotomy and drainage and vagotomy and antrectomy became widely accepted by surgeons throughout the world for the surgical treatment of peptic ulcer disease by the late 1950s and throughout the 1960s and 1970s. However, there still was some dissatisfaction with the nonselective nature of these procedures. Selective gastric vagotomy, with preservation of the hepatic branch of the anterior vagus nerve supplying the liver and biliary tract and the celiac branch of the posterior vagus trunk supplying the rest of the upper abdominal viscera, had been introduced by 1948 [27]. The rationale was to prevent some of the side effects of truncal vagotomy, especially postvagotomy diarrhea. However, this procedure was technically tedious, and the purported advantages were minimal, so that selective vagotomy was not widely performed. Eventually, though, an even more selective operation was gradually accepted by surgeons, first in Europe and later worldwide.

G.   Parietal Cell Vagotomy

Griffith and Harkins in 1957 had demonstrated that the vagal innervation to the parietal region of the stomach came from branches derived from the vagal trunks along the lesser curvature, the so-called nerves of Latarjet [28]. Thus, these branches could be divided, vagally denervating the parietal cells while preserving the motor nerves to the gastric antrum. They considered that this operation might be potentially useful in the surgical treatment of peptic ulcer disease but were discouraged from applying the procedure clinically by prominent surgeons of the time, who raised concerns about leaving the antral mucosa vagally innervated [29].

A decade later, Holle and Hart [30] demonstrated that parietal cell vagotomy combined with a drainage procedure was effective in reducing gastric acid secretion, and proposed parietal cell vagotomy as an elective operation for duodenal ulcer. Two years later, in 1969, Johnson and Wilkinson [31] demonstrated that a concomitant drainage procedure was unnecessary. Parietal cell vagotomy without a drainage procedure has gradually come to be accepted in the surgical community as an alternative to truncal vagotomy and pyloroplasty or truncal vagotomy and antrectomy, although questions regarding its efficacy remain.

III.   CURRENT SURGICAL THERAPY

A.   Duodenal Ulcer

Currently there are three major operations that are widely used to treat duodenal ulcer: vagotomy and drainage (V&D), vagotomy and antrectomy (V&A), and proximal gastric or parietal cell vagotomy (PCV).

1. Vagotomy and Drainage

Truncal vagotomy accomplishes an approximately 80–90% diminution in basal acid output (BAO), with a 50–60% decrease in maximal acid output (MAO) (Fig. 2) [32]. This results in a cure rate of generally greater than 90% for duodenal ulcer. We reported a nearly 6% recurrence rate at long-term follow-up [33]. Most duodenal ulcer recurrences occur within 5 years postoperatively, but gastric ulcers may occur in the late postoperative period, possibly secondary to gastric stasis.

Because the gastric phase of acid secretion is maintained, it is mandatory that the vagotomy be complete. Almost all patients with recurrence following vagotomy and drainage will be found at reoperation to have an intact vagal trunk, usually the posterior [32,34]. The major advantage of vagotomy and pyloroplasty is that it can be performed expeditiously with very low morbidity and mortality. A relative disadvantage of truncal vagotomy, however, is its nonselective nature. The entire gastrointestinal tract is vagally denervated from the gastroesophageal junction to the midtransverse colon. Side effects are common but are generally well tolerated. Dumping, bile vomiting, and diarrhea have been reported in up to 50% of patients but generally are considered severe in only 5–10% [35].

These side effects result from unwanted effects of truncal vagotomy as well as from the accompanying drainage procedure. Gastric vagal denervation, although it diminishes acid secretion, also impairs gastric motility. Dragstedt et al. found that nearly one-third of patients developed intractable gastric stasis if a concomitant drainage procedure was not added [23]. The addition of a drainage procedure results in nearly normal gastric emptying of solids. However, gastric emptying of liquids is generally sped, secondary to multiple factors, including decreased resistance to outflow at the pylorus, loss of the so-called duodenal brake, and increased intragastric pressure secondary to loss of vagally mediated fundal reflexes [36]. Vagal denervation of the small bowel may result in postvagotomy diarrhea.

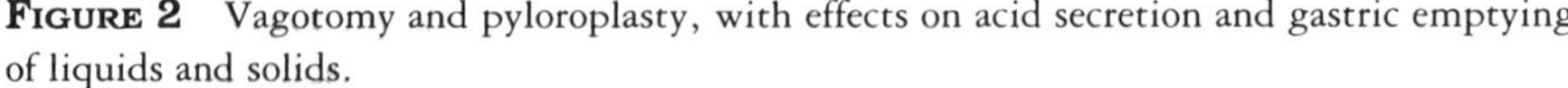

FIGURE 2 Vagotomy and pyloroplasty, with effects on acid secretion and gastric emptying of liquids and solids.

The major utilization of vagotomy and drainage currently is in the emergency therapy of acute upper gastrointestinal hemorrhage. Under these circumstances, the pyloroplasty provides direct access for suture ligation of the ulcer, and a concomitant truncal vagotomy can be performed expeditiously. We also consider vagotomy and pyloroplasty useful to treat a duodenal ulcer complicated by pyloric stenosis. Under these circumstances, we would add a temporary gastrostomy, with a simultaneous feeding jejunostomy through a separate enterotomy, or with a combined gastrostomy tube/jejunostomy tube. Whereas some surgeons would avoid a vagotomy with a preoperative diagnosis of gastric outlet obstruction, we have not found an increased risk of postoperative gastric retention if the stomach is adequately decompressed for at least 72 hr prior to surgery.

2. Vagotomy and Antrectomy

Antrectomy, with the ablation of the gastric phase of acid secretion, combined with truncal vagotomy (Fig. 3) results in an approximately 90% reduction in both basal and maximal acid output [32]. At first glance, this would seem somewhat surprising, as gastrin secretion is normal in duodenal ulcer disease. However, Jordan has demonstrated that a reduction in circulating gastrin levels markedly reduces the sensitivity of the parietal cell to vagal stimulation [37]. This is because of the striking synergism between the stimulants of gastric secretion: histamine, acetylcholine, and gastrin. Thus, both basal and maximal acid output are lower following vagotomy and antrectomy than following truncal vagotomy alone. This profound acid reduction results in a very low recurrence rate, approaching 1% [32,34,38]. In addition, antrectomy provides protection against an incomplete vagotomy [32,38].

The trade-off, however, is an increased operative morbidity and mortality due to the longer intraoperative time required, as well as increased blood loss secondary to performing the distal gastrectomy. In addition, following vagotomy and antrectomy

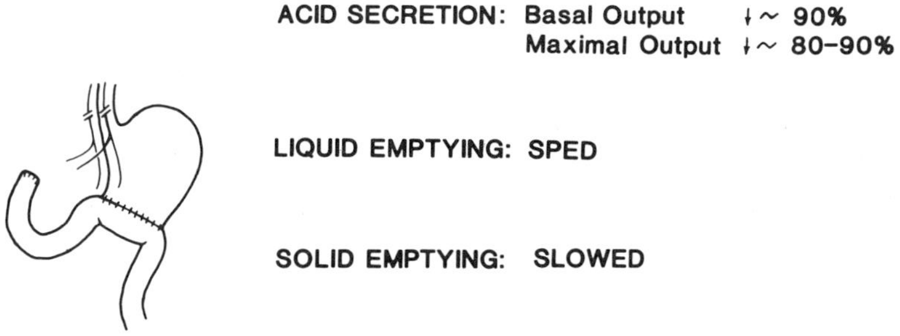

FIGURE 3 Vagotomy and antrectomy with gastrojejunostomy (Billroth II), with effects on acid secretion and gastric emptying of liquids and solids.

with gastrojejunostomy, a duodenal stump is created, with leaks and fistulas reported in up to 5–6% of patients so treated [39]. Another major disadvantage of vagotomy and antrectomy is the relatively high incidence of postgastrectomy symptoms.

The combination of truncal vagotomy and partial gastrectomy results in a profound disruption of gastric function. Gastric emptying of liquids is sped, secondary to loss of fundal reflexes, partial removal of the gastric reservoir, loss of the duodenal brake, and decreased resistance to outflow through the gastroenterostomy or gastroduodenostomy [36]. Gastric emptying of solids is generally slowed [40,41]. The distal gastrectomy effects a loss of the major contractile force of the stomach, while the vagotomy results in a weakening and disorganization of any remaining peristalsis. This is compensated for to a greater or lesser degree by the decreased resistance to outflow through the new gastroenterostomy. Loss of the pylorus and terminal antrum also results in gastric incontinence, with premature emptying of solids of increased particle size. In turn, this may result in impaired absorption of fat and other nutrients [42]. Although controversial, the incidence of postgastrectomy symptoms is probably higher following vagotomy and antrectomy than that seen following vagotomy and drainage [34]. Because of the low ulcer recurrence rate, these symptoms are the most frequent reason for surgical failures.

There is no objective evidence to support gastroduodenostomy (Billroth I) versus gastrojejunostomy (Billroth II) following vagotomy and antrectomy, although many surgeons prefer the former because of a desire to preserve a more "normal" pathway for digestion [32]. Recently, Roux-en-Y gastrojejunostomy has been advocated as a primary reconstruction following vagotomy and antrectomy [43,44]. This procedure prevents reflux of pancreatic and biliary content into the gastric remnant and may also ameliorate dumping symptoms [45]. However, the trade-off may be an increased incidence of gastric retention postoperatively. We urge caution with this approach and reserve Roux-en-Y gastrojejunostomy as a secondary procedure [46,47].

Because of the potential increase in operative morbidity and mortality, the latter approaching 2% in the elective setting, we feel that vagotomy and antrectomy has little role in the emergency treatment of duodenal ulcer. Instead, we consider this procedure ideally suited for a patient who has recuperated from a massive upper gastrointestinal hemorrhage secondary to duodenal ulcer. Ulcer recurrence in these patients is usually heralded by recurrent hemorrhage, and in an elective setting the slightly higher morbidity rate seems a worthwhile trade-off for a lower chance of ulcer recurrence. While vagotomy and antrectomy has also been advocated in the emergency treatment of upper gastrointestinal hemorrhage, if adopted by the general surgical community, this recommendation would inevitably lead to an increase in morbidity and mortality rates. The surgeon's first priority must always be to ensure the patient's survival, and secondarily to treat the ulcer disease.

Vagotomy and antrectomy is also acceptable in the treatment of pyloric or prepyloric ulcers, or duodenal ulcers complicated by gastric outlet obstruction. As with vagotomy and drainage, attention must be paid to adequate preoperative decompression, and intraoperative gastrostomy would seem prudent. Surgical judgment must be exercised when dealing with a badly scarred duodenum. In the face of severe scarring, it would seem prudent to perform a truncal vagotomy with pyloroplasty or, better yet, a gastrojejunostomy. In our opinion, the vast surgical literature on dealing with a difficult duodenal stump should be summarized in three words: don't create one!

3. Parietal Cell Vagotomy

Parietal cell vagotomy (PCV) consists of vagal denervation of the parietal cell area of the stomach, with preservation of the vagal innervation of the antrum and pylorus. Despite continued vagal innervation of the antral G cells, gastric acid reduction is similar to that seen following truncal vagotomy. Basal acid output is reduced by approximately 70–80% of preoperative values, with MAO decreased by 50–60% in the early postoperative period (Fig. 4) [48]. Thus, theoretically the ulcer recurrence rate should be similar to that reported following truncal vagotomy and drainage. There is, however, some tendency to an increase in acid production in the late postoperative period [5,49]. Serum gastrin levels also rise in the late postoperative period, but this does not seem to correlate with the increased acid output [50].

Reported recurrence rates following PCV have been highly variable, with the individual surgeon being the biggest risk factor in many series [35,51]. The surgical technique is not easily mastered, and a learning curve is seen. Clearing of at least the distal 7 cm of the esophagus appears to be of primary importance.

The main advantage of parietal cell vagotomy is its low morbidity and mortality. Because the gastric lumen is not entered, operative mortality is generally less than 1% [48,52]. Side effects are minimal. Gastric emptying of solids is generally normal postoperatively. Gastric emptying of liquids is slightly accelerated secondary to loss of fundal reflexes, with resulting increased intragastric pressure, but clinical dumping is rare, and postvagotomy diarrhea is almost nonexistent [36,48,52]. Postgastrectomy side effects are seen in probably less than 5% of patients [48,51,52].

Most clinicians consider that the low incidence of postgastrectomy symptoms

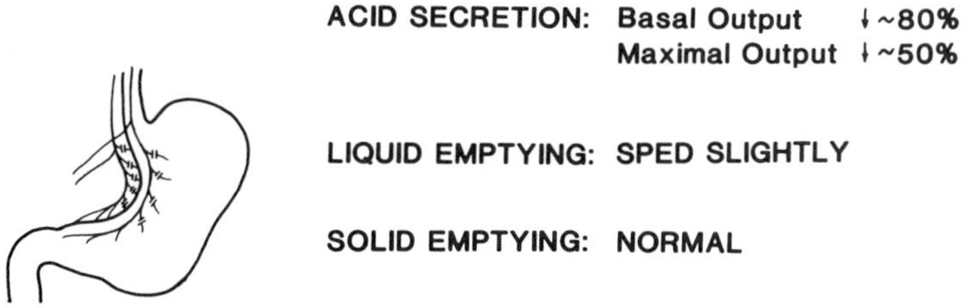

FIGURE 4 Parietal cell vagotomy with effects on gastric acid secretion and gastric emptying of liquids and solids.

outweighs the increased risk of recurrence and have therefore been proponents of parietal cell vagotomy, especially in the elective setting. We feel that this procedure is ideally suited for the treatment of a medically intractable duodenal ulcer. In addition, this procedure has been advocated in the setting of a perforated ulcer when peritoneal contamination is minimal and the patient is stable [53]. Again, the surgeon's top priority has to be patient survival and not cure of the ulcer disease. Factors that predict an increase in operative morbidity and mortality include preoperative shock, delay in operation of greater than 48 hr, and patient age greater than 60 [54]. If these risk factors are absent, a parietal cell vagotomy may be safely performed. Clearly, parietal cell vagotomy is beneficial in the setting of a chronic perforated ulcer, but it also appears to be valuable even in the situation of a perforated ulcer of recent onset with no antecedent ulcer history [53].

Parietal cell vagotomy is also acceptable in the setting of upper gastrointestinal hemorrhage, where the patient will tolerate the additional operative time required [55]. In this setting, the pylorus is preserved and the duodenal ulcer is approached through a duodenotomy, which is closed transversely. Again, good surgical judgment must be exercised, as vagotomy and pyloroplasty can be accomplished much more expeditiously. The use of parietal cell vagotomy in the face of prepyloric or pyloric channel ulcer or an ulcer complicated by gastric outlet obstruction is currently controversial. Although some studies show no increased recurrence rate in this setting, many others document an increased risk of recurrence [56–59]. There is some evidence that these ulcers have a different pathophysiology, with a lower acid secretion and hypertrophy of the pyloric and antral muscle layers [51,58]. Abnormal pyloric motility may play a role [48]. Parietal cell vagotomy combined with a drainage procedure may possibly result in a lower recurrence rate [58,60]. For the present, however, we would urge caution with the use of PCV in this setting.

B. Gastric Ulcer

Advances in the understanding of the pathophysiology of gastric ulcer have lagged behind those of duodenal ulcer. The basis for the surgical therapy of gastric ulcer remains largely empirical [61]. Gastric ulcers may be subdivided into type I, type II, and type III [62]. Type I ulcers are corporal ulcers that are typically located along the lesser curvature of the stomach in the antrum. Type II gastric ulcers are those associated with a concomitant duodenal ulcer, and type III ulcers are prepyloric ulcers located in proximity to the pylorus. The latter two types of ulcers behave as duodenal ulcers and should be treated accordingly. For type I ulcers, distal gastrectomy remains the mainstay of therapy, with vagotomy and drainage reserved for high-risk patients and PCV being evaluated.

1. Gastric Resection

Unlike duodenal ulcer patients, patients with type I gastric ulcers tend to be hyposecretors of gastric acid. Antrectomy (Fig. 5) results in a 50% decrease in basal

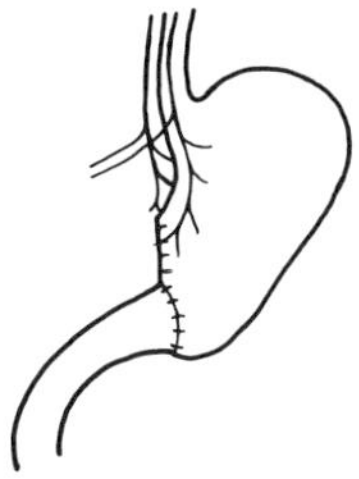

ACID SECRETION: Basal Output   ↓~50–60%

Maximal Output ↓~50–60%

LIQUID EMPTYING: SPED SLIGHTLY

SOLID EMPTYING: SPED SLIGHTLY

FIGURE 5   Gastric resection, with gastroduodenostomy (Billroth I), with effects on acid secretion and gastric emptying of liquids and solids.

acid output secondary to a decreased gastrin level and may speed gastric emptying [63,64]. In addition, as most gastric ulcers lie along the lesser curvature in the distal stomach, distal gastrectomy removes the gastric ulcer and the mucosa that seems most prone to develop an ulceration. Long-term cure is reported in approximately 95% of patients [63,64]. Operative mortality is usually in the 2% range [64]. In the relatively rare situation where the ulcer lies in the proximal stomach, the Kelling-Madlener technique may be used, in which a distal gastrectomy is combined with biopsy of the gastric ulcer, which is left in situ [65,66]. Alternatively, a Pauchet gastrectomy may be performed, resecting a tongue of antral tissue along the lesser curvature up to just below the gastroesophageal junction [67].

Preservation of the vagi results in a lowered incidence of side effects. In one series the incidence of postgastrectomy syndromes was reported as 12% following vagotomy and antrectomy versus 3% following antrectomy alone [63]. We consider antrectomy with gastroduodenostomy as the procedure of choice for the elective surgical treatment of a distal gastric ulcer. If the ulcer is located proximally, we have obtained good results with the Kelling-Madlener technique, leaving the ulcer in situ. Attempts to resect the ulcer in this location may result in an inadvertent vagotomy, and thus the ulcer should probably be left in situ. Biopsies of the ulcer should be performed, as there have been occasional reports of an occult gastric carcinoma, even following preoperative endoscopic biopsies [64].

Distal gastrectomy has also been advocated for hemorrhage or perforation secondary to a type I gastric ulcer. In this setting, even with the use of surgical staplers, a distal gastrectomy will almost invariably lead to increased morbidity and mortality. As with the treatment of emergency complications of a duodenal ulcer, the number one priority has to be to save the patient's life. Recently, simple undersewing of a bleeding gastric ulcer has been recommended, with a low operative mortality and only a 5% rehemorrhage rate [68]. Again, good surgical judgment must be used.

2.   Vagotomy and Drainage

Vagotomy and drainage has also been used to treat gastric ulcers, predominantly in high-risk patients. As gastric ulcer patients do not generally hypersecrete acid, the rationale has largely been empirical [64]. The overall ulcer recurrence is slightly higher than that reported following antrectomy and gastroduodenostomy, in the 10% range [64,69]. The main advantage of vagotomy and drainage over that of distal gastrectomy is that it can probably be performed in the emergency setting with a lower operative morbidity and mortality [69]. It also may be of benefit in the elective setting with a high-lying gastric ulcer [64]. The incidence of postgastrectomy symptoms is similar to that following antrectomy and gastroduodenostomy. As with distal gastrectomy, if the ulcer is left in situ, intraoperative biopsies should be obtained. Endoscopic biopsies have been reported to have a greater than 90% accuracy, but again, occasional reports of a missed malignancy suggest that rebiopsy or excision of the ulcer is prudent [64]. Currently, we would utilize vagotomy and drainage in the emergency setting, such as a perforated gastric ulcer or gastric hemorrhage in a high-risk patient. Again, with an extremely high risk or unstable patient, simple undersewing of a bleeding gastric ulcer or omental patching of a perforated ulcer is acceptable, with postoperative administration of H_2 blockers [68].

3.   Parietal Cell Vagotomy

Parietal cell vagotomy has been proposed for the surgical treatment of type I gastric ulcers [59,61,64,70,71]. However, the reported recurrence rate has been relatively high, and PCV may be technically difficult in the face of scarring and edema associated with a lesser curvature ulcer [61,70]. In addition, the incidence of postgastrectomy symptoms has not been decreased [70]. Therefore, at the present time, this procedure would have to be considered experimental for the treatment of gastric ulcer disease and is not recommended for routine use.

IV.   FUTURE TRENDS IN THE SURGICAL THERAPY OF PEPTIC ULCER DISEASE

A.   Declining Incidence of Duodenal Ulcer Disease

Is the surgical treatment of peptic ulcer disease a topic of historical interest only? Whereas the incidence of gastric ulcer has been relatively stable, the same cannot be said for duodenal ulcer [72]. The declining incidence of duodenal ulcer, along with decreasing rates for hospitalization and surgical treatment, has been well documented in Western countries, although the same is not true worldwide [72–76]. The most dramatic decline has been in the incidence of elective operations for duodenal ulcer. In several series, however, the incidence of emergency surgical treatment of duodenal ulcer complications is unchanged, or indeed has risen [73,76]. Interestingly, the use of H_2 blockers has also increased [74]. Most studies, however, conclude that the trend of decreased operative intervention preceded the introduction of H_2 blockers, and most patients with emergency complications of peptic ulcer disease have not previously been on H_2 blockers [72–76]. Although previously the number of males with duodenal ulcer far exceeded the number of females, the male/female ratio is now approximately 1 [72,76]. The surgical treatment of duodenal ulcer has changed from primarily elective operations in young, healthy men to predominantly emergency surgery in older men and women with multiple medical problems. Surgeons must change their operative approaches accordingly.

A major problem with the decrease in elective surgical experience is the potential difficulty in training young surgeons to treat duodenal ulcers [51]. This is most critical in terms of the newer techniques, such as parietal cell vagotomy, which are inevitably associated with a learning curve. The ultimate effect may be to have a large cadre of surgeons in clinical practice with extremely limited exposure to the surgical treatment of peptic ulcer disease. Thus, ironically, advances in medical therapy are threatening concomitant gains in the surgical treatment of duodenal ulcer. The end result may be an increasing referral of such patients to "ulcer centers" with surgeons at such institutions doing enough surgery to maintain their competence as well as having adequate clinical material to perform clinical trials.

B. Indications for Surgery

The other aspect of this declining incidence of elective surgical treatment is to define what is a failure of medical therapy. The current general view is that elective surgical treatment should be reserved for patients resistant to H_2 blockers or with frequent recurrences during maintenance therapy. Although there is no doubt that medical therapy has improved dramatically over the past two decades, there is still the question of long-term side effects of continual medical therapy, as well as the substantial costs involved. Interestingly, the few studies that have compared medical therapy to parietal cell vagotomy have generally favored the latter [77–79]. This, of course, is controversial and depends on one's viewpoint! As our societies become increasingly cost-conscious regarding medical care, we may find pressure for early elective surgical therapy of peptic ulcer disease, especially in young patients. In this regard, parietal cell vagotomy has the advantage of being extremely safe, as well as having minimal long-term side effects.

C. Long-Term Results of Parietal Cell Vagotomy

If we are to advocate parietal cell vagotomy, especially as an elective procedure in young patients, however, we need to have better information regarding the long-term results. Somewhat disconcerting is a recent report by one of the pioneers in the use of PCV demonstrating a 30% proven ulcer recurrence rate with an additional 9% of patients with suspected ulcers at 16–18-year follow-up [80]. This puts parietal cell vagotomy on a par with the first procedure widely used to treat peptic ulcer disease, gastroenterostomy, which also was safe but had an unacceptable late failure rate [5].

The reasons for the high recurrence following PCV are unknown. Unlike truncal vagotomy and drainage, recurrences following parietal cell vagotomy appear to increase linearly with time [5,80,81]. Possible reasons include vagal reinnervation, antral hyperfunction, motility disturbances, or inhibition of release of a fundal inhibitory substance [5,81]. Initially negative Hollander tests become positive with time, suggesting that vagal nerve regeneration occurs. However, an alternative explanation is that some of the initial decrease in acid production is secondary to devascularization of the lesser curvature, which of necessity accompanies parietal cell vagotomy and can recover with time [82]. Another concern is that parietal cell vagotomy may have an even higher failure rate in patients who are medically intractable, that is, have failed to respond to H_2 blockers [83].

To solve the recurrence problem, modifications of parietal cell vagotomy have been advocated. Intraoperative tests for completeness of vagotomy have been proposed, including the endoscopic Congo red test [84]. These tests have demonstrated the need to divide the gastroepiploic nerves to ensure a complete denervation of the parietal cell area [84,85]. However, follow-up studies have shown no advantage in terms of ulcer recurrence [85].

D. Newer Operations

As one of the disadvantages of parietal cell vagotomy has been the tediousness of the procedure, as well as the learning curve involved, several authors have attempted to simplify the procedure. The currently most popular variation is anterior lesser curve seromyotomy with posterior truncal vagotomy (ASPTV) (Fig. 6) [86–88]. This procedure is based on the fact that both the anterior and posterior antral walls contract following preservation of only the anterior nerve of Latarjet. The operation involves interruption of the posterior vagal trunk, with division of the superficial layers of the

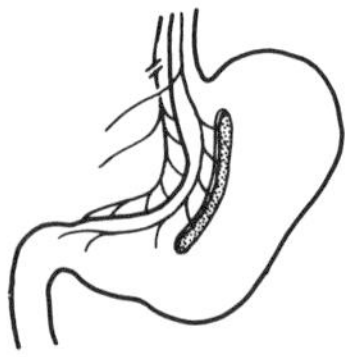

ACID SECRETION:	Basal Output	↓ ~60–80%
	Maximal Output	↓ ~40–50%
LIQUID EMPTYING:	SPED SLIGHTLY	
SOLID EMPTYING:	NORMAL	

FIGURE 6 Anterior lesser curve seromyotomy with posterior truncal vagotomy, with effects on acid secretion and gastric emptying of liquids and solids.

anterior gastric wall along the lesser curvature. Average operative time has been decreased by approximately 50% compared to PCV, which is the major advantage of this technique. However, theoretical objections are that there may be an increased incidence of gastric stasis, as well as postvagotomy diarrhea, as the posterior vagal trunk supplies parasympathetic innervation to the small bowel. In addition, high fundal branches from the anterior vagal trunk may be missed. Apart from these theoretical objections, the posterior vagal trunk is the one most commonly missed when truncal vagotomy is performed, so that the incidence of incomplete vagotomy may be increased. Furthermore, this procedure is essentially similar to parietal cell vagotomy in terms of abolishing only the cephalic phase of gastric acid secretion, and therefore the ultimate ulcer recurrence rate should be no better than that seen following PCV. Preliminary reports have been encouraging, but further follow-up is necessary before ASPTV can be recommended for use other than in clinical trials.

Another proposed procedure could result in an extremely low ulcer recurrence rate, with minimal side effects. This procedure is combined parietal cell vagotomy and mucosal antrectomy (PCV&MA) (Fig. 7) [89,90]. Although technically more challenging, PCV&MA theoretically combines the low incidence of side effects seen after parietal cell vagotomy with the high cure rate seen following vagotomy and antrectomy. Studies of gastric emptying in experimental animals show nearly normal gastric emptying of liquids and nondigestible solids with a slight delay in the gastric emptying of digestible solids [89,90]. Thus, postoperative side effects should be minimal. PCV&MA has been advocated in patients with recurrent ulcers following parietal cell vagotomy and could also be of benefit in patients with a predicted high recurrence rate following PCV, such as pyloric or prepyloric ulcers, or possibly patients with a high preoperative secretory rate, although the latter is controversial as a predictor of postoperative recurrence [5,82]. No clinical trials have yet been reported with PCV&MA.

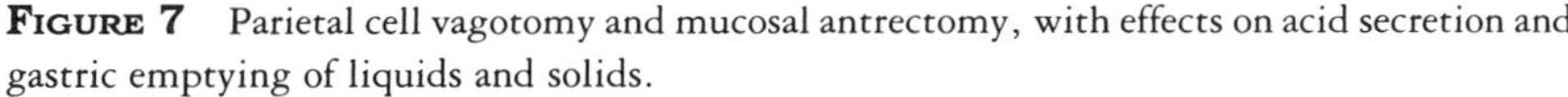

FIGURE 7   Parietal cell vagotomy and mucosal antrectomy, with effects on acid secretion and gastric emptying of liquids and solids.

E.   Recurrent Ulcers

While traditionally it has been stated that recurrent ulcers following parietal cell vagotomy are easily managed medically, Jensen and coworkers, in their long-term follow-up study, reported that almost 90% of recurrent ulcers following PCV required either surgical intervention or prolonged medical therapy [80]. In terms of surgical therapy for recurrent ulcers, antrectomy has generally been advocated [91]. This procedure can be performed with a fairly low mortality but a high immediate postoperative morbidity as well as a high incidence of postgastrectomy symptoms [92]. In this regard, mucosal antrectomy may present an acceptable alternative.

V.   SUMMARY

The ideal operation for the surgical therapy of peptic ulcer disease has yet to be introduced. Over the past 100 years, the pendulum of surgical therapy has swung from conservative (gastroenterostomy) to radical (subtotal gastrectomy) to conservative (vagotomy and drainage) to radical (vagotomy and antrectomy) back to conservative (parietal cell vagotomy) again (Fig. 8). If other studies confirm the high recurrence rates that Jensen and his colleagues have reported, there will be strong pressure on surgeons to adopt a new, more radical surgical procedure, such as PCV&MA (see

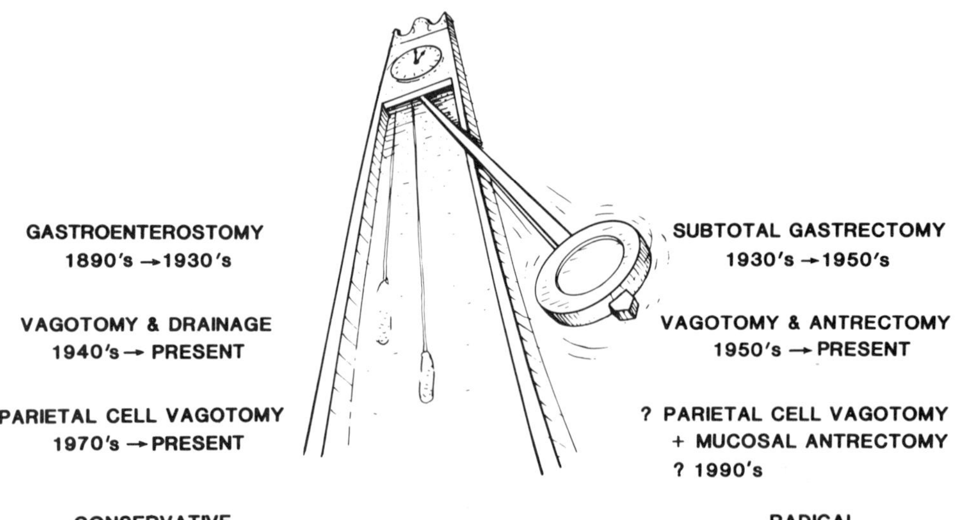

FIGURE 8   Evolution of the surgical therapy of duodenal ulcer, demonstrating how the "pendulum" has swung between "conservative" and "radical" procedures.

Table 1 Overall Results and Potential Advantages and Disadvantages of Current and Proposed Operations for Duodenal Ulcer

Operation	Morbidity[a]	Mortality[b]	Recurrence	Advantage	Disadvantage
Parietal cell vagotomy	<5%	<1%	>15%	Minimal morbidity and mortality	High recurrence; time-consuming; learning curve
Vagotomy and drainage	5–10%	1%	5–10%	Can be performed expeditiously	Nonselective; intermediate recurrence
Vagotomy and antrectomy	10–20%	1.5–2%	<2%	Low recurrence	Operative mortality; relatively high morbidity
Anterior lesser curve sero-myotomy with posterior truncal vagotomy	<5%	<1%	Unknown	Decreased operative time	Possible increased morbidity relative to parietal cell vagotomy
Parietal cell vagotomy with mucosal antrectomy	Unknown	Unknown	Unknown	Should combine low recurrence with low morbidity	Technical difficulty

[a]Postgastrectomy symptoms.
[b]Elective.

Table 2 Overall Results and Potential Advantages and Disadvantages of Current Operations for Gastric Ulcer

Operation	Morbidity[a]	Mortality[b]	Recurrence	Advantage	Disadvantage
Partial gastrectomy	<5%	2%	5%	Removes ulcer	Morbidity and mortality, especially in emergency setting
Vagotomy and drainage	5–10%	1%	10%	Can be performed expeditiously	Slightly higher recurrence and morbidity; ulcer not resected
Parietal cell vagotomy	<5%	<1%	Unknown	Antropyloric mechanism preserved	Technical difficulty; higher recurrence; ulcer not resected

[a]Postgastrectomy symptoms.
[b]Elective.

Table 3 First-Line, Second-Line, and Potential Future Operations for Peptic Ulcer Disease

Indication	First Choice	Alternative	Future
Duodenal ulcer			
Intractable	PCV	V&P, V&A	? PCV&MA
Perforation	Closure ± PCV[a]	Closure ± V&P	Closure ± ASPTV
Hemorrhage	V&P w/oversewing	V&A[b] or PCV[b] and oversewing	ASPTV and oversewing
Obstruction	V&P or V&GE	V&A	? PCV + drainage
Pyloric or prepyloric ulcer	V&P	V&A	? PCV + drainage; PCV&MA
Gastric ulcer			
Intractable	PG	V&P	? PCV
Perforation	Closure ± V&P[a]	Closure ± PG[a]	?
Hemorrhage	Oversewing ± V&P[b]	Oversewing ± PG[b]	?

PCV = parietal cell vagotomy; V&P = vagotomy and pyloroplasty; V&A = vagotomy and antrectomy; V&GE = vagotomy and gastroenterostomy; ASPTV = anterior lesser curve seromyotomy with posterior truncal vagotomy; PCV&MA = parietal cell vagotomy and mucosal antrectomy; PG = partial gastrectomy.

[a] If patient stable, without shock, perforation < 48°, age < 60, no associated severe medical conditions.

[b] If patient stable, without shock, age < 60, no associated severe medical conditions.

Sec. IV.D). If this procedure lives up to its promise as an effective operation with a low incidence of side effects, it may ultimately become the operation of choice for the elective treatment of duodenal ulcer. Along with this trend will be an increasing trend for surgeons to operate on complications of peptic ulcer disease in elderly, high-risk patients rather than in the elective setting on young healthy patients. The operative mortality will inevitably rise, especially as surgeons are being exposed to fewer ulcer operations. Thus, newer procedures that require less of a learning curve and can be performed more expeditiously, such as ASPTV, may find a role.

Tables 1 and 2 list the overall results, with the relative advantages and disadvantages, of the current and proposed operations for duodenal and gastric ulcers, respectively. Table 3 gives our suggestions for the first-line and second-line operations, as well as potential future operations, related to the preoperative indications for surgery. Our contention is that no *one* operation can or should be used in *all* patients with peptic ulcer. The operation used should be selected on the basis of the particular situation. For the forseeable future, parietal cell vagotomy, vagotomy and drainage, and vagotomy and antrectomy will continue to have a role in the surgical treatment of duodenal ulcer. For gastric ulcer, distal gastrectomy will remain the procedure of choice, with vagotomy and drainage reserved for the emergency setting. Because of technical difficulties and lack of a clear-cut benefit, it is unlikely that PCV will be widely used for gastric ulcer.

These are simultaneously exciting and frustrating times for the gastric surgeon. Both the medical and surgical therapy of peptic ulcer disease are clearly evolving, and the gastrointestinal surgeon must adapt his/her treatment to these changing conditions.

REFERENCES

1.   Billroth T. Offenes schreiben an herrn Dr. L. Wittelshofer. Wein Med Wochenschr 1881; 31:162–5.
2.   Wolfer A. Gastro-enterostomie. Zentralbl F Chir 1881; 8:705–8.
3.   McNealy RW, Lichtenstein ME. Evolution and present technique of gastrojejunostomy. Surg Gynecol Obstet 1935; 60:1003–5.
4.   Woodward WW. Brief history of peptic ulcer surgery. Aust NZ J Surg 1958; 28:81–95.
5.   Taylor TV. Parietal cell vagotomy: long term followup studies. Br J Surg 1987; 74:971–2.
6.   Kelly KA. Which operation for duodenal ulcer? Mayo Clin Proc 1980; 55:5–9.
7.   Olch PD, Harkins HN. A history of gastric surgery. In: Harkins HN, Nyhus LM, eds. Surgery of the stomach and duodenum, 2nd ed. Boston: Little Brown, 1969.
8.   Fischer AB. The long-term results following Billroth II resection for duodenal ulcer. Dan Med Bull 1986; 33:319–35.
9.   Edkins JS. The chemical mechanism of gastric secretion. J Physiol 1906; 34:133–44.
10.   Lewisohn R. The frequency of gastro-jejunal ulcer. Surg Gynecol Obstet 1925; 40:70–6.

11. Berg AA, Klein E, Crohn BB. The radical surgical cure of gastric and duodenal ulcer. Surg Clin North Am 1925; 5:49–91.

12. Pribram BO. Die gastroenterostomia als krankheit. Klin Wochenschr 1923; 2:1542–5.

13. Walters W, Chance DP, Berkson J. A comparison of vagotomy and gastric resection for gastrojejunal ulceration: a followup study of 301 cases. Surg Gynecol Obstet 1955; 100:1–10.

14. Zubiram JM, Kark AE, Montalbetti AJ, Morel CJL, Dragstedt LR. Quantitative studies on the effect of gastrojejunostomy on gastric secretion. Arch Surg 1952; 65:239–49.

15. Fisher AB. Twenty-five years after Billroth II gastrectomy for duodenal ulcer. World J Surg 1984; 8:293–302.

16. Dinbar A, Avigad I, Shafir R, Tulchinsky DB. Long-term results of subtotal gastrectomy for duodenal ulcer. World J Surg 1980; 4:625–33.

17. McCrea ED. The nerves of the stomach and their relation to surgery. Br J Surg 1926; 13:621–47.

18. Dragstedt LR, Owens FM. Supra-diaphragmatic section of the vagus nerves in treatment of duodenal ulcer. Proc Soc Exp Biol Med 1943; 53:152–4.

19. Dragstedt LR, Woodward ER, Neal WB Jr, Harper PV Jr, Storer EH. Secretory studies on the isolated stomach. Arch Surg 1950; 60:1–20.

20. Dragstedt LR. Peptic ulcer: an abnormality in gastric secretion. Am J Surg 1969; 117:143–56.

21. Moore JG, Englert E Jr. Circadian rhythm of gastric acid secretion in man. Nature 1970; 226:1261–2.

22. Moore JG, Wolfe M. The relation of plasma gastrin to the circadian rhythm of gastric acid secretion in man. Digestion 1973; 9:97–105.

23. Dragstedt LR, Harper PV Jr, Tovee EB, Woodward ER. Section of the vagus nerves to the stomach in the treatment of peptic ulcers. Ann Surg 1947; 126:687–708.

24. Farmer DA, Smithwick RH. Hemigastrectomy combined with resection of vagus nerves. N Engl J Med 1952; 247:1017–22.

25. Edwards LW, Herrington JL Jr. Vagotomy and gastroenterostomy—vagotomy and conservative gastrectomy: a comparative study. Ann Surg 1953; 137:873–83.

26. Woodward ER, Bigelow RR, Dragstedt LR. Quantitative study of effect of antrum resection on gastric secretion in Pavlov pouch dogs. Proc Soc Biol Med 1948; 68:473.

27. Franksson C. Selective abdominal vagotomy. Acta Chir Scand 1948; 96:409–12.

28. Griffith CA, Harkins HN. Partial gastric vagotomy: an experimental study. Gastroenterology 1957; 32:96–102.

29. Griffith CA. Long-term results of selective vagotomy plus pyloroplasty: 12 to 17 year followup. Am J Surg 1980; 139:608–15.

30. Holle VF, Hart W. Neue wege der chirurgie des gastrodudenalulkus. Med Klin 1967; 62:441–50.

31. Johnston D, Wilkinson AR. Selective vagotomy with innervated antrum without drainage procedure for duodenal ulcer. Br J Surg 1969; 56:626. Abstract.

32. Schrock TR. Vagotomy in the elective treatment of duodenal ulcer. Gastroenterology 1981; 68:1615–28.

33. O'Leary JP, Woodward ER, Hollenbeck JI, Dragstedt LR. Vagotomy and drainage procedure for duodenal ulcer: the results of seventeen years' experience. Ann Surg 1976; 183:613–8.

34. Mulholland M, Morrow C, Dunn DH, Schwartz ML, Humphrey EW. Surgical treatment of duodenal ulcer. A prospective randomized study. Arch Surg 1982; 117:393–7.

35. Clark CG, Fresini A, Aroyjo JGC, Boulos PB. Proximal gastric vagotomy or truncal vagotomy and drainage for chronic duodenal ulcer? Br J Surg 1986; 73:298–300.

36. Kelly KA. Effect of gastric surgery on gastric motility and emptying. In: Akkermans LMA, Johnson AG, Read NW, eds. Gastric and gastroduodenal motility. East Sussex, UK: Praeger, 1984:241–62.

37. Jordan PH Jr. Relationship between stimulating mechanisms of gastric secretion in dogs. JAMA 1967; 199:149–55.

38. Jordan PH Jr. A followup report of a prospective evaluation of vagotomy-pyloroplasty and vagotomy-antrectomy for treatment of duodenal ulcer. Ann Surg 1974; 180:259–64.

39. Ahmad W, Harbrecht PJ, Polk HC Jr. Leaks and obstruction after gastric resection. Am J Surg 1986; 152:301–7.

40. Yamagishi T, Debas HC. Control of gastric emptying: interaction of the vagus and pyloric antrum. Ann Surg 1978; 187:91–4.

41. Vogel SB, Vair DB, Woodward ER. Alterations in gastrointestinal emptying of 99m-technetium-labelled solids following sequential antrectomy-truncal vagotomy and Roux-en-Y gastroenterostomy. Ann Surg 1983; 198:506–15.

42. Doty JE, Meyer JH. Vagotomy and antrectomy impairs canine fat absorption from solid but not liquid dietary sources. Gastroenterology 1988; 94:50–6.

43. Herrington JL Jr, Scott WH Jr, Sawyer JL. Experience with vagotomy-antrectomy and Roux-en-Y gastrojejunostomy in surgical treatment of duodenal, gastric, and stomal ulcer. Ann Surg 1984; 199:590–7.

44. Karlquist PA, Anderberg B, Olaison G, Sjodahl R. Early and late results after antrectomy, selective vagotomy and Roux-en-Y reconstruction for severe peptic ulcer disease. Acta Chir Scand 1986; 152:357–61.

45. Vogel SB, Hocking MP, Woodward ER. Clinical and radionuclide evaluation of Roux-en-Y diversion for post-gastrectomy dumping. Am J Surg 1988; 155:57–62.

46. Boren CH, Way LW. Alkaline reflux gastritis: a re-evaluation. Am J Surg 1980; 14:40–6.

47. Hocking MP, Vogel SB, Falasca CA, Woodward ER. Delayed gastric emptying of liquid and solids following Roux-en-Y diversion. Ann Surg 1981; 194:494–9.

48. Selking O, Krause U, Nilsson F, Thoren L. Parietal cell vagotomy and truncal vagotomy as treatment of duodenal ulcer. Acta Chir Scand 1981; 147:561–7.

49. Von Holstein CS, Graffner H, Oscarson J. One hundred patients ten years after parietal cell vagotomy. Br J Surg 1987; 74:101–3.

50. Busman DC, Brombacher PJ, Munting JDK. Highly selective vagotomy and serum gastrin levels. Surg Gynecol Obstet 1987; 165:397–403.

51. Peptic ulceration: the eye of the cyclone. Editorial. Lancet 1986; ii:1015–6.

52. Hershlag A, Argov S. Parietal cell vagotomy II: the first decade: clinical considerations. Curr Surg 1983; March-April:93–104.

53. Boey J, Branicki FJ, Alagarathnam TT, Fok PJ, Poon A, Wong J. Proximal gastric vagotomy: the preferred operation for perforations in acute duodenal ulcer. Ann Surg 1988; 208:169–74.

54. Klein SR, Wethe JD, Rose DM, Long JB, White RA. Selective surgical management of perforated duodenal ulcer. Am Surg 1986; 52:500–3.

55. Hoak BA, Tiley E, Kusminsky R, Boland JP. Parietal cell vagotomy for bleeding duodenal ulcers. Ann Surg 1988; 54:249–52.

56. Adami H-O, Enander L-K, Enskog L, Ingvar C, Rydberg B. Recurrences 1 to 10 years after highly selective vagotomy in prepyloric and duodenal ulcer disease: frequency, pattern, and predictors. Ann Surg 1984; 199:393–9.

57. Graffner HO, Liedberg GF, Oscarson JEA. Recurrence after parietal cell vagotomy for peptic ulcer disease. Am J Surg 1985; 150:336–40.

58. Muller C, Liebermann-Meffert D, Allgower M. Pyloric and prepyloric ulcers. World J Surg 1987; 11:339–44.

59. Heberer G, Teichmann RK. Recurrence after proximal gastric vagotomy for gastric, pyloric, and prepyloric ulcers. World J Surg 1987; 11:283–8.

60. Andersen D, Amdrup E, Hostrup H, Sorensen FH. The Aarhus County vagotomy trial: trends in the problem of recurrent ulcer after parietal cell vagotomy and selective gastric vagotomy with drainage. World J Surg 1982; 6:86–92.

61. Jordan PH. Treatment of gastric ulcer by parietal cell vagotomy and excision of the ulcer: rationale and early results. Arch Surg 1981; 116:1320–3.

62. Johnson HD. Gastric ulcer, classification, blood group characteristics, secretion patterns, and pathogenesis. Ann Surg 1965; 162:996–1004.

63. Rehnberg O. Antrectomy and gastroduodenostomy with or without vagotomy in peptic ulcer disease. A prospective study with a 5 year followup. Acta Chir Scand 1983; 515(Suppl):1–63.

64. Greenall MJ, Lehnert T. Vagotomy or gastrectomy for elective treatment of benign gastric ulcerations. Dig Dis Sci 1985; 30:353–61.

65. Kelling G. Ueber die operative behandlung des chronischen ulces ventriculi. Arch Klin Chir 1918; 109:775–813.

66. Madlener M. Ueber pylorektomi bie pylorusfernem magengeschwir. Zentralbl Chir 1923; 50:131–7.

67. Donahue PE, Nyhus LM. Surgical excision of gastric ulcer near the gastroesophageal junction. Surg Gynecol Obstet 1982; 155:85–8.

68. Rogers PN, Murray WR, Shaw R, Brar S. Surgical management of bleeding gastric ulceration. Br J Surg 1988; 75:16–7.

69. Kraft RO. Long-term results of vagotomy and pyloroplasty in the treatment of gastric ulcer disease. Surgery 1984; 95:460–6.

70. Reid DA, Duthie HL, Branson CJ, Johnson AG. Late results of highly selective vagotomy with excision of the ulcer compared with Billroth I gastrectomy for treatment of benign gastric ulcer. Br J Surg 1982; 69:605–7.

71. Emas S, Hammarberg C. Prospective, randomized trial of selective proximal vagotomy with ulcer excision and partial gastrectomy with gastroduodenostomy in the treatment of corporeal gastric ulcer. Am J Surg 1983; 146:631–4.

72. Mulholland MW, Debas HT. Chronic duodenal and gastric ulcer. Surg Clin North Am 1987; 67:489–507.

73. Jensen MO, Bubrick MP, Onstad GR, Hitchcock CR. Changes in the surgical treatment of acid peptic disease. Am Surg 1985; 51:556–8.

74. Larson GM, Davidson PR. The decline in surgery for peptic ulcer disease. J Ky Med Assoc 1986; May:233–6.

75. Alagaratnam TT, Wong J. No decrease in duodenal ulcer surgery after cimetidine in Hong Kong. J Clin Gastroenterol 1988; 10:25–7.

76. Walker LG Jr. Trends in the surgical management of duodenal ulcer: a fifteen year study. Am J Surg 1988; 155:436–8.

77. Gear MWL. Proximal gastric vagotomy versus long-term maintenance treatment with cimetidine for chronic duodenal ulcer: a prospective randomized trial. Br Med J 1983; 286:98–9.

78. Strom M, Lindhagen J, Bodemar G, Sjodahl R, Walan A. Cimetidine or parietal-cell vagotomy in patients with juxtapyloric ulcers. Lancet 1984; ii:897.

79. Harling H, Balslev I, Bentzen E. Parietal cell vagotomy or cimetidine maintenance therapy for duodenal ulcer? A prospective controlled trial. Scand J Gastroenterol 1988; 20:747–50.

80. Hoffmann J, Olesen A, Jensen H-E. Prospective 14- to 18-year follow-up study after parietal cell vagotomy. Br J Surg 1987; 74:1056–9.

81. Debas HT. Proximal gastric vagotomy interferes with a fundic inhibitory mechanism: a hypothesis for the high recurrence rate of peptic ulceration. Am J Surg 1983; 146:51–6.

82. Wittebol P, Akkermans LMA, Hulstaert PF. Prognostic factors in surgery for duodenal ulcer. Surg Annu 1985; 17:235–47.

83. Primrose JN, Axon ATR, Johnston D. Highly selective vagotomy and duodenal ulcers that fail to respond to H_2 receptor antagonist. Br Med J 1988; 296:1031–5.

84. Donahue PE, Bombeck CT, Yoshida Y, Nyhus LM. Endoscopic Congo red test during proximal gastric vagotomy. Am J Surg 1987; 153:249–55.

85. Braghetto I, Csendes A, Lazo M, Rebolledo P, Diaz A, Bardavid A, Bahamonde A, Thomet G. A prospective, randomized study comparing highly selective vagotomy and extended highly selective vagotomy in patients with duodenal ulcer. Am J Surg 1988; 155:443–6.

86. Lygidakis NG. Posterior truncal vagotomy and anterior curve superficial seromyotomy as an alternative for the surgical management of chronic ulcer of the duodenum. Surg Gynecol Obstet 1984; 158:251–4.

87. Taylor TV, Gunn AA, MacLeod DAD, et al. Mortality and morbidity after anterior lesser curve seromyotomy with posterior truncal vagotomy for duodenal ulcer. Br J Surg 1985; 72:950–1.

88. Oostvogel HJM, VanVroonhoven JMV. Anterior lesser curve seromyotomy with posterior truncal vagotomy versus proximal gastric vagotomy. Br J Surg 1988; 75:121–4.

89. Becker JM, Kelly KA, Haddad AC, Zinsmeister AR. Proximal gastric vagotomy and mucosal antrectomy. A possible operative approach to duodenal ulcer. Surgery 1983; 94:58–64.

90. Olinde AJ, Maher JW, McGuigan JE, Patel BR. Proximal gastric vagotomy and mucosal antrectomy: a comparative physiologic examination. J Surg Res 1985; 38:350–5.

91. Jordan GL Jr. Recurrence after highly selective vagotomy should be treated by gastric resection. Am J Surg 1986; 152:312–3.

92. Hoffman J, Shokouh-Amiri MH, Klarskov P, Madsen OG, Jensen HE. Gastrectomy for recurrent ulcer after vagotomy: five- to nineteen-year follow-up. Surgery 1986; 99:517–22.

HUMAN INVESTIGATION

18

Statistical Methods in Trials of Anti-Ulcer Drugs

JANET D. ELASHOFF

University of California, Los Angeles, and
Cedars-Sinai Medical Center, Los Angeles, California

GARY G. KOCH

School of Public Health, University of North Carolina,
Chapel Hill, North Carolina

I. INTRODUCTION

This chapter is intended to be helpful to people involved in planning and conducting a clinical trial of an anti-ulcer drug or in reviewing the results of published trials. For these clinical trials, the range of research questions includes the following.

1. What degree and duration of acid suppression are achieved by a drug?
2. How does the proportion of patients with acute peptic ulcer who heal within a fixed period of time (usually 2–8 weeks for duodenal ulcer and 6–14 weeks for gastric ulcer) compare with the proportion healed on placebo or another active drug?
3. What degree and/or duration of symptom relief is achieved with a drug for relief of "ulcer pain," relief of "heartburn," relief of symptoms attributed to reflux esophagitis, or other related conditions?
4. How long do treated patients remain free of symptoms and/or ulcers after short-term healing?
5. Does the use of a drug in a maintenance regimen increase the time to

symptomatic recurrence, reduce ulcer prevalence, prevent ulcer recurrence, and/or prevent ulcer complications such as rebleeding?

6.   Is a drug safe for use in the intended population?

We outline statistical issues that merit attention in the design, conduct, analysis, and reporting of clinical trials in general and specifically emphasize methods appropriate in trials of anti-ulcer drugs. We consider these statistical issues first in the context of trials to assess short-term ulcer healing, and then we deal with issues and methods for maintenance or recurrence trials and touch briefly on studies of acid suppression or *Helicobacter pylori* inhibition. The reader will find more complete discussion of the topics in this chapter in the accompanying references; in particular, see references 1–7.

We encourage readers planning their own trial protocols to make use of the previous experience of others, to read reports of well-conducted trials, and to convene an Advisory Committee during the planning stages. The Advisory Committee should include members with statistical expertise as well as members with experience in conducting the type of trial under consideration. If drug approval is one goal of the trial, consulting the relevant regulatory agency during protocol development can often be worthwhile. In general, regulatory agencies require well-defined, well-documented scientific studies, but what is considered sufficient for approval may change as knowledge in a specific area increases.

II.   STATISTICAL CONSIDERATIONS FOR ULCER HEALING TRIALS

In a typical ulcer healing trial, we study patients with endoscopic evidence of acute ulcer disease to compare a test drug and a control drug for the proportion of patients who show endoscopic evidence of healing after a fixed treatment period. The control drug is either placebo or another active drug according to the objectives of the study. In this section, we discuss methods for the design, conduct, analysis, and reporting of these ulcer healing trials.

A.   Design

The design of a clinical trial for an anti-ulcer drug should be based on specification of the goals of therapy. Different goals or different models for the disease process will suggest different trial designs. Important design areas include specification of study population, treatment groups, and response variables; determination of sample size; and plans for any interim analyses.

1.   Study Population and Generalizability

Selection of the patient group to study involves a balance between generalizability (i.e., making the group studied as representative as possible of the potential end-user population) and homogeneity (i.e., reducing between-patient variability in the study). Conducting the study at multiple centers will increase generalizability but may also weaken homogeneity and present more management and analytic problems. Marked differences in placebo healing rates across sites within a study are frequently observed; in particular, placebo healing rates for studies conducted in the United States are often higher than for studies in other countries.

Inclusion and exclusion criteria must be carefully considered with respect to the trade-offs between generalizability and homogeneity and clearly stated in the study protocol. Typically, entry criteria are stated with respect to age, women of child-bearing age, ulcer diagnosis (duodenal, gastric, prepyloric), number and size of ulcers at entry, patient use of other medications such as NSAIDs, presence of multiple medical problems, recent treatment with other anti-ulcer drugs, and previous ulcer surgery or complications. Decisions such as whether to allow patients concomitant antacid use also affect the generalizability of study results.

Since inclusion and exclusion criteria as well as patient willingness to participate can markedly restrict patient entry, it is good practice to maintain and report a log of those patients screened for the study and not enrolled, with the reasons for their exclusion. The case report forms for the data from enrolled patients should include information on demographic and background variables so that the study population can be described in the report and the comparability of the treatment groups assessed.

2. Comparability

The major basis for assuming comparability of the treatment groups in trials of anti-ulcer drugs is provided by blinded and random assignments of patients to groups. Moreover, the use of random assignment for this purpose is even more important when it is difficult or impossible to maintain double blinding during treatment. In acute ulcer healing trials of anti-ulcer drugs, treatment assignments are typically made through coded medications that have been prepared with a blocked randomization scheme within each site. The block size should be small enough to ensure balance at an early stage but large enough to prevent guessing of the next assignment. Blocks of size 6 are often used for studies with two treatment groups, and blocks of size 9 for those with three treatment groups. It is occasionally desirable to vary the block size within a study.

Treatment assignments may be stratified on factors known to be important in prediction of patient healing. Stratification ensures balance between the treatment groups on these factors but leads to increased management and analytic complexity. At this time, the major factors worth considering as stratifying variables are smoking and severity of ulcer disease.

Clinical trials of anti-ulcer drugs should be double-blind. Neither the patient, the person dispensing the medication to the patient, nor the person(s) assessing patient symptoms and endoscopic healing should be aware of the treatment assignment. Typically the medications are prepared in coded bottles or packs by a pharmacist unconnected with the conduct of the study. Placebo medication should be identical in taste and appearance to the active medication. In studies with two active treatments that cannot be made to appear identical, a double dummy technique can be used; that is, a placebo identical to each active treatment is prepared and patients are randomly assigned to receive one active treatment and the placebo counterpart of the other active treatment (e.g., see Gough et al. [8]). Trials of bismuth present problems of maintaining the blind for the patient and for the endoscopist because of the mucosal and stool blackening that occurs in many patients. In such circumstances, it is important to ensure that study outcomes are as objectively measured as possible and to consider approaches such as using an endoscopist not involved in other aspects of the trial.

The treatment groups should receive identical management in every respect aside from the administered drug, and the methods for their evaluation should be identical also. Equivalence of study procedures for all patients is more assured when double blinding is effective. Lack of equivalence can cause bias, which can undermine the validity of a study.

3. Choice of Treatment Groups

For simplicity of management and analysis, an ulcer healing trial would compare an optimum dose of the test drug with a placebo. For a trial that compares a test drug only to another active drug to demonstrate equivalence, the precision necessary for results to be convincing will require more patients than a trial comparing an active drug to placebo (see Sec. II.A.5). Moreover, whether a trial can validly demonstrate efficacy without a placebo group is an important question (see references 9,10).

Inclusion of multiple doses of the test drug enlarges the trial and leads to issues of multiplicity of comparisons (see Sec. II.C.5). In multiple-dose studies where the group sizes are relatively small, the relationship between dose and response may remain unclear even after thorough analysis of results.

Some studies are now being designed to evaluate combination therapies. A question that often requires attention in the design of these studies is whether the combination is more effective than either component. Thus, a study for a combination therapy requires sufficiently many groups for this purpose (e.g, a 2×2 factorial design for combinations with two active components); see [11] and [12] for additional discussion.

4. Response Variables

The primary response variable in acute ulcer healing trials has been the time at which ulcer healing was first observed, where endoscopic assessments of healing status were made on a fixed schedule, for example, at one or more of the times 2, 4, 6, and 8 weeks. Typically, patients have been withdrawn from further assessment after initial healing. However, due to the possibility of misclassification and early relapse, we note that a patient with endoscopic healing at 2 weeks cannot strictly be considered as "healed at 4 weeks" but rather as "first healed prior to 4 weeks." A formal assessment of healing prevalence at 4 weeks would require that all patients be endoscoped at 4 weeks regardless of their healing status at 2 weeks.

An important issue in planning an ulcer healing trial is selection of the time points at which patient symptom status and endoscopic healing status will be evaluated. Time points should be chosen with regard to matching other studies, maximizing information about the healing rate, and minimizing the number of procedures a patient must face. The maximum difference in percentages healed on different treatments is typically seen after 4 weeks for duodenal ulcer and at 8 weeks for gastric ulcer. Measurements of ulcer size or assessments of percent of the ulcer healed are currently too unreliable to qualify as a primary outcome measure. Should this situation change, their analysis would require different procedures than those for healing rates, and reduction in the necessary sample size might be possible.

Typical secondary outcome measures in healing trials are patient-reported symptoms and antacid use. Data for symptoms are usually obtained through questions about frequency, duration, and severity of ulcer-related pain during the day and night, with the ones for severity involving a choice among adjectives such as mild, moderate, or severe relative to normal daily activities or a marking of a 10-cm analogue scale. In general, the additional information potentially available when patients fill in symptom diaries is not sufficient to outweigh the logistic complications involved in trying to ensure completion of the diaries, coding the extensive resulting data, developing an arbitrary weighting and summarization of the daily scores, and dealing with missing data. Even the effort to measure frequency, severity, and duration of ulcer pain separately may not generally provide much extra information, because they are usually markedly skewed and fairly highly correlated; consideration of summary variables such as their product is usually sufficient.

A problem of definition in symptoms is that some patients may report no "ulcer" symptoms even though they have other noteworthy conditions such as severe nausea. Additional problems for the analysis and interpretation of data for symptoms as well as antacid usage come from their repeated measures character and its incomplete nature for patients who leave the trial because of early healing or withdrawal for some other reason. An issue for those lost to follow-up is their tendency to consist largely of patients either with no symptoms or with severe symptoms, and so any resulting bias has unclear direction.

Patient compliance is typically assessed by counting pills returned at follow-up visits; such methods can lead to much missing data when patients forget to bring in the unused pills, and patients can easily fake good compliance if they wish. Alternatively, measurements of blood levels at intervals of two or more weeks may not be very representative of overall compliance. Better quality for compliance data may require developing technological devices for unobtrusive measurement of medication usage.

Outcome criteria concerned with safety include complications, adverse events, and abnormal laboratory values (e.g., liver function tests) or vital signs.

5. Sample Size

Substantial consideration must go into planning the sample size for a clinical trial. If the sample size is larger than necessary, both time and effort are wasted. Too large a sample size, however, is seldom a problem—most trials are too small. A trial with a sample size that is too small can end inconclusively or can result in misleading conclusions. A promising new drug may be erroneously discarded because it did not test significantly different from placebo, or a new drug may be considered equivalent to the standard when in fact there are noteworthy differences. In determining sample size for an ulcer healing trial, we must distinguish between trials in which a new active drug is being tested against a placebo and "equivalence trials" in which a new active drug is being tested against a standard active drug.

Consider first the case in which a new active drug is being tested against a placebo and the primary outcome is duodenal ulcer healing at 4 weeks. On the basis of past experience, 40–50% of patients on placebo and 70–80% on the standard dose of an H_2 blocker such as cimetidine or ranitidine might be expected to be healed in 4 weeks (see [4]). A simple table (see [13, pp. 260–280] or [14]) can be used to find out what sample sizes will be necessary. If the new drug is at least as effective as an H_2 blocker, 45–50 patients per group will be needed to obtain an 80% chance that the study will yield a significant difference between the new drug and the placebo at the two-sided $p \leq .05$ level.

The comparison of a new active drug to a standard active drug presents a different problem. A clinician may prefer the new drug if it is definitely more effective than the standard and may disregard it if it is definitely worse. Often the investigator will be interested in using the new drug for some subjects if it is "at least as good" as the standard. Thus, a trial might be planned in which the new drug would be accepted for future use if it is not significantly worse than the standard. This is a very weak conclusion, however, especially if sample sizes are small. For example, suppose a duodenal ulcer healing trial comparing a new drug to a standard drug was conducted with 40 patients per group and approximately 70% of the subjects in each treatment group were observed to have a healed ulcer by 4 weeks. How firm is the conclusion from the equivalent results in this study that the new drug will prove in the future to be at least as good as the standard? In this case, a 95% confidence interval for the difference between treatments would run from -23% to $+23\%$ (see [13, p. 29]); that is, one can reasonably conclude that the new drug would result in healing rates no more than 23% lower than those for the standard drug. Is this close enough to conclude that the two drugs are equivalent? Probably not, because H_2 blockers typically yield healing rates only 30–40% higher than placebo.

Suppose that we assume that the standard active drug will result in 70% healing at 4 weeks. Blackwelder and Chang [15] show how to set up null and alternative hypotheses for testing equivalence. Here, we will consider the two drugs equivalent if the difference in favor of the standard drug is $\leq 15\%$, that is, a healing rate $\geq 55\%$ for the new drug is compatible with equivalence. We test this alternative hypothesis versus the null hypothesis that the standard drug is better than the new drug by $\geq 15\%$ (i.e, the healing rate for the new drug is $\leq 55\%$). A one-sided test at the 0.025 significance level and with 80% power against the alternative that the difference is zero (i.e., both healing rates are 70%) would require 160–175 subjects per group [13, pp. 33–49; 14]; a one-sided test at the 0.05 level would require 125–140 subjects per group.

Determinations of sample size must also depend on practical issues. These include how long it will take a subject to complete the trial, what rates of subject accrual can be expected, and what the dropout rate is likely to be. In this regard dropout rates of 10–20% are typical in duodenal ulcer healing trials. If we were to allow for 15% dropout in the previously discussed sample size projections, we might specify a total of 56 subjects per group for a trial with placebo and 200 patients per group for a trial to show equivalence at the one-sided 0.025 level.

An additional sample size problem arises in stratified or multicenter trials. A minimum sample size per center should be specified to allow at least informal evaluation of between-strata homogeneity for treatment differences, for example, at least five patients per treatment in each center of a multicenter study. To obtain reasonable power in a test of center by treatment interaction (i.e., lack of homogeneity), 20–30 subjects per treatment per center would be necessary. Some pooling of centers may be desirable when sample sizes per center are small, but it should be specified prior to analysis. In addition, one should avoid the situation where only one center has a reasonably large sample size and dominates the study, because of difficulties in interpretation if the results for this center conflict with those for the other centers.

When a study has two or more time points for response evaluation, sample size determination is usually based on the one that is considered primary. However, if more than one is of interest, then the corresponding multiplicity can be taken into account by use of a Bonferroni adjustment [16, p. 337]; that is, use $\alpha/$(number of time points) as the significance level in the sample size determination, although this will necessitate larger sample sizes. If only a combined test across time points will be made, some strength and power will be gained from analyses of this ordered outcome measure as primary.

For studies with more than two treatment groups, several methods for sample size determination are available. A straightforward strategy is to consider all pairwise comparisons and use the maximum sample size per group obtained using the previously described methods. The p value for each comparison can be chosen on the basis of Bonferroni adjustments for multiple comparisons. When the multiple treatments are multiple doses, such adjustments are not required when the primary objective is a test of linear or monotonic relationship. Studies with multiple treatment groups not only have the logistical problems of a more complex study design, but their large sample sizes may also require the inclusion of more centers or extension of the period of patient recruitment. This can introduce more heterogeneity into the study, which can further increase sample size. Another consideration when comparisons between doses are of interest is that the smaller differences expected between doses can make the required sample sizes for each group more comparable to those for testing for equivalence than to those for comparisons with placebo.

6. Interim Analyses

If data for a clinical trial are to be analyzed during the course of the trial and a decision to stop or to continue is to be made on the basis of results for the primary outcome, a formal stopping rule and plan for the interim analysis should be developed as part of the trial design [17–19]. For example, the O'Brien and Fleming [19] rule specifies that a significance test at the 0.005 level is used after half the planned number of patients have completed the trial. If results are significant, the trial is stopped; if results are not significant, the trial is completed and the final significance tests are conducted at the 0.0475 level.

An interim analysis might be planned not to focus on the primary outcome but to verify data entry and analysis procedures and to focus on safety issues. Here control of the type I error is not the central issue, and testing of adverse event or side-effect frequencies for higher rates with the test drug might be done each time at the one-sided 0.05 level. A monitoring committee should be appointed to review the results of the interim analyses. Since ulcer disease is usually not life-threatening and one generally knows about what to expect in terms of healing rates before the trial begins, planned interim analyses are often not included in the design of acute ulcer healing trials.

B. Conduct of Trial, Data Collection, and Management

Before beginning an ulcer healing trial, it is important to develop a clear, detailed protocol spelling out inclusion and exclusion criteria and detailing what to do in the case of protocol violations. A multicenter trial will require meetings between the principals (including endoscopists and research nurses) to review the details of the protocol and data forms both before the trial begins and again soon after the trial starts to go over questions and problems.

Construction of good case report forms that include all the necessary information with no excess and are easy to use and interpret is a demanding task that may require many iterations. In view of the many ulcer healing trials that have been conducted, new trials should build on forms already developed for past trials. Before the trial begins, forms should be pilot tested on a few patients by those expected to use them. If it is expected or later discovered that a variable will frequently be unrecorded, its later usefulness is likely to be so limited that it should be deleted from data collection efforts.

Plans should be made for prompt data entry and error checking. This will facilitate early discovery of protocol deviations, problems in filling in the form, and identification of missing, out-of-range, or logically incorrect data. Edited files should be constructed for statistical analysis. It is useful to organize these files according to background characteristics of patients, response variables for efficacy, and adverse events and laboratory tests for safety.

C. Analysis

The statistical evaluation of data from a clinical trial has several components. These include the specification of the population(s) for inference, description of the demographic and pretreatment characteristics of the patient population, comparisons among treatments for efficacy variables (e.g., ulcer healing rates), exploration of the sensitivity of efficacy findings to aspects of the patient population (e.g., heterogeneity across centers or subgroups) or to the conduct of the trial (e.g., patterns of patient withdrawal from the study or of missing data), and comparisons among treatments for safety variables (e.g., adverse event prevalences). In this section, we outline some appropriate methods for addressing these components of analysis for acute ulcer healing trials. To illustrate these methods, we apply them to data adapted from an actual clinical trial. As a convenience for presentation, we occasionally illustrate more than one method with different adaptations of the same data; however, the reader should note that in practice the appropriate analyses are determined by the actual study design.

1. Specification of Population(s) for Inference

If all patients entered into a clinical trial complete the trial with no protocol violations and no missing data, then they comprise one population for the analyses of efficacy and safety. Most studies, however, have patients who withdraw before completion, are in violation of the protocol because of poor compliance (use of excluded concomitant medications, for example), or are missing data for primary response variables because of missed visits, visits at times outside the scheduled limits, or missing determinations at a visit. Because of these inconsistencies, statistical analysis may need to be done for two or more populations. These populations usually include:

1. A *safety population* of all patients who took at least one dose of the assigned treatment
2. An *intent-to-treat population* of all patients who took at least one dose of the assigned treatment and have minimal efficacy data (e.g., at least one endoscopy during treatment)
3. A *protocol-compatible population* of all patients who took at least one dose of the assigned treatment, have minimal efficacy data, and have no noteworthy protocol violations

The reader should note that intent-to-treat and protocol-compatible populations can each have more than one definition. For example, for the intent-to-treat population, minimal efficacy data may range from none to complete; and for the protocol-compatible population, exclusions due to protocol violations can range from major violations to any violation. In view of the many definitions that are possible, we recommend that the ones chosen be stated a priori in the statistical analysis section of the study protocol. At a minimum, they should be defined before the unblinding of treatments. When the intent-to-treat population contains only a few more patients than the protocol-compatible population, it is usually sufficient to report the analysis only for the population in which results favor the test treatment the least. Consideration of both types of populations is of the most interest when they differ as much as reasonably possible—that is, with a less restrictive criterion for minimal efficacy data to maximize the number of patients in the intent-to-treat population and a more restrictive criterion for protocol violations to minimize the number of patients in the protocol-compatible population.

2.   Description of the Patient Population

For the safety population and any inferential population that is more than a few patients smaller, the distributions of patient demographic and pretreatment characteristics are described for each of the randomized groups. Frequency tables and percentages are used to describe the distributions of categorical variables (e.g., gender, ethnic origin, smoking history, alcohol consumption, previous ulcer history, ratings of baseline pain symptoms). The distributions of continuous variables (e.g., age, weight, duration of ulcer history, etc.) are often described with means, standard errors, and minimum and maximum values.

These pretreatment characteristics are often evaluated for the degree of equivalence between the randomized groups. In a study with two treatments and no stratification, the usual methods for these comparisons are Fisher's exact test for dichotomous variables (e.g., gender), the Wilcoxon rank-sum test (with midranks to manage ties) for ordered categorical variables (e.g., baseline pain), and two-sample t-tests for continuous variables with relatively symmetrical distributions. For continuous variables with strongly asymmetrical distributions, comparisons between randomized groups can be made using two-sample t-tests after appropriate transformations such as square roots or logarithms, or using Wilcoxon rank-sum tests. For a study with stratification, the counterparts to these methods are the Mantel-Haenszel test for dichotomous variables, the extended Mantel-Haenszel test for ordered categorical variables, and two-way analysis of variance relative to treatments and strata for continuous variables. Some references for the previously mentioned methods are [5], [13], [16], and [20].

In a study with more than two treatments and at least moderately large sample sizes for each (e.g., $n \geq 30$), the evaluation of pretreatment equivalence of the randomized groups might be based on applying the previously described methods to all possible pairwise comparisons (or perhaps on only the subset of primary interest for efficacy). Overall comparisons can be made with multigroup extensions of the methods for two-group comparisons. For a study with no stratification, these are the chi-square test (as an approximation to the multigroup Fisher's exact test) for dichotomous variables, the Kruskal-Wallis test for ordered categorical variables, and one-way analysis of variance for continuous variables. Stratified counterparts of these methods are multigroup versions of the extended Mantel-Haenszel test [5, pp. 418–421] and two-way analysis of variance.

Since some multidose studies have small sample sizes at each of many doses, comparisons among the randomized groups do not provide much information about pretreatment equivalence. The Spearman rank correlation test [5, p. 414] for dose versus any demographic or pretreatment variable that is dichotomous, ordered categorical, or continuous is an effective method for a study with no stratification. For stratified studies, extended Mantel-Haenszel counterparts of this method are applicable.

The results of analyses of pretreatment equivalence between treatment groups require careful interpretation. Since, for the safety population, the groups have been formed by randomization, any "statistically significant" results are presumably due to chance. For other populations, however, differences between groups could also result from factors related to early study withdrawal, noncompliance, etc. In any case, to assess the degree to which any imbalance in pretreatment characteristics may favor one treatment over the other, it is helpful to contrast the results of analyses in which treatment groups are compared after adjustment for differences in pretreatment variables to the results of analyses in which no adjustments are made. The conservative approach is to base conclusions on the analysis that results in the smallest apparent effect of the test drug. When sample sizes are appropriately large and stratification has been used for factors with strong relationships to response variables, the results of adjusted and unadjusted analyses should be similar.

3. Comparisons of Efficacy Variables among Treatments

For acute ulcers, primary treatment efficacy is evaluated with endoscopic assessments of healing status at one or more scheduled visits. We illustrate the structure of this information in Table 1 with data adapted from a report by Hirschowitz et al. [21] for a 6-week trial for the healing of benign gastric ulcer.

This multicenter, randomized, double-blind trial for the comparison of a test drug and placebo had scheduled endoscopic assessments of patient healing at 2 weeks and 6 weeks. All patients continued on treatment up to the endoscopy at 6 weeks whether healed at 2 weeks or not. Since Hirschowitz et al. [21] reported only data pooled over the centers, we analyze data from Table 1 using methods for a single-center study. In this setting, the number of patients in the two groups provide about 80% power for the detection of 20% differences at the two-sided 0.05 significance level.

Note that in Table 1 the healing status of 19 patients was nonevaluable at 2 weeks, and for 46 patients it was nonevaluable at 6 weeks. Hirschowitz et al. [21] indicate that the reasons patients were nonevaluable included patient dropout because of

Table 1   Data for Endoscopic Assessments in 6-Week Trial for Healing Benign Gastric Ulcer

Treatment	Number healed		Number nonevaluable		Number not healed, 6 wk[a]	Total
	2 wk[a]	6 wk[a]	2 wk[a]	6 wk[a]		
Placebo	12	40	11	27	35	102
Test drug	18	56	8	19	26	101

[a]2 weeks encompasses 14 ± 4 days, and 6 weeks encompasses 42 ± 8 days.
Source: Adapted from Hirschowitz et al. [21].

worsening ulcer disease, adverse event, unrelated illness or some other reason, invalid endoscopy because of omission or excessively early or late performance, and protocol violations. The presence of nonevaluable patients for any reason always complicates the analysis and interpretation of the data for ulcer healing, because the healing status of these patients is unclear or unknown. Moreover, the ambiguity in conclusions resulting from a high prevalence of patients classified as nonevaluable (e.g., $\geq 50\%$) can undermine the validity of a study.

a. **Analysis of Healing at 6 Weeks.** One way to manage patients classified as nonevaluable is to designate them as "not healed." This convention has an intent-to-treat spirit, because analysis of healing can then include all patients who received treatment. For the primary endpoint of 6 weeks, the healing rates are 39.2% (40/102) for placebo and 55.4% (56/101) for test drug. We use Fisher's exact test for (2 × 2) contingency tables to compare these rates [5, pp. 405–409]; the resulting two-sided p-value is 0.025. Alternatively, the moderately large sample sizes in this study make the continuity-corrected chi-square test [13, pp. 19–24] nearly equivalent to Fisher's exact test. For this test, we compute

$$Q = \frac{\left\{ \left| \left(\frac{56}{101} - \frac{40}{102} \right) \right| - \frac{1}{2}\left(\frac{1}{101} + \frac{1}{102} \right) \right\}^2}{\left\{ \left(\frac{96}{203} \right)\left(\frac{107}{203} \right)\left(\frac{1}{101} + \frac{1}{102} \right) \right\}} = 4.73$$

and determine its two-sided $p = 0.030$ from the chi-square distribution with one degree of freedom. Since $p \leq .05$ for both of these methods, we interpret the difference between test drug and placebo as statistically significant. We further describe the extent of this difference with a two-sided, continuity-corrected, 95% confidence interval [13, pp. 29–30]

$$\left(\frac{56}{101} - \frac{40}{102}\right) \pm \left\{1.96\left[\frac{(56)(45)}{(101)^3} + \frac{(40)(62)}{(102)^3}\right]^{\frac{1}{2}} \right.$$

$$\left. + \frac{1}{2}\left(\frac{1}{101} + \frac{1}{102}\right)\right\} = .162 \pm .145$$

$$= (.017, .307) \text{ or } (1.7\%, 30.7\%)$$

This confidence interval supports the conclusion that the test drug has a significantly higher rate of healing at 6 weeks than placebo, but its wide range expresses some uncertainty about the magnitude of this treatment effect. A larger sample size would have provided a narrower confidence interval, but usually the principal objective of a placebo-controlled study is only to demonstrate that the test drug is better than placebo, and not to define how much better.

A limitation of designating nonevaluable patients as not healed is that it causes underestimation of healing rates. Moreover, for the data in Table 1, the underestimation is probably greater for placebo, because 26.5% (27/102) of the placebo group were nonevaluable at 6 weeks compared to 18.8% (19/101) for the test drug. Another approach is to manage nonevaluable classifications as missing data. This convention has a protocol-compatible spirit because it excludes patients with nonevaluable healing status from analyses as protocol violators. Excluding patients nonevaluable at 6 weeks, we obtain healing rates of 53.3% (40/75) for placebo and 68.3% (56/82) for test drug; and for Fisher's exact test to compare these rates, two-sided $p = .071$. The results for this analysis are similar to those obtained by managing nonevaluable healing status as not healed, because the prevalences of nonevaluable healing status at 6 weeks are similar for the two treatment groups (Fisher's exact test comparing these prevalences yields two-sided $p = .241$).

   b.   **Analysis of Healing at 2 Weeks.**   Analyses of healing at 2 weeks would be the same as those for healing at 6 weeks. However, their role would be descriptive rather than inferential, because healing at 2 weeks is a secondary response variable in the study of Hirschowitz et al. [21]. If both were considered primary response variables, analyses of healing at 2 weeks and healing at 6 weeks could be adjusted for multiplicity of testing by using the .025 level rather than the .05 level.

   c.   **Analysis of Time to First Healing.**   An effective way to use the information for both 2 weeks and 6 weeks without any adjustment for multiple comparisons is to specify time to first healing as the primary response variable. This criterion has an ordinal nature, with first healing at 2 weeks as the best response, first healing at 6 weeks as the second best response, and not healed at either 2 or 6 weeks as the worst response. However, when patients are nonevaluable at either 2 or 6 weeks, only partial orderings are possible. For example, a patient who is not healed at 2 weeks and is not evaluable at 6 weeks has a poorer response than a patient who is healed at 2 weeks, but has unknown ordering relative to both a patient who is not healed at 2 weeks and is known to be unhealed at 6 weeks and a patient who is not healed at 2 weeks and is known to be healed at 6 weeks. We use the Mantel-Haenszel statistic [5, pp. 436–442; 22] to compare treatments in a way that accounts for this partial ordering. We consider the healing status of two "risk sets" of patients: (1) 2-week healing for all those entering the study and (2) 6-week healing for those not healed at 2 weeks. The first row in Table 2 shows the healing status at 2 weeks for those patients evaluable at 2 weeks (91 placebo and 93 test drug patients). Deleting those healed at 2 weeks, $102 - 12 = 90$ placebo patients and $101 - 18 = 83$ test drug patients were at risk for healing at 6 weeks; $90 - 27 = 63$ were evaluable in the placebo group, and $83 - 19 = 64$ were evaluable in the test drug group. Assuming for the sake of this example that all the patients known to have healed at 2 weeks were evaluated and shown to be healed also at 6 weeks (although this may not be strictly true), we find that of these numbers 28 in the placebo group and 38 in the test drug group were healed at 6 weeks but not at 2 weeks.

To obtain the Mantel-Haenszel statistic, we proceed as shown in Table 2 to determine within each risk set the number of patients healed on test drug together with its expected value and its variance under the hypothesis of no difference between treatments, and then we add these quantities across the risk sets. The Mantel-Haenszel statistic is

$$Q_{\mathrm{MH}} = \frac{(\text{observed sum healed} - \text{expected sum healed})^2}{\text{variance}}$$

$$= (56 - 48.5)^2/14.30 = 4.02$$

and has approximately the chi-square distribution with one degree of freedom. Two-sided $p = .045$ for Q_{MH} indicates that the difference between test drug and placebo is statistically significant.

The Mantel-Haenszel test is also applicable when patients classified as nonevalu-

Table 2   Data Structure and Results for Analysis of Time to First Healing in 6-Week Trial for Benign Gastric Ulcer

Risk set	Placebo		Test drug		Expected healed for test drug	Variance of healed for test drug
	Healed	Total	Healed	Total		
2 weeks	12	91	18	93	$93(30)/184 = 15.2$	$\dfrac{15.2(91)(154)}{184(183)} = 6.31$
6 weeks	28	63	38	64	$64(66)/127 = 33.3$	$\dfrac{33.3(63)(61)}{127(126)} = 7.99$
Total			56		48.5	14.30

able are analyzed as not healed. In this case, $Q_{MH} = 5.31$ with $p = .021$ reinforces the conclusion of a significant treatment difference.

d.   Analysis of Symptoms and Antacid Use.   Data for symptoms of ulcer pain and antacid use are obtained from patients at each of the visits of an ulcer healing study, for example, at 1, 2, 4, and 6 weeks in the study reported by Hirschowitz et al. [21]. The data for symptoms are typically dichotomous classifications for presence versus absence of pain; or ordinal scores for frequency, duration, severity of pain; or a pain index composed of some combination, such as the product, of these ordinal scores. The data for antacid use are typically estimates of tablets used per day based on counts of unused tablets at each visit. Appropriate methods for comparison between treatment groups in accordance with these differing measurement scales have been outlined in Section II.C.2.

The common practice of comparing symptom scores at all visits and displaying time curves for average symptom scores is undesirable in two respects. First, in a typical study, patients leave the study after healing, and many drop out for a variety of reasons; thus the groups being compared are changing markedly at each visit. Second, such comparisons involve multiplicity of testing. Comparisons might reasonably be made at the first- and second-week visits or at the patient's last visit. In addition, symptom data can be used to address questions such as the relationship between healing and the presence or absence of symptoms or to provide additional information for ranking patient outcomes.

To illustrate aspects of the analysis of symptom data, we consider results from Hirschowitz et al. [21] adapted as shown in Table 3. For patients with pain at baseline, we compare symptom status at 6 weeks between the test drug and placebo for those healed at 6 weeks and those not healed at 6 weeks. Fisher's exact test can be used to confirm that among those not healed at 6 weeks the percentage of asymptomatic patients is higher for the test drug than for placebo and that more of those healed at 6 weeks are asymptomatic than of those not healed at 6 weeks.

Table 3   Data for Absence of Symptoms among Patients with Baseline Pain in 6-Week Trial for Healing Benign Gastric Ulcer

Subgroups	Placebo No symptoms (%)	Total	Test drug No symptoms (%)	Total	Fisher's exact test two-sided p value
Not healed at 6 weeks	6 (18%)	34	10 (43%)	23	0.041
Healed at 6 weeks	18 (50%)	36	26 (54%)	48	0.826
Total	24 (34%)	70	36 (51%)	71	0.061

Occasionally, a combined analysis of data for healing status and symptoms is of interest. One reasonable strategy for these situations is the Mantel-Haenszel test. For its application to the data for healing status at 6 weeks in Table 1 (with nonevaluable managed as missing) and the data for no symptoms in Table 3 for the subgroups of healed and not healed patients, we obtain

$$Q_{MH} = \frac{(56 + 10 + 26 - 50.1 - 6.5 - 25.1)^2}{9.37 + 2.82 + 5.19} = 6.06$$

by computations like those shown in Table 2. The corresponding two-sided $p = .014$ from a chi-square approximation with one degree of freedom indicates that the status of patients for healing or symptoms at 6 weeks was significantly more favorable for test drug than for placebo.

e. Methods for Multicenter (or Stratified) Studies.   Studies with separate randomization of patients within centers or such pretreatment factors as smoking status have a stratified structure that analyses need to take into account. A method for comparing healing rates for two treatments with adjustment for a set of strata (e.g., centers) is the Mantel-Haenszel test [5, pp. 415–418]. It is computed for a dichotomous variable such as healing status at 6 weeks through a data structure analogous to Table 2 with the respective strata being the risk sets. Similarly, for a partially ordered variable like time to first healing, risk sets would be based on cross-classification of the strata with the subsets of eligible patients at the successive visits. For ordinal or continuous variables like symptom scores or antacid use, a counterpart to the Wilcoxon test for stratified studies is the van Elteren version of the extended Mantel-Haenszel test [5, pp. 418–421].

In stratified studies, homogeneity of treatment differences across strata should be evaluated for the primary response variable. At a descriptive level, one can present estimated treatment differences for each stratum and discuss their consistency. For example, in a placebo-controlled study, do differences favor the test drug in most strata? Or, in a study designed to demonstrate equivalence, do similar numbers of strata favor each treatment? More formal assessment of homogeneity of treatment differences across strata is possible through tests of treatment by strata interactions based on statistical models describing variation in responses as a function of treatment and stratum effects. These analyses may be based on logistical regression for dichotomous response variables, ordered logistical (proportional odds) regression for ordinal response variables, linear regression (or two-way analysis of variance) for continuous variables with relatively symmetrical distributions (either directly or after transformation), and proportional hazards regression for continuous variables with skewed distributions (or censoring in the sense that only a lower bound for a value is available). For these models, lack of significance (e.g., $p > .100$) of the test of treatment–strata interaction can be interpreted as supporting homogeneity of treatment differences across strata. References for the previously mentioned models include Koch and Edwards [5], Fleiss [20], Kleinbaum et al. [23], and Lee [24].

When there is no treatment—strata interaction, we can use the models cited above to test for treatment effects after adjustment for stratum effects. The results from these tests should generally agree with those from the Mantel-Haenszel test or its extensions. However, Mantel-Haenszel methods are more directly applicable when there is some heterogeneity of treatment differences across strata, although the presence of heterogeneity weakens their ability to detect treatment differences and complicates interpretation.

For studies with fewer than 10 strata, each with enough patients (e.g., >20) to stand on its own as a substudy, analyses with the previously described methods are relatively straightforward. However, many studies of anti-ulcer drugs have a large number of small strata, many with very few patients (e.g., ≤6), and this structure complicates analysis. In essence, the Mantel-Haenszel test for such studies essentially excludes from analysis strata in which all patients have the same response or received the same treatment. In some statistical models, small strata either cannot be included (e.g., logistical regression) or complicate the conclusions (e.g., multiple linear regression). One strategy for dealing with small strata is to pool them into clusters that are then managed as large strata in the analysis. Centers can be pooled on the basis of geographical region or some other objective criteria, although these criteria should be specified in the study protocol or at least prior to breaking the treatment blinding.

   f.   **Methods for Studies with More than Two Treatments.**   The inclusion of more than two treatments in a study yields a wide range of potential comparisons for analysis. When the sample sizes per treatment are moderately large, say greater than 30, the methods discussed in the previous subsections can be used for the two-group comparisons of interest. Adjustment for multiple comparisons might be achieved by making overall comparisons with multigroup extensions of methods for two-group comparisons, for example, chi-square tests for dichotomous variables, Kruskal-Wallis tests for ordinal variables, and multigroup analysis of variance for continuous variables (or their stratified counterparts for multicenter studies). Some references for these methods are [5], [16], [20], and [23].

For multidose studies with small sample sizes at each of many doses, analyses must focus on description of the dose—response relationship. The Spearman rank correlation test [5, p. 414] can be used to evaluate whether a dichotomous, ordinal, or continuous response variable has a monotonic (e.g., increasing) relationship with dose. For stratified studies, its extended Mantel-Haenszel counterpart [5, pp. 418–421] is similarly applicable. Alternatively, model-based methods such as logistic regression [5, pp. 421–428] for dichotomous variables or multiple linear regression [20,23] for continuous variables are useful for describing dose—response relationships and can accommodate stratification factors such as center.

4.   Methods to Explore the Influence of Patient Factors on Response

Patient background characteristics such as age and smoking status as well as patient compliance may be related to patient response to treatment. Evaluation of how such factors are related to outcome is of interest for several reasons: It may help to elucidate the nature of ulcer disease, it may help to characterize the patients who are most likely to benefit from treatment, it may suggest variables for which stratification in future studies would enhance clarity of findings, it sheds light on the sensitivity of the results to any differences between treatment groups on these factors, and it identifies factors with noteworthy heterogeneity of treatment effects across subgroups through corresponding treatment–factor interactions for response.

Lack of equivalence between treatment groups for factors of importance to outcome such as smoking status or patient compliance are potential sources of bias for comparisons of treatment efficacy. Methods for comparing treatment groups for patient background characteristics were discussed in Section II.C.2. These methods can also be used for comparisons for compliance, prevalences of protocol violations, duration of study participation, reasons for study discontinuation, and other aspects of the conduct of a trial. Since these latter factors pertain to patient experiences subsequent to randomization, they may differ between treatment groups. If there are marked differences between treatments for any of these variables, it will be necessary to assess how sensitive efficacy results are to potential bias from the degree of these differences.

One way of dealing with factors that are potential sources of bias for treatment efficacy comparisons is to analyze patient response using a statistical model that includes treatment effects, stratification variables, and relevant patient factors. For example, when the response variable is dichotomous, logistic regression [5, pp. 421–428] can be used to provide tests of treatment comparisons adjusted for patient factors that are possible sources of bias; multiple linear regression [20,23] is applicable when the response variable is continuous. If these results agree with the results of unadjusted treatment comparisons, they provide mutual support; conflict between adjusted and unadjusted results can suggest that the validity of the study has been undermined by bias.

To address such questions as whether the treatment effect is smaller among smokers than among nonsmokers, analyses of whether there are interactions between patient factors and treatment can be made. Tests for treatment by factor interactions can be included in the statistical models outlined above. If there are any significant treatment by factor interactions, treatment differences can be examined in each of the relevant subgroups.

5. Comparisons among Treatments for Safety Variables

Safety variables include determinations from laboratory tests, presence and severity of adverse events, and vital signs. Analyses for these variables are usually descriptive, with methods like those summarized in Section II.C.2 for background characteristics; for example, frequency tables and percentages for categorical variables, and means, standard errors, and minimum and maximum values for continuous variables. Occasionally, treatment comparisons are made for those safety variables with enough information for this to be meaningful. Methods for these comparisons include Fisher's exact test for dichotomous variables, the Wilcoxon test for ordinal variables, and the t-test for continuous variables. Discussion of limitations concerning the scope of analyses for safety variables is given in Section IV.

D. Reporting

The completed report of the clinical trial should contain details on each of the issues discussed here—in particular, the basis on which the sample size was selected, details of exclusions and inclusions, a log of patients screened and not enrolled, and a detailed tabulation of dropouts should be supplied. The analysis should contain confidence intervals and enough information about outcome to support future meta-analyses. The effects of predictor variables should be included (these are typically discussed so cryptically that it is impossible to assess direction of result across studies let alone size). Chalmers et al. [1] provide a list of items that should be included in a thorough report of clinical trial results.

III. MAINTENANCE AND RECURRENCE TRIALS

Although anti-ulcer drugs clearly speed the healing of acute duodenal ulcers, as many as 50% of patients may have ulcer recurrences within 6 months after treatment stops. For this reason, low maintenance doses of anti-ulcer drugs are often given, with the goal of preventing rapid recurrence of ulcers and thus alleviating the pain and inconvenience of symptomatic ulcer recurrences and lowering the risk of dangerous and expensive complications such as bleeding, obstruction, and perforation. In addition, one might expect that a truly effective drug for healing ulcers would prolong the time to recurrence without further treatment after its use. To evaluate the protective effects of healing with an anti-ulcer drug or of maintenance therapy, we consider studies in which patients with healed ulcers are followed until ulcer recurrence.

A. Design

For ulcer healing trials, study designs have been reasonably well defined for some time. This is not the case for maintenance or recurrence trials. Initially, the typical maintenance study was a one-year randomized double-blind trial comparing patients treated with half the short-term dose of the active compound to patients treated with placebo. Patients entered with healed ulcers. When patients presented with symptoms and an ulcer crater was seen at endoscopy, they were removed from the trial as treatment failures. Patients underwent scheduled endoscopies at regular intervals of 4 or 6 months to detect possible asymptomatic recurrences. The results of such maintenance trials were thought to demonstrate prevention of active recurrence by the treatments. However, simulation studies by Elashoff et al. [4] demonstrated that for a

4-month trial with one exit endoscopy, more rapid ulcer healing or a lower fraction of symptomatic ulcers in the active treatment group can cause a reduction in observed ulcer recurrences even if the active treatment does not affect recurrence rates. Moreover, in the case where maintenance therapy reduces the recurrence rate, these factors can result in an observed treatment effect markedly weaker than the actual treatment effect. In summary, trials with only a few widely spaced scheduled endoscopies may have little ability to discriminate between null and alternative hypotheses with respect to the prevention of recurrence. On the other hand, such trial designs can support conclusions about reduction in symptomatic recurrences or reduction in ulcer prevalence at fixed time points and also provide information about the long-term safety of a treatment. Thus, it is important to define the research question carefully before designing a "maintenance" study.

1.   Research Questions

We distinguish several possible research questions relevant to trials for maintenance therapy:

1.   Does an active drug reduce the frequency of symptomatic recurrences?
2.   Does an active drug reduce ulcer prevalence (either by prevention of recurrence or by more rapid healing of ulcers that do recur)?
3.   Does continuous maintenance therapy lower the risk of treatment failure or improve quality of life more than the treatment of acute ulcers on an as-needed basis?
4.   Does an active drug prevent ulcer recurrence?
5.   Does an active drug reduce the frequency of ulcer complications?
6.   Is long-term maintenance therapy safe?

The standard maintenance trial design outlined previously can address question 1 for whether the active drug reduces the time to first symptomatic recurrence. No scheduled endoscopies are necessary to address this specific goal. On the other hand, it is the scheduled endoscopies that allow us to address question 2 concerning reductions in ulcer prevalence.

A design addressing question 3 was reported by VanDeventer et al. [25]. In this 2-year double-blind maintenance study, patients with documented ulcer recurrences received up to 8 weeks of active therapy to heal their acute ulcers and returned to the trial medication after ulcer healing. Patients underwent endoscopies annually, and asymptomatic recurrences were treated the same as symptomatic recurrences. Patients who failed to heal, had a complication, or had two recurrences within 6 months left the trial as treatment failures.

To address question 4 for prevention of ulcer recurrence, it is necessary to have frequent scheduled endoscopies. In the trial design reported by Bynum and Koch [26], patients were given endoscopies at monthly intervals for a total of 4 months.

For question 5 concerning prevention of complications, one could consider designing a very large maintenance trial in which patients with recurrences are treated with active drugs to heal their acute ulcers and are returned to the trial after ulcer healing. No scheduled endoscopies are used, and complication is the endpoint. Alternatively a trial could be directed at recurrence of a complication such as bleeding (see Jensen et al. [27]).

A virtue of maintenance studies for addressing question 6 about safety is their capacity to shed light on moderately prevalent adverse effects during relatively long treatment periods. However, as discussed in Section IV, the information concerning safety from these studies is critically limited by their sample size.

2. Sample Size

For maintenance studies for which the primary endpoint for treatment comparisons is the recurrence rate at some fixed time such as 1 year, sample size considerations are similar to those discussed for ulcer healing studies in Section II.A.5. Thus, for an expected difference in recurrence rates such as 20–30% for test drug versus 50–60% for placebo, one can note from available tables [13, 14] that 45–50 patients per group provides 80% power for a significant finding at the two-sided $p \leq .05$ level. However, because the follow-up periods for maintenance studies are relatively long, dropout rates can be as high as 20–40%. Thus, in this example, the sample size might be adjusted to 70–80 patients.

Another endpoint of interest for maintenance studies is time to first recurrence. For this continuous variable, an approximation for the sample size n necessary for each group is

$$n = \frac{(z_\alpha + z_\beta)^2 2(\mathrm{CV})^2}{(\ln R)^2}$$

where z_α and z_β are values from the normal distribution for α-level significance and $100(1 - \beta)$ power, CV is the coefficient of variation (i.e., standard deviation/mean) for time to recurrence, and ln R is the natural logarithm of the ratio of the mean survival times for treatments. For example, if $\mathrm{CV} = 1$ on the basis of previous studies of a similar nature and $R = 2.0$, this method gives $n = 33$ for two-sided $\alpha = .05$ and 80% power (via $\beta = .20$); this number might be inflated to about 42 patients per group to allow for a dropout rate of 30%. Discussions of other methods for determining sample size for time to event variables are given in [16], [28], and [29].

B. Conduct

The conduct of maintenance and recurrence trials requires planning, organization, and activities similar to those discussed for healing trials in Section II.B. Additional issues requiring careful consideration for maintenance and recurrence studies are a relatively long period of follow-up (e.g., 1 year) over which subjects may discontinue for many reasons, a mixture of scheduled and unscheduled visits for assessment of whether ulcer recurrences are present, and possible inclusion of a phase for treatment of recurrent ulcers. The structure of case report forms also needs to account for these components of maintenance and recurrence trials. In particular, both visit forms for scheduled evaluations and event forms for unscheduled ones are needed.

C. Analysis

Many components of the statistical analysis of maintenance and recurrence trials are similar to those discussed for healing trials in Section II.C. For this reason, attention in this section is primarily restricted to methods for describing and comparing patterns of recurrence for treatments. For more complete discussion of statistical methods for analysis of maintenance studies, see [30].

1. Analysis of Recurrence Prevalences in a Maintenance Study

The typical design of an ulcer maintenance study provides information concerning ulcer recurrence like that shown in Table 4 for data adapted from a report by Gough et al. [8] for a 12-month trial. In this multicenter, randomized, double-blind study for the comparison of a test drug and an active control, endoscopic assessments for ulcer recurrence were made for patients with previously healed ulcers during scheduled visits at 4, 8, and 12 months and during unscheduled visits prompted by symptoms or other matters.

Patients with documented ulcer recurrences were classified as treatment failures and had no further follow-up. Patients with no observed ulcer recurrences consisted of those who completed 12 months of follow-up without an observed recurrence and those who discontinued the study before 12 months for some reason (e.g., protocol violation, poor compliance, lost to follow-up). Gough et al. [8] report only the pooled data for the centers, and so we focus our discussion of analyses for Table 4 on methods for a single-center study. In this setting, the two treatment groups have sufficient

Table 4 Data for Endoscopic Assessment in 12-Month Maintenance Trial for Duodenal Ulcer

Treatment	Number with recurrence first seen in interval[a]			Number withdrawn from risk during interval			Number with no recurrence seen by 12 mo	Total
	0–4 mo	4–8 mo	8–12 mo	0–4 mo	4–8 mo	8–12 mo		
Active control	40	24	6	44	12	5	110	241
Test drug	17	11	16	36	14	7	142	243

[a]Includes recurrences at both scheduled and unscheduled visits during time intervals.
Source: Data adapted from Gough et al. [8].

sample size for at least 90% power to detect 15% differences at the two-sided .05 significance level and 60–70% power for detection of 10% differences.

An issue that complicates the analysis of maintenance studies with data like those in Table 4 is how to deal with patients who are withdrawn from risk prior to study completion (i.e., 12 months) without having an observed ulcer recurrence. These patients with unknown recurrence status subsequent to their last endoscopy can cause ambiguity in the study conclusions in much the same way as nonevaluable patients in ulcer healing studies discussed in Section II.C.3. Accordingly, analyses of maintenance studies may need to use more than one method for managing withdrawals to assess their impact on conclusions.

Analysis of Crude Recurrence Rates.   An intent-to-treat approach to patients who are withdrawn from risk is to regard them as having no recurrence through the end of the study. This convention leads to the definition of the crude recurrence rate during a time period as

$$\text{Crude rate} = \frac{\text{total number of patients with recurrence during period}}{\text{total number of patients}}$$

For the data in Table 4, the crude rates for 1 year of follow-up are 29.0% (70/241) for the active control drug and 18.1% (44/243) for the test drug. These rates are compared with a continuity-corrected chi-square statistic (see Sec. II.C.3) because the sample sizes are large. Its result, $Q = 7.42$, is significant with two-sided $p < .01$. The difference between the recurrence rates for the active control and the test drug is described by a continuity-corrected 95% confidence interval (see Sec. II.C.3) extending from (3.0%, 18.8%), which supports the conclusion that ulcer recurrences are less prevalent for test drug than active control by a small to moderate amount.

A limitation of the crude rate is its understatement of the prevalence of recurrence. The degree of understatement depends on how many of the withdrawn patients would have had an observed recurrence if they had remained in the study. From Table 4, we note that the withdrawal rate for active control was 25.3% (61/241) and that for test drug was 23.5% (57/243). Thus, the actual recurrence rates in the study could have been as high as 54% and 42%, respectively. This potential extent of understatement merits some concern because it exceeds the 11% difference between the crude recurrence rates for the two treatments. In this situation, however, the withdrawal rates for the two treatments are nearly the same; and so for treatment comparisons concerning recurrence, bias from withdrawal might be minimal.

Another way to manage withdrawal patients is to exclude them as protocol violations from analyses for any time period that ends after their last endoscopy. This protocol-compatible convention leads to the definition of the adjusted crude recurrence rate as

$$\text{Adjusted crude rate} = \frac{\text{total number of patients with recurrences during period}}{\text{total number of patients} - \text{number of patients who withdraw before end of period}}$$

For the data in Table 4, the adjusted crude recurrence rates for 1 year of follow-up are 38.9% (70/180) for active control and 23.7% (44/186) for test drug. The difference between these rates is significant ($p < .01$) on the basis of the continuity-corrected chi-square statistic $Q = 9.18$. A 95% confidence interval for this difference is (5.3%, 25.1%). Thus, for the data in Table 4, the conclusions from treatment comparisons with adjusted crude rates are similar to those with crude rates. For descriptive purposes, however, one can note that adjusted crude rates are higher than crude rates, because their definition essentially presumes that withdrawals would have had the same observed recurrence rate if they had remained in the study as patients who completed the study. A limitation of this posture is that the direction of any bias in these adjusted rates is unclear.

Life Table Analysis of Recurrence Rates. Although withdrawals have unknown status at the study endpoint (e.g., 1 year), they provide information through the time of their last endoscopy. We can estimate recurrence rates in a manner that accounts for this incomplete information by using life table methods [24,30]. Computation of life table estimates for recurrence rates are illustrated in Table 5. As shown there, risk sets are constructed for the time intervals between scheduled endoscopies. For each interval, the fraction with no recurrence is determined in the middle columns of Table 5 as

$$\text{No recurrence rate for interval} = \frac{\text{number of patients completing interval with no observed recurrence}}{\text{number of patients at risk for observed recurrence during interval}}$$

In this expression, the denominator is the numerator plus the number of patients with observed recurrences during the interval. Cumulative nonrecurrence rates during the

Table 5 Computation of Recurrence Rates by Life Table Methods

Interval	No recur. seen in interval	At risk for interval	No recur. rate for interval	Cumulative no-recur. rate by end of interval	Cumulative recur. rate by end of interval
			Active control		
0–4 mo	157	197	0.797	0.797	0.203
4–8 mo	121	145	0.834	0.834(0.797) = 0.665	0.335
8–12 mo	110	116	0.948	0.948(0.665) = 0.631	0.369
			Test drug		
0–4 mo	190	207	0.918	0.918	0.082
4–8 mo	165	176	0.938	0.938(0.918) = 0.861	0.139
8–12 mo	142	158	0.899	0.899(0.861) = 0.773	0.227

time from study entry to the end of an interval are obtained by multiplying the successive recurrence rates for the intervals within this period, and corresponding results are shown in the penultimate column of Table 5.

Subtraction of these cumulative rates of nonrecurrence from 1.000 provides the cumulative rates for observed recurrences, which are shown in the last column of Table 5. Thus, by life table methods, the recurrence rates for 1 year of follow-up are 36.9% for the active control drug and 22.7% for the test drug. With standard errors for life table estimates from methods available in such references as [16, pp. 445–452] and [24], we can form confidence intervals for the difference between two treatments.

A method for comparing sets of life table estimates for two treatments is the Mantel-Haenszel statistic [5, pp. 436–442; and 30]. It is obtained from the information in the second and third columns of Table 5 by the computations described in Section II.C.3 relative to Table 2. Here we have

$$Q_{\text{MH}} = \frac{(40 + 24 + 6 - 27.8 - 15.8 - 9.3)^2}{12.26 + 7.75 + 4.96} = 11.71$$

which is significant with two-sided $p < .01$.

The principal advantage of life table methods is that they make use of the information from withdrawals for those intervals in which they are at risk. However, life table methods are based on the assumption that withdrawals would have had recurrence at the same rate as patients remaining in the trial. For this reason, results from life table analyses must be interpreted cautiously when withdrawal rates are high.

2. Point Prevalence Analysis of Recurrence Rates

When one of the treatments in a maintenance study is more effective in reducing the severity of ulcer symptoms, then patients with observed ulcer recurrences at an unscheduled endoscopy are a potential source of bias for treatment comparisons. Since asymptomatic ulcers can reheal before detection at a scheduled endoscopy, two treatments with equal recurrence rates and equal rehealing rates could have different observed prevalences because the treatment with better reduction of symptoms would have fewer ulcers detected by endoscopic evaluations of unscheduled visits.

One way to evaluate the impact of this source of bias is to manage patients with ulcers detected at an unscheduled visit as withdrawals during the corresponding time interval. The resulting point prevalence analyses include only the observed recurrences at scheduled visits. Their application to a 4-month study with scheduled endoscopies at the end of each month is discussed by Bynum and Koch [26]. In that study, the conclusions from point prevalence analyses agreed with those from analyses that did not exclude patients with ulcers detected at unscheduled visits; that is, such conclusions were not sensitive to possible bias resulting from more masking of symptoms by one treatment than by the other. On the other hand, if conclusions from these two analyses had not agreed, then both types of analyses would require cautious interpretation, because excluding patients with "symptomatic" recurrences from point prevalence analyses leads to bias against the treatment with better symptom reduction.

3. Analysis of Recurrence Rates for Symptomatic Ulcer Recurrences

For studies in which symptomatic ulcer recurrence is the outcome of interest, the times of detection at unscheduled visits provide the principal information for analysis; the intervals for life table analysis are defined as the time periods between successive symptomatic recurrences. The life table estimates for symptomatic recurrence rates from this data structure are sometimes called Kaplan-Meier estimates [16, pp. 445–448; 31]. Patients with asymptomatic ulcer observed at scheduled visits can be managed as withdrawals. The Mantel-Haenszel statistic can be used for treatment comparisons. A study with symptomatic ulcer recurrence rates analyzed as outlined here is reported in VanDeventer et al. [25].

IV. SAFETY ISSUES

The typical ulcer healing or maintenance trial enrolls from 50 to 150 patients in the active treatment group. Such trials are able to detect only marked increases in relatively common events. In particular, a side effect or adverse event observed to occur in 10% of patients will have a 95% confidence interval running from 1% to 19% for $n = 50$, or from 5% to 15% for $n = 150$. Also, there would only be 6–29% power to detect doubling in the side-effect rate from 5% to 10%. For side effects or adverse events not observed in the trial, we can conclude with 95% confidence only that the true rate for the population studied is below 5.8% for $n = 50$ or below 2% for $n = 150$. However, when a drug can be expected to be used by millions of people, a serious adverse event with a rate of only 0.1% will result in thousands of cases.

Due to the typical exclusion of elderly patients or patients with multiple medical problems from clinical trials, it is likely that most clinical trials underestimate the side-effect and adverse-event rates to be expected in their general use. In addition, such designs are unlikely to detect potentially important adverse interactions of the anti-ulcer drug with other patient medications.

Postmarketing surveillance studies are conducted to provide additional safety information. However, since it is often not clear what kinds of side effects or adverse events are likely to occur, such events, unless they are very unusual, may not be attributed to the drug. The extreme rarity of diethylstilbestrol (DES) syndrome before the advent of DES led to its attribution to the drug, but an increase in myocardial infarctions in an elderly population may not attract attention. Even when certain kinds of events are reported in association with the drug sufficiently often to be alarming, the lack of any adequate comparison group often leaves it unclear whether these actually represent an increase over the expected background rate in the population taking the drug. Additional discussion of safety issues is given in [32] and [33].

V.   ACID SUPPRESSION, *HELICOBACTER* KILLING, AND INJURY PROTECTION

As an aid in dose selection, full-scale healing trials of anti-ulcer drugs are often preceded by short-term trials focused on immediate efficacy issues.

A.   Acid Suppression

Generally, the acid-suppressing capabilities of a drug are assessed in small crossover studies in volunteers; each subject receives a placebo and several different doses of the drug in question, and for each dose a time course of acid output is measured. Generally, such trials should be designed using a Latin square to balance order and sequence effects (see [20]). To avoid multiple testing problems, it is important to summarize across the time course (first 4 hr, second 4 hr, etc). Typically the analysis will involve repeated measures analysis of variance with adjustment for order effects and evaluation of carryover effects. For specific discussion of such methods of analysis, see [34] and [35].

B.   Mucosal Protection and Inhibition of *Helicobacter pylori*

These studies present new issues that are largely due to the nature of the outcome measures. Measurement of mucosal protection involves assessment of ordered endoscopic scores (see [36]), and the success of *Helicobacter pylori* inhibition is assessed by estimating the number of bacteria per high-power field. An issue for the analysis of such measures is the skewness of their distributions. It can be addressed for comparisons between two treatments by the use of nonparametric rank methods such as the Wilcoxon rank-sum test or the logrank test [37] or by the use of a transformation (e.g., logarithm) prior to a two-sample t-test.

VI.   META-ANALYSIS

Rarely must conclusions about the efficacy of an anti-ulcer drug be based on the results of only one study. Conclusions about overall efficacy are usually based on consideration of the results of several trials. A review of the relevant studies should include a meta-analysis, that is, a comprehensive examination of the data from a collection of related studies.

Before making conclusions about the results of the relevant studies obtained by a literature search, the reviewer must consider several major issues. First we will want to establish criteria for which studies are relevant and of high enough quality to merit inclusion. Chalmers et al. [1] provide a useful checklist for evaluating the quality of clinical trials.

Second, should the various studies actually be combined; are the results sufficiently homogeneous to warrant combination? Similarity of studies strengthens clarity of findings. When one combines the results of several studies, one makes the implicit assumption that the therapeutic effect is homogeneous across such study characteristics as dosage and other aspects of protocol design or patient population. If the therapeutic effect differs widely between individual studies, then the combination of results may not make sense. The reviewer can begin by looking at the results of each study in relation to the details of the study. Each study can be categorized in terms of features potentially important to outcome such as treatment dose, duration of treatment, definition of treatment response, and such patient characteristics as age, sex, diagnosis, and severity of disease. If the therapeutic effect appears to depend heavily on some study characteristic, then there is not "one" result. In fact, such differences may suggest questions on which further studies should focus. If the various study characteristics are homogeneous among the separate studies, or are inhomogeneous but appear to make little consistent difference in the effect of therapy, one may examine whether the results themselves look homogeneous by comparing the observed variability between study results to that expected on the basis of the sample sizes. For dichotomous outcomes like ulcer healing or recurrence rates, tests of treatment–study interactions in logistic regression models can be used. Another possible approach described by Gilbert et al. [38] is illustrated by Elashoff [39] for an early review of ulcer healing studies with cimetidine.

Has the new therapy been compared with placebo (or another active drug) in a sufficient variety of circumstances to warrant a conclusion about what is best overall? Diversity of studies strengthens generalizability of findings. The wider the variety of study characteristics and the more homogeneous the results across the studies, the more secure one is in making generalizations such as "Active drug in doses of x mg per day increases percentage healed at 2 to 4 weeks for duodenal ulcer patients."

After the reviewer decides on a set of studies to combine, he must consider how to combine the results. The first step is specification of response criteria in an objective and comparable way for all studies. Any method for combining results must be based on study-by-study differences between active drug and standard or placebo. Simply adding up cases across studies can obscure a therapeutic effect obvious in individual studies. A variety of methods exist for analysis of differences in percentages. The choice of method for testing the significance of combined results depends on how the reviewer wishes to weight the results from each study. If the reviewer wishes to weight large studies more heavily than smaller studies, the Mantel-Haenszel method provides a test of significance based on looking at standardized differences in proportions. On the other hand, one could argue that a study with a large sample size only provides a better assessment of therapeutic efficacy in that study population under those study conditions, and therefore, in generalizing across populations and conditions, constitutes a sample of size 1. This suggests using the sign test or a Wilcoxon signed rank test [16,20]. Approaches that take into account other potentially relevant factors such as dose or length of treatment include logistic regression. For a thorough discussion of statistical methods for combining results across studies, see [40] and [41].

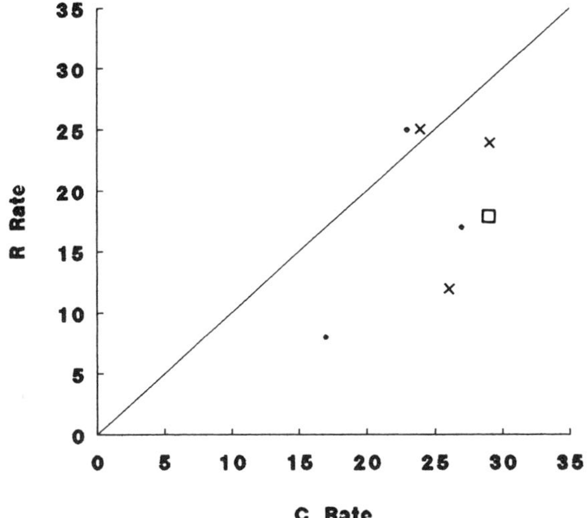

FIGURE 1   Crude 12-month recurrence rates for ranitidine and cimetidine from seven studies by Kurata et al. [42]. Minimum sample size per group: (•) <30; (×) $30-100$; (□) >100.

A useful way to display results from several studies is illustrated in Figure 1. There, a scatterplot is given for crude recurrence rates observed in seven studies of 12 months of maintenance therapy with treatment C versus treatment R in a meta-analysis reported by Kurata et al. [42]. Visually, it is clear that treatment C rates are consistently higher than those for treatment R by about 8%. Analyses reported in Kurata et al. [42] indicate a combined estimate of ulcer recurrence prevalence by 12 months of 27% for treatment C and 19% for treatment R. In addition, this type of display can illustrate the differences in patterns of variability for the results of the larger studies versus the results of the smaller studies.

A limitation for the interpretation of meta-analysis is that its scope includes only studies through a particular time. Thus, to have continuing usefulness, meta-analyses require updating as the results of new studies become available.

VI.   SUMMARY

We have presented an outline of statistical considerations for the design, conduct, and analysis of data from clinical trials of anti-ulcer drugs. Table 6 summarizes the analytical methods most likely to be appropriate for various types of outcome variables and provides references for readers desiring more details.

Table 6 Summary of Useful Statistical Methods

Measurement type	Tests for comparisons		Model-based methods
	Single-center study	Multicenter, or stratified study	
Dichotomous	Fisher's exact test, chi-square tests [5, 13, 16]	Mantel-Haenszel test [5, 13,16]	Logistic regression [5, 20]
Nominal categories	Chi-square tests [5, 13, 16]	Extended Mantel-Haenszel test [5]	Log-linear models [5]
Ordinal categories or discrete counts	Rank-sum tests [5, 16]	Extended Mantel-Haenszel test [5]	Proportional odds model [5]
Time to events (e.g., healing, recurrence)	Logrank tests [5, 16, 24, 37]	Extended Mantel-Haenszel (logrank) test for survival data [5, 16, 24, 37]	Proportional hazards regression [5, 24]
Continuous	Rank sum tests, t-tests [16, 20]	Van Elteren test [5]	Multiple linear regression and analysis of covariance [20, 23]

In addition, we have emphasized that statistical considerations apply throughout the multiple stages of a clinical trial:

    I.   Clarifying the research question
   II.   Designing the trial
       1.   Choosing the study population
       2.   Ensuring comparability of groups
       3.   Selecting treatments and doses
       4.   Defining the response variables
       5.   Computing the necessary sample size
       6.   Detailing interim analysis plans
  III.   Planning the conduct of the trial (protocol, data entry, and management)
  IV.   Analyzing the results
       1.   Specifying inference populations
       2.   Describing entry characteristics of the treatment groups
       3.   Comparing efficacy of the treatments
       4.   Exploring the impact on efficacy results of patient characteristics
   V.   Reporting the results
  VI.   Understanding the limitations of safety data
 VII.   Combining the results of several different studies

REFERENCES

1. Chalmers TC, Smith H, Blackburn B, Silverman B, Schroeder B, Reitman D, Ambroz A. A method for assessing the quality of a randomized control trial. Controlled Clin Trials 1981; 2:31–49.
2. Elashoff JD. Statistical considerations in drug trials of peptic ulcer. J Clin Gastroenterol 1981; 3(Suppl 2):135–40.
3. Elashoff JD. Trial designs to demonstrate cost-benefit claims for antiulcer drugs. Drug Inf J 1988; 22:385–93.
4. Elashoff JD, Koch GG, Chi GYH. Designing a clinical trial to demonstrate prevention of ulcer recurrence: modelling simulation approaches. Stat Med 1988; 7:877–88.
5. Koch GG, Edwards S. Clinical efficacy trials with categorical data. In: Peace KE, ed. Biopharmaceutical statistics for drug development. New York: Marcel Dekker, 1988: 403–57.
6. Koch GG, Sollecito WA. Statistical considerations in the design, analysis, and interpretation of comparative clinical studies. Drug Inf J 1984; 18:131–51.
7. Pocock SJ. Clinical trials: a practical approach. New York: Wiley, 1983.
8. Gough KR, Bardhan KD, Crowe JP, et al. Ranitidine and cimetidine in prevention of duodenal ulcer relapse. Lancet 1984; ii:659–62.
9. Temple R. Difficulties in evaluating positive control trials. American Statistical Association 1983 Proceedings from the Biopharmaceutical Section.
10. Pledger G. The role of a placebo-treated control group in combination drug trials. Controlled Clin Trials 1989; 10:97–107.
11. Laska E, Morris M. Testing whether an identified treatment is best. Biometrics 1990; in press.
12. Snapinn SM. Evaluating the efficacy of combination therapy. Stat Med 1987; 6:657–65.
13. Fleiss JL. Statistical methods for rates and proportions. 2nd ed. New York: Wiley, 1981.
14. Machin D, Campbell MJ. Statistical tables for the design of clinical trials. Oxford: Blackwell, 1987.
15. Blackwelder WC, Chang MA. "Proving the null hypothesis" in clinical trials. Control Clin Trials 1982; 3:345–53.
16. Woolson RF. Statistical methods for the analysis of biomedical data. New York: Wiley, 1987.
17. Elashoff JD, Reedy TJ. Two-stage clinical trial stopping rules. Biometrics 1984; 40: 791–5.
18. Pocock SJ, Geller NL. Interim analyses in randomized clinical trials. Drug Inf J 1986; 20:263–9.
19. O'Brien PC, Fleming TR. A multiple testing procedure for clinical trials. Biometrics 1979; 35:549–56.
20. Fleiss JL. The design and analysis of clinical experiments. New York: Wiley, 1986.
21. Hirschowitz BI, DeLuca V, Graham D, Lorber S, Bright-Asare P, Keaton R. Treatment of benign chronic gastric ulcer with ranitidine. A randomized, double-blind, and placebo-controlled six week trial. J Clin Gastroenterol 1986; 8:371–6.
22. Mantel N. Evaluation of survival data and two new rank order statistics arising in its consideration. Cancer Chemother Rep 1966; 50:163–70.
23. Kleinbaum DG, Kupper LL, Muller KE. Applied regression analysis and other multivariate methods. Boston: PWS-KENF, 1988.

24. Lee ET. Statistical methods for survival data analysis. Belmont, Calif.: Lifetime Learning Publications, 1980.

25. VanDeventer GG, Elashoff JD, Reedy TJ, Schneidman D, Walsh JH. A randomized study of maintenance therapy with ranitidine to prevent the recurrence of duodenal ulcer. N Engl J Med 1989; 320:1113–9.

26. Bynum TE, Koch GG. Sucralfate tablets 1 g twice a day for the prevention of duodenal ulcer recurrence. Am J Med 1989; 86:127–32.

27. Jensen D, You F, Jensen ME, et al. Randomized controlled study of ranitidine maintenance for patients with a recent severe duodenal ulcer hemorrhage. Gastroenterology 1990; in press.

28. Donner A. Approaches to sample size estimation in the design of clinical trials—a review. Stat Med 1984; 3:199–214.

29. Freedman LS. Table of the number of patients required in clinical trials using the log-rank test. Stat Med 1982; 1:121–9.

30. Koch GG, McCanless I, Ward JF. Interpretation of statistical methodology associated with maintenance trials. Am J Med 1984; 77(Suppl 5B):43–50.

31. Kaplan EL, Meier P. Nonparametric estimation from incomplete observations. J Am Stat Assoc 1958; 53:457–81.

32. Edwards S, Koch GG, Sollecito WA. Summarization, analysis, and monitoring of adverse experiences. In: Peace KE, ed. Statistical issues in drug research and development. New York: Marcel Dekker, 1990:19–170.

33. O'Neill RT. Assessment of safety. In: Peace KE, ed. Biopharmaceutical statistics for drug development. New York: Marcel Dekker, 1988:543–604.

34. Elashoff JD. Analysis of repeated measures designs. BMDP technical report 83. Los Angeles: BMDP Statistical Software, 1986.

35. Koch GG, Elashoff JD, Amara IA. Repeated measurements—design and analysis. In: Kotz S, Johnson NL, eds. Encyclopedia of statistical sciences. Vol. 8. New York: Wiley, 1988:46–73.

36. Lanza FL, Aspinall RL, Swabb EA, Davis RE, Rack MF, Rubin A. Double-blind, placebo-controlled endoscopic comparison of the mucosal protective effects of misoprostal versus cimetidine on tolmetin-induced mucosal injury to the stomach and duodenum. Gastroenterology 1988; 95:289–94.

37. Koch GG, Sen PK, Amara IA. Logrank scores, statistics and tests. In: Johnson NL, Kotz S, eds. Encyclopedia of statistical sciences. Vol. 5. New York: Wiley, 1985:136–42.

38. Gilbert JP, McPeek B, Mosteller F. Progress in surgery and anesthesia: benefits and risk of innovative therapy. In: Bunker JP, Barnes BA, Mosteller F, eds. Costs, risks and benefits of surgery. New York: Oxford Univ. Press, 1977:124–69.

39. Elashoff JD. Combining results of clinical trials. Gastroenterology 1978; 75:1170–2. Editorial.

40. Hedges LV, Olkin I. Statistical methods for meta-analysis. San Diego: Academic, 1985.

41. Chalmers TC, Buyse ME. Meta-analysis. In: Chalmers TC, ed. Data analysis for clinical medicine: the quantitative approach to patient care in gastroenterology. New York: International Univ. Press, 1988:75–84.

42. Kurata JH, Koch GG, Nogawa AN. Comparison of ranitidine and cimetidine ulcer maintenance therapy. J Clin Gastroenterol 1987; 9(6):644–50.

19

Meta-Analyses in Ulcer Disease

Karl E. Peace

Biopharmaceutical Research Consultants, Inc.,
Ann Arbor, Michigan

I. INTRODUCTION

Hedges and Olkin [1] regard meta-analysis as a rubric used to describe quantitative methods for combining evidence across experiments. DerSimonian and Laird {2] define meta-analysis as the statistical analysis of a collection of analytic results for the purpose of integrating the findings. Although neither Cochran [3–5] nor Yates and Cochran [6] used the rubric, their methods for combining results from series of experiments are clearly meta-analysis methods.

Numerous applications of meta-analysis techniques to agricultural experiments were reported in the decades of the 1930s, 1940s, and 1950s. The 1970s saw a branching out of the techniques to many applications in the social sciences, whereas the 1980s, particularly the latter half, were witness to a virtual explosion of the techniques to many areas of medical research.

The purpose of this chapter is to review applications of meta-analysis techniques in the study of ulcer disease. The results are presented in Section IV. To facilitate the review, statistical methods are reviewed in Section II; and investigations using meta-analysis techniques, viewed as a scientific research process, are discussed in Section III.

II. STATISTICAL METHODS

Classical statistical inferential methods about population parameters are categorized either as methods for testing statistical significance or as methods for estimation. It is not surprising, then, that statistical methods for synthesizing individual experimental results across experiments are categorized similarly. Significance-testing methods for combining experimental results are reviewed in Section 2.1. Estimation methods for combining experimental results are presented in Section 2.2.

In the statistical and applied literature, the phrases "significance testing" and "hypothesis testing" often appear and are often used interchangeably. A distinction between these phrases is warranted. We use "significance testing" to refer to statistical testing methods performed in an a posteriori or ad hoc manner. We use "hypothesis testing" to refer to statistical testing methods performed on data collected in an experiment designed a priori to address a question of interest (hypothesis). Therefore, in this context, statistical, meta-analytic testing methods are significance-testing rather than hypothesis-testing methods.

In conducting meta-analyses, we assume that we have available a finite collection of independent experiments (say K) that address the same question, that were reasonably well designed and conducted, and that were analyzed appropriately using similar outcome measures. The question each (or ith, $i = 1, 2, \ldots, K$) experiment was designed to address will be symbolized as the statement about some parameter $@$ in the alternative hypothesis ($H_{a,i}$). The alternative hypothesis $H_{a,i}$ is the logical negation to the null hypothesis ($H_{0,i}$) in the hypothesis-testing specification framework:

$$
\begin{array}{llllll}
H_{0,i}: & @i = 0 & \quad H_{0,i}: & @i \le 0 & \quad H_{0,i}: & @i \ge 0 \\
H_{a,i}: & @i \ne 0 & \quad H_{a,i}: & @i > 0 & \quad H_{a,i}: & @i < 0
\end{array}
$$

Which of the three specifications obtains will depend upon the directionality of the research question [7]. We assume that certain summary information that could be used to make inferences about $H_{a,i}$ in each experiment is also available. Such information includes the test statistic T_i, its distribution under $H_{0,i}$, and its corresponding p value:

$$
p_i = \text{Prob}[T_i \text{ is as extreme as or more extreme than } t_i]
$$

where t_i is the value of T_i obtained from the data in the ith experiment. In addition, estimates of $@$ such as means, differences between means, medians, correlations, their standard errors, and the associated sample sizes are asssumed to be known. In some cases, although rare, the raw data originally analyzed in each experiment may be available.

A. Significance Tests for Combined Results

Methods for testing statistical significance summarized here are methods based on combining p values, on combining test statistics, or on models and vote counting. These methods provide tests of statistical significance of the "global" or "omnibus" null hypothesis H_0 versus a global or omnibus alternative hypothesis H_a:

$$H_0: \quad \theta_1 = \theta_2 = \ldots = \theta_K = 0$$

versus

$$H_a: \quad \text{Not all the } \theta_i = 0, \qquad i = 1, 2, \ldots, K.$$

The particular form of H_a will depend upon the original research question embodied as the individual $H_{a,i}$.

1. Combining p Values

Methods for combining p values date back to the early 1930s. Tippitt [8] appears to have been the first to publish such a method. Fisher [9] and Pearson [10] soon followed with independent work on another method. Others contributing yet different methods were Wilkinson [11], Edgington [12,13], George [14] and Mudholkar and George [15]. Methods based upon p values require that the p values be one-tailed or one-sided, and that the direction be selected a priori and independent of the data [1]. For emphasis, the p values from the K experiments, each addressing the common question embodied in the alternative hypothesis of each experiment, are denoted as $p_1, p_2, \ldots, p_K$.

Numerous other methods have been proposed for combining p values from independent studies. Pearson [10] proposed a method based upon the product of the complement of the p values: $(1 - p_1)(1 - p_2) \ldots (1 - p_K)$. David [16] proposed a method for combining two-sided p values based upon the statistics $m_1, m_2, \ldots, m_K$, where $m_i = $ minimum of p_i and $(1 - p_i)$, $i = 1, 2, \ldots, K$. Good [17] proposed an extension of Fisher's method that involves weighting the individual p values. Zelen and Joel [18] and Pape [19] explored the use of optimal weights and the power of the weighted Fisher method. Strube [20] studied the general problem of the power of methods for combining p values. Littell and Folks [21,22] established that Fisher's method is asymptotically optimal among all methods for combining p values. Berk and Cohen [23] showed that Fisher's procedure also satisfied the criterion of Bahahur efficiency. Brown [24] and Strube [25] address combining p values when the independence of experiments assumption is relaxed. Others addressing various aspects of combining p values are Brozek and Tiede [26], Rosenthall [109], and Rosenthall and Rubin [27,28]. The first paper by Rosenthall and Rubin [27] is an excellent review of the methods and includes worked numerical examples.

2. Combining Test Statistics or Summary Measures

The procedures just discussed used the p values available from the individual studies. Tippett's, Wilkinson's, and Edgington's procedures made direct use of the p values. Fisher's procedure and that of George and Mudholkar made use of transformations of the p values. Fisher's procedure started with the product of the p values and then required the natural logarithmic transformation of the product, whereas the procedure of George and Mudholkar transformed the individual p values into logits and then required their sum. Neither of these procedures explicitly transformed the individual p values into a corresponding random variable whose distribution is known.

A p value is produced through knowledge of the distribution of the test statistic under the null hypothesis. Therefore it should be possible to produce the value of the test statistic from knowing the p value. In addition, the value of the test statistic may be known directly if studies are properly reported. Since the more common distributions of test statistics are the normal, Student's t, chi-square, and F, we review the procedures in this section based upon combining results of individual studies by the use of linear combination of the values of their test statistics. In addition, the procedures of Cochran [5], Mantel and Haenszel [29], DerSimonian and Laird [2], and Peto [30], which combine summary measures, are reviewed.

The test procedure can be characterized in the same manner in each situation:

1. Select the significance level α for the omnibus test of H_0.
2. Determine the critical point C of the test such that there is area α to the right of C, in the upper tail of the distribution of the test statistic.
3. Compute the value of the test statistic T.
4. Compare the value of T to C.
5. If $T \geq C$, then reject H_0.

Methods Combining Normal Statistics. The procedure based upon combining normal statistics was first proposed by Stouffer et al. [31] and later independently by Liptak [32]. The procedure requires transforming each p value into its corresponding standard normal deviate (for example, if $p = .05$, then the standard normal deviate $= 1.645$), then summing the deviates, and then dividing the sum by the square root of the number of deviates, to produce the test statistic T. The distribution of the test statistic under H_0 is the standardized normal with mean 0 and variance 1. This procedure is often referred to as the *inverse normal method*.

If the values of the individual test statistics of the studies are given and have a distribution that is the standard normal, they can be summed and the sum divided by the square root of the number of statistics to produce the value of the test statistic [33]. Mostellar and Bush [34] proposed a variation of the inverse normal procedure that allowed weighting each standard normal deviate.

Methods Combining t Statistics. Oosterhoff [35] and Winer [36] proposed methods for combining independent test statistics, each of which has a Student's t distribution with d_i degrees of freedom. Since the mean and variance of the t distribution with d_i degrees of freedom are 0 and $d_i/(d_i - 2)$, respectively, and the distribution is symmetric about the mean, it is closely approximated by the standardized normal when the number of degrees of freedom is large. Therefore, when sample sizes are rather large for each study, the test statistic can be produced as in the inverse normal case. However, when the sample sizes are small for each study, then the test statistic for each study, providing its distribution is Student's t with degrees of freedom d_i, should be standardized by dividing by the square root of the variance, then summing these quotients and dividing the sum by the number of quotients to produce the test statistic T. The distribution of the test statistic is then closely approximated by the standard normal or by the Student's t statistic with degrees of freedom being the sum of the d_i.

Methods Combining Chi-Square Statistics. Lancaster [37] proposed methods for combining test statistics that each have a chi-square distribution with d_i degrees of freedom. Basically, the unweighted test statistic T is obtained by summing the individual test statistics. The distribution of the test statistic T is a chi-square distribution with number of degrees of freedom equal to the sum of the numbers of degrees of freedom of the individual chi-squares. Each chi-square statistic from each individual study can also be weighted appropriately, before summing, to produce the test statistic T.

Koziol and Perlman [38,39] and Marden [40] have also investigated combining results of independent studies through the use of linear combinations of individual chi-square statistics. It should be noted that Fisher's method can be considered a special case of this type of procedure.

Methods Combining F Statistics. Zelen [41], Pape [19], and Marden [40] proposed methods for combining statistics that have F distributions with n_i and d_i degrees of freedom for numerator and denominator, respectively. These procedures are similar to those used with chi-square statistics, particularly for individual test statistics that follow an F distribution with denominator degrees of freedom that is large. When the denominator degrees of freedom is sufficiently large, the F distribution is closely approximated by the chi-square distribution with degrees of freedom equal to the numerator degrees of freedom.

Popular Methods for Combining Summary Measures. Among the more popular methods to examine the statistical significance of the aggregate results from a series of experiments are those of Cochran [5], Mantel and Haenszel [29], Peto's [30] modification of the Mantel-Haenszel method, and DerSimonian and Laird's [2] modification of Cochran's method. These methods require the identification of a summary measure reflecting the experimental objective that can be computed from the known individual experimental results. Pooling the experimental results, in general, to assess their statistical significance is then facilitated through defining a mathematical function that combines the individual summary measures in a meaningful way. For the four methods mentioned, the function is a simple sum, an unweighted average, or a weighted average (of the individual summary measures). Statistical significance is then assessed from the exact (sampling) distribution of the function (or a transformation thereof) or by drawing on asymptotic normal theory. In the latter case, the variance of the function (or transformation) has to be determined.

For the Cochran method, the summary measure is the standardized mean difference, whereas DerSimonian and Laird consider three summary measures: the risk difference, the relative risk, and the relative odds. For the Mantel-Haenszel method and Peto's method, the summary measure is the deviation between observed and expected frequencies of results. Berlin et al. [42] compare the Peto and DerSimonian and Laird methods.

3. Other Methods

Various other methods for combining and assessing the significance of results across independent experiments have been considered. These include a model-based approach, vote-counting methods, Bayesian methods, and likelihood ratio methods.

The procedures of Cochran [5], Mantel and Haenszel [29], DerSimonian and Laird [2], and Peto [30] can be considered model-based methods. Others who have studied model-based approaches are Hedges and Olkin [1], Katz et al. [43], and Jones and Fiske [44]. The book by Hedges and Olkin [1] provides an excellent treatment of a linear models approach as well as a summary of vote-counting methods. Vote-counting methods were also considered earlier by Hedges and Olkin [45]. Whereas Katz et al. [43] consider nonparametric model-based procedures, Raudenbush and Bryk [46] consider empirical Bayesian methods, and Goodman [47] and Zucker and Yusuf [48] discuss methods based upon the likelihood ratio of the collection of experimental results.

B. Estimation Methods

In addition to p values and test statistics, the summary information available on individual studies may consist of means, medians, their standard errors, and the corresponding sample sizes. Such information or measures may reflect an individual group or two or more groups, depending on the objective of each study. For example, if the objective of a study is to compare two groups in terms of some specified endpoint, the comparison may be facilitated by the mean difference between the two groups, the ratio or some transformation of the means of the two groups, a measure of correlation between the two groups, or any of these methods standardized to account for variation. In studies of two or more groups, the summary measure may be the regression slope or some other contrast across all groups. Such measures are point estimates of parameters of interest in the studies. When meta-analyses are performed, such estimates are increasingly referred to as *study effect sizes.* Ideally, consideration would have been given at the design stage of each study as to the choice of summary measure or study effect size that most appropriately reflects the study objective.

Various authors—Glass [49], Hedges [50], Hedges and Olkin [1,51], Kraemer and Andrews [52], Kraemer [53], Lund [54], Matt [55], Orwin [56], Rosenthall and Rubin [28], and Thomas [57] consider various definitions of study effect sizes. Standardized study effect sizes permit meta-analyses of studies where the measurement scale of the data may not be uniform across studies.

As indicated in Section II.A, an objective of meta-analysis is to assess the statistical significance of the individual study findings taken as an aggregate. Assessing statistical significance is important, but providing a "pooled" estimate of the parameter embodying the objective of the studies by using the individual estimates from all studies may be more informative. This is particularly true when the pooled estimate is accompanied by a confidence interval.

The functions of the summary measures for the four procedures discussed in Section II.B.2 are pooled point estimates. For example, the pooled estimate from Peto's method is the pooled odds ratio. This is obtained by dividing the sum of the summary measures in the Mantel-Haenszel procedure by the variance of the sum and exponentiating the results. Confidence intervals based on the pooled estimates can be obtained from knowledge of the associated sampling distribution and/or their standard errors by drawing on asymptotic normal theory.

III.   RESEARCH METHODS

Meta-analysis as defined in Section I pertains to statistical methods for combining results from a collection of studies. The methods may be applied to a collection of small, moderate, or large size, and regardless of rules that define the collection or how valid the measurement processes or techniques are that produced the individual study results. If the results of meta-analyses are to be credible, then they must be only part of an investigative research process reflecting good science. Simply put, a protocol should be developed prior to beginning any meta-analyses that reflects the process. Attention should be given to the objective of the investigation, endpoints reflecting the objective, how studies are to be identified and included, procedures for investigating bias, and statistical methods.

There exist numerous papers by authors who discuss shortcomings of meta-analysis investigations and/or criteria for viewing investigations using meta-analyses as a scientific research process. Some of these are: Berlin and Chalmers [58], Boissel et al. [59], Chalmers [60], Chalmers et al. [61,62], Einarson et al. [63], Ellenberg [64], Fitz-gibbon [65], Gerbarg and Horwitz [66], Hunter et al. [67], Jenicek [68], Kurata [69], L'abbe et al. [70], Light and Smith [71], Orwin and Cordray [72], Pignon [73], Rockette and Redmond [74], Sacks et al. [75], and Smith [76]. The papers by Chalmers et al. [61,62], L'abbe et al. [70], and Sacks et al. [75] are particularly noteworthy and in my opinion have greatly influenced the improved quality of meta-analysis investigations seen recently in the literature. Authors who have looked specifically at assessing the bias that may arise from failure to publish negative studies (publication bias or "the file drawer problem") are Begg and Berlin [77], Berlin et al. [78], Dickerson et al. [79], Iyengar and Greenhouse [80], and Simes [81].

IV.   META-ANALYSES OF ULCER DISEASE

To assess the degree to which meta-analysis techniques have been used to synthesize research results from studies of ulcer disease, 36 literature searches, using the sources MEDLINE, RINGDOC, Biosis Previews, EMBASE/Excerpta Medica, MATHSCI, and Comprehensive Core Medical Library were conducted (July 12, 1989). The searches are characterized as follows:

1. S1 AND S2
2. S1 AND S3
3. S1 AND S3 AND S4
4. S1 AND S3 AND S5
5. S1 AND S3 AND S6
6. S1 AND S7
7. S1 AND S7 AND S4
8. S1 AND S7 AND S5
9. S1 AND S7 AND S6
10. S1 AND S2 AND S8
11. S1 AND S3 AND S8
12. S1 AND S3 AND S4 AND S8
13. S1 AND S3 AND S5 AND S8
14. S1 AND S3 AND S6 AND S8
15. S1 AND S7 AND S8
16. S1 AND S7 AND S4 AND S8
17. S1 AND S7 AND S5 AND S8
18. S1 AND S7 AND S6 AND S8

where

S1 = meta-analysis (or meta-analyses)
S2 = ulcer
S3 = duodenal ulcer
S4 = healing (or healed)
S5 = maintenance
S6 = relapse (or recurrence)
S7 = gastric ulcer

and

S8 = randomized controlled trials

After the above 18 searches were run, they were repeated with S1 = combined analysis (or combined analyses). The searches produced 15 abstracts or articles of meta-analyses of clinical trials of ulcer disease. Nine of these reflected investigations of duodenal ulcer; one, an investigation of gastric ulcer; one, an investigation of ulceration from nonsteroidal anti-inflammatory drugs (NSAIDs); two, investigations of stress-related ulcer; one, an investigation of management of variceal bleeding; and one, an investigation of reflux esophagitis.

Three other investigations I know of but did not find in the searches were added to those from the literature search. In addition, a review of the references of the articles produced by the searches revealed three other publications. All of these investigations

were also in the area of duodenal ulcer disease. These six investigations together with
the 15 identified by the searches provide 21 meta-analysis investigations in the area of
ulcer disease. Of these, 15 are the area of duodenal ulcer disease, one is in the area of
benign gastric ulcer disease, four are in the general area of gastrointestinal hemorrhage, and one is in the area of reflux esophagitis.

A.   Meta-Analyses of Duodenal Ulcer Disease

Of the 15 meta-analysis investigations in the area of duodenal ulcer disease, 10 are
articles, two are abstracts, and three are technical reports. All three technical reports
were peer reviewed. These investigations addressed five general questions:

(i)   Is there an association between duodenal ulcer disease and urinary pepsinogen phenotypes?

(ii)   Is there an association between acute duodenal ulcer therapy used for healing
and subsequent relapse rates?

(iii)   Is there an association between gastric acid suppression and duodenal ulcer
healing?

(iv)   Is there a difference between ranitidine and cimetidine in terms of acute
duodenal ulcer healing rates?

(v)   Does potency of maintenance therapy following duodenal ulcer healing
count?

1.   Association Between Duodenal Ulcer Disease and Urinary Pepsinogen Phenotype

Ellis and McConnell [82] address the question of whether there exists an association
between duodenal ulcer disease and urinary pepsinogen phenotypes A and B. They
present individual and combined results of two studies that investigated the association. The individual studies were retrospective involving 437 duodenal ulcer patients
and 1605 controls. Little information is provided about the selection of controls.
Whereas the authors do not use the term meta-analysis, it is clear that the combined
analysis presented is a meta-analysis of the relative risk of the presence of phenotype A
in duodenal ulcer patients compared to controls. The combined analysis from a
methods point of view is sound. Homogeneity of the relative risk across the two
studies is explored using a chi-square test ($.6 < p < 1.0$). The combined relative risk
estimate is 1.74 (chi-square $= 8.01, p < .005$) with a corresponding 95% confidence
interval of (1.19;2.55). It therefore appears that phenotype A is significantly increased in duodenal ulcer patients compared to controls.

2.   Association Between Acute Duodenal Ulcer Therapy and Relapse Rates

McClean et al. [83], Miller and Faragher [84], Peace [85], Peace and Dickson
[86,87], Dobrilla et al. [88], Hunt et al. [89], and Chiverton and Hunt [90] consider
the question of whether there is an association between the acute duodenal ulcer
healing regimen used and subsequent relapse rates. Basically, these eight investiga-

tions reflect four published meta-analysis studies: McClean et al. [83], who report the combined results of 18 trials; Miller and Faragher [84], who report the combined results of six trials; Dobrilla et al. [88], who report the combined results of 25 trials; and Hunt et al. [89], who report the results of 14 trials. These four studies are further summarized and critiqued by Chiverton and Hunt [90], who also explore possible acid secretory mechanisms. These studies suggest strongly that relapse rates differ according to the drug used for acute healing. In particular, the rate of relapse following healing with H_2 receptor antagonists appears greater than that with alternative agents.

A variety of meta-analytic statistical methods were employed in the four studies. These included chi-square tests for homogeneity of association between acute duodenal ulcer therapy and subsequent relapse rates across individual trials, the Mantel-Haenszel [29] test for significance of association when combining the trials, a binomial probability analysis of the sign of the difference in relapse rates between short-term therapies, which is an example of vote-counting methods [1,45], Fisher's [9] inverse chi-square method for combining p values, and 95% confidence intervals based upon the weighted difference between therapies.

The abstract by Dickson and Peace [87] reflects the two technical reports by Peace [85] and Peace and Dickson [86]. These results are also reported in Hunt et al. [89] as one of 14 studies contributing to that meta-analysis. The meta-analysis methods used to produce the results differ from those typically seen in the meta-analysis literature. Since raw data were available on patients, these data were analyzed using life table methods that pooled data across individual trials rather than pooling estimates across trials. Analysis of variance and covariance procedures as well as chi-square procedures were used to assess poolability and to identify factors other than acute therapy that might be associated with relapse. These investigations revealed that previous ulcer history was correlated ($p < .05$) with relapse. Among patients without a history of duodenal ulcer, 6-month relapse rates of 21%, 33%, and 56% were observed among those treated on a short-term basis with placebo, misoprostol 200 μg four times daily, and cimetidine 300 mg four times daily, respectively. Further, in this subset of patients, median time to relapse was 288, 365, and 169 days for patients treated with placebo, misoprostol, and cimetidine, respectively. Comparisons of cimetidine to placebo and to misoprostol revealed statistically significant differences ($p < .05$). These results therefore suggest that relapse following short-term treatment with the H_2-receptor antagonist cimetidine occurs more rapidly and with greater frequency than with placebo or misoprostol and should warrant a large-scale prospective confirmatory clinical trial.

3. Association Between Gastric Acid Suppression and Duodenal Ulcer Healing

Jones et al. [91] and Chiverton et al. [92] considered the question of whether there is an association between acid suppression and duodenal ulcer healing of gastric antisecretory drugs. From a computer-assisted MEDLINE search, Jones et al. [91] identified 18 studies that used aspiration techniques and satisfied Goldman and Feinstein's [93] criteria for pooling. These studies, which were undertaken in duodenal ulcer patients in remission, represented 17 different dosage regimens involving seven drugs. Four of the drugs were H_2-receptor antagonists, one was a proton pump inhibitor, one was a synthetic prostaglandin, and one was antacid. Of the 17 different dosage regimens, 11 involved the H_2-receptor antagonists, four involved the proton pump inhibitor, one involved prostaglandin, and one involved antacid. An additional review of published clinical trials that were double-blinded, randomized, and endoscopically controlled, reflecting the 17 dosage regimens, was undertaken. This review identified 141 trials representing a total of 11,578 patients. Of these trials, 103 involved H_2-receptor antagonists and represented 9469 patients.

Weighted means of suppression of 24-hr acidity (%), suppression of nocturnal acidity (%), and suppression of daytime acidity (%) were computed for the 17 dosage regimens from the 18 gastric antisecretory studies. Weighted healing rates (%) were also computed from the duodenal ulcer healing studies corresponding to the 17 dosage regimens. This effectively produced three derived data sets of 17 paired observations each, on two variables. Percent ulcer healing was considered the dependent variable, and percent suppression was considered the independent variable and subjected to simple and stepwise linear regression analyses.

The results of these analyses revealed that for the H_2-receptor antagonists alone, the most significant correlation was between percent healing and the suppression of nighttime intragastric acidity ($n = 11$, $r = .926$, $p = .001$). Among all 17 regimens, the closest correlation was between percent healing and the suppression of 24-hr intragastric acidity ($r = .911$; $p < .001$). These results, particularly for the H_2-receptor antagonists, enable one to predict the healing rate for a dosage regimen of an antisecretory drug from a knowledge of its effect on intragastric acidity.

The study by Jones et al. [91] is commendable. It is an excellent example of the objective of meta-analysis, which is to answer a medically meaningful question by synthesizing available research results. The analysis, however, is based upon treating averages as analysis units. Effectively, data from 141 clinical trials of duodenal ulcer healing involving 11,578 patients and 18 trials of intragastric acidity have been reduced to 17 paired observations. Although rather large correlation coefficients and corresponding percents of variability in average healing rates explained by a linear relationship with suppression of intragastric acidity were produced, a linear relationship between these two variables is intuitively unappealing—a point with which Rune [94] appears to agree. An alternative analysis would be to perform a weighted regression analysis of the healing rates of individual studies corresponding to each gastric antisecretory regimen and suppression of intragastric acidity. Such an analysis would incorporate study-to-study variation and would enable one to explore other models, including higher order polynomials and piecewise linear regression models, and to assess their goodness of fit.

It would also be interesting to consider only those placebo-controlled trials involving a subset of the dosage regimens. The therapeutic gain (above placebo) in healing rates could be computed for each trial using a standardized effect size as defined in Glass [49]. A meta-analysis of weighted effect sizes could be performed of the trials of each dosage regimen, and confidence intervals on the combined effect size computed. These intervals could then be plotted against dosage regimen to produce confidence bands portraying the relationship between standardized therapeutic gain and suppression of intragastric acidity. A regression analysis of individual standardized study effect sizes on suppression of intragastric acidity could also be performed. Since it is known that more than 40% of duodenal ulcer patients on placebo from randomized controlled clinical trials will experience ulcer healing, the healing rates attributed to the dsoage regimens in Jones et al. [91] do not reflect the effect of the regimens. Therefore, an attraction of either of the alternative approaches using standardized effect sizes is the incorporation of placebo response.

Chiverton et al. [92] studied the relationship between the percent of patients healed on various dosage regimens of intragastric antisecretory drugs and their duration of suppression and length of therapy. Using search procedures and inclusion criteria similar to those of Jones et al. [91], 201 clinician trials of duodenal ulcer healing were identified. Seven investigators were contacted, and raw data were obtained on suppression of intragastric acidity of the dosage regimens. Response surface methodology [95,96] with polynomial regression models was then used to examine the relationship between percent healing and the two predictor variables duration of suppression and length of therapy and to predict ulcer healing rates as a function of these two variables.

The study by Chiverton et al. [92] is an abstract of a presentation made on behalf of an international study group at the DDW meetings in New Orleans. I have long been an advocate of the use of response surface methods to more objectively guide the choice of dose and frequency of dosing in clinical drug development. In fact, I made a presentation on the use of such methods to the International Study Group at its meeting in Deerhurst, Ontario, in March 1987. Such methods are ideally suited to determine dose and frequency of dosing of intragastric antisecretory agents based upon prospective phase I or phase II antisecretory trials. The use of randomized factorial designs of various doses and frequency of dosing should enable one to determine the optimal combination of dose and frequency to suppress a clinically desirable percent of intragastric acidity. This combination could then be used in pivotal phase III clinical efficacy trials to assess healing. In a meta-analysis of 30 published studies of the clinical pharmacology of gastric antisecretory agents in normal volunteers and duodenal ulcer patients, Howden et al. [97] conclude that the expected antisecretory effect of a particular dosage regimen in patients with duodenal ulcer can be predicted mathematically from data derived from studies in normal volunteers. If this is indeed the case, then the phase I and II trials using response surface designs and methods referenced above could be conducted in normal volunteers rather than in duodenal ulcer patients.

4. Comparison of Duodenal Ulcer Healing Rates

McIsaac et al. [98] considered the question of whether there is a real difference between the H_2-receptor antagonists ranitidine and cimetidine in terms of acute duodenal ulcer healing rates. An exhaustive search of the literature (to February 1987) and internal Glaxo databases identified 50 trials that directly compared ranitidine to cimetidine. A review of these trials revealed that six were duplicate publications, and the duplications were therefore eliminated. Of the 44 trials, all appear to have been randomized; 36 favored ranitidine; and 31 had endoscopy at 4 weeks, of which four were double-blinded and 27 were single-blinded.

Meta-analyses comparing ranitidine to cimetidine were performed on six subsets of the 44 trials. These were: (i) All 44 trials; (ii) only those 25 trials in which the cimetidine regimen was 1.0 g/day and endoscopy was performed at 4 weeks; (iii) a further subset (15) of the previously mentioned 25 trials in which the ranitidine dose was 150 mg twice daily; (iv) only those six trials in which the cimetidine dose was 400 mg twice daily and endoscopy was performed at 4 weeks; (v) a further subset (5) of the previously mentioned six trials (one trial was a three-arm study and contained insufficient data); and (vi) the 13 remaining trials $(44 - 25 - 6)$. The Breslow-Day [99] test was used to assess homogeneity of the odds ratio of ranitidine to cimetidine in terms of percent of patients healed, across trials. The Mantel-Haenszel [29] procedure was used to assess the statistical significance of the difference in combined healing rates across the trials.

The results of the meta-analyses are summarized in Table 1.

It appears, on the basis of results of this investigation, that there is a statistically

Table 1

Subset	Percentage healed (healed/total) Ranitidine	Cimetidine	Treat. diff. $(R - C)$ (%)	Homogeneity treat. diff. χ^2	p
i	77.7	70.4	7.3	45.8	(0.33)
	(1702/2191)	(1536/2183)		32.4	(<0.01)
ii	—	—	—	—	
	—	—		11.7	(<0.01)
iii	75.8	70.0	5.8	5.39	(0.98)
	(847/1117)	(767/1096)		8.62	(<0.01)
iv	—	—	—	—	
	—	—		14.8	(<0.01)
v	81.0	69.5	11.5	2.32	(0.68)
	(294/363)	(246/354)		12.9	(<0.01)
vi	—	—	7.6	—	
	—	—		11.9	(<0.01)

significant difference in healing rates in favor of ranitidine and that this difference appears to be consistent across the trials. On average, ranitidine would be expected to induce healing in 7% more patients than cimetidine.

Apparently no placebo-controlled trials were included in the investigation by McIsaac et al. [98], if indeed any trials that also included both ranitidine and cimetidine have been conducted. It is widely thought that positive controlled trials in many disease areas may reflect an upward bias. If trials are double-blinded, one would expect the bias to be the same for both treatment groups and to therefore cancel out when looking at the difference between the two groups. Nevertheless, it would be of interest to see whether the results of the McIsaac investigation are corroborated when the therapeutic gain of ranitidine (compared to placebo) is compared to the therapeutic gain of cimetidine (compared to placebo).

5. Relationship Between Duodenal Ulcer Maintenance and Potency of Maintenance Therapy

Dickson et al. [100] considered the question of whether there is a relationship between duodenal ulcer relapse and the potency of maintenance regimens. All published studies available in the literature (March 1986) were reviewed. After deleting multiple reports of the same studies and reports for which numerator and/or denominator and/or relapse percentage could not be determined, 79 studies were identified. These studies represented over 4000 patients and 16 dosage regimens of anti-ulcer agents. The agents included placebo, sucralfate, bismuth, antacid, pirenzipine, cimetidine, and ranitidine. The potency of each of the 16 regimens was rated on a scale from 1 to 16 in terms of suppression of nocturnal gastric acidity and in terms of suppression of 24-hr gastric acidity. Concordance between ratings was good. Placebo received the lowest rating, and ranitidine 150 mg twice daily received the highest rating.

Meta-analyses including and excluding placebo were then performed that addressed the association between relapse rates at 3, 6, and 12 months and potency. Several measures of association—Kendall's τ, Spearman's ρ, Pearson's r, Pearson's r weighted according to study size, and Pearson's r applied to the ranks of the relapse rates weighted according to study size—were used. There was close agreement between results using the various measures of association. When placebo was included, a significant negative correlation was observed at 3, 6, and 12 months. A maximum of 56% ($r = -.75$; $p < .0001$) of the variation among relapse rates was explained by a linear relationship between relapse and potency. When placebo was excluded, there was no evidence (maximum $r^2 = 8\%$; $p = .42$) of an association. The significance of an association with the inclusion of placebo likely reflects a corroboration of the fact that most nonplacebo regimens were statistically significant ($p < .05$) compared to placebo at 3, 6, and 12 months. The authors therefore concluded, on the basis of the analyses conducted, that there was little or no evidence to support an association between duodenal ulcer relapse and potency of maintenance regimens.

B.   Meta-Analysis of Gastric Ulcer Disease

The single investigation by Howden et al. [101] in the area of benign gastric ulcer disease addressed the general question of whether healing of gastric ulcer was correlated with either the suppression of intragastric acidity or the duration of medical treatment. Previously Jones et al. [91] reported a relationship between healing of duodenal ulcer and suppression of intragastric acidity, particularly for suppression of nocturnal acidity. The investigation by Howden et al. [101] was carried out to see whether a similar relationship existed in gastric ulcer healing.

A computer-generated MEDLINE search from 1974 onwards identified 56 published clinical trials of antisecretory drugs in benign gastric ulcer. A further search produced 10 published studies of 24-hr or nocturnal intragastric acidity. Regression analyses similar to those reported in Jones et al. [91] were used to assess correlation. The analyses were conducted including and excluding the placebo arm from the gastric ulcer trials. Analyses of trend were also performed using the methodology of Williams [102]. This analysis permits the assessment of a monotonic increase in healing rates according to the increasing order of their observed gastric antisecretory potencies.

The results of the analyses revealed no significant correlations or trends between healing rates and suppression of intragastric acidity unless placebo was included in the analysis. When placebo was included, the correlation was stronger for suppression of 24-hr than for nocturnal acidity. The authors [101] conclude that duration of treatment with gastric antisecretory drugs appears to be the most important factor in predicting gastric ulcer healing rates. Placebo and all drug regimens showed a consistent increase with prolongation of treatment.

C.   Meta-Analysis in Gastrointestinal Hemorrhage

Four meta-analytic investigations were in the general area of gastrointestinal hemorrhage. Of these, one was an abstract and three were articles. These investigations addressed four questions:

1.   Do critically ill patients derive benefit from antacid or cimetidine therapy as stress ulcer prophylaxis?
2.   What is the estimate of rare gastrointestinal complications, particularly hemorrhage, in patients requiring nonsteroidal anti-inflammatory drugs (NSAIDs)?
3.   Are fibrinolytic inhibitors of value when given to patients with upper gastrointestinal hemorrhage?
4.   What is the role of variceal sclerotherapy in the management of variceal bleeding?

1. The Benefit of Prophylaxis Therapy in Critically Ill Patients at Risk for Stress Ulcer

Kussin et al. [103] examined the first question. Eleven randomized controlled trials of stress ulcer prophylaxis in the critically ill were identified. These trials, in which the regimens were no prophylaxis or antacid or cimetidine as prophylactic agent, ranged in size from 27 to 320 patients, with a broad range of diseases. Pooling the 11 trials, 1174 patients produced rates of gastrointestinal bleeding of 30%, 8%, and 4% for the no prophylaxis, cimetidine, and antacid groups, respectively. No prophylaxis was found to be statistically significantly ($p < .001$) inferior to both cimetidine and antacid, whereas cimetidine was found to be statistically significantly ($p < .01$) inferior to antacid.

Kussin et al. recognize that the 11 trials are generally of poor quality and assess the quality by a previously developed mean quality score. The trials were particularly deficient in the areas of blinding, randomization process, determination of sample size, and discussion of power. Nevertheless, the authors conclude that the results of the combined analysis strongly suggest that prophylaxis is beneficial and that antacid therapy is superior to cimetidine therapy.

Since this investigation was reported as an abstract, space was limited. This could explain why no mention was made of literature search procedures, the assessment of homogeneity across trials, or the methodology for combining results across trials.

2. The Incidence of Rare Gastrointestinal Complications in Patients Requiring NSAIDs

Chalmers et al. [104] addressed the second question. They conducted an investigation aimed at estimating the incidence of rare gastrointestinal complications in patients from randomized controlled clinical trials (RCTs) requiring NSAID therapy. The investigation is one of the most rigorous meta-analyses yet conducted. Prior to commencing the investigation, a protocol was developed detailing methods for finding studies, selection of studies for inclusion, and analyses. Care was taken to minimize bias in each of these areas that might influence results and conclusions from the investigation.

From an initial MEDLINE search that revealed 54,730 papers, selection criteria permitted inclusion on only 140 RCTs, which were subjected to meta-analyses. These trials were such that the control to which the NSAID was compared was placebo, no drug, or a drug with no anti-inflammatory property. The 140 trials permitted separation of the comparisons into those in which the NSAID was aspirin or a non-aspirin nonsteroidal drug (NANSAID). This resulted in 44 comparisons of aspirin to control and 123 comparisons of NANSAID to control.

Analysis methods included crude pooling and unweighted averaging of the rate differences between control and treated groups for each study. Those comparisons for which the unweighted mean difference was two or more standard deviations away from zero were pooled using the DerSimonian and Laird (D&L) [2] modification of the

Cochran [5] procedure. Finally, logistic regression procedures were used to assess whether any factors seemed to be more associated with side effects than others.

The results of the analyses for the 44 aspirin-to-control comparisons showed that the unweighted rate difference was $0.6 \pm 0.3\%$ for ulcer, $3 \pm 1\%$ for unspecified gastric symptoms, and $0.6 \pm 0.2\%$ for hemorrhage. Analysis results for the 123 NANSAID-to-control comparisons showed that the unweighted rate difference was $0.05 \pm 0.03\%$ for ulcer, $2 \pm 0.5\%$ for unspecified gastric symptoms, and $0.7 \pm 0.4\%$ for hemorrhage. Further, the conservative D&L method revealed that only the unspecified gastric symptoms associated with NANSAIDs and hemorrhage associated with aspirin were statistically significant.

3. The Value of Fibrinolytic Inhibitors on Mortality in Patients with Upper Gastrointestinal Hemorrhage

Henry and O'Connell [105] addressed the third question. They conducted an investigation aimed at assessing the effects of fibrinolytic inhibitors on rebleeding, the need for surgery, and mortality in patients with upper gastrointestinal hemorrhage. The investigation is an example of the best features of meta-analyses. Prior to commencing the investigation, a protocol was developed specifying the objective of the investigation, identification of endpoints, detailing methods for the literature search, selection of studies for inclusion, and analyses. Care was taken to minimize bias in each of these areas that might influence results and conclusions from the investigation. The manuscript is well written, with results and discussion succinctly presented.

From an initial MEDLINE search that revealed 11 publications, selection criteria permitted inclusion of only six RCTs, which were subjected to meta-analyses. These trials all compared tranexamic acid to placebo and represented a total patient population of 1212. Data on 55 additional patients were obtained directly from authors of two of the trials.

Analysis methods included computing the odds ratios of the endpoints in patients assigned to tranexamic acid to those assigned to placebo for each trial. Two methods were then used to assess homogeneity of the odds ratios and to combine them across trials. These methods were the D&L [2] modification of Cochran's [5] procedure, and Peto's [30] modification of the Mantel-Haenszel [29] procedure.

The results of the analyses are summarized in Table 2 (a version of Table 4 in Henry and O'Connell [105]). The authors conclude that treatment with tranexamic acid may be of value to patients considered to be at risk of dying after an upper gastrointestinal hemorrhage.

4. The Role of Variceal Sclerotherapy in the Management of Patients with Variceal Hemorrhage

Infante-Rivard et al. [106] addressed the fourth question. They conducted an investigation aimed at assessing the effect of repeated endoscopic variceal sclerotherapy on

Table 2

Endpoint	Pooled odds ratio	95% CI	*p*-Value for treatment	*p*-Value for homogeneity
		D & L method		
Rebleed	0.72	(0.5;1.1)	0.14	0.09
Operation	0.58	(0.3;1.8)	0.13	0.01
Mortality	0.60	(0.4;0.9)	0.02	0.78
		Peto method		
Rebleed	0.80	(0.6;1.1)	0.13	0.08
Operation	0.72	(0.5;1.0)	0.05	0.01
Mortality	0.60	(0.4;0.9)	0.01	0.82

Source: Adapted from Henry and O'Connell [105].

the long-term survival of patients with variceal hemorrhage. The investigation is another example of sound principles of meta-analyses as described by Sacks et al. [75] and L'abbe et al. [70]. Prior to initiating the investigation, a protocol was developed detailing methods for the literature search, selection of studies for inclusion, and analyses. Care was taken to minimize bias in each of these areas that might influence results and conclusions from the investigation, including sensitivity analyses and attention to the impact of possible unpublished results. The manuscript is well written, with results and discussion concisely and succinctly presented.

An initial search utilizing MEDLINE and a manual search of the references from review articles revealed nine publications. Selection criteria permitted inclusion of seven RCTs that were subjected to meta-analyses. These trials compared serial sclerotherapy to standard therapy (tamponade or vasopressin or both) and represented a total patient population of 748.

Analysis methods included the computation of total mortality risk difference between patients assigned to sclerotherapy and those assigned to standard therapy for each trial. DerSimonian and Laird's [2] modification of Cochran's [5] procedure was then used to assess homogeneity of the risk differences and to combine them across trials.

The results of the analyses revealed risk differences to be consistent with the hypothesis of homogeneity across trials ($p = .12$). The overall weighted risk difference of -0.15 was statistically significant ($p < .0005$) with 95% confidence limits of -0.21 to -0.08. These results indicate that sclerotherapy may reduce overall mortality by 25% compared to standard therapy. The authors therefore conclude that repeated sclerotherapy may be beneficial in patients with variceal bleeding requiring long-term management.

It appears that these analyses ignored the time of death. If this information were known, then meta-analysis life table methods could be used to provide a more precise and informative analysis. Care must be exercised, however, in applying such methods [107].

D.   Meta-Analysis of Reflux Esophagitis

The single investigation by Stalnikowicz-Darvasi [108] addressed the general question of whether H_2-receptor antagonists are clinically beneficial in the management of patients with reflux esophagitis. The investigation describes in detail methods for finding studies and subsequent selection for inclusion. However, selection criteria may have been too rigid, and the investigation appears lacking in appropriate attention to statistical methods.

From an initial *Index Medicus* search and review of bibliographic resources of textbooks, 20 articles were reviewed for inclusion. Of these, 10 satisfied the inclusion criteria (i) randomization, (ii) similarity of control and experimental groups, (iii) definition of criteria for diagnosis or of endoscopic criteria for esophagitis and patient characteristics, (iv) definition of criteria for assessment of outcome, (v) blind outcome assessment, (vi) determination of both type I and type II errors, and (vii) thorough follow-up with all patients who entered accounted for at study conclusion. The studies compared either cimetidine or ranitidine to placebo and represented a patient population of 411.

The range of symptomatic improvement across studies was 43–63% among patients treated with H_2-receptor antagonists as contrasted to a range of 9–35% among patients receiving placebo. The range of endoscopic improvement across studies was 60–88% among patients treated with H_2-receptor antagonists as contrasted to a range of 26–28% among patients receiving placebo. Overall endoscopic improvement rates were 62% and 31% for the H_2-receptor antagonists and placebo ($p < .01$), respectively. I conclude that H_2-receptor antagonists are an effective treatment for reflux esophagitis.

REFERENCES

1.   Hedges LV, Olkin I. Statistical methods for meta-analysis. Orlando, Fla.: Academic, 1985:1–369.
2.   DerSimonian R, Laird N. Meta-analysis in clinical trials. Controlled Clin Trials 1986; 7(3):177–88.
3.   Cochran WG. Problems arising in the analysis of a series of similar experiments. J Roy Stat Soc 1937; 4:102–18.
4.   Cochran WG. The comparison of different scales of measurement for experimental results. Ann Math Stat 1943; 14:205–16.
5.   Cochran WG. The combination of estimates from different experiments. Biometrics 1954(Mar):101–29.
6.   Yates F, Cochran WG. The analysis of groups of experiments. J Agric Sci 1938; 28:556–80.

7.   Peace KE. The alternative hypothesis: One-sided or two-sided? J Clin Epidemiol 1989; 42(5):473–6.

8.   Tippett LHC. The method of statistics. London: WIlliams and Norgate, 1931.

9.   Fisher RA. Statistical methods for research workers. 4th ed. London: Oliver and Boyd, 1932.

10. Pearson K. On a method of determining whether a sample of given size n supposed to have been drawn from a parent population having a known probability integral has probably been drawn at random. Biometrika 1933; 25:379–410.

11. Wilkinson B. A statistical consideration in psychological research. Psych Bull 1951; 48:156–8.

12. Edgington ES. An additive method for combining probability values from independent experiments. J Psychol 1972; 80:351–63.

13. Edgington ES. A normal curve method for combining probability values from independent experiments. J Psychol 1972; 82:85–9.

14. George EO. Combining independent one-sided and two-sided tests—some theory and applications. Doctoral Dissertation, Univ. of Rochester, 1977.

15. Mudholkar GS, George EO. The logit method for combining probabilities. In: Rustagi J, ed. Symposium for optimizing methods in statistics. New York: Academic, 1979:345–66.

16. David FN. On the P test for randomness: remarks, further illustrations and table for P. Biometrika 1934; 26:1–11.

17. Good IJ. On the weighted combination of significance tests. J Roy Stat Soc Ser B 1955; 17:264–5.

18. Zelen M, Joel LS. On the weighted compounding of two independent significance tests. Ann Math Stat 1959; 30:885–95.

19. Pape ES. A combination of F-statistics. Technometrics 1972; 14:89–99.

20. Strube MJ. Power analysis for combining significance levels. Psychol Bull 1985; 98: 595–9.

21. Littell RC, Folks JL. Asymptotic optimality of Fisher's method of combining independent tests. J Am Stat Assoc 1971; 66(336):802–6.

22. Littell RC, Folks JL. Asymptotic optimality of Fisher's method of combining independent tests II. J Am Stat Assoc 1973; 68(341):193–4.

23. Berk RH, Cohen A. Asymptotically optimal methods of combining tests. J Am Stat Assoc 1979; 74(368):812–4.

24. Brown MB. 400: a method for combining non-independent, one-sided tests of significance. Biometrics 1975; 31:987–92.

25. Strube MJ. Combining and comparing significance levels from nonindependent hypothesis tests. Psychol Bull 1985; 97:334–41.

26. Brozek J, Tiede K. Reliable and questionable significance in a series of statistical tests. Psych Bull 1952; 49:559–74.

27. Rosenthall R, Rubin DB. Comparing significance levels of independent studies. Psych Bull 1979; 86:1165–8.

28. Rosenthall R, Rubin DB. Comparing effect sizes of independent studies. Psych Bull 1982; 92:500–4.

29. Mantel N, Haenszel W. Statistical aspects of the analysis of data from retrospective studies of disease. J Natl Cancer Inst 1959; 22:719–48.

30. Yusuf S, Peto R, Lewis J, Collins R, Sleight P. Beta blockade during and after myocardial infarction: an overview of the randomized trials. Prog Cardiol Dis 1985; 27(5):335–71.

31. Stouffer SA, Suchman EA, DeVinney LC, Star SA, Williams RM Jr. The american soldier: adjustment during army life. Vol. 1. Princeton, NJ: Princeton Univ. Press, 1949.

32. Liptak T. On the combination of independent tests. Mat Kut Intez Kozl 1958; 3:1971–7.

33. Schaafsma W. A comparison of the most stringent and the most stringent somewhere most powerful test for certain problems with restricted alternative. Ann Math Stat 1968; 39:531–46.

34. Mosteller FM, Bush RR. Selected quantitative techniques. In: Lindzey G, ed. Handbook of social psychology. Vol. I. Theory and method. Cambridge, Mass.: Addison-Wesley, 1954.

35. Oosterhoff J. Combination of one-sided statistical tests. Amsterdam: Mathematical Centre Tracts, 1969:28.

36. Winer BJ. Statistical principles in experimental design. 2nd ed. New York: McGraw-Hill, 1971.

37. Lancaster HO. The combination of probabilities: an application of orthonormal functions. Aust J Stat 1961; 3:20–33.

38. Koziol JA, Perlman MD. Combining independent Chi-square tests. Tech Report 19, Dept of Statistics, Univ. of Chicago, 1976.

39. Koziol JA, Perlman MD. Combining independent chi-square tests. J Am Stat Assoc 1978; 73:753–63.

40. Marden JI. Combining independent noncentral chi-squared or F tests. Ann Stat 1982; 10(1):266–77.

41. Zelen M. The analysis of incomplete block designs. J Am Stat Assoc 1957; 52:204–17.

42. Berlin JA, Laird NM, Sacks HS, Chalmers TC. A comparison of statistical methods for combining event rates from clinical trials. Stat Med 1989; 8(2):141–51.

43. Katz BM, Marascuilo LA, McSweeney M. Nonparametric alternatives for testing main effects hypotheses: a model for combining data across independent studies. Psychol Bull 1985; 98:200–8.

44. Jones LV, Fiske DW. Models for testing the significance of combined results. Psych Bull 1953; 50:375–82.

45. Hedges LV, Olkin I. Vote counting methods in research synthesis. Psych Bull 1980; 88:359–69.

46. Raudenbush SW, Bryk AS. Empirical Bayes meta-analysis. J Educ Stat 1985; 10:75–98.

47. Goodman SN. Meta-analysis and evidence. Control Clin Trials 1989; 10:188–204.

48. Zucker D, Yusuf S. The likelihood ratio versus the p value in meta-analysis: where is the evidence? Control Clin Trials 1989; 10:205–8.

49. Glass GV. Primary, secondary and meta-analysis of research. Educ Res 1976; 10:3–8.

50. Hedges LV. Estimation of effect size under nonrandom sampling: the effects of censoring studies yielding statistically insignificant mean differences. J Educ Stat 1984; 9:61–85.

51. Hedges LV, Olkin I. Nonparametric estimators of effect size in meta-analysis. Psych Bull 1984; 96:573–80.

52. Kraemer HC, Andrews G. A nonparametric technique for meta-analysis effect size calculation. Psychol Bull 1982; 91:404–12.

53. Kraemer HC. Theory of estimation and testing of effect sizes: use in meta-analysis. J Educ Stat 1983; 8:93–101.

54. Lund T. Some metrical issues with meta-analysis of therapy effects. Scand J Psychol 1988; 29(1):1–8.

55. Matt GE. Decision rules for selecting effect sizes in meta-analysis: a review and reanalysis of psychotherapy outcome studies. Psychol Bull 1989; 105(1):106–15.

56. Orwin RG. A fail-safe N for effect size in meta-analysis. J Educ Stat 1983; 8:157–9.

57. Thomas H. Effect size standard errors for the non-normal non-identically distributed case. J Educ Stat 1986; 11:293–303.

58. Berlin JA, Chalmers TC. Commentary on meta-analysis in clinical trials. Hepatology 1988; 8(3):690–1.

59. Boissel JP, Sacks HS, Leizorovicz A, Blanchard J, Panak E, Peyrieux JC. Meta-analysis of clinical trials: summary of an international conference. Eur J Clin Pharmacol 1988; 34(6):535–8.

60. Chalmers TC. Meta-analysis in clinical medicine. Trans Am Clin Climatol Assoc 1987; 99:144–50.

61. Chalmers TC, Berrier J, Sacks HS, Levin H, Reitman D, Nagalingam R. Meta-analysis of clinical trials as a scientific discipline. I. Control of bias and comparison with large co-operative trials. Stat Med 1987; 6(3):315–28.

62. Chalmers TC, Berrier J, Sacks HS, Levin H, Reitman D, Nagalingam R. Meta-analysis of clinical trials as a scientific discipline. II. Replicate variability and comparison of studies that agree and disagree. Stat Med 1987; 6(7):733–44.

63. Einarson TR, Leeder JS, Doren G. A method for meta-analysis of epidemiological studies. Drug Intell Clin Pharmacol 1988; 22(10):813–24.

64. Ellenberg SS. Meta-analysis: the quantitative approach to research review. Semin Oncol 1988; 15(5):472–81.

65. Fitz-Gibbon CT. In defence of randomised controlled trials, with suggestions about the possible use of meta-analysis. Br J Disord Commun 1986; 21(1):117–24.

66. Gerbarg ZB, Horwitz RI. Resolving conflicting clinical trials: guidelines for meta-analysis. J Clin Epidemiol 1988; 41(5):503–9.

67. Hunter JE, Schmidt FL, Jackson GB. Review of meta-analysis: cumulating research findings across studies. Studying organizations: innovations in methodology, Vol. 4. Contemp Psychol 1983; 28:835–6.

68. Jenicek M. Meta-analysis in medicine. Where we are and where we want to go. J Clin Epidemiol 1989; 42(1):35–44.

69. Kurata JH. Ulcer epidemiology: an overview and proposed research framework. Gastroenterology 1989; 96(2.2 Suppl):569–80.

70. L'abbe KA, Detsky AS, O'Rourke K. Meta-analysis in clinical research. Ann Intern Med 1987; 107:224–33.

71. Light RJ, Smith PV. Accumulating evidence: procedures for resolving contradictions among different research studies. Harvard Educ Rev 1971; 41:429–71.

72. Orwin RG, Cordray DS. Effects of deficient reporting on meta-analysis: a conceptual framework and reanalysis. Psychol Bull 1985; 97:134–47.

73. Pignon JP. La meta-analyse en recherche clinique. Presse Med 1988; 17(44):2328–30.

74. Rockette HE, Redmond CK. Limitations and advantages of meta-analysis in clinical trials. Recent Results Cancer Res 1988; 222:99–104.

75. Sacks HS, Berrier J, Reitman D, Ancona-Berk VA, Chalmers TC. Meta-analyses of randomized controlled trials. N Engl J Med 1987; 316(8):450–5.

76. Smith MC. Meta-analysis. NLN Publ 1988; 15:77–91.

77. Begg CB, Berlin JA. Publication bias and dissemination of clinical research. J Natl Cancer Inst 1989; 81(2):107–15.

78. Berlin JA, Begg CB, Louis TA. An assessment of publication bias using a sample of published clinical trials. J Am Stat Assoc 1989; 84(406):381–92.

79. Dickerson K, Chan S, Chalmers TC, Sacks HS, Smith H Jr. Publication bias and clinical trials. Controlled Clin Trials 1987; 8(4):343–53.

80. Iyengar S, Greenhouse JB. Selection models and the file-drawer problem. Tech Report 394, Carnegie-Mellon Univ, Pittsburgh, Pa, 1987:1–27.

81. Simes RJ. Confronting publication bias: a cohort design for meta-analysis. Stat Med 1987; 6(1):11–29.

82. Ellis A, McConnell RB. Duodenal ulcer and urinary pepsinogen phenotypes. Gastroenterology 1982; 83(6):1261–3.

83. McClean AJ, Harrison PM, Ioannides-Demos L, Byne AJ, McCarthy P, Dudley FJ. The choice of ulcer healing agent influences duodenal ulcer healing rate and long term clinical outcome. Aust MZ J Med 1985; 15:367–74.

84. Miller JP, Faragher EB. Relapse of duodenal ulcer: does it matter which drug is used in initial treatment? Br Med J 1986; 293:1117–8.

85. Peace KE. An analysis of GD Searle in-house data on spontaneous duodenal ulcer recurrence. Tech Rept S81-87-07-001. GD Searle & Co, Skokie, Ill., February 1987.

86. Peace KE, Dickson B. Meta-analysis of duodenal ulcer relapse using actual patient data: a comparison of the effect of acute treatment with cimetidine, misoprostol and placebo. Tech Rept. GD Searle & Co, Skokie, Ill., June 1987.

87. Dickson B, Peace KE. The effect of acute treatment with misoprostol, cimetidine and placebo on spontaneous duodenal ulcer recurrence. Gastroenterology 1987; 92(5):1370.

88. Dobrilla G, Vallaperta P, Amplatz S. Influence of ulcer healing agents on ulcer relapse after discontinuation of acute treatment: a pooled estimate of controlled clinical trials. Gut 1988; 27:181–7.

89. Hunt RH, Chiverton S, Burget DW, Peace KE, Dickson B. Effect of initial treatment for duodenal ulcer on subsequent relapse rates. Post Grad Med 1988:27–31.

90. Chiverton SG, Hunt RH. Initial therapy and relapse of duodenal ulcer: possible acid secretory mechanisms. Gastroenterology 1989; 96(2.2 Suppl):632–9.

91. Jones DB, Howden CW, Burget DW, Kerr GD, Hunt RH. Acid suppression in duodenal ulcer: a meta-analysis to define optimal dosing with antisecretory drugs. Gut 1987; 28(9):1120–7.

92. Chiverton SG, Burget DW, Hunt RH. A meta-analysis to predict duodenal ulcer healing from acid suppression. Gastroenterology 1988; 94(5 part 2).

93. Goldman L, Feinstein AR. Anticoagulants and myocardial infarction: the problems of pooling drowning and floating. Ann Intern Med 1979; 90:92–4.

94. Rune SJ. The relationship between acid reduction and rate of ulcer healing. Scand J Gastroenterol Suppl 1988; 155:12–5.

95. Myers RH. Response surface methodology. Boston: Allyn and Bacon, 1971.

96. Peace KE. Response surface methods in anti-anginal drug development. In: Peace K, ed. Statistical issues in pharmaceutical drug research and development. New York: Marcel Dekker, 1989:285–303.

97. Howden CW, Jones DB, Burget DW, Hunt RH. Comparison of the effects of gastric antisecretory agents in healthy volunteers and patients with duodenal ulcer. Gut 1986; 27(9):1058–61.

98. McIsaac RL, McCanless I, Summers K, Wood JR. Ranitidine and cimetidine in the healing of duodenal ulcer meta-analysis of comparative trials. Aliment Pharmacol Ther 1987; 1(5):369–82.

99. Breslow NE, Day NE. Statistical methods in cancer research. Vol. 1. The analysis of case control studies. Lyon: International Agency for Research in Cancer; 1980.

100. Dickson B, Peace KE, Dixon W, Braverman A. Duodenal ulcer maintenance: does potency count? Tech Rept., Smith Kline and French Laboratories, June 1986.

101. Howden CW, Jones DB, Peace KE, Burget DW, Hunt RH. The treatment of gastric ulcer with antisecretory drugs: relationship of pharmacological effect of healing rates. J Dig Dis Sci 1987.

102. Williams DA. A test for differences between treatment means when several dose levels are compared with a zero dose control. Biometrics 1971; 27:103–17.

103. Kussin P, Sacks HS, Chalmers TC. Stress ulcer prophylaxis in the critically ill: quality assessment and meta-analysis of randomized control trials (RCT's). Gastroenterology 1985; 88(5.2):1715.

104. Chalmers TC, Berrier J, Hewitt P, Berlin J, Reitman D, Nagalingam R, Sacks H. Meta-analysis of randomized controlled trials as a method of estimating rare complications of non-steroidal anti-inflammatory drug therapy. Aliment Pharmacol Ther 1988; 2(Suppl 1):9–26.

105. Henry DA, O'Connell DL. Effects of fibrinolytic inhibitors on mortality from upper gastrointestinal haemorrhage. Br Med J 1989:1142–6.

106. Infante-Rivard C, Esnaola S, Villeneuve JP. Role of endoscopic variceal sclerotherapy in the long-term management of variceal bleeding: a meta-analysis. Gastroenterology 1989; 96(4):1087–92.

107. Abel UR, Edler L. A pitfall in the meta-analysis of hazard ratios. Controlled Clin Trials 1988; 116(1.1):149–51.

108. Stalnikowicz-Darvase R. H_2 Antagonists in the treatment of reflux esophagitis: a critical analysis. Am J Gastroenterol 1989; 84(3):245–8.

109. Rosenthall R. Combining results of independent studies. Psych Bull 1978; 85:185–93.

20

An Academic Investigator's Perspective

SHIU-KUM LAM

University of Hong Kong Queen Mary Hospital,
Hong Kong

I. INTRODUCTION

Therapeutic advances have outpaced scientific attempts to understand the etiology of peptic ulcer. In this respect, research in peptic ulcer follows the same evolution as that in diabetes mellitus and hypertension. It is likely that future research in ulcer therapy will concentrate on fine-tuning of treatment strategies, while that in etiology will, because of the well-known heterogeneity of peptic ulcer, focus on identification of pathogenetic processes responsible for subsets of peptic ulcers.

II. THERAPEUTIC PERSPECTIVES

A. What Do We Know About Ulcer Healing?

Ulcer Heals "Spontaneously."   It is fair to assume from placebo studies that ulcers heal spontaneously, and the healing rate varies in different parts of the world, ranging from 0 to 79% for duodenal ulcers [1]. In general, placebo healing rates are about half the rates achieved by most therapeutic agents. The fact that spontaneous healing occurs suggests that either the precipitating cause of ulceration has been removed or there has been readjustment of the gastric milieu to a state that favors healing. Because we do not know the cause of ulcer, we are not clear what would precipitate ulcer formation. However, we have some clues as to the states of gastric environment that would favor healing.

Hypochlorhydria Favors Healing.   This is well documented for both duodenal and gastric ulcers. The healing rates, in fact, are positively related to the degree of acid inhibition, as has been reviewed [2]. The observations that omeprazole, the most potent acid inhibitory agent available on the market, achieves healing rates similar to those of H_2-receptor antagonists, but in half the time, further attest to this view. We thus have a situation in which the 2-week healing rate of duodenal ulcer is about 25% for placebo, 50% for H_2-receptor antagonists, and 75% for omeprazole. It would seem from these observations that placebo is able to reduce acidity to some extent, which obviously cannot be true. One explanation is that the stomach reacts to the ulcer-precipitating factor by readjusting its milieu, and one way to achieve this is to down-regulate its parietal cells, making them less sensitive to stimulation. There is recent evidence that physiological down-regulation may indeed occur [3]. This may help to facilitate spontaneous healing or healing in the absence of pharmacological alteration of gastric acidity.

A Nonsmoking Environment Favors Healing.   Cigarette smoking consistently delays duodenal ulcer healing by placebo, and the effect is highly significant if studies are pooled together (Table 1). Although this effect is less consistently seen in patients treated with potent acid-reducing agents such as H_2-receptor antagonists and large doses of antacids, the effect remains highly significant when trials are pooled together (Table 2). Even in patients treated with omeprazole, the most potent acid-reducing agent known, a significant delay in healing at 2 weeks but not at 4 weeks could be observed in patients who smoked (Table 2). These results suggest that very

Table 1   Cigarette Smoking and Duodenal Ulcer Healing by Placebo

Study	Year	Smokers		Nonsmokers	
		n	% healed	n	% healed
Peterson et al. [4]	1977	25	32	13	69
Hetzel et a. [5]	1978	30	37	12	42
Bardhan et al. [6]	1979	33	24	13	38
Bianchi Porro et al. [7]	1980	55	31	15	53
Massarrat and Eisenmann [8]	1981	56	48	24	75
Sonnenberg et al. [9]	1981	26	38	23	57
Strom et al. [10]	1982	14	14	10	60
Barakat et al. [11]	1984	19	16	20	20
Frederiksen et al. [12]	1984	65	52	26	69
Dyck et al. [13]	1987	64	35	37	17
Gitlin et al. [14]	1987	59	42	38	50
Total		446	35	231	48

$p < .0005.$

Table 2 Cigarette Smoking and Duodenal Ulcer Healing by Conventional Acid-Reducing Agents (H_2 Antagonists, Antacids, Anticholinergics) and by Omeprazole

		Smokers		Nonsmokers	
Study	Year	*n*	% healed	*n*	% healed
Conventional acid-reducing agents					
Peterson et al. [4]	1977	28	75	8	89
Hetzel et al. [5]	1878	30	86	15	80
Lam et al. [15]	1979	17	59	34	91
Bardhan et al. [6]	1979	93	65	41	68
Marks et al. [16]	1980	18	78	10	60
Bianchi Porro et al. [7]	1980	63	71	27	81
Korman et al. [17]	1981	23	44	27	85
Sonnenberg et al. [9]	1981	29	59	25	72
Strom et al. [10]	1981	32	88	11	91
Gugler et al. [18]	1982	69	68	30	93
Barr et al. [19]	1982	25	72	25	64
Korman et al. [20]	1983	71	63	64	95
Ippoliti et al. [21]	1983	66	52	95	77
Ireland et al. [22]	1984	59	85	43	95
Barakat et al. [11]	1984	19	74	21	76
Collin-Jones et al. [23]	1984	59	85	43	95
Lam et al. [24]	1985	23	78	20	95
Farley et al. [25]	1985	68	81	21	100
Lee et al. [26]	1986	272	79	152	84
Hamilton et al. [27]	1986	25	68	14	86
Dyck et al. [13]	1987	144	59	70	66
Simon et al. [28]	1987	434	78	343	84
Gitlin et al. [14]	1987	162	81	104	87
Bardhan et al. [29]	1987	100	69	24	75
Merki et al. [30]	1988	103	61	31	71
Bardhan et al. [31]	1988	18	94	15	80
Weberg et al. [32]	1988	101	75	49	73
Total[a]		2151	73	1362	83
Omeprazole (2 week healing)					
Classen et al. [33]	1985	92	66	54	81
Lauritsen et al. [34]	1985	46	74	21	71
Prichard et al. [35]	1985	37	65	29	66
Hui et al. [36]	1989	64	63	114	95
Total[b]		239	67	218	85

[a]$p < .0005$.
[b]$p < .0005$.

significant reduction in acid secretion is necessary to reduce satisfactorily the harmful effects of cigarette smoking on duodenal ulcer healing.

Ulcers Heal Faster in the Duodenum Than in the Stomach.   It is well known that the time taken by a therapeutic agent to heal a gastric ulcer is double that necessary to heal a duodenal ulcer. Given the vast differences in the physiology and structure of duodenal and gastric mucosa and in the pathophysiology of the two conditions, no clear explanation is available. The well-known larger size of gastric ulcer relative to duodenal ulcer, which as yet remains unexplained, appears to be one logical reason, but some salient differences are worthy of note. First, the duodenum has Brunner's glands, and Brunner's glands contain epidermal growth factor. Second, the proximal duodenum secretes about five times as much bicarbonate as the stomach [37]. Third, the blood flow requirement by the duodenum is only half that of the stomach [38]. The role played by epidermal growth factor, bicarbonate, and mucosal blood flow in ulcer healing is unclear. Epidermal growth factor heals experimental ulcer [39], and mucosal blood flow at ulcer edge improves with healing [40].

Helicobacter pylori **Does Not Affect Healing.**   Many studies have shown that the occurrence and density of *Helicobacter pylori* (formerly *Campylobacter pylori*) remain unchanged before and after healing with H_2-receptor antagonists [41–44]. Furthermore, "spontaneous" healing with placebo is unaffected by the presence of the bacteria [41]. These findings strongly suggest that the organisms do not affect ulcer healing.

B.   Can We Achieve Better Control of Acid Secretion?

1.   Control of Nocturnal and Meal-Stimulated Acid Secretion

The efficacy of controlling nocturnal acid secretion in the healing of duodenal ulcer using a single bedtime dose of H_2-receptor antagonists has been established by a placebo-controlled study [24] and comparative studies against standard regimens of H_2-receptor antagonists [23,25,26]. The efficacy of controlling meal-stimulated acid secretion in the healing of duodenal ulcer is likewise undoubted, as shown by six placebo-controlled and six comparative studies against H_2-receptor antagonists, all of which employed a regimen that aimed at controlling meal-stimulated acid secretion, following the concept of Fordtran [45] and Deering [46] that antacids given 1 and 3 hr after a meal significantly reduce for 4 hr the acid response to the meal.

Thus, reduction of either nocturnal or meal-stimulated acid secretion works better than placebo in the healing of duodenal ulcer. One question that follows is how these two strategies compare with each other in terms of efficacy. A recent study from Hong Kong [47] on 120 patients with duodenal ulcer compared cimetidine 400 mg three times daily with meals and 1200 mg at bedtime; a reference regimen of 200 mg three times daily and 600 mg at bedtime was also used. The use of endoscopic assessment at 2-week intervals for 12 weeks permitted point assessment in time as well as overall assessment using the life-table method. The results indicated that the mealtime

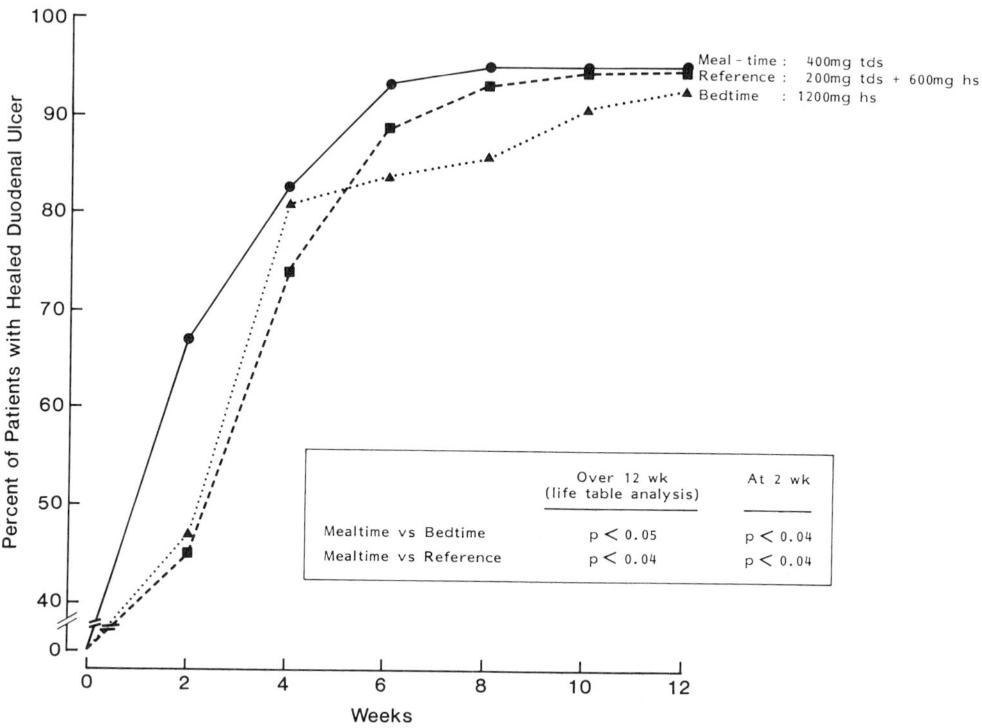

FIGURE 1 Cumulative endoscopic healing rates of 141 patients with duodenal ulcer randomized to receive one of three cimetidine regimens: bedtime, 1200 mg at bedtime; mealtime, 400 mg with breakfast, lunch, and dinner; reference, 200 mg with meals + 600 mg at bedtime.

regimen was significantly better than the other two in the overall assessment as well as at point assessment at 2 weeks (Figure 1). This study shows that during the design of any antisecretory regimen for patients, the control of meal-stimulated acid secretion should not be ignored.

Since the control of nocturnal and meal-stimulated acid secretion is important, another question is whether controlling *both* these secretions will lead to better healing rates. There has been no direct comparison. However, the trials so far conducted with omeprazole, which significantly suppresses acid secretion over 24 hr, have shown that the healing rates of duodenal ulcer achieved in 4 weeks have been consistently greater than 90%, whereas the corresponding rates for cimetidine and ranitidine are usually between 75 and 80% [33–36,48,49]. These results strongly suggest that controlling acid secretion throughout the 24-hr period achieves the best healing rates.

2.   Maintaining a Physiological Level of Acid Secretion

In diabetes mellitus, it will be to the patient's advantage if insulin can be administered from instant to instant according to the blood sugar level, and a device for this is now available. In patients with duodenal ulcer, should gastric acidity be controlled from instant to instant according to the gastric pH? A device for this is not available but should be possible. For short-term peptic ulcer treatment, this approach will not be satisfactory, because in all antisecretory regimens, effective treatment can be achieved only if gastric acidity is lowered to physiologically abnormal levels. The more abnormal it is, the better the healing rate. In this respect, treatment of peptic ulcer is different from that for diabetes and hypertension. For peptic ulcer, acid is clearly nonpermissive to healing.

For long-term maintenance treatment, achieving a physiological level of gastric acidity appears logical, but the approach obviously needs be tested.

C.   What Can We Gain with Cytoprotective and Mucosal Protective Agents?

1.   Prostaglandin-Dependent and Prostaglandin-Independent Mechanisms

Cytoprotective mechanisms are conventionally assumed to equate with the actions of prostaglandin. It should be realized that cytoprotective mechanisms can occur in the absence of prostaglandin secretion. Mucus secretion as stimulated by sucralfate is one example [50]. Dose–response studies also showed that sucralfate achieves a significantly higher gastric mucosal blood flow than misoprostol [51]. The beneficial effects of these enhanced mechanisms are not known. Furthermore, sucralfate improves the contact of epidermal growth factor with mucosa [52,53].

2.   Avoiding the Adverse Effects of Smoking on Healing

The use of prostaglandin appears to promote duodenal ulcer healing as much in smokers as in nonsmokers [54–56], although these results have not been consistent (Table 3). Interestingly, identical healing rates between smokers and nonsmokers have been consistently observed with the use of the mucosal protective agents sucralfate and colloidal bismuth (Tables 3 and 4). Through what mechanisms these agents help the smokers is entirely unknown. Cigarette smoking impairs the release and synthesis of prostaglandins [71,72], and nicotine impairs mucosal blood flow [73]. More research is clearly needed in this area.

3.   Longer Ulcer Remission Than Acid-Reducing Agents

By pooling all reports [64,66,74–76] in the literature, it can be shown that duodenal ulcers healed with sucralfate ($n = 279$) relapsed slower than ulcers healed with H_2-receptor antagonists ($n = 299$), in the same manner as ulcers healed with bismuth ($n = 171$) had slower relapse than ulcers healed with H_2-receptor antagonists ($n = 155$) [44,69,70,77–80]. In fact, the sucralfate curve and the bismuth curve completely overlap each other (Fig. 2). A recent study showed that following withdrawal

Table 3 Duodenal Ulcer Healing in Smokers and Nonsmokers: Prostaglandins vs. Sucralfate

	Smokers		Nonsmokers	
	n	% healed	n	% healed
Prostaglandins (4–6 wk)				
Misoprostol				
Sontag et al. [57]	75	57	36	80
Nicholson [58]	138	53	93	71
Brand et al. [54]	60	75	47	78
Bright-Asare et al. [59]	53	59	48	73
Lam et al. [55]	25	65	51	72
Enprostil				
Bright-Asare et al. [60]	19	58	14	86
Thomson et al. [61]	26	60	16	73
Carling et al. [62]	24	88	27	96
Lam (unpublished data)	30	77	67	81
Total	450	62%	399	77%
Sucralfate (4 wk)				
Marks et al. [16]	20	90	9	67
Brandstaetter [63]	40	78	34	74
Lam et al. [64]	35	86	17	76
Marks et al. [65]	49	76	16	75
Lam et al. [66]	38	82	93	78
Coste et al. [67]	119	74	103	80
Total	301	78.4%	272	77.6%

after 1 year of maintenance treatment, patients maintained on sucralfate relapsed significantly more slowly than patients maintained on cimetidine [81]. The same phenomenon has been observed for gastric ulcers following withdrawal after 6 months of maintenance treatment with sucralfate and ranitidine [82]. The explanation for these observations can only be either that withdrawal of antisecretory agents speeds up relapse or that cytoprotective mechanisms are associated with longer lasting remission, or both. Indeed, histological normality of the duodenal mucosa is better achieved with sucralfate than with cimetidine [81], and up-regulation of parietal cells occurs after treatment with H_2-receptor antagonists as has recently been reviewed [83]. The observation that carbenoxolone sodium may prolong remission [84] sup-

Table 4 Duodenal Ulcer Healing in Smokers and Nonsmokers:
Colloidal Bismuth vs. H$_2$-Antagonist (4 wk)

	H$_2$-antagonist				Colloidal bismuth			
	Smokers		Non-smokers		Smokers		Non-smokers	
	n	%	n	%	n	%	n	%
Harley [68]	9	55	17	59	15	87	13	77
Shreeve [69]	18	50	6	66	14	79	10	70
Hamilton et al. [70]	78	68	14	86	26	81	15	80
Total	52	60	37	70	55	82	38	76

$p < .01$

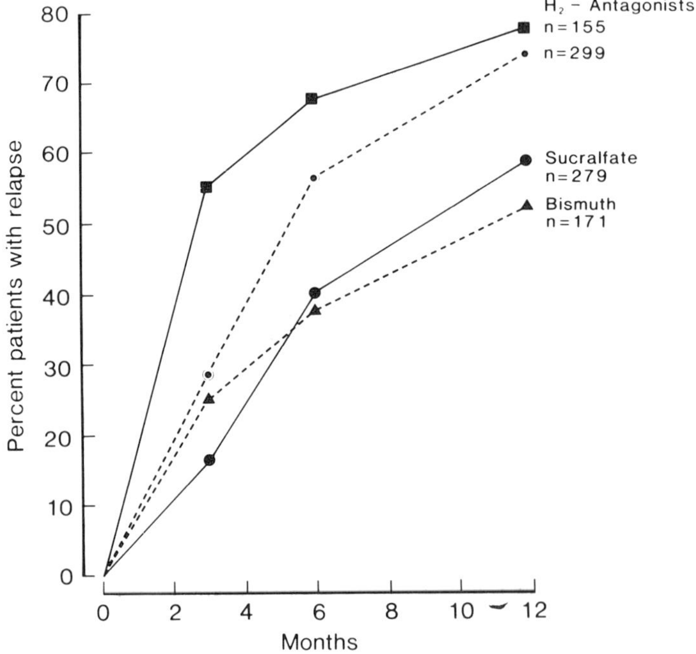

FIGURE 2 Combined posttreatment relapse rates of duodenal ulcer: colloidal bismuth subcitrate versus H$_2$-receptor antagonists [44,77–80] and sucralfate versus H$_2$-receptor antagonists [64,66,74–76] at 3, 6, and 12 months. The corresponding curves are significantly separated from each other, whereas the bismuth and sucralfate curves overlap.

ports "the better-healed ulcer" theory. On the other hand, the findings that anticholinergics may do the same [85,86] would support the "up-regulation" theory, since anticholinergics may theoretically down-regulate the parietal cells and therefore may not shorten the remission as acid-reducing agents, including H_2-receptor antagonists, omeprazole, and antacids would [83]. The proposed role of *Helicobacter pylori* [80], the existence of which is unaffected by sucralfate, anticholinergics, or carbenoxolone sodium, in the shortening of ulcer remission is exciting but cannot be accepted as established at this time [87].

D.   Should We Use Combination Therapy?

Combination therapy theoretically increases potency and efficacy and may lessen side effects.

1.   Combining Acid-Reducing Agents

Antacids and Anticholinergics.   This empirical approach is still the prescriber's favorite. Its efficacy has been confirmed recently [85]. Interestingly, while antacid healing alone does not lead to longer remission compared with H_2-receptor antagonists, the combination prolongs subsequent remission [85,86]. Once again, do anticholinergics give rise to down-regulation of parietal cells, or do they lead to better-healed ulcers? In this respect it is of interest to note that anticholinergics have been shown to be cytoprotective [88,89].

Antacids and H_2-Receptor Antagonists.   Antacids taken 1 and 3 hr after meals and at bedtime plus 300 mg cimetidine with meals and at bedtime were more effective than cimetidine alone in the reduction of daytime gastric acidity [90]. The efficacy of this complicated regimen in ulcer healing has not been tested. Sequential use of daytime antacids and bedtime cimetidine has similar duodenal ulcer healing rates as mealtime and bedtime cimetidine [91]. This regimen may be of value in countries where H_2-receptor antagonists are expensive.

Antacids and Neuroleptics.   Antacids plus sulpiride, a hypothalamic neuroleptic and possibly dopamine antagonist, do not appear to confer a significant advantage over antacids alone [15].

2.   Combining Acid-Reducing and Mucosal Protective Agents

In view of the unique advantages of each of these two groups of drugs, combination appears logical. Unfortunately, the adherence of the available mucosal protective agents, sucralfate and colloidal bismuth, to the mucosa is pH-dependent, so that raising the pH with, for example, H_2-receptor antagonists may impede the mucosal binding affinity of the protective agents. Perhaps it is for this reason that the combined use of cimetidine and sucralfate has not been shown to be of advantage over either drug alone in duodenal ulcer healing [92].

Future studies should perhaps examine the feasibility of using daytime sucralfate or colloidal bismuth with bedtime H_2-receptor antagonists.

3.   Sequential Use of Acid-Reducing and Mucosal Protective Agents

A possible advantage of this approach is that subsequent ulcer remission may be prolonged. One short-term study using a full dose of cimetidine for 4 weeks followed by a full dose of sucralfate for another 4 weeks has indeed suggested that this may well be the case [66]. It is not clear, however, whether the use of a maintenance dose of sucralfate—half that of the short-term treatment dose—following short-term treatment with a full dose of H_2-receptor antagonist may be of any advantage over sequential therapy using single drugs. This is because if up-regulation of parietal cells indeed occurs, the half-strength dose of sucralfate may not be able to deal with the heightened acid secretion after cessation of the short-term H_2-receptor antagonist.

E.   Do Refractory Ulcers Occur?

In a recent consensus meeting in Rome, it was agreed that refractory ulcers do occur but that they occur rarely—in about 5% of patients with duodenal ulcer, for example—and may vary from population to population [93]. The usual definition of refractory ulcer is one that fails to heal after at least 8 weeks of treatment with H_2-receptor antagonists or persists at the same size after 4 weeks of similar treatment. The accepted treatment for such ulcers includes colloidal bismuth [94,95] and omeprazole [96]. Duodenal ulcers may also be refractory to mucosal protective agents and may benefit from a course of H_2-receptor antagonists [66]. Whether duodenal ulcers are ever resistant to omeprazole is not clear. They probably are [33,34], and it is obviously important to establish this, because if they are never resistant to omeprazole it would mean that hypochlorhydria facilitates healing of all duodenal ulcers. Refractory gastric ulcers are seldom discussed and probably occur more frequently. Gastric ulcers associated with duodenal ulcers are the most difficult to heal, and they do not respond to sucralfate [97] or colloidal bismuth [98]; in fact, no medical treatment has been established for this type of gastric ulcer.

F.   Is Maintenance Treatment Cost-Effective?

It is generally accepted that ulcers that relapse infrequently should be treated with intermittent therapy, that is, by a full course of short-term treatment every time they recur, and that ulcers that relapse frequently should be given maintenance treatment, possibly for life, because it is likely that a very small percentage of ulcers will truly burn out. The safety of lifelong treatment with any agent is clearly not known. Furthermore, the efficacy of maintaining remission on a lifelong basis and whether drug tolerance will later develop is not clear. Because long-term maintenance treatment is costly to any society, and because uncomplicated ulcers generally run a benign course, long-term maintenance treatment should not be accepted until all other options have been explored.

With the availability of superpotent acid-reducing agents, such as the proton pump inhibitors, the length of short-term treatment can be shortened by half, and likewise, therefore, that of intermittent treatment, which should in theory reduce costs.

Furthermore, ulcers can be treated or treatment can be supplemented with a course of mucosa-protective agents to lengthen the remission period, which may be as long as twice that achieved with acid-reducing agents [66]. In this way, some frequent relapsers may be turned into infrequent relapsers and may be more cost-effectively treated with intermittent therapy.

It is hoped that a decreasing proportion of patients will require long-term maintenance treatment in the future and that such treatment will be used for patients for whom intermittent treatment fails or for whom surgical treatment carries unwarranted risk or is unlikely to be cost-effective, such as the elderly.

III.   ETIOLOGICAL PERSPECTIVES

A.   Are There Subsets of Duodenal Ulcers?

1.   Genetic and Environmental Heterogeneity

Hyperpepsinogenemia I is a known genetic marker [99], and G-cell hyperfunction [100] and G-cell hyperplasia [101] may be others. Parietal cell hyperplasia as reflected by an abnormally high maximal output may be familial [102]. These suggest that some patients may be genetically predisposed to hypersecretion of acid in response to appropriate stimuli. Acquired hypersecretion of acid probably also occurs; for example, chronic smokers are more often hypersecretors of acid [103,104]. The distribution of these subsets of hypersecretors is not known. However, it has been estimated that approximately 60% of patients have increased acid response to meals, and a similar percentage of patients have increased acid secretion at night [105]. These appear to fit in with clinical observations that a major proportion of patients will respond to the control of either meal-stimulated acid secretion or nocturnal acid secretion (see above).

2.   Clinical Subsets

Early-Onset Patients.   Patients whose symptoms start while they are young ($\leq$30 years of age) often have familial dyspepsia and do not have blood group O predilection [106,107]. Their maximal acid output is often increased [102], and they have been reported to respond readily to acid-reducing agents [15].

Cigarette Smokers.   As discussed earlier, smokers are frequently hypersecretors, may have impaired prostaglandin synthesis, and respond less readily to acid-reducing agents.

B.   Are There Subsets of Gastric Ulcers?

1.   Genetic and Environmental Heterogeneity

The genetic basis of gastric ulcer is weak, but environmental factors play a strong role.

In one study, cigarette smoking and habitual use of analgesics could account for over 80% of the ulcers [108].

2. Clinical Subsets

The classification of gastric ulcers by Johnson [109] into three types is still useful. More evidence has become available to indicate that prepyloric ulcers are different from duodenal and corpus ulcers both pathogenetically [110–112] and in clinical behavior [113]. Prepyloric ulcers generally heal more slowly than duodenal ulcers and faster than corpus ulcers. The best treatment of gastric ulcers associated with duodenal ulcers is probably surgery.

Evidence that smokers with gastric ulcers respond less readily to treatment is, interestingly, weak [97]. Some believe that analgesic ulcers respond less well to medical treatment, but good evidence is still forthcoming.

C. Is There a Role for *Helicobacter pylori?*

Evidence is strong that *Helicobacter pylori* is closely associated with chronic *active* histological antral gastritis, although clearance of the organisms does not improve the chronicity [114]. Evidence is also strong that active histological antral gastritis occurs closely with active or healed duodenal ulcer (about 95%) and with active or healed gastric ulcer (about 70%). A crucial question is, what can be a possible link between peptic ulcer and antral gastritis, which occurs irrespective of the activity of the ulcer? There are three possibilities. First, both may be caused by one common denominator, and this would fit in with the hypothesis that *H. pylori* causes both. However, the close association would require that *H. pylori* cause practically all ulcers, which does not appear to be likely, in view of the gross heterogeneity of ulcers and in view of the observations that spontaneous [41] and drug-induced [42,44,115] ulcer healing occurs in the presence of the organisms; still, *H. pylori* may be a contributing factor. Second, antral gastritis may cause ulcers. This requires that the inflammation spread distally to the duodenum and proximally to the fundus. The latter is known to occur. Spreading to the duodenum is compatible with the occurrence of gastric metaplasia in the duodenal mucosa, which, according to the literature, occurs in 30–90% of duodenal ulcer patients (generally cited at about 50%). Antral gastritis is not specific to ulcers and occurs in 60% of asymptomatic Finns [116] and in 50% of non-ulcer dyspepsia patients. It improves with ulcer healing by placebo and can be further improved by nonantibacterial agents such as misoprostol [117] and sucralfate [118]; still, mucosal inflammation may be a contributing factor to ulceration. Third, an ulcer may be the cause of the antral gastritis. This requires that antral gastritis occur as a protective phenomenon, its spread to the body and fundus being a favorable process, because this would lead to less acid secretion (and would, in fact, lead to secondary hypergastrinemia as a result of decreased inhibition by acid, hence also another possible explanation of the "gastrin link" [119] between *H. pylori* and ulcer), and that *H. pylori* inhabit and activate chronic antral gastritic mucosa. More work is clearly required to establish any of these three possibilities. Meantime, investigators and clinicians should keep an open mind.

IV. CONCLUSION

It should be realized that certain facts concerning ulcer healing are established, such as that placebo heals ulcers, that hypochlorhydria and a nonsmoking environment favor healing, that ulcer healing is faster in the duodenum than in the stomach, and that *H. pylori* does not affect healing. A better control of acid secretion to include both nocturnal and meal-stimulated acid secretion should speed up healing. Cytoprotective substances can be categorized as prostaglandin-dependent and prostaglandin-independent. It is likely that they help to overcome the adverse effects of cigarette smoking on ulcer healing and lead to a longer remission compared with acid-reducing agents. Combination and sequential drug therapy should be considered in the future to make the best use of acid reduction and cytoprotection in ulcer healing. Other than safety, cost-effectiveness should be a major concern in putting patients on lifelong maintenance therapy. Multiple subsets of peptic ulcers exist, and it is likely that more will be recognized in the future. Investigators should keep an open mind with respect to *Helicobacter pylori* in determining its clinical significance.

REFERENCES

1. Wormsley KG. Short-term treatment of duodenal ulceration. In: Baron JH, ed. Cimetidine in the 80s. New York: Churchill Livingstone, 1981:3–8.
2. Jones DB, Howden CW, Burget DW, Kerr GD, Hunt RH. Acid suppression in duodenal ulcer: a meta-analysis to define optimal dosing with antisecretory drugs. Gut 1987; 28:1120–7.
3. Marks IN, Young GO, Tigler-Wybrandi NA, Bridger S, Newton KA. Acid secretory response and parietal cell sensitivity in patients with duodenal ulcer before and after healing with sucralfate or ranitidine. Am J Med 1989; in press.
4. Peterson WL, Sturdevant RAL, Frankl HD, Richardson CT, Isenberg JI, Elashoff JD, Jones JQ, Gross RA, McCallum RW, Fordtran JS. Healing of duodenal ulcer with an antacid regimen. N Engl J Med 1978; 297:341–6.
5. Hetzel DJ, Hansky J, Shearman DJC, Korman MG, Taggart GJ, Jackson R, Jabb BW. Cimetidine treatment of duodenal ulceration: clinical trial and a maintenance study. Gastroenterology 1978; 74:389–92.
6. Bardhan KD, Saul DM, Edwards JL, Smith PM, Haggie SJ, Wyllie JH, Duthie HL, Fussey IV. Comparison of two doses of cimetidine and placebo in the treatment of duodenal ulcer: a multicentre trial. Gut 1979; 20:68–74.
7. Bianchi Porro G, Petrillo M, Grossi E, Lazzaroni M. Smoking and duodenal ulcer. Gastroenterology 1980; 79:180–1.
8. Massarrat S, Eisenmann A. Factors affecting the healing rate of duodenal and pyloric ulcers with low-dose antacid treatment. Gut 1981; 22:97–102.
9. Sonnenberg A, Muller-Lissner SA, Vogel E, Schmid P, Gonvers JJ, Peter P, Stroh-

meyer G, Blum AL. Predictors of duodenal ulcer healing and relapse. Gastroenterology 1981; 81:1061–7.

10. Strom M, Gotthard R, Bodemar G, Walan A. Antacid/anticholinergic, cimetidine, and placebo in treatment of active peptic ulcers. Scand J Gastroenterol 1981; 16:593–602.

11. Barakat MH, Menon KN, Badawi AR. Cigarette smoking and duodenal ulcer healing. An endoscopic study of 97 patients. Digestion 1984; 29:85–90.

12. Frederiksen H-JB, Matzen P, Madsen P, Kragelund E, Krag E, Christiansen PM, Bonnevie O. Spontaneous healing of duodenal ulcers. Scand J Gastroenterol 1984; 19:417–21.

13. Dyck WP, Cloud ML, Offen WM, Matsumoto C, Chernish SM. Treatment of duodenal ulceration in the United States. Scand J Gastroenterol 1987; 22(Suppl 136):47–55.

14. Gitlin N, McCullough AJ, Smith JL, Mantell G, Berman R. A multicenter, double-blind, randomized, placebo-controlled comparison of nocturnal and twice-a-day famotidine in the treatment of active duodenal ulcer disease. Gastroenterology 1987; 92:48–53.

15. Lam SK, Lam KC, Lai CL, Yeung CK, Yam LY, Wong WS. Treatment of duodenal ulcer with antacid and sulpiride. A double-blind controlled study. Gastroenterology 1979; 76:316–22.

16. Marks IN, Wright JP, Denyer M, Garish JAM, Lucke W. Comparison of sucralfate with cimetidine in the short-term treatment of chronic peptic ulcers. S Afr Med J 1980; 57:567–73.

17. Korman MG, Shaw RG, Hansky J, Schmidt GT, Stern AI. Influence of smoking on healing rate of duodenal ulcer in response to cimetidine or high-dose antacid. Gastroenterology 1981; 80:1451–3.

18. Gugler R, Rohner HG, Kratochril P, Brandstatter G, Schmitz H. Effect of smoking on duodenal ulcer healing with cimetidine and oxmetodine. Gut 1982; 23:866–71.

19. Barr GD, Paris CH, Middleton WRJ, Piper DW. Comparison of ranitidine and cimetidine in duodenal ulcer healing. Med J Aust 1982; 2:83–5.

20. Korman MG, Hansky J, Eaves ER, Schmidt GT. Influence of cigarette smoking on healing and relapse in duodenal ulcer disease. Gastroenterology 1983; 85:871–4.

21. Ippoliti A, Elashoff J, Valenzuela J, Cano R, Frankl H, Samloff M, Koretz R. Recurrent ulcer after successful treatment with cimetidine or antacid. Gastroenterology 1983; 85:875–80.

22. Ireland A, Colin-Jones DG, Gear P, Golding PL, Ramage JK, Williams JG, Leicester RJ, Smith CL, Ross G, Bamforth J, DeGara CJ, Gledhill T, Hunt RH. Ranitidine 150 mg twice daily vs 300 mg nightly in treatment of duodenal ulcers. Lancet 1984; ii:274–5.

23. Collin-Jones DG, Ireland A, Gear P, Golding PL, Ramage JK, Williams JG, Leicester RJ, Smith CL, Ross G, Bamforth J, DeGara CJ, Gledhill T, Hunt RH. Reducing overnight secretion of acid to heal duodenal ulcers. Comparison of standard divided dose of ranitidine with a single dose administered at night. Am J Med 1984; 77(Suppl 5B):116–22.

24. Lam SK, Lai CL, Lee LNW, Fok KH, Ng MMT, Siu KF. Factors influencing healing of duodenal ulcer: control of nocturnal secretion by H_2 blockade and characteristics of patients who failed to heal. Dig Dis Sci 1985; 30:45–51.

25. Farley A, Levesque D, Pare P, Thomson ABR, Sherbaniuk R, Archambault A, Maho-

ney K. A comparative trial of ranitidine 300 mg at night with ranitidine 150 mg twice daily in the treatment of duodenal and gastric ulcer. Am J Gastroenterol 1985; 80:665–8.

26. Lee FI, Reed PI, Crowe JP, McIsaac RL, Wood JR. Acute treatment of duodenal ulcer: a multicentre study to compare ranitidine 150 mg twice daily with ranitidine 300 mg once at night. Gut 1986; 27:1091–5.

27. Hamilton I, O'Connor HJO, Wood NC, Bradbury I, Axon ATR. Healing and recurrence of duodenal ulcer after treatment with tripotassium dicitrato bismuthate (TDB) tablets or cimetidine. Gut 1986; 27:106–10.

28. Simon B, Cremer M, Dammann HG, Hentschel E, Keohane PP, Mulder H, Muller P, Sarles H. 300 mg nizatidine at night versus 300 mg ranitidine at night in patients with duodenal ulcer. A multicentre trial in Europe. Scand J Gastroenterol 1987; 22(Suppl 136):61–70.

29. Bardhan KD, Thompson M, Bose K, Hinchliffe RFC, Crowe J, Weir DG, McCarthy C, Walters J, Thompson TJ, Thompson MH, Gait JE, King C, Prudham D. Combined anti-muscarinic and H_2 receptor blockade in the healing of refractory duodenal ulcer. A double blind study. Gut 1987; 28:1505–9.

30. Merki H, Witzel L, Huttemann W, Ansari A, Panijel M, Harre K, Heim J, Wolbergs E, Neumann HJ, Rohmel J. Early evening ranitidine administration promotes faster duodenal ulcer healing. Am J Gastroenterol 1988; 83:362–4.

31. Bardhan KD. UK frimoprostil study collaborative group. A multicentre comparison of trimoprostil and cimetidine in the treatment of duodenal ulcer. Scan J Gastroenterol 1988; 23:134–8.

32. Weberg R, Aubert E, Dahlberg O, Dybdahl J, Ellekjaer E, Farup PG, Hovdenak N, Lange O, Melsom M, Stallemo A, Vetvik KR, Berstad A. Low-dose antacids or cimetidine for duodenal ulcer. Gastroenterology 1988; 95:1465–9.

33. Classen M, Dammann HG, Domschke W, Hengels KJ, Hüttemann W. Short-duration treatment of duodenal ulcer with omeprazole and ranitidine: results of a multi-centre trial in Germany. Dtsch Med Wochenschr 1985; 110:210–5.

34. Lauritsen K, Rune SJ, Bytzer P, Kelbaek H, Jensen KG. Effect of omeprazole and cimetidine on duodenal ulcer. A double-blind comparative trial. N Engl J Med 1985; 312:958–61.

35. Prichard PJ, Rubinstin D, Jones DB, Dudley FJ, Smallwood RA, Louis WJ, Yeomans ND. Double blind comparative study of omeprazole 10 mg and 30 mg daily for healing duodenal ulcers. Br Med J 1985; 290:601–3.

36. Hui WM, Lam SK, Lau WY, Branicki FJ, Lok ASF, Ng MMT, Lai CL, Poon GP. Omeprazole and ranitidine in duodenal ulcer healing and subsequent relapse—a randomized double-blind study with weekly endoscopic assessment. J Gastroenterol Hepatol 1989; 4(Suppl 2):35–44.

37. Simson JNL, Merhav A, Silen W. Alkaline secretion by amphibian duodenum: I. General characteristics. Am J Physiol 1981; 240:G401–8.

38. Christoforidis EC, Horendal C, Bjerring P, Kruse A. Continuous measurement of gastric blood flow by laser-Doppler flowmetry during gastroscopy. Scand J Gastroenterol 1989; 24:16–20.

39. Olsen PS, Poulsen SS, Therkelsen K, Nexo E. Oral administration of synthetic human urogastroine promotes healing of chronic duodenal ulcers in rats. Gastroenterology 1988; 90:911–7.

40. Kamada T, Kawano S, Sato N, et al. Gastric mucosal blood distribution and its changes in the healing process of gastric ulcer. Gastroenterology 1983; 84:1541–6.

41. Ho J, Lui I, Hui WM, Ng MMT, Lam SK. A study on the correlation of duodenal-ulcer healing with *Campylobacter*-like organisms. J Gastroenterol Hepatol 1986; 1:69–74.

42. Hui WM, Lam SK, Chau PY, Ho J, Lui I, Lai CL, Lok ASF, Ng MMT. Persistence of *Campylobacter pyloridis* despite healing of duodenal ulcer and improvement of accompanying duodenitis and gastritis. Dig Dis Sci 1987; 32:1255–60.

43. Humphreys H, Bourke S, Dooley C, McKenna D, Power B, Keane CT, Sweeney EC, O'Morain C. Effect of treatment on *Campylobacter pylori* in peptic disease: a randomized prospective trial. Gut 1988; 29:279–83.

44. Marshall BJ, Goodwin CS, Warren JR, Murray R, Blincow ED, Blackbourn SJ, Philips M, Waters TE, Sanderson CR. Prospective double-blind trial of duodenal ulcer relapse after eradication of *Campylobacter pylori*. Lancet 1988; ii:1437–41.

45. Fordtran JS. Reduction of acidity by diet, antacids and anticholinergic agents. In: Sleisenger MH, Fordtran JS, eds. Gastrointestinal diseases. Philadelphia: WB Saunders, 1973:718–42.

46. Deering TB, Malagelada J-R. Comparison of an H_2 receptor antagonist and a neutralising antacid on postprandial acid delivery into the duodenum in patients with duodenal ulcer. Gastroenterology 1977; 73:11–4.

47. Lam SK, Hui WM, Ng MMT, Lok ASF, Lai CL, Branicki F, Lau WY, Poon GP. Reducing meal-stimulated acid secretion versus reducing nocturnal acid secretion for the healing of duodenal ulcer. Dig Disc Sci 1989; 34:1544–51.

48. Bardhan KD, Bianchi Porro G, Bose K, et al. A comparison of two different doses of omeprazole versus ranitidine in treatment of duodenal ulcers. J Clin Gastroenterol 1986; 8:408–13.

49. Barbara L, Blasi A, Chali R, et al. Omeprazole vs ranitidine in the short-term treatment of duodenal ulcer: an Italian multicenter study. Hepatogastroenterology 1987; 34:229–32.

50. Quadros E, Ramsamvoj E, Wilson DE. Role of mucus and prostaglandins in the gastric mucosal protective actions of sucralfate against ethanol-induced injury in the rat. Am J Med 1987; 83(Suppl 3B):19–23.

51. Chen BW, Hui WM, Lam SK, Ng MMT, Cho CH, Luk CT. Effect of sucralfate on gastric mucosal blood flow in rats. Gut 1989; 30:1544–51.

52. Nexo E, Poulssen SS. Does epidermal growth factor play a role in the action of sucralfate? Scand J Gastroenterol 1987; 22(Suppl 127):45–9.

53. Konturek SJ, Bielanski W, Brzozowski T, Drozdowics D. Role of epidermal growth factor in gastroprotective and ulcer healing effects of sucralfate. Am J Med 1989; 86(Suppl 6A):32–7.

54. Brand DL, Ronfail WM, Thomson ABR, Tapper EJ. Misoprostol, synthetic PGE_1 analogue, in the treatment of duodenal ulcers: a multicenter double-blind study. Dig Dis Sci 1985; 30:147–58S.

55. Lam SK, Lau WY, Choi TK, et al. Prostaglandin E_1 (misoprostol) overcomes the adverse effect of chronic cigarette smoking on duodenal ulcer healing. Dig Dis Sci 1986; 31:68–74S.

56. Carling L, Unge P, Hagg S, Almstrom C, Cronstedt J. A comparison of enprostil and cimetidine in the treatment of duodenal ulcer. Abstracts of Proceedings, Symposium on

protective and therapeutic effects of gastrointestinal prostaglandins, Toronto, 1985:54–5.

57. Sontag SJ, Mazure PA, Pontes JF, Beker SG, Dajani EZ. Misoprostol in the treatment of duodenal ulcer: a multicenter double-blind placebo-controlled study. Dig Dis Sci 1985; 30(Suppl):59–63S.

58. Nicholson PA. A multicenter international controlled comparison of two dosage regimes of misoprostol and cimetidine in the treatment of duodenal ulcer in outpatients. Dig Dis Sci 1985; 30(Suppl):171–7S.

59. Bright-Asare P, Sontag SJ, Gould RJ, Brand DL, Roufail WM, et al. Efficacy of misoprostol (twice daily dosage) in acute healing of duodenal ulcer—a multicentre double-blind controlled trial. Dig Dis Sci 1986; 31(Suppl):63–7S.

60. Bright-Asare P, Grdjs GJ, Santangelo WC, et al. Treatment of duodenal ulcer with enprostil, a prostaglandin E_2 analogue. Am J Med 1986; 81(2A):64–8.

61. Thomson ABR, Navert H, Halvorsen L, Maxton D, Archambault A, Sutherland LR, Lee SP, Sevelius H. Treatment of duodenal ulcer with enprostil, a synthetic prostaglandin E_2 analogue. Am J Med 1986; 81(2A):59–63.

62. Carling L, Unge P, Almstrom C, Cronstedt J, Ekstrom P, Hagg S, Hansson B. Enprostil and cimetidine: comparative efficacy and safety in patients with duodenal ulcer. Scand J Gastroenterol 1987; 22:325–31.

63. Branstaetter G. Comparison of two sucralfate dosages (2 g twice a day versus 1 g four times a day) in duodenal ulcer healing. Am J Med 1985; 79(Suppl 2C):36–8.

64. Lam KT, Lai ST, Kan YS, Chan AYT. Sucralfate compared with ranitidine in the short-term healing of duodenal ulcers. J Intern Med Res 1985; 13:338–41.

65. Marks IN, Wright JP, Glinsky NH, et al. A comparison of sucralfate dosage schedule in duodenal ulcer healing. Two grams twice a day vs one gram four times a day. J Clin Gastroenterol 1986; 9:419–23.

66. Lam SK, Hui WM, Lau WY, et al. Sucralfate overcomes adverse effect of cigarette smoking on duodenal ulcer healing and prolongs subsequent remission. Gastroenterology 1987; 92:1193–1201.

67. Coste T, Rautureau J, Beaugrand M, et al. Comparison of two sucralfate dosages presented in tablet form in duodenal ulcer healing. Am J Med 1987; 83(Suppl 3B):83–90.

68. Harley H, Alp MH. Treatment of chronic duodenal ulceration. Effectiveness of colloidal bismuth subcitrate tablets compared with cimetidine. Med J Aust 1983; 2:627–8.

69. Shreeve DR, Klass HJ, Jones PE. Comparison of cimetidine and tripotassium dicitrato bismuthate in healing and relapse of duodenal ulcers. Digestion 1983; 28:96–101.

70. Hamilton I, O'Connor HJ, Wood NC, Bradbury I, Axon ATR. Healing and recurrence of duodenal ulcer after treatment of dicitrato bismuthate (TDB) tablets or cimetidine. Gut 1986; 27:105–10.

71. McCready DR, Clark L, Cohen MM. Cigarette smoking reduces human gastric luminal prostaglandin E_2. Gut 1985; 26:1192–6.

72. Quimby GF, Bonnice CA, Burstein SH, et al. Active smoking depresses prostaglandin synthesis in human gastric mucosa. Ann Intern Med 1986; 104:616–9.

73. Leung FW, Guth PH. Tobacco smoke and nicotine infusion induce significant reduction in duodenal mucosal blood flow in anaesthetized rats. Gastroenterology 1984; 86:1160.

74. Marks IN, Wright JP, Lucke W, et al. Relapse rates following initial ulcer healing with sucralfate and cimetidine. Scand J Gastroenterol 1982; 17:429–32.
75. Hentschel E, Schuelze K, Dufek W. Recurrence of duodenal ulcers following treatment with sucralfate or cimetidine. Wien Klin Wochenschr 1984; 96(4):153. In German.
76. Hallerback B, Solhaug JH, Carling L, et al. Recurrent ulcer after treatment with cimetidine or sucralfate. Scand J Gastroenterol 1987; 22:791–7.
77. Martin DF, Hollanders D, May SJ, et al. Difference in relapse rates of duodenal ulcer after healing with cimetidine or tripotassium dicitrato bismuthate. Lancet 1981; i:7–10.
78. Kang JY, Piper DW. Cimetidine and colloidal bismuth in treatment of chronic duodenal ulcer comparison of initial healing and recurrence after healing. Digestion 1982; 23:73–9.
79. Lee FL, Samloff IM, Hardman M. Comparison of tripotassium dicitrato bismuthate tablets with ranitidine in healing and relapse of duodenal ulcers. Lancet 1985; i:1299–1302.
80. Coghlan JG, Gilligan D, Humphries H, et al. *Campylobacter pylori* and recurrence of duodenal ulcers—12 months follow-up study. Lancet 1987; ii:1107–11.
81. Tovey FI, Husband EM, Yiu YC, Baker L, McPhail G, Lewin MR, Jayaraj AP, Clark CG. Comparison of relapse rates and of mucosal abnormalities after healing of duodenal ulceration and after one year's maintenance with cimetidine or sucralfate: a light and electron microscopy study. Gut 1989; 30:586–93.
82. Takamoto T, Kimura K, Okita K, Tsuneoka K, Ohshiba S, Namiki M, Fukuchi S, Miyake T, Fukutomi H, Okazaki Y, Tanaka T. Efficacy of sucralfate in the prevention of recurrence of peptic ulcer—double blind multicenter study with cimetidine. Scand J Gastroenterol 1987; 22(Suppl 140):49–60.
83. Lam SK. Implications of sucralfate-induced ulcer healing and relapse. Am J Med 1989; 86:122–6.
84. Cook PJ, Vincent-Brown A, Lewis SI, et al. Carbenoxolone (Duogastrone) and cimetidine in the treatment of duodenal ulcer—a therapeutic trial. Scand J Gastroenterol 1980; 15(Suppl 65):93–101.
85. Strom M, Gotthard R, Bodemar G, Walan A. Antacid/anticholinergic, cimetidine and placebo in the treatment of active peptic ulcers. Scand J Gastroenterol 1981; 16:593–602.
86. Tomassetti P, Stanghellini E, Bonorag, Vezzadini P, Labo G. Comparative trial on healing and relapse of duodenal ulcer treated with trithiozine or cimetidine. Curr Ther Res 1981; 29:517–24.
87. Lam SK. Duodenal ulcer relapse after eradication of *Campylobacter pylori.* Lancet 1989; i:384(C).
88. Guth PH, Aures D, Paulsen G. Topical aspirin plus HCl gastric lesions in the rat. Cytoprotective effect of prostaglandin, cimetidine, and probanthine. Gastroenterology 1979; 76:88–93.
89. Konturek SJ, Kwiecien N, Obtulowicz W, Olesky J. Cytoprotective effects of pirenzepine. Proceedings satellite symposium on pirenzepine: Advances in gastroenterology with selective antimuscarinic compounds. Stockholm: June 17, 1982.
90. Peterson WL, Barnett C, Feldman M, Richardson CT. Reduction of twenty-four hour gastric acidity with combination drug therapy in patients with duodenal ulcer. Gastroenterology 1979; 77:1015–20.

91. Berstad A, Bjerke K, Carlsen E, Aaland E. Treatment of duodenal ulcer with antacids in combination with trimipramine or cimetidine. Scand J Gastroenterol 1980; 15(Suppl): 46–52.

92. Van Deventer GM, Schneidman D, Walsh JH. Sucralfate and cimetidine as single agents and in combination for treatment of active duodenal ulcers: a double-blind placebo controlled trial. Am J Med 1985; 79(Suppl 2C):39–44.

93. Domschke W, Lam SK, Pounder RE, Andersen D. H_2-Blocker-resistant duodenal ulceration. Gastroenterol Int 1989; 2:85–91.

94. Lam SK, Lee NW, Koo J, Hui WM, Ng M. Randomized crossover trial of tripotassium dicitrato bismuthate versus high dose cimetidine for duodenal ulcers resistant to standard dose of cimetidine. Gut 1984; 25:703–6.

95. Bianchi Porro G, Parente F, Lazzaroni M. Tripotassium dicitrato bismuthate (TDB) versus two different dosages of cimetidine in the treatment of resistant duodenal ulcers. Gut 1987; 28:907–11.

96. Tytgat GNJ, Lamers CBHW, Hameeteman W, Jansen JMBJ, Wilson JA. Omeprazole in peptic ulcers resistant to histamine H_2-receptor antagonists. Aliment Pharmacol Ther 1987; 1:31–8.

97. Lam SK, Lau WY, Lai CL, Lee NW, Poon GP, Hui WM, Lok A, Ng MMT, Fok KH, Yu HC. Efficacy of sucralfate in corpus, prepyloric, and duodenal-ulcer associated gastric ulcers. A double-blind, placebo-controlled study. Am J Med 1985; 79(2C):24–31.

98. Koo J, Lam SK. Discriminant factors of gastric ulcer healing by colloidal bismuth. J Gastroenterol Hepatol 1987; 2:473–83.

99. Rotter JI, Sones JQ, Samloff IM, et al. Duodenal ulcer disease associated with elevated serum pepsinogen I. An inherited autosomal disorder. N Engl J Med 1979; 300:63–6.

100. Lam SK, Ong GB. Identification of two subgroups of familial early-onset duodenal ulcers. Ann Intern Med 1980; 93:540–4.

101. Taylor I, Calam J, Rotter JI, et al. Family studies of hypergastrinemic, hyperpepsinogenemic I duodenal ulcer. Ann Intern Med 1981; 95:421–5.

102. Lam SK, Hasan M, Sircus W, Wong J, Ong GB, Prescott RJ. Comparison of maximal acid output and gastrin response to meals in Chinese and Scottish normal and duodenal ulcer subjects. Gut 1980; 21:324–8.

103. Guo FL, Chen GZ, Liu SQ, et al. The effects of smoking and nicotine on the parietal cell mass of human beings and rats. J Gastroenterol Hepatol 1986; 1:45–54.

104. Parente F, Lazzaroni M, Sangaletti O, et al. Cigarette smoking, gastric acid secretion, and serum pepsinogen I concentrations in duodenal ulcer patients. Gut 1985; 26: 1327–32.

105. Lam SK. Pathogenesis and pathophysiology of duodenal ulcer. In: Isenberg JI, Johanssen C, eds. Peptic ulcer disease. Clinics in gastroenterology. Philadelphia: WB Saunders, 1984; 13:447–72.

106. Lam SK, Ong GB. Duodenal ulcers: early and late onset. Gut 1976; 17:169–79.

107. Jirasek V. Hereditary factors in the aetiology of peptic ulcer. Acta Univ Carolinea: Med (Praha) 1971; 17:383–455.

108. McIntosh JH, Byth K, Piper DW. Environmental factors in aetiology of chronic gastric ulcer: a case control study of exposure variables before the first symptoms. Gut 1985; 26:789–98.

109. Johnson HD. Gastric ulcer: classification, blood group characteristics, secretion patterns and pathogenesis. Ann Surg 1965; 162:996–1004.

110. Lam SK, Lai CL. Gastric ulcers with and without associated duodenal ulcer have different pathophysiology. Clin Sci Mol Med 1978; 55:97–102.

111. Gotthard R, Bodemar G, Tjadermo M, et al. High gastric bile acid concentration in prepyloric ulcer patients. Scand J Gastroenterol 1985; 20:439–46.

112. Leth R, Elander B, Fellenius E, et al. Acid secretion in isolated gastric glands from healthy subjects and ulcer patients. Scand J Gastroenterol 1985; 20:6.

113. Lauritsen K, Bytzer P, Hansen J, et al. Comparison of ranitidine and high-dose antacid in the treatment of prepyloric or duodenal ulcer: a double-blind controlled trial. Scand J Gastroenterol 1985; 20:123–8.

114. Glupczynski Y, Burette A, Labbe M, Deprez C, De Reuck M, Deltenre M. *Campylobacter pylori*-associated gastritis: a double-blind placebo-controlled trial with amoxycillin. Am J Gastroenterol 1988; 83:365–72.

115. Hui WM, Lam SK, Chau PY, Ho J, Lau WY, Poon KP, Lai CL, Lok ASF, Lui IOL, Ng MMT. Pathogenetic role of *Campylobacter pyloridis* in gastric ulcer. J Gastroenterol Hepatol 1987; 2:309–16.

116. Maaroos HI, Salupere V, Uibo R, et al. Seven-year follow-up study of chronic gastritis in gastric ulcer patients. Scand J Gastroenterol 1985; 20:198–204.

117. Hui WM, Lam SK, Ho J, Ng MMT, Lui I, Lai CL, Lok A, Lau WY, Poon GP, Choi S, Choi TK. Chronic antral gastritis in duodenal ulcer—natural history and treatment with prostaglandin E. Gastroenterology 1986; 91:1095–101.

118. Hui WM, Lam SK, Ho J, Ng I, Lau WY, Branicki FJ, Lai CL, Lok ASF, Ng MMT, Fok PJ, Poon GP, Choi TK. The effect of sucralfate and cimetidine on duodenal ulcer associated antral gastritis and *Campylobacter pylori*. Am J Med 1989; 86(Suppl 6A):60–5.

119. Levi S, Beardshall K, Haddad G, Playford R, Ghosh P, Calam J. *Campylobacter pylori* and duodenal ulcers: the gastrin link. Lancet 1989; i:1167–8.

21

The Role of an Independent Clinical Research Organization in the Development of New Drugs for Treating Gastrointestinal Disorders

Roland A. Sauer* and Joe A. Bollert

Institute for Biological Research and Development, Inc.,
Irvine, California

I. INTRODUCTION

In the United States, the last two decades have seen the advent and growth of an industry serving a critical need in the development of new pharmaceutical agents. This service industry has grown to the point where the federal government in the Code of Federal Regulations refers to them as clinical research organizations (CROs) and specifically allows the CRO to accept any or all of the responsibilities of a "sponsor." Today, there are more than 200 CROs providing services to the pharmaceutical industry, all but a handful being limited to the conduct of small-scale clinical trials. From this handful, there has emerged a select subgroup of organizations that are capable of conducting complete drug development programs. Their services are used throughout the spectrum of the pharmaceutical industry for a variety of reasons:

1. The pharmaceutical company may find itself in an overcapacity situation, whereby their clinical development staff members are relegated to other projects and the patent life of a promising agent is waning.
2. The agent in need of development is in a clinical area in which the pharmaceutical company has little or no expertise.

---

*Present affiliation: Pacific Research Network, San Diego, California.

3. The pharmaceutical company may have limited clinical development capability or none at all.
4. The clinical development capability may exist within the pharmaceutical company, yet their internal cost and/or time to completion may be significantly greater than if they used the services of a CRO.

Over these same two decades, the development and marketing of new drug therapies for the treatment of gastrointestinal disorders has increased markedly, becoming one of the largest worldwide pharmaceutical markets. In 1988, the United States had sales of anti-ulcer products alone of $1.3 billion. The development of new agents capable of capturing a portion of this market has gained considerable attention within the pharmaceutical industry.

The following gastrointestinal disorders are currently in the spotlight of the U.S. pharmaceutical industry's research and development activities:

Duodenal ulcers
Gastric ulcers (including nonsteroid-induced)
Gastroesophageal reflux disease
Nonulcerative dyspepsia
Zollinger-Ellison syndrome
Crohn's disease

II. OVERVIEW OF U.S. DRUG DEVELOPMENT

To develop a new drug to treat any of these disorders, stringent regulations and guidelines of the U.S. Food and Drug Administration (FDA) must be followed. The FDA is committed to getting safe and effective new drugs to the public in the shortest time possible. On the average this process takes more than 8 years to accomplish; however, with the aid of CROs this time can be significantly reduced. The drug development process is divided into three basic stages: manufacturing, preclinical, and clinical, as depicted in Figure 1.

The manufacturing process begins with the initial synthesis of the agent, either chemically or via recombinant technology. Initially, only small amounts of the new agent are needed for basic animal screening tests. However, as the agent travels further and further down the developmental pathway, greater amounts of compound are needed, and benchtop synthesis must move through a scale-up process into a final manufacturing process that will supply sufficient amounts for the clinical studies and hopefully for the newly marketed product. The final product is the result of formulating the manufactured bulk drug to maximize bioavailability and the duration of therapeutic activity. Typically, the manufacturing is conducted by the pharmaceutical company that initially synthesized the agent, although, if needed, a full-service CRO can arrange for contract manufacturing services.

The preclinical studies are conducted in animals to ascertain the pharmacological

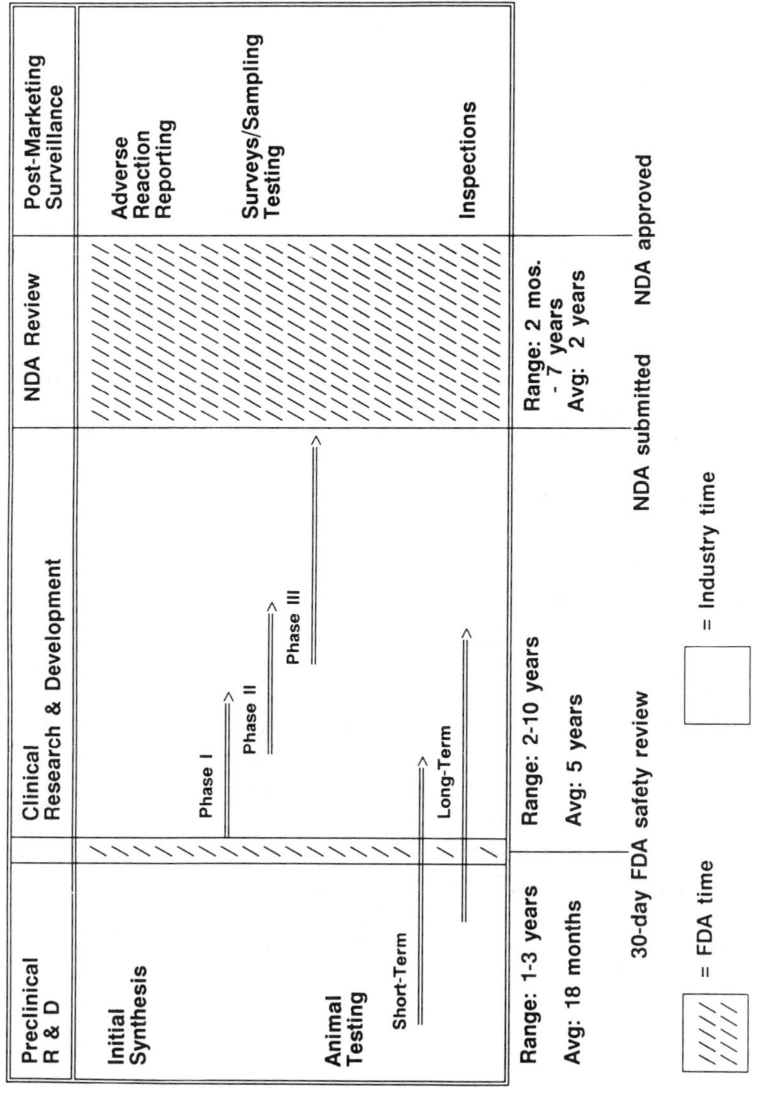

FIGURE 1 New drug development.

activity of the agent. As the agent begins to look promising, acute toxicity studies are conducted. Assuming that the drug continues to demonstrate a positive safety profile, a prerequisite amount of preclinical animal pathological and toxicological work must be completed and provided to the FDA before the clinical (human) studies are begun. This preclinical animal work takes, on average, 18 months to complete. Once the clinical studies are under way, long-term animal safety studies continue. There are animal pathology and toxicology laboratories available for either the "sponsor" or the full-service CRO to contract with.

The sponsor, usually a pharmaceutical company, although increasingly commonly a CRO or even a governmental agency or an individual, must file an Investigational New Drug (IND) application with the FDA before initiating the clinical studies, which are divided into phases I, II, and III. The phase I studies represent the initial introduction of the agent into humans. These studies use healthy normal volunteers to assess only the safety of the drug. Once the phase I studies are completed, usually totaling less than 100 volunteers, and the FDA has reviewed the data and given approval, phase II clinical studies can begin.

Phase II represents the first time that the drug has been given to subjects with the disease it is intended to treat. Early phase II studies are used primarily to determine the proper dose and regimen. Safety is still the primary endpoint, although efficacy is now being assessed as well. These studies are almost all conducted in a double-blind design using either a placebo, a standard, or both as controls, such that neither the patient nor the investigator knows which medication is being used, thus eliminating most evaluation biases. The phase II studies normally involve a few hundred patients. Upon completion, summaries of the safety and efficacy data from these studies are submitted to the FDA for approval to initiate the phase III studies.

Phase III studies are similar in design but are more extensive than phase II, both in the number of patients, sometimes several thousand, and in the duration of treatment, sometimes several years if the drug is intended for long-term therapy. These studies are geared to more closely reflect the manner in which the drug will be used by physicians once it is approved for marketing. Assuming the drug has continued to demonstrate sufficient safety and efficacy, the sponsor will compile all the manufacturing, preclinical, and clinical data and file a New Drug Application (NDA) with the FDA. On the average, the combined phase I, II, and III clinical studies will have taken 5 years to complete. The FDA will take another 2 years, on average, to review the NDA, making the entire drug development process from synthesis to NDA approval in excess of 8 years.

III. CRO FACILITATION OF GASTROINTESTINAL DRUG DEVELOPMENT

The phase II and III clinical studies consume both the most time and the most money in the overall drug development process. Coincidentally, phases II and III also offer the greatest opportunity for CROs to reduce developmental time and cost. As previously mentioned, CROs are numerous and run a continuum from providing all the services needed to take a new chemical entity from the chemist's bench to the marketplace, to serving as a single investigational site conducting one of the many studies needed for NDA approval. Agents under development for treatment of gastrointestinal disorders may present a unique opportunity in utilizing a CRO to significantly reduce the time and cost of the phase II and III clinical programs. Historically, treatments such as histamine-receptor blockers, prostaglandins, and proton pump inhibitors have been developed for multiple gastrointestinal indications. Typically, this multiple indication development process is sequential, one indication after another, or staggered, one indication started when the previous one is almost completed. The merit of a sequential or staggered development program is twofold. It requires a minimum amount of manpower, albeit over an extended period of time, and places a minimal amount of capital at risk in the event that one of the indications is problematic.

In the development of pharmaceuticals, time is money. Money is lost to competitive products already on or quicker to reach the market, money is lost to a shrinking patent life, and money is lost to waiting years for NDA approval of additional indications.

The use of a CRO with the combined capability to conduct large-scale clinical studies and considerable experience with documented performance in gastrointestinal drug studies, coupled with the willingness to integrate its experience and capability into the specific needs of a pharmaceutical company's clinical development program, can generate significant savings. For example, if an agent were under development that could be used to treat multiple indications such as duodenal and gastric ulcers, gastroesophageal reflux disease, and nonulcerative dyspepsia, and these programs could be run concurrently at sites throughout the country, the benefits would be numerous.

First of all, when symptomatic patients are screened for entry into any one of the four studies, most patients end up qualifying for one of the studies, resulting in very few screen failures. The referral of potential study patients is increased for the same reason; that is, the patient has four times the chance of qualifying, resulting in the speed of patient accrual being substantially increased. The use of similar protocols and case report forms for all studies speeds data collection and reduces error rates. The shorter the clinical program, the greater the continuity of investigators and nursing and research support staff. This also permits the economy of monitoring four studies at each site per monitoring visit. Most important, it reduces the total clinical development time, allowing NDAs for multiple indications to be filed sooner, all for significantly less cost than if the indications had been pursued sequentially or in a staggered development program. Thus designing a program in this fashion and utilizing an appropriate CRO to conduct it in concert with the pharmaceutical company results in substantial savings of time and money.

IV.   WHY DO PHYSICIANS PARTICIPATE
IN CLINICAL STUDIES?

Physicians become involved in conducting clinical studies for a variety of reasons. For some the overriding reason is scientific curiosity or the desire to be at the forefront of therapeutics or to reap the benefits of the added education they receive. Others enjoy the satisfaction of giving their patients the latest therapeutic advancement that cannot be gotten anywhere else in town. For some the main attraction is the diversion from the standard day-to-day medical practice or the altruism of helping others. For some it is an opportunity to build a practice or increase the revenue generated from their ongoing practice. Or it may be a combination of any of these factors. Whatever their motivations, the clinicians all share in the knowledge that there is not a single gastrointestinal disorder for which the existing therapy could not be improved.

V.   WHY DO PATIENTS PARTICIPATE
IN CLINICAL STUDIES?

Typically, patients want one thing from their physicians: more time with them. By virtue of participation in a clinical study, patients will receive more intensive medical care than they would normally receive, resulting in greater exposure to physicians, nurses, and the research staff. This increased exposure to the research team translates into patients who are considerably more knowledgeable about their disease and the therapy they are receiving than they were before their involvement. Some patients participate because the cost of normal care is beyond their means. Others become involved in the hope that if they do not directly benefit from the therapy, as it may be ineffective or they might receive placebo, at least others with their disease may benefit.

VI.   FACTORS IN CONDUCTING SUCCESSFUL PHASE II OR III
CLINICAL STUDIES IN GASTROINTESTINAL DISORDERS

The more knowledgeable about a study the participants of that study are, the more efficiently the study will operate. The investigator, subinvestigators, local referring physicians, nursing staff, support and technical staff, research coordinators, and whoever schedules appointments must all know the study in general and their role in detail. In addition, the more knowledgeable the subjects become about the program, the more likely they are to participate, the more compliant they will be in keeping appointments and taking their medication correctly, and the more astute they will become in assessing potential adverse reactions.

Sponsors of clinical studies must be willing to fund the entire costs for patient participation. In addition to providing the medications being studied, they should provide any other medications that may be required or preferred. For example, when background antacids are used in a placebo-controlled study for relief of pain or acetominophen is to be used in place of nonsteroidal drugs as an analgesic, then these should be provided to the patients to maximize compliance. In addition to funding the costs of all the visits and procedures, honoraria should be given to patients whenever they are required to undergo time-consuming or unpleasant procedures such as endoscopies, to compensate them for the inconvenience, time lost from work, and travel expenses. All costs of screening a patient should be assumed by the sponsor, even for those patients who end up failing to qualify. If the costs of the workups on patients who fail to qualify for a study are not funded by the sponsor, the sponsor can expect the time for enrollment of patients to be greatly increased. After all, why should a physician refer a patient into a study for a more costly workup than he would normally provide if a reasonable chance exists that the patient will not qualify and then have to go out of pocket for it? Only under unusual circumstances should there be any charges to a patient as a direct result of his or her participation in a clinical research study.

When the study is completed and the sponsor has analyzed the data, a conscious effort should be made to provide the investigators with the results obtained from their patients and to inform them of which therapy each patient was given during the course of the study.

Often investigators in gastrointestinal studies are unable to identify and enroll a sufficient number of patients from their own practice. As a result, they are dependent upon subjects being referred from other sources such as subinvestigators or local physicians or self-referrals from advertising. Physicians willing to refer patients into the program should be educated about the program so that they can recruit and refer qualified patients. When the patient's participation in the study is completed, the patient should be scheduled to see the referring physician for future care.

Many patients who would qualify for participation in a reflex esophagitis or ulcer study would normally be seen by a primary care physician, not a gastroenterologist. Often the primary care physician will treat the patient's symptoms with an anti-ulcer agent, and then if the patient does not respond, send him or her to the gastroenterologist for an endoscopy. In order for such patients to become potential candidates for study participation, the primary care physician needs to be educated about the study and think about the study when the patient presents with symptoms indicative of the disease being studied. In some settings, it is more efficient for the gastroenterologist, who is the principal investigator, to serve as the overseer of the study and provider of endoscopies and have the primary care physician who knows the patient complete the physical exams and assess any potential side effects.

VII. CONCLUSION

Pharmacological treatment for gastrointestinal disorders represents one of the largest pharmaceutical markets worldwide. The clinical development of agents to treat a variety of gastrointestinal disorders is ongoing at a rapid pace. The advent and popularity of CROs as full-service providers can be incorporated into the drug development plans of pharmaceutical companies to their benefit. Substantial savings in time and cost can be achieved by this interaction.

22

Pharmaceutical Industry Perspectives on Human Investigation and Development of Anti-Ulcer Drugs

Esam Z. Dajani

G.D. Searle & Co. and Chicago Medical School,
Chicago, Illinois, and
University of California, Los Angeles, California

Hugo E. Gallo-Torres

Food and Drug Administration, Rockville, Maryland

I. INTRODUCTION

The most critical issue for research-based pharmaceutical companies is the maintenance of a continuous flow of innovative drugs that ensure survival of the corporation in the marketplace. Most large pharmaceutical companies are committed to the challenge of the discovery and development of new innovative products. However, drug development is an extremely costly, time-consuming, and difficult endeavor. By some current estimates, the average new chemical entity (NCE) taken to market in the United States requires approximately 10–12 years to develop, at a total cost sometimes exceeding $200 million [1,2].

To discover new drugs, research scientists must synthesize thousands of novel compounds, which are then tested for efficacy and safety in laboratory animals. Very few compounds survive preclinical tests and go on to clinical trials, and only a very small fraction of these compounds become medically successful marketed drugs. For example, in the search for a drug that can inhibit the action of gastrin, no fewer than 1000 compounds were synthesized and tested over the course of 7 years at G. D. Searle and Co. without success. Similarly, more than 700 new compounds were synthesized

The opinions expressed by the authors represent their own views on the subject. These are not official statements of either G.D. Searle & Co. or the U.S. Food and Drug Administration.

as potential histamine (H_2) receptor antagonists at Smith, Kline and French Laboratories, among which burimamide and metiamide were not successful, prior to the discovery of cimetidine [3]. Extensive use of human resources and financial commitment were essential ingredients to the success of this program. Thus, industrial pharmaceutical research, although geared to be very efficient, is expensive. The industry as a whole must finance the cost of research in the hope of recovering the investment in the form of successful drugs. Thus, business opportunities and profit incentives are essential factors affecting the ultimate success of the pharmaceutical industry. This economic motivation is no different from that of any other type of business.

In an attempt to improve the efficiency of drug discovery and development, companies are adopting global strategies using state-of-the-art technologies. This chapter describes one aspect of drug development, namely, the human investigation and development of anti-ulcer drugs. Special emphasis will be placed on the U.S. regulatory aspects concerning anti-ulcer drugs. We have had extensive experience in the characterization and development of anti-ulcer drugs, namely misoprostol [4–9] and trimoprostil [10–12]. This chapter reflects personal perspectives on the development of anti-ulcer drugs from a global perspective.

Guidelines for the clinical evaluation of anti-ulcer drugs were issued by the Food and Drug Administration in 1985 [13]. This chapter will also attempt to integrate recommendations made in those guidelines.

II. PRECLINICAL RESEARCH AND DEVELOPMENT

There are three major sources of obtaining new drugs: in-house research discoveries, licensing from other companies or groups, and joint ventures with other companies. Irrespective of the origin of the drugs, certain preclinical pharmacological and toxicological studies are required in most western countries before a manufacturer can obtain regulatory approval to begin human investigations. The following is a brief outline of the types of preclinical studies that are necessary for the development of any anti-ulcer drug.

A. Pharmacological Characterization

The pharmacological class of the test drug must be identified, and the mechanism of action must, whenever possible, be established. The sponsor should conduct these types of studies in order to determine the relation between the mechanism of action and the potential use of the drug for the treatment of peptic ulcer disease. For example, if a drug is a gastric secretory inhibitor, the mechanism of this inhibition, insofar as acid secretion, should be well established [4,5]. Should this drug belong to well-established pharmacological classes of gastric secretory inhibitors such as anti-cholinergics, histamine (H_2) receptor antagonists, proton-pump inhibitors, or prostaglandins, then comparative preclinical studies should be performed with reference standards to determine potential advantages and disadvantages with respect to these standards. It is important to determine if acid inhibition is reversible or irreversible and whether it is competitive or noncompetitive.

Should a drug inhibit acid secretion by one or more mechanisms unrelated to those of well-known inhibitors of gastric secretion, studies should be conducted to characterize effects of the drug on other gastroduodenal physiological functions of the mucosa. Similar considerations should apply to drugs acting mainly via cytoprotective mechanisms [6]. For example, it would be useful to establish the type of gastroduodenal cells being protected and perhaps other organ cells that are protected by the drug in addition to the stomach and duodenum [7].

For compounds possessing pharmacological actions other than inhibition of acid secretion, such as somatostatin analogues, the relative degree of specificity of these effects should be established. With superactive secretory inhibitors, we would need to establish whether the compound inhibits gastric acid secretion in response to low and high doses of histamine and gastrin, whether there is a tachyphylactic response, or whether there is interference with cholinergic transmission.

In all these studies, investigations of a dose–response relationship with respect to the primary mechanism of action should be established. Pharmacokinetic and metabolic studies should also be conducted to provide an idea of the extent of absorption, distribution, metabolism, and excretion in one or more species that is more relevant to humans.

B. Broad Pharmacological and Toxicological Characterization

The potential toxicity and/or effects on other organ systems (cardiovascular, renal, hepatic, respiratory, etc.) should be identified during the pharmacological characterization of the drug. A thorough investigation of all the known properties of this class of compound should be made. In particular it is important to identify a dose–response relationship for these properties in relation to the potential therapeutic effects. Calculations of the therapeutic index (a measure of the degree of specificity of the test drug derived from the division of ED_{50} value of the undesirable action by the ED_{50} value of the desirable action) can provide an idea of the risk/benefit ratio for a given therapeutic entity. The higher the therapeutic index, the better the specificity for the primary anti-ulcer action. The dose used in the broad pharmacological studies should be a sufficiently large multiple of the effective gastric antisecretory, cytoprotective, and anti-ulcer dosages. Should an undesirable activity be found, then dose titration evaluation is needed to establish either a minimum effective dose or an ED_{50} value for this activity. Again, should the therapeutic index be near unity, the wisdom of further development of such a nonpromising compound should be carefully considered. There are no uniform rules among pharmaceutical organizations in regard to the termination of early development of a drug candidate unless rather serious pharmacological and/or toxicological findings are encountered. In such a case, all organizations would promptly discontinue the development. The difficulty, however, arises when the preclinical findings are not very clear or are of dubious clinical relevance. Likewise, appropriate safety studies including mutagenicity and teratogenicity examinations are required. Because anti-ulcer drugs are usually administered for long periods of time, long-term, 2-year toxicity and carcinogenicity studies are also required for phase II/III of clinical development, but these studies are not needed for early clinical investigations, which are usually short-term (4–12 weeks of treatment).

C. Proposed Clinical Doses

Information on the previously described therapeutic indices, as well as metabolic and pharmacokinetic considerations, permits the establishment of a dose range to be explored in humans. The choice of a rational dosage is most important to reduce the cost and speed the time of development of an effective agent. For companies that are not very firmly committed to the development of NCEs, inappropriate dose selection can have a significant negative psychological impact on company scientists and can prematurely result in the discontinuation of the development of many good drugs. This is one of the reasons that a good preclinical characterization is essential for a rational proposal of a dose range expected to be effective in human patients.

III. CLINICAL RESEARCH AND DEVELOPMENT

Since peptic ulcer disease is a chronic relapsing disease, the goals of pharmacological intervention are:

1. To promote the acute healing of an ulcer (short-term use of medication)
2. To provide relief of dyspeptic pain (short-term use of medication)
3. To establish whether short-term therapy (4–8 weeks of treatment) would alter the natural history of peptic ulcer disease.

There is not a drug marketed in the United States that has convincingly been found to alter the natural course of peptic ulcer disease. Also, it has not been convincingly shown whether short-term treatment with some therapeutic modalities may result in fewer recurrences than with others. This information, however, appears to be irrelevant to practicing physicians in this country, because immediately after the ulcer is healed on short-term treatment, physicians commonly prescribe maintenance doses of these drugs. Therefore, to prevent the inevitable ulcer recurrences, physicians would need to administer the drug continuously after healing to maintain an ulcer-free state. The value of maintenance therapy is most controversial in regard to continuous vs. intermittent therapy. It seems important to determine, first, if the drug has value in accelerating the healing of gastric and duodenal ulcers prior to examining the effect on ulcer recurrence; however, due to difficulties in accruing patients, most placebo-controlled acute ulcer studies include a follow-up maintenance phase.

The question of which type of ulcer claim is to be obtained first is also an important consideration on the basis of the market size. The preponderance of patients with duodenal ulcers compared to the population of patients with gastric ulcers would justify the effort to determine a duodenal ulcer claim first, but, depending upon a number of factors and circumstances, this may not be the best path. In the past, many companies have opted for obtaining an initial claim for the treatment of duodenal ulcer, then at a later time filing a claim for gastric ulcer or other indication. Table 1 lists some of the potential claims to be investigated. However, not all classes of pharmacological agents could prove effective for all these claims. Depending on their pharmacological profile, some drugs would certainly be more effective in some claims than others. It is logical, therefore, to formulate a clinical development plan for the drug considering all pharmacological goals in the therapy of peptic ulcer disease. It is very useful for the pharmaceutical company to assemble a multidisciplinary task force consisting of basic scientists, clinicians, and business development personnel to plan

Table 1 Potential Medical Claims for Antiulcer Drugs

Primary claims
    Short-term treatment of active duodenal ulcer
    Short-term treatment of active benign gastric ulcer
Secondary claims
    Aspiration pneumonitis
    Gastritis/nonulcer dyspepsia
    Hypersecretory states, e.g., Zollinger–Ellison syndrome, multiple endocrine adenomas
    Maintenance therapy for duodenal ulcer
    Maintenance therapy for gastric ulcer
    Prevention of NSAID-induced gastric ulcer
    Prevention of NSAID-induced duodenal ulcer
    Prevention of ulcer recurrence
    Treatment of reflux esophagitis
    Treatment of refractory or poorly responsive peptic ulcer
    Prevention and/or treatment of stress ulcer
    Treatment of NSAID-induced gastric ulcer
    Treatment of NSAID-induced duodenal ulcer
    Prevention and/or treatment of upper gastrointestinal bleeding
    Treatment of alkaline reflux gastritis

Note: The denomination primary or secondary claim is relative, since a secondary claim may become the most important and perhaps the only claim for which a certain drug is approved.

the future development of the anti-ulcer drug given what is known about the preclinical pharmacology, toxicology, and potential commercial opportunities in the marketplace.

IV. CLINICAL PHARMACOLOGY (PHASE I)

To permit clinical investigation with a new substance or possibly a new use for a substance approved for a use other than the proposed use, the sponsor must file with the FDA an IND (Investigational New Drug) application, synonymous with "notice of claimed investigator exemption for a new drug." Briefly, the sponsor will provide all the data previously discussed in addition to a proposed protocol for the first investigation in human subjects. The FDA has 30 calendar days in which to review the IND application. If no objections are received by the sponsor within that time frame, clinical studies may commence. For definitions and interpretations and other details of the content and format of an IND, the reader is referred to pages 64–91, Part 312, 21 CFR Ch. I of the April 1, 1987, edition of the Code of Federal Regulations.

In essence, an IND is a request for FDA authorization to administer an investigational drug to humans. The request may originate from a pharmaceutical firm or from an individual sponsor-investigator. The essential components of an IND are listed in Table 2, and the reader is encouraged to review additional details cited in the federal regulations.

There are four major phases in the clinical development program (Fig. 1). In

Table 2   Essential Components of an IND

Form FDA 1571
Table of contents
Introductory statement
General investigational plan
Investigator's brochure
Protocol(s)
   Study protocol(s)
   Investigatory data or completed form(s) (FDA 1572)
   Facilities data or completed form(s) FDA 1572
   Institutional Review Board data or completed form(s) FDA 1572
Chemistry, manufacturing, and control data
   Environmental assessment or claim for exclusion
Pharmacology and toxicology data
Previous human experience
Additional information

Note: Treatment INDs and treatment protocols are special cases.

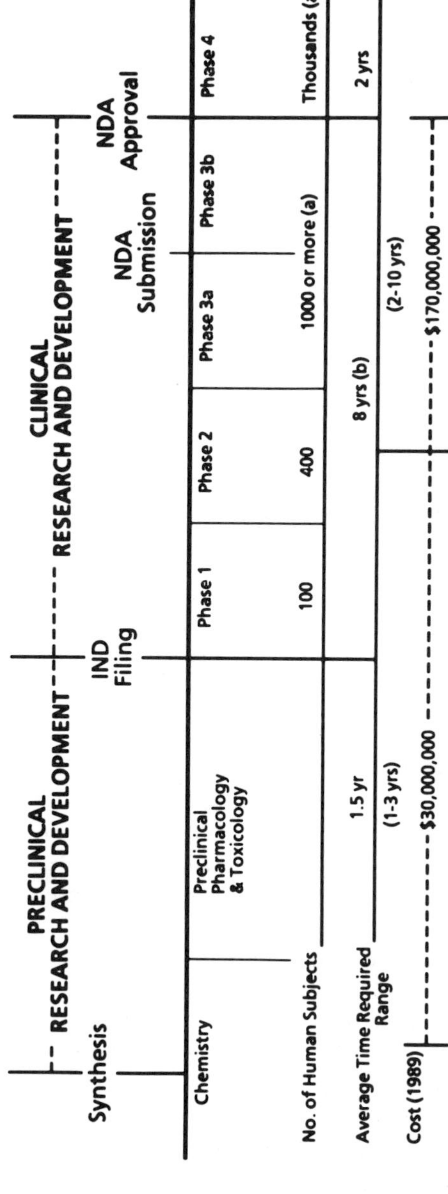

FIGURE 1 Drug Development in the United States. (a) The number of human subjects in phase IIIb and phase IV depends in some cases on business considerations and in other cases on FDA requirements. (b) The average time for the FDA to approve a drug after submission of the NDA is about 32 months.

Figure 1, phase III is divided into subphases IIIa and IIIb to accommodate those unusual circumstances of drugs for which NDAs are submitted for an initial indication. While this information is under review, further research (phase IIIb) may show utility for a different indication for which approval may be granted even though no decision may have been rendered regarding the initial application. This section will provide an overview of the phase I clinical development program for an anti-ulcer drug. The goals of this phase of development are:

1. To establish the range of doses that have potential therapeutic benefits and those that are likely to produce adverse effects.
2. To correlate dose administered with blood levels. This provides data on absorption, metabolism, half-life ($T_{1/2}$), volume of distribution, maximum plasma concentration (C_{max}), and time to maximum plasma concentration (T_{max}).
3. To establish steady-state kinetics to permit detection of accumulation of drug or its metabolites.
4. To assess rate and route(s) of excretion.
5. To assess interindividual variability.
6. To evaluate the relationship between blood concentration and pharmacological action.

The accomplishment of phase I objectives entails conducting studies in predominantly healthy human subjects. Typical core studies to be performed during phase I development are shown in Table 3. The following is a brief discussion of these studies.

A.   Dose–Response and Time Effect Studies

The initial study in phase I development will examine the safety and tolerance of the test drug by studying the effect of single escalating doses in order to achieve a dose that produces definitive adverse effects.

Although the trial can be performed as an open-label study, it is definitely better to conduct a double-blind, placebo-controlled study in pairs of subjects to rule out the contribution of placebo to a given adverse event. Placebo effects are very well documented, and in some trials almost half of the subjects treated with the placebo complain of some type of adverse event. The placebo provision would provide a good baseline for the drug-treated group, especially if performed in pairs of subjects.

Following the completion of the single-dose tolerance study, a multidose tolerance study is recommended to rule out potential cumulative effects that cannot be established from the single-dose acute study. However, in our opinion the conduct of a multidose tolerance study should be delayed until some specific information is obtained to confirm some aspect of the pharmacology that is relevant to peptic ulcer disease. For example, in the case of a drug that is believed to work via an inhibitory

Table 3 Typical Core Studies Conducted During Phase I Clinical Development of an Anti-Ulcer Drug[a]

Single-dose acute safety and tolerance study in healthy subjects, usually sequential-ascending groups

Multidose tolerance study in healthy subjects

Dose-ranging nocturnal gastric antisecretory study in healthy subjects

Dose-ranging gastric antisecretory study against meal-stimulated gastric secretion in healthy subjects

Dose-ranging gastric antisecretory study against histamine-stimulated gastric secretion in healthy subjects

Meal-stimulated gastric antisecretory studies in patients with duodenal ulcers

Absolute bioavailability study in healthy subjects

Dose-proportionality bioavailability studies

Drug interaction studies (see text for details)

Miscellaneous studies (see text for details)

---

[a]For a drug presumably acting through a cytoprotective mechanism of action, most of the antisecretory studies could be replaced by properly designed cytoprotective studies [9].

effect on gastric acid secretion, it would be useful to determine the dose levels and the intervals between doses that had varying and graded effects on acid production at various times during a single 24-hr period. It would be very useful to establish the nature of the gastric antisecretory action against different physiological stimuli of gastric acid secretion, such as gastrin-, histamine-, and cholinergic-mediated secretory responses. Furthermore, studies on basal and nocturnal gastric acid secretion are also important to provide the dose needed to inhibit nocturnal gastric acid secretion [8]. Inhibition of nocturnal gastric secretion is thought to be very important in the healing of duodenal ulcers, although there is a debate on whether the drugs should be administered with the evening meal or just before retiring at night.

It is also recommended by the FDA that a dose-ranging antisecretory study be conducted in patients with quiescent duodenal ulcer. In the case of a drug that acts primarily through a cytoprotective mechanism of action, most of the antisecretory studies should be replaced by properly designed cytoprotective studies [9]. These would confirm the preclinical observations and would improve the likelihood of observing a positive finding in humans. Since it is possible to heal duodenal ulcers with drugs that have little or no gastric antisecretory effects (e.g., sucralfate, organic bismuth salts), the most convincing way of showing efficacy is via clinical trials in patients with duodenal ulcers (see below).

B. Pharmacokinetics and Characterization of Dosage Form

For some drugs that seem to act locally on the gastroduodenal mucosa and thus are not absorbed except for a small amount of aluminum and bismuth in drugs such as sucralfate and organic bismuth salts, standard pharmacokinetic studies are obviously not relevant. On the other hand, for drugs acting systemically, pharmacokinetics and characterization of the bioavailability of the dosage form should be performed in accordance with the guidelines established by the Division of Biopharmaceutics at the FDA. These guidelines do not deal with drugs that have a partial systemic activity such as prostaglandins. In this situation, it is suggested that these agents be treated as systemic drugs. Briefly, the pharmacokinetic investigations should generate the following information:

1. Provide absolute bioavailability of the test formulation. This is dervied from plasma level values as a function of time for both oral and intravenous formulations of the test drug. The relevant pharmacokinetic parameters T_{max}, C_{max}, and AUC (area under the plasma concentration–time curve) should be obtained. It is of interest to mention that for the majority of systemically available pharmacological agents, the site of action "follows the plasma/serum in sequence." However, some drugs, such as cimetidine, are handled metabolically differently by critically ill patients in comparison to noncritically ill subjects. This emphasizes the importance of regular monitoring of the gastric pH in these patients [14].
2. Provide information on the pharmacokinetic model (linear versus nonlinear kinetics) of drug action. This would include studies of dose proportionality. For example, for a drug exhibiting linear kinetics, a 100-mg dose would be associated with an AUC value that is twice the value obtained with the same drug administered at a 50-mg dose. For a drug that exhibits nonlinear kinetics, bioavailability should be determined during multiple-dose regimens, at steady-state.

It is important to note that it is sometimes necessary to change drug formulations during the conduct of clinical trials. When this is done, the dissolution kinetics of the various drug formulations used in proving clinical efficacy should be compared to the original data provided to the FDA.

C. Drug Interaction Studies

Should a drug have an obvious drug interaction profile derived from preclinical data (protein binding, an effect on liver metabolizing enzymes, an effect on renal excretion, etc.), it would be important to conduct initial drug interaction studies in healthy subjects to confirm the preclinical data and to provide an understanding of the type of patients to be selected in phases II and III of clinical development. More important, it is of value to establish the degree of drug interaction and the possible adverse effects, if any, from such interaction.

D. Miscellaneous Studies

In the clinical pharmacology workup of a new drug, although not mandated by health authorities, it is advisable to conduct studies to obtain good characterization of the pharmacological profile of the test drug. The scope of these studies is obviously compound-dependent and very much influenced by the preclinical characterization. For example, in the case of a drug that inhibits gastric acid secretion, it would be important to know if there is an effect on intrinsic factor secretion or if there is any interference with various hormones or if there is increased bacterial colonization or increased formation of gastric nitrosamines secondary to prolonged and continuous inhibition of gastric acid secretion. Some of these studies are needed for phase II clinical development, while the vast majority of them could be performed when convenient during the course of the development of the compound.

It is advisable to plan ahead for these studies. As knowledge obtained during drug development evolves, the need for this type of study should be reviewed as appropriate.

V. CLINICAL EFFICACY TRIALS (PHASES II AND IIIa)

The goals of phase II and IIIa studies are:

1. To establish that the new drug is safe and effective in managing patients with the disease being studied
2. To establish the dose–response relationship and the best dose regimen for the test drug
3. To permit risk/benefit analysis, especially when the test drug is being compared with existing (already approved) drugs

Establishing these ends is accomplished by the conduct of properly designed double-blind, randomized trials comparing the efficacy of test drug to either placebo or another dose of the same drug or some known established therapy that may not have been approved by the FDA although it is widely used in clinical practice (i.e., vasopressin for the treatment of upper gastrointestinal bleeding). In spite of intensive research, the exact pathophysiology and the amount and duration of inhibition of acid and pepsin secretion or mucosal protective activity needed to heal peptic ulcers are not fully known. For this reason, the efficacy of a new therapeutic modality can be shown only during controlled clinical trials with peptic ulcer patients. Among the many questions that the sponsor must consider when assessing the efficacy and safety of new drugs are:

1. Is this drug more effective than placebo?
2. What doses and what length of exposure are needed to achieve effectiveness?
3. How does the effectiveness of the new drug compare to already established therapeutic modalities for the same indication?
4. What is the safety profile of the new drug?
5. Does the drug produce side effects of concern, and if so, would these preclude its use in the general population at risk?

A full-scale development program should be designed to provide concrete answers to these essential questions.

Phase II clinical studies are intended to determine safety and efficacy in a small population of patients who exhibit only either duodenal or gastric ulcer without any other significant concomitant systemic disease that could confound the interpretation of the data for the new drug. Phase IIIa clinical studies are designed to recruit a larger population of patients who may have other medical problems in addition to peptic ulcer disease. Sometimes it is difficult to establish clear demarcation between phase II and phase III clinical development. Many phase II studies are being telescoped into phase III studies. It is our recommendation that drug sponsors meet regularly with FDA representatives to discuss the study protocols and other relevant issues concerning the clinical development. The following discussion is a narrative description of the proposed FDA guidelines for the clinical evaluation of anti-ulcer drugs [13].

A. Investigators

The drug sponsor must recruit investigators who are skilled in the conduct of clinical trials and who are knowledgeable in all aspects of peptic ulcer disease. Specifically, the trials must be performed by clinical investigators who are endoscopists of recognized competence in gastroenterology. It is important to stress that the subinvestigators should not be responsible for the endoscopic diagnosis or follow-up. Careful inspection of the stomach, esophagus, and duodenum must be done, with the findings recorded in a validated format.

There is a need for standardization of the experimental conditions and identification of what variables (factors) are to be controlled. Because the majority of the trials will need to enroll a very large number of patients, these trials would have to enroll several investigators from several centers. A meeting of potential investigators before the start of the trial may be useful in the standardization of definitions and procedures. For a multicenter study, the protocol should establish, a priori, a minimum number of subjects to be enrolled at each center. This approach may result in fewer protocol violations, thereby improving the quality of the data and allowing the assessment of intercenter variability. If a set number of patients at each center is prospectively determined, the study should not be halted until each center's quota of patients is filled; in this way, internal consistency can be measured in the multicenter trial. The possibility of using a linked computer system, whereby monitoring can be rapidly conducted, should be considered. This approach may result in fewer protocol violations, thereby improving the quality of the data.

B.   Number of Trials Needed to Determine Efficacy

The purpose of multiple trials is to ensure valid and reliable results to prove clinical efficacy. The exact number of trials depends on endpoints evaluated and the consistency of the results, although as a minimum, two well-controlled, double-blind, randomized trials are usually necessary for establishing the safety and efficacy of a drug. However, in instances where the endpoint is survival, only one trial may suffice.

Because the target population will be patients residing in the United States and because there may be significant differences in ulcer healing rates between U.S. and other populations, it is recommended that at least one major pivotal trial be conducted in a U.S. population. Supporting information can be gained from proper trials conducted outside the United States if they are conducted in compliance with the provisions of good clinical practice and are adequately monitored. In fact, the FDA has recently accepted several foreign clinical trials as pivotal studies in support of NDA submissions of cardiovascular and gastrointestinal drugs. The principal problems encountered by the FDA in accepting data from foreign studies relate to institutional review boards, informed consent, record keeping, and monitoring. In addition, storage conditions encountered during the transportation of drugs from the United States to Europe and other continents may not be ideal to maintain the therapeutic efficacy of the test drug. It is thus very important to stipulate methods to ensure product quality. Furthermore, on-site inspection by FDA personnel must be carried out to validate the foreign data.

C.   Placebo-Controlled Trials

The need for clear demonstration of activity of the new drug cannot be avoided. This is best done when the test drug is compared to a placebo. The composition of the placebo should be the same as the test drug without the presumably active ingredient. The placebo must be indistinguishable from the test drug and administered on the same predetermined dose schedule. Despite the fact that there is known effective therapy for the healing of acute duodenal and gastric ulcers, placebo-controlled trials are still reasonable because of the known high and variable placebo response rate. In addition, the use of placebo is ethical because there appears to be no risk (increase in complications related to either gastric or duodenal ulcer) in treating patients with a placebo in a controlled, carefully monitored setting [15].

In clinical practice today there are several well-established effective drugs for the short-term treatment of duodenal and gastric ulcer. It is therefore most difficult to recruit patients to the study if the patient is aware of the possibility that he or she might receive a placebo in place of an effective drug. Furthermore, institutional review boards or hospital ethical committees in many countries, including the United States, may not sanction the conduct of placebo-controlled peptic ulcer trials even if these trials are conducted in a carefully monitored setting. In the United States, most of the placebo-controlled studies have been conducted in patients recruited from either Veterans Administration or city or county hospitals. These types of patients may not be totally representative of the general population of peptic ulcer patients. These dissimilarities may be due to the degree of the disease or the presence of concomitant medical problems, or they may represent possible differences in life styles that are known to aggravate peptic ulcer disease (e.g., smoking habits, alcohol consumption).

Ethical questions are not usually raised about the importance of including a placebo arm in ulcer recurrence trials examining the effect of treatment on the natural history of peptic ulcer disease. One reason for this may be that patients in these studies do not exhibit endoscopically proven ulcer lesions. Another is that the value of maintenance therapy is becoming more and more controversial. Despite these limitations, placebo-controlled trials have important value in the evaluation of new therapeutic agents in peptic ulcer disease and therefore should be carried out whenever possible.

Although alternative study designs to be considered include comparison with an active drug or dose–response studies, preference should be given to including a placebo arm in these studies. Incidentally, it is not a good idea to compare the test drug to an active drug that has not yet been approved, because one would be comparing two experimental drugs, and the efficacy of the comparator is not recognized by the FDA. If the new drug is to be compared to a known effective and approved treatment, and if the new drug is clinically and statistically superior to such established treatment, there would be no question as to agreeing to its efficacy. The problem arises when the new drug is not significantly different from an approved drug. In fact, this is the case with many drugs of diverse pharmacological classes that have been studied and approved for ulcer healing. Adequate sample sizes to limit type II error are helpful, but careful attention to the allowable differences in responses should be made before initiation of the study.

The ideal study recommended by the FDA draft guideline would consist of four arms: placebo, active control drug, and two dose levels of the test drug. However, for practical reasons and from our own experience in planning and managing clinical studies, this type of trial is difficult to implement. An alternative approach is to split such a trial into two studies, similar to what was done in the case of misoprostol: a two-arm placebo-controlled study (placebo and one dose of the test drug) and a second three-arm study (two doses of test drug and an active control). Investigators who do not wish to include their patients in the placebo-controlled trial are given the option of including their patients in an active-control trial.

D.   Dose–Response Studies

Because a direct correlation between a pharmacological effect (i.e., acid suppression or cytoprotection) and drug efficacy (i.e., healing an ulcer) cannot yet be made, only through clinical efficacy trials in which varying doses of the study drug are used can a dose–response relationship for healing ulcer be determined. It is very important to find an optimal dose, which can be defined as the dose above which no additional efficacy occurs and below which efficacy is unlikely. This has practical regulatory and clinical implications. The approval of the use of a drug without substantial knowledge of its maximum or minimum effective dose may result in patients receiving doses that are either larger than necessary or smaller than effective. Thus, it is important to know the clinical effect and the pharmacokinetic fate of higher doses of the test drug, because in clinical practice physicians usually increase the dose to maximize efficacy results, especially if the drug being used is perceived as safe. When empirically done, this approach may result in patients experiencing adverse drug reactions.

In addition to possibly minimizing adverse drug reactions, characterization of the dose response and time course of healing is essential in determining other aspects of the risk/benefit ratio (drug interactions, convenience to the patient) and in giving adequate prescribing information to the practicing physician. Furthermore, dose–response efficacy trials offer a viable alternative to a strictly placebo-controlled trial in determining drug efficacy as long as there is no evidence that at high doses the drug exerts a deleterious effect and that at least the lowest and highest doses can be differentiated from each other in the clinical trial.

E.   Patient Population

The number and diversity of the patients studied in clinical efficacy trials should be broad enough that adequate information can be obtained in terms of both efficacy and safety in as wide a patient range as possible. It is important to mention that even within the United States the study population must be carefully chosen. Some organizations that conduct contract clinical research on behalf of pharmaceutical companies enroll investigators in geographical areas where certain types of patients (e.g., Hispanics) may be overrepresented. The findings in these patients may not be applicable to the general U.S. population. Patients selected for entry should not only have evidence of an ulcer but also have associated symptoms so that determinations can be made during the trial of symptom response as well as ulcer healing. It is well recognized, however, that dyspeptic symptoms do not always correlate with the presence of an ulcer, and this inclusion requirement may slow the enrollment rate. Therefore, in early phase II studies this requirement should be upheld, whereas in phase IIIa studies it should be optional, although the endoscopy of an asymptomatic patient may raise ethical concerns.

In order to determine if trials are of comparable ulcer populations, the FDA draft guideline suggests that a minimum ulcer size of 0.5 cm be required for entry into the studies. It should be stressed, however, that a smaller ulcer size (0.3 cm) has been used in most controlled trials with the provision that what is seen by the endoscopist was truly an ulcer, not just an erosion. That is, the experienced endoscopist must observe mucosal depth and not just a superficial erosion (see Section VIII).

Consideration should also be given to certain baseline demographic factors that influence ulcer formation and healing. These factors include cigarette consumption, alcohol or antacid use, and ulcer size. Ideally, treatment groups should be comparable at entry with respect to these factors, and in large trials the randomization of the test subjects should ensure equal distribution of risk factors among the patients. In certain instances, stratification based on certain baseline demographics should be considered. The inference is that baseline imbalances may explain the result observed. But in reality, these are "soft data," as exemplified in the case of cigarette consumption. Some trials stratify patients on the basis of smoking status, the definition of which is not standardized. The real issue arises for those patients considered not to be smokers on the basis of self-reports, given the fact that there is no biochemical confirmation of absence of smoking status. The other point, which is difficult to control, is that some investigators counsel patients to stop smoking during the trial. But again, the outcome of such an approach is usually not well documented. These issues with respect to smoking may explain the confusing literature on this risk factor. Some investigators [16–18] established that smoking is a major factor associated with frequent recurrences. Others, however, such as Penston and Wormsley [19] in their study with continuous maintenance therapy with ranitidine and the Bardhan [20] maintenance study with cimetidine, reported that smoking exerts no influence on the relapse of ulcers during maintenance therapy. Also, inconsistent results have been reported with regard to healing and initial size of the ulcer.

F.   Endpoint for Clinical Trials

The protocol should prospectively incorporate adequate operational criteria to measure primary (i.e., ulcer healing) and secondary (i.e., changes in symptoms) endpoints of efficacy. Assessment of the kinetics of the healing process in response to treatment in the first 2–8 weeks is also of interest. The FDA draft guideline indicates that the primary reliable evidence of efficacy should be based on total endoscopic healing as defined by visual reepithelialization without evidence of erosions. We fully agree with the FDA recommendations that ulcer healing should be the principal efficacy parameter for an anti-ulcer drug. However, the observation concerning erosions is most controversial, as detailed below:

1.   Erosions are not considered to be ulcers from endoscopic and histological appearance.
2.   The natural history of erosions does not suggest a progression toward the formation of ulcers.
3.   The drug is being advocated for healing ulcers but not erosions.

4. The inclusion criteria would not permit the enrollment of patients with *only* erosions and not true ulcers.

5. There is a considerable database derived from a large number of clinical studies with diverse pharmacological agents in which erosions were not considered as evidence for lack of healing.

On these grounds, most of these trials would have to be repeated to provide a comparable basis for efficacy among these diverse drugs. Until firm data regarding the meaning and evolution of erosions become available (see Section VIII), it would be useful to conduct a subgroup analysis of the data on the basis of total healing (ulcers and erosions) and on the basis of healing only the ulcers and not erosions. Endoscopic videography/photography to provide actual documentation may assist in resolving a discrepancy concerning interpretation of the observations, but this technique is not yet standardized. Clear instructions as to the withdrawal of patients because of worsening condition (e.g., an ulcer that enlarges in size by more than 20%) should be given to protect the patients and to ensure consistency among the investigators.

In clinical trials using upper gastrointestinal bleeding as an endpoint, it may be important to characterize bleeding rates on the basis of the amount of blood loss. The bleeding could therefore be massive (blood loss of 1000 mL or more in 24 hr); brisk (blood loss of 500–1000 mL or more in 24 hr), or slow (up to 250 mL in 24 hr). Each of these rates is accompanied by a suggestive set of clinical manifestations. In addition to the complete cessation of bleeding, it is of interest to establish efficacy on the basis of other clinical parameters. These include decrease in the number of units and volume of blood transfused, prevention of the need for surgery, shortening of the hospital stay, and perhaps improvement of survival. It is also important to remember that it is nearly impossible to be certain whether the patient continues to bleed if there is no nasogastric tube in place. On the other hand, a little bit of bright red blood in the nasogastric aspirate plus coffee grounds is of questionable clinical relevance.

G. Length of Trial

For peptic ulcer trials, the time of exposure to a therapeutic modality is entirely arbitrary. Short-term treatments have included anywhere from 1 to 12 weeks. Since efficacy for approved products has been demonstrated for certain fixed periods, it is important to use such fixed periods for comparative purposes. For example, a customary and appropriate single time interval for duodenal ulcer is 4 weeks and for gastric ulcer, 8 weeks. Consideration of other time periods should be approached carefully and only after adequate justification is agreed upon.

H. Data Analysis and Presentation

A detailed statistical report including tables and graphic display of data is extremely helpful in analyzing efficacy trials. A list of dropouts with indications of when and why is essential.

It is essential to realize that effective reporting of the gathered data should be an integral component of adequate research of a test drug's effectiveness and safety profiles. Before beginning the study, specific plans on how the data will be analyzed (e.g., what statistical tests and what levels of significance will be used) should be clearly described in the protocol. The handling of dropouts must be carefully planned and be provided for prospectively. An analysis of all patients entered (intent-to-treat) should always be done in addition to any other contemplated analyses. Early stopping (by acceptable and prespecified statistical methods) should be justified on the basis of ethical concerns or instances where a new drug might be significantly inferior to a proven drug. However, in general, interim analyses are not helpful, are difficult to justify, and can lead to a variety of biases, thereby jeopardizing the validity of the trial.

I. NDA Submission and Approval

The compilation of an NDA is achieved with the collaborative efforts of many scientists and clinicians. The essential components of an NDA are listed in Table 4, but a detailed discussion of these is beyond the scope of this review. We will only mention that according to FDA guidelines, the following constitutes a good NDA:

1. The submission is consistent with published guidelines, has acceptable format, and is complete.
2. The data are presented in a manner to facilitate a critical review.
3. The document clearly provides evidence that the drug is safe and effective.
4. The material is well organized, paginated, and cross-referenced where appropriate.

As an example of the complexity of the NDA document, the initial NDA submission on misoprostol for the treatment of duodenal ulcer included 120 volumes with more than 30,000 pages. In addition to the many volumes describing all the technical sections, there is also a complete master summary in which everything that is important is succinctly described and integrated into a meaningful document. The drug sponsor is required by law to submit not only analyses and summaries of all scientific data but also the actual raw data, which constitute the bulk of the NDA submissions.

The FDA review of the NDA is prioritized in accordance with the importance of the NCE using the FDA classification described in Table 5. Thus, new compounds with little or no therapeutic value are assigned low priority (1C) and would require a longer review time compared to compounds in the 1A/1AA class. During the 1980s, the mean approval time for an NCE was 32.3 months [21].

We have already stressed that it is essential to assemble a good NDA with special attention to the organization and presentation of the data. The latter should be of such

Table 4 Essential Components of an NDA

Index
Summary
Chemistry, manufacturing, and control section
Samples (submit only upon FDA's request)
Methods validation package
Labeling
    Draft labeling (4 copies)
    Final printed labeling (12 copies)
Nonclinical pharmacology and toxicology section
Human pharmacokinetics and bioavailability section
Microbiology section
Clinical data section
Safety update report
Statistical section
Case report tabulations
Case report forms (deaths, withdrawals)
Patent information on any patent that claims the drug
A patent certification with respect to any patent that claims the drug
Other (specify)

Note: The proper, complete, and organized submission should allow the following types of NDA reviews: chemistry, pharmacology-toxicology, medical, biopharmaceutics, statistics, and microbiology.

Table 5 Priority of the NDA Review Process by the FDA

Types	Therapeutic value[a]
NMA (new molecular entity)	Important (A)[b]
NCE (new chemical entity)	Modest (B)
New salt	Little or none (C)
New formulation	Orphan drug candidate (D)
New combination	
Already marketed drug product duplication	
New claim for already marketed drug product	

[a]Other less important classifications (e.g., M, P, R, S, T, U) have also been assigned by the FDA, and the reader is encouraged to review additional details on these classifications.
[b]The 1AA priority was established for AIDS drugs.

quality that there should be little difficulty in establishing the evidence of safety and effectiveness. The long approval time for many drugs is usually the result of FDA requests for additional data or classifications. These may originate from any of the six types of NDA reviews (chemistry, pharmacology, medical, biopharmaceutics, statistics, and microbiology). The FDA may also wish to convene a meeting of an advisory committee to review the NDA submission with the sponsor. It is important to realize that the recommendations of the advisory committee are not binding. The purpose of the NDA review is to establish the safety and effectiveness of a new drug. To be approved, a drug must show substantial evidence of effectiveness. The latter is defined as evidence consisting of adequate and well-controlled investigations by qualified scientific experts proving that the drug will have the effect claimed in the labeling.

It is a well-known fact that all drugs have certain and often definable risks inherent in their use. To assist the FDA in its review of the NDA, a risk/benefit assessment should examine the positive and negative contributions of the test drug, especially in relation to other marketed products. Because we already have several safe and effective agents for the treatment of uncomplicated duodenal or gastric ulcer, it would be prudent from regulatory and marketing standpoints to establish whether the drug has certain advantages with possibly little or no adverse attributes in comparison to standard treatments. For example, neither a proton-pump inhibitor nor prostaglandins were approved by the FDA for the treatment of duodenal ulcer, because of potential adverse reactions (carcinoid and entrochromaffin-like (ECL) cell hyperplasia with omeprazole in animals and uterotonic effects with prostaglandins). However, recognizing these potential risks, these drugs were approved by the FDA for the treatment of disease states not amenable to therapy with standard drugs. Thus, omeprazole was approved for severe erosive esophagitis or in poorly responsive patients with gastroesophageal reflux disease (GERD) and pathological hypersecretory conditions (e.g., Zollinger-Ellison syndrome). Misoprostol was approved by the FDA for the prevention of nonsteroidal anti-inflammatory drug-induced gastric ulcer.

It should also be emphasized that none of the marketed anti-ulcer drugs have been found to alter the natural history of peptic ulcer disease, although several studies have shown promising findings for prostaglandins and bismuth-containing drugs. Should a sponsor conduct the appropriate trial in support of this claim, approval of the drug, even one having certain undesirable attributes, may be favored because of a shift in the benefit/risk profile in favor of an important, unique new benefit.

VI.   CLINICAL EFFICACY TRIALS (PHASE IIIb)

In this review, phase IIIb is defined as a stage in the drug development process that occurs sometimes after the formal submission of a New Drug Application (NDA) and before FDA grants approval for the original NDA. There are two principal goals served by phase IIIb trials:

1.   To obtain a large-scale database supporting the safety and efficacy of the drug. This would permit obtaining labeling changes, or new dosage reformulation,

or even making a new claim not originally made in the initial submission of the NDA.

2. To obtain marketing support for the product, especially with office-based physicians who may not have been involved in the clinical development of the product, thereby identifying a medical/marketing position for the product prior to launch. This large physician-user base could very well help market the product.

It is important to mention that there could be a potential disadvantage for the conduct of phase IIIb studies, because this program is sometimes inadequately funded and this can lead to inadequate monitoring of the trials. All of this could in turn significantly delay the NDA review process. Although the phase IIIb program is initially driven by the interests of the marketing groups in obtaining early product acceptance in the marketplace, there is also considerable interest by the clinical researchers in uncovering adverse reactions reports (ADRs), especially for drugs that have a very low incidence of a major adverse reaction that would not be evident from an NDA submission based on 1500–2000 patients but would indeed be evident when 10,000 or more patients are exposed to the product. The larger the population, the higher the probability of uncovering risks that are not so common. For example, chloramphenicol has a risk of inducing agranulocytosis in 1 out of 20,000 exposed patients, and the initial NDA application could not have predicted this risk. Thus, if the safety data of an NDA submission is well supported by the data obtained from phase IIIb studies, this may result in an expedited approval, especially for drugs that may have no therapeutic advantages over drugs currently on the market, such as an additional nonsteroidal anti-inflammatory drug (NSAID).

More important, phase IIIb studies could also uncover a new claim that was not sought in the original NDA filing. For example, the NDA on misoprostol was originally submitted to the FDA in 1984 for the treatment of duodenal ulcer. Phase IIIb studies uncovered a more important clinical utility of this drug for the prevention of NSAID-induced gastric ulcer, for which FDA approval was granted in late 1988. It is of interest to note that in addition to the studies carried out under phases I, II, and III, clinical trials can also be conducted under a treatment use protocol. These studies involve patients with life-threatening or terminal illness such as AIDS and cancer, for which alternative treatments are either not available or not effective.

From this discussion, it is obvious that for certain drugs, phase IIIb studies do have a place in the drug development process, providing that these studies are adequately conceived and monitored.

VII. POSTMARKETING STUDIES (PHASE IV) AND SURVEILLANCE

Postmarketing research is to a large extent an extension of the phase IIIb studies and has several potential advantages:

1. It may establish the product in the marketplace. This is usually accomplished by the use of seeding trials with a large number of physicians.
2. From a scientific point of view, postmarketing research permits us to learn more about the beneficial therapeutic effects and also about potential undesirable effects of a drug.

Postmarketing research studies are usually designed to be simple and easily performed by the investigators, because the sponsor is mostly interested in physician experience with the drug and not in proving efficacy as in phases I–III. The simplicity of the protocols for the phase IV studies must be designed to yield good information about ADRs. The heterogeneity and volume of data produced in postmarketing surveillance require a major effort to ensure a minimum quantity of data of acceptable quality in every case report or in every study [22]. Another requirement is the wider use of generally accepted terminologies for given ADRs. Without these prerequisites, much of the information would become lost or possibly misinterpreted and therefore useless.

Some of the most important advances in therapeutics have occurred only through observations of patients receiving drugs for completely different indications than those approved for marketing. Such discoveries cannot be planned for, but careful observation and vigilance are essential for postmarketing discoveries [23]. Examples of such discoveries include the use of beta-blockers in hypertension, glaucoma, anxiety, thyroid disease, migraine headaches, and coronary death; the use of the antihypertensive drug minoxidil for the promotion of hair growth; and the antihistamine drugs for motion sickness. Should a marketed drug exhibit any unpredictable beneficial action, such action would require clinical confirmation of the safety and efficacy of the drug for this particular property. That is, the sponsor would have to go through the NDA process again to prove safety and efficacy for this new indication.

VIII.   FUTURE RESEARCH

Listed below are certain areas where, in our opinion, research is needed. These are not listed in order of priority.

(1)   One important yet unresolved research issue is how to unmistakenly define a small ulcer so that, upon endoscopy, it can be distinguished from an erosion. With the existing endoscopic techniques, an accurate measurement of the lesion depth is not possible. It is easy to say that an ulcer should possess depth. However, how deep the lesion should be and how depth should be measured are in need of research and standardization.

(2)   Characterization is needed for the meaning and evolution of acute and chronic gastritis and duodenitis and their relationship to ulcer formation and development. In other words, there is need for extension of the pioneering work of Kreuning [24] and the suggestion that chronic nonspecific duodenitis probably represents the

early phase of development of a duodenal ulcer or the later stage of the healing of such an ulcer. Similarly, do acute ulcers become chronic ulcers?

(3) A prostaglandin (misoprostol) has been approved for the prevention of NSAID-induced ulcers in one part of the gastrointestinal tract (the stomach). Do other areas of the gut need to be protected? If so, to what extent? NSAIDs also seem to injure, although to a much lesser extent, the mucosa of the duodenum [25,26], the esophagus [27], the small intestine [28], and even the colon [29,30]. We need to establish the exact incidence and clinical relevance of these injuries in patients receiving NSAIDs. Furthermore, are different therapeutic modalities needed to prevent injuries in areas other than the stomach? For example, a cimetidine–antacid regimen was reported to afford superior protection to the duodenum but not to the stomach [31]. Several other studies with the H_2 antagonists consistently demonstrated that these drugs do not protect the gastric mucosa against NSAID-induced gastric ulcer [32–36]. These results suggest a fundamental difference in the pathology and pharmacology of NSAID-induced ulcer in stomach and duodenum.

(4) Further characterization is needed of the relationship between the erosion- and ulcer-inducing action of NSAIDs and their antiplatelet effects.

(5) Is it possible that the scarring or healing process of the gastroduodenal mucosa is different depending on the therapeutic agent employed? If so, what factors influence these differences? Do endogenously produced prostaglandins or peptides synthesized by gastroduodenal mucosa, or other known or even unknown substances at the local level, play a role in these events? Thus, can one differentiate between histamine blockers, prostaglandins, peptides, proton pump inhibitors, and locally acting substances (sucralfate, bismuth compounds, alone or in combination with antibiotics or with antacids) on the basis of quality of ulcer healing? If so, do these differences have clinical relevance?

Researching these issues requires an expanded use of biopsy of the gastroduodenal mucosa in patients whose duodenal or gastric ulcer has been healed with a certain therapeutic agent. In other words, it would be of interest to expand the initial observations made by Sakita and Fukutomi and those of Miwa, who have proposed a six-stage classification of gastric ulcers based on endoscopy/biopsy findings: active stage 1 (A_1), active stage 2 (A_2); healing stage 1 (H_1), healing stage 2 (H_2); and two scarring stages: S_1, during which the regeneration region is markedly red and, on close observation, many capillaries are seen (red scar); and S_2, which occurs in several months to a few years and during which the redness is reduced to the color of the surrounding mucosa ("white scar"). We suggest that confirmation and extension of this or similar classification systems may prove helpful in interpreting and characterizing the salutary effects of the variety of agents beneficial in the treatment of peptic ulcer disease.

(6) In clinical trials designed to test the effectiveness of prescription drugs for use under over-the-counter (OTC) conditions, it is becoming fashionable to enrich the population of "responders" or patients in need of true therapeutic intervention. This

is thought to be accomplished by a 1–2-week screening phase during which the patients receive placebo. Noninclusion of these placebo reactors (placebo responders) is an accepted means of improving the chances of obtaining more meaningful results, because this process eliminates from the trial those patients with a high proclivity for reacting to placebo. However, this issue has not been properly researched. The little available evidence [37] does not support the concept that either a placebo reactor or nonreactor really exists as a separate or distinct entity. In an experiment measuring vomiting (an objective phenomenon) or nausea (a subjective phenomenon), the intraindividual variation in response to placebo was found to be as great as the interindividual variation. Similarly, it is not known whether or not the placebo responders in peptic ulcer trials are always the same patients. Also, it is not known if the likelihood of predicting placebo responses may be enhanced by increasing the number of placebo tests performed on any individual patients. This kind of information may be useful in determining the true effectiveness of an anti-ulcer drug.

(7)   More research is needed on the proposed association of potent acid reduction and risk of enteric infection [38]. This information may be of practical importance, because such enteritis is preventable. However, wider experience with these potent and very effective antisecretory drugs is needed to determine with certainty whether this effect is a real hazard or merely coincidence [39].

(8)   The use of a placebo antacid—a tablet that has the appearance of an antacid but with no neutralizing capacity—should be considered in some trials where the consumption of a true antacid is suspected of confounding the results of an effective therapy.

(9)   Is the clinical picture of peptic ulcer disease in the elderly substantially different from that in younger patients? Are surrogate measures (i.e., ulcer healing and prevention) in clinical trials adequate to study elderly populations, or should one depend on results from observations of ulcer complications (i.e., bleeding, perforation, stenosis) to better define the therapeutic needs in this population?

(10)   What type of ulcer is more likely to relapse upon the withdrawal of active medication? What factors play a role, and to what extent?

(11)   In addition to more frequent endoscopies, what is the best design to show that a drug prevents ulcer recurrence? What are the most appropriate statistical analyses? Among the models in need of further validation are those of Sontag [40], Pounder [41], and Boyd et al. [42] discussed at the January 17, 1986, meeting of the GI Advisory Committee to the FDA.

IX.   SUMMARY AND CONCLUSIONS

An attempt has been made to highlight some aspects of the pharmaceutical industry perspective on human investigation and development of anti-ulcer drugs. The research necessary to support the registration and marketing of new chemical entities is complex, expensive, and time-consuming. Only a few of the thousands of compounds survive preclinical testing, and of these even fewer compounds become successfully marketed drugs. During preclinical research and development, pharmacological characterization—including determinations of the mode of action, toxicological profile, effect on organs other than the gastrointestinal tract, mutagenicity and teratogenicity, pharmacokinetics, and pharmacodynamics—yields estimates for a clinical dose. Approval of an IND is needed to start studies in humans.

The clinical research and development is carried out in sequential phases. Briefly, the primary purpose of phase I studies is to establish the safety and tolerance, clinical pharmacology, and pharmacodynamics in healthy subjects. Initial efficacy studies are performed in phase II utilizing controlled trials in 50–200 patients with peptic ulcer disease. Phase III studies consisting of both controlled and open trials further establish the safety and efficacy in up to 1000 or more additional patients. This information is used to arrive at proper labeling for the drug. Phase IV studies consist of postmarketing surveillance, with reporting of adverse reactions, survey sampling, testing, and inspection.

In this chapter emphasis was placed on the overall design of clinical trials to show substantial evidence of effectiveness. Discussions centered on the use of the best comparators, dose–response studies, patient populations, clinically meaningful endpoints (i.e., total healing and length of exposure), data analysis, and data presentation. Finally, some areas of needed clinical and experimental investigations were discussed.

The cost for the development of a new NCE may be as much as $200 million. One critical consideration for gaining approval for the drug in a timely fashion is the organization of the NDA according to FDA guidelines and is consistent with FDA regulations. Poorly organized applications for inadequately studied drugs are wasteful in effort, energy, and money.

The uncertainties of drug development coupled with increased costs have the potential for reducing incentives for many U.S. drug companies to conduct basic research and development of new drugs. This is particularly evident in the field of anti-ulcer drugs. With the exception of misoprostol, which was discovered in the United States, no major discoveries during the past 25 years were made in the United States. However, the development and eventual approval of drugs such as misoprostol, omeprazole, and more potent H_2-receptor antagonists is a powerful incentive to continue the search for better drugs.

We wish to thank Dr. Alphonso Perez for reviewing the manuscript and Dr. Jeffrey Staffa for his critical and helpful comments on the manuscript.

REFERENCES

1. Hansen RW. The pharmaceutical development process: estimates of development cost and times and effects of proposed regulatory changes. In: Chien RF, ed. Issues in pharmaceutical economics. Lexington, Mass.: D.C. Heath, 1979:151–81.

2. Grabowski H. Research and development cost. FDC reports January 1, 1990.

3. Black JW, Duncan WAM, Durant CJ, Ganellin CR, Parsons EM. Definition and antagonism of histamine H_2 receptors. Nature 1972; 236:385–90.

4. Dajani EZ. Perspectives on the pharmacology of misoprostol. In: Szabo S, Pfeifer C, eds. Ulcer disease: new aspects of pathogenesis and pharmacology. Boca Raton, Fla.: CRC Press, 1989:Chap. 27, 321–34.

5. Dajani EZ, Driskill DR, Bianchi RG, Collins PW, Pappo R. SC-29333, a potent inhibitor of canine gastric secretion. Dig Dis Sci 1976; 21:1049–57.

6. Dajani EZ, Callison DA, Bertermann RE. Effects of E-prostaglandins on canine gastric potential difference. Dig Dis Sci 1978; 23:436–42.

7. Dajani EZ. Mucosal defense and concept of cytoprotection. An editorial. Mod Pathol 1990; 3:3–4.

8. Dajani EZ. Perspective on the gastric antisecretory effects of misoprostol in man. Prostaglandins 1987; 33(Suppl):68–77.

9. Dajani EZ. Overview of the mucosal protective effects of misoprostol in man. Prostaglandins 1987; 33(Suppl):117–29.

10. Brozinsky S, Koss MA, Isenberg JI, Sandersfeld MA, Gallo-Torres H, Given S. Dose ranging antisecretory activity of trimoprostil in patients with peptic ulcer disease. Clin Pharmacol Ther 1984; 35(2):230.

11. Wills RJ, Rees MMC, Rubio F, Gibson DM, Parsonnet M, Gallo-Torres HE. Influence of antacids on the bioavailability of trimoprostil. Eur J Clin Pharmacol 1984; 27:251–2.

12. Berkowitz JM, Adler SN, Posse S, Gallo-Torres H. An endoscopic evaluation of the effect of trimoprostil on aspirin induced gastroduodenal mucosal injury. Gastroenterology 1985; 88:1322. Abstract.

13. Anonymous. Proposed guidelines for the clinical evaluation of antiulcer drugs. Washington, DC: Food and Drug Administration [Draft] 1985.

14. Martin LF, Staloch DK, Simonowitz DA, Dellinger EP, Max MH. Failure of cimetidine prophylaxis in the critically ill. Arch Surg 1979; 114:492–6.

15. Schiller LR, Fordtran JS. Ulcer complications during short-term therapy of duodenal ulcer with active agents and placebo. Gastroenterology 1986; 90:478–81.

16. Sonnenberg A, Müller-Lissner SA, Vogel E, Schmid P, Gonvers JJ, Peter P, Strohmeyer G, Blum AL. Predictors of duodenal ulcer healing and relapse. Gastroenterology 1981; 81:1061–7.

17. Sontag S, Graham DY, Belsito M, Weiss J, Farley A, Grant R, Cohen N, Kinnear D, Davis W, Archambault A, Achord J, Thayer W, Gillies R, Sidorov J, Sabesin SM, Dyck W, Fleshler B, Cleater I, Wenger J, Opekum A. Cimetidine, cigarette smoking and recurrence of duodenal ulcer. N Engl J Med 1984; 311:689–93.

18. Massarrat A, Eisenman A. Factors effecting the healing rate of duodenal and pyloric ulcers with lose-dose antacid treatment. Gut 1981; 22:97–102.

19. Penston JG, Wormsley K. Long term treatment of duodenal ulcers. Gastroenterology 1988; 94:A349.

20. Bardhan KD. Treatment of duodenal ulceration: reflections, recollections and reminiscences. Gut 1989; 30:1647–55.

21. Anonymous. Approval time for 1989 new molecular entities is under three years; December approval rush is still fact of life at FDA, but is less pronounced in 1989. FDC Rep January 8, 1990, pp. 3–7.

22. Venulet J. Potential role of postmarketing research. Drugs Exp Clin Res 1987; 13(11): 673–83.

23. Wardell WM, Sheck LE. Is pharmaceutical innovation declining? Interpreting measures of pharmaceutical innovation and regulatory impact in the USA, 1950–1980. Pharmacol Physicians 1983; 17:1–5.

24. Kreuning J. Chronic non-specific duodenitis. A clinical and histopathological study. World Congress of Gastroenterology, Madrid, Spain, 1978.

25. Lanza FL. Endoscopic studies of gastric and duodenal injury after the use of ibuprofen, aspirin and other nonsteroidal anti-inflammatory drugs. Am J Med 1984; 77(1A):19–24.

26. Semple EL, Wu WC. Anti-inflammatory drugs and gastric mucosal damage. Semin Arthritis Rheum 1987; 16:271–86.

27. Tympner F. Gastroscopic findings after therapy with nonsteroid anti-rheumatic drugs. Z Rheumatol 1981; 40:179–81.

28. Bjarnasson I, Zanelli G, Smith T, Pronse P, Williams P, Smethurst P, Delany G, Gumpel MT, Levi AJ. Nonsteroidal antiinflammatory drug-induced intestinal inflammation in humans. Gastroenterology 1987; 93:480–9.

29. Rampton DS. Nonsteroidal anti-inflammatory drugs and the lower gastrointestinal tract. Scand J Gastroenterol 1987; 22:1–4.

30. Langman MJS, Morgan L, Worrall A. Use of anti-inflammatory drugs by patients admitted with small or large bowel perforations and hemorrhage. Br Med J 1987; 290:347–9.

31. Lanza FL, Royer GL, Nelson RS. Effect of a cimetidine-antacid regimen on the gastric and duodenal mucosal injury seen with aspirin and other nonsteroidal antiinflammatory agents. Gastroenterology 1983; 84:1223.

32. Stalnikowicz R, Goldin E, Fich A, Wengrower D, Eliakim R, Ligumsky M, Rachmilewitz D. Indomethacin induced gastroduodenal damage is not affected by co-treatment with ranitidine. J Clin Gastroenterol 1989; 11:178–82.

33. Ehsanulla RSB, Page MC, Tildesley, Wood JR. Prevention of gastroduodenal damage induced by nonsteroidal anti-inflammatory drugs: controlled clinical trial of ranitidine. Br Med J 1988; 29:1017–21.

34. Lanza F, Robinson M, Bowers J, et al. A multi-center, double-blind comparison of ranitidine vs placebo in the prophylaxis of nonsteroidal anti-inflammatory drug (NSAID) induced gastric and duodenal mucosa. Gastroenterology 1988; 94:A250. Abstract.

35. Bianchi Porro G, Pace F. Ulcerogenic drugs and upper gastrointestinal bleeding. Bailliere Clin Gastroenterol 1988; 2(2):309–27.

36. Roth SH, Bennett RE, Mitchell CS, et al. Cimetidine therapy in nonsteroidal anti-inflammatory drug gastropathy: double-blind, long-term evaluation. Arch Intern Med 1987; 147:1798–801.

37. Wolf S, Doering CR, Clark ML, Hagans JA. Chance distribution and the placebo "reactor." J Lab Clin Med 1957; 49:837–41.

38. Littman A. Potent acid reduction and risk of enteric infection. Lancet 1990;

39. Wingate DL. Acid reduction and recurrent enteritis. Lancet 1990;

40. Sontag SJ. Current status of maintenance therapy in peptic ulcer disease. Am J Gastroenterol 1988; 83:607–17.

41. Pounder RE. Model of medical treatment for duodenal ulcer. Lancet 1981; i:29–30.

42. Boyd EJS, Penston JG, Johnston DA, Wormsley KG. Does maintenance therapy keep duodenal ulcers healed? Lancet 1988; i:1324–7.

23

Principles and Practices in the Clinical Investigation of Anti-Ulcer Drugs in Japan

TAKESHI MIWA

Tokai University School of Medicine,
Isehara, Japan

I. INTRODUCTION

The methods for investigating anti-ulcer medications, although generally similar to those for other drugs, nevertheless must recognize a number of characteristics of ulcer disease. Ulcers may recur on a chronic basis, requiring long-term treatment. Subjective symptoms of ulcers usually disappear rapidly during therapy. Gastric acid and pepsin are major aggressive factors, especially in duodenal ulcer. Mucosal bicarbonate and mucus secretions as well as mucosal microcirculation are defensive factors. Poor gastric emptying or bile reflux impair ulcer healing. Nonsteroidal anti-inflammatory drugs (NSAIDs) can induce and aggravate ulcers. Various types of stressors and chemicals, such as ethanol and smoking, may induce or aggravate ulcers. When medical therapy of ulcers fails, surgery should be used if necessary.

There are a number of important desirable characteristics of new anti-ulcer medications. The toxicity of the drug when it is administered chronically must be minimal. The dosage form and method of administration should be easy for the patient to use. Drugs that inhibit gastric acid secretion, improve mucosal microcirculation, stimulate bicarbonate and mucus secretion, and promote the motility of the alimentary tract are recommended. Drugs that heal ulcers even when NSAIDs are administered concurrently are desirable, as are drugs that inhibit ulcers due to stress factors. Surgery should be avoided, if possible; however, if it is necessary, it must be undertaken at the proper time.

Essentially all Japanese investigations of anti-ulcer agents employ a unique, highly descriptive grading system for the evaluation of ulcer healing. This system will be described later in the section on phase II studies.

II.   PRECLINICAL PHASE

The following preclinical studies serve as the essential scientific basis for the clinical assessment of new anti-ulcer drugs.

A.   Pharmacology

For drugs intended to reduce aggressive factors, the antisecretory effects on gastric acid and pepsin and the value of serum gastrin should be measured using canine Heidenhain pouches and rat Schild and Shay preparations, etc. For defensive-factor-enhancing agents, pharmacological data on the improvement in gastric mucosal blood flow, increase in mucoprotein synthesis, and mucosal resistance to acid are required.

B.   Pharmacokinetics

The pharmacokinetics of single and multiple doses administered by various routes should be studied, and the potential for drug accumulation should be evaluated. Data are required not only for mice and rats but also for larger animals. In addition, comparative pharmacokinetic data of other anti-ulcer drugs are very useful.

C.   Efficacy

Chronic gastric and duodenal ulcer models [1] in various animals, such as rats, guinea pigs, cats, dogs, and miniature swine, are used for efficacy assessment. Generally, a drug that exerts effects on chronic ulcer models is appropriate for the treatment of gastric and duodenal ulcers in humans. A drug that exerts effects on acute ulcer models tends to be effective for inflammatory mucosal lesions.

D.   Toxicology

Since anti-ulcer drugs are administered for long durations, the results of chronic toxicity studies are required as well as those of acute and subacute toxicity studies.

E.   Determination of Clinical Dose

It is not easy to determine the clinical dose from the results of preclinical pharmacology and toxicity studies. However, the effective single dose in grams per kilogram in animals (in particular, rats) is converted to grams per person per day and multiplied by some factor to obtain the clinical dose using Okabe's method [2]. Doses around this calculated dose are used in the dose-determination (phase II) study. Doses for rats

Table 1 Animal and Clinical Doses of Recently Marketed Anti-Ulcer Drugs[a]

Generic name (product name)	Indications	Dose for Rats (mg/kg)	Clinical Dose (mg/day/person)
Cetraxate HCl (Neuer S)	GU	300–1000	800
Sofalcone (Solon)	GU	100–300	150
Teprenone (Selbex)	GU	100–200	150
Pirenzepine HCl (Gastrozepin)	GU/DU	30–100	75
Cimetidine (Tagamet)	GU/DU	50–100	800
Ranitidine (Zantac)	GU/DU	30–200	300
Famotidine (Gaster)	GU/DU	20–60	40

GU, gastric ulcer; DU, duodenal ulcer.
[a]Oral administration.

and clinical doses of recently approved anti-ulcer drugs are shown in Table 1. The results tend to be similar to those calculated using Okabe's method.

III. PHASE I

Single- and multiple-dose clinical pharmacological studies follow the preclinical confirmation of the safety of single and multiple doses of the investigational drug.

Clinical pharmacological studies to be stressed vary depending on the type of investigational drug—that is, on whether the aggressive-factor-depressing effect is stronger than the defensive-factor-enhancing effect or vice versa. However, since aggressive-factor-depressing and defensive-factor-enhancing effects work together to heal ulcers, both categories of effect will often be investigated.

Specific clinical pharmacological studies typically conducted for anti-ulcer drugs are as follows:

1. Gastric antisecretory study: inhibition of basal secretion, nocturnal secretion, and gastrin-, histamine-, insulin-, and meal-stimulated secretions
2. Gastric mucosal hemodynamic study
3. H^+ back-diffusion study, potential difference study, and bicarbonate secretory study
4. Measurement of mucosal prostaglandin content
5. Measurement of gastric mucus secretion
6. Study of gastric-emptying activity
7. Fluctuations of plasma gastrin and secretion
8. Fluctuations of collagen in ulcer margin

Although in the phase I study, anti-ulcer drugs are usually administered repeatedly for five days, the safety of long-term use must also be confirmed. Thus, a phase I study will sometimes be prolonged using subjects leading everyday lives. Additional phase I studies of anti-ulcer drugs are conducted in the same manner as for other drugs, for example, single and multiple ascending dose tolerance and studies of drug absorption, distribution, metabolism, and excretion (ADME).

IV.   PHASE II

A.   Dosage and Administration Method

As previously mentioned, the starting clinical dose is estimated and increased (usually by a factor of 2) or decreased (usually by a factor of ½) to make three different dose regimens for investigation. The method of administration will be chosen on the basis of results of clinical pharmacological and pharmacodynamic studies.

Since the plasma concentration of anti-ulcer drugs does not always correlate with efficacy, the daily fluctuation of pH in the stomach and the life pattern of the patients must be considered in determining the dosage and method of administration. Thus, in phase II studies, various methods need to be tried to find the most effective dosage and method of administration.

During the development of many anti-ulcer agents, it was found that a regimen of three times daily, which was formerly often used, was not necessarily the most effective method of administration. For some drugs, two times daily (in the morning and before bedtime) and once daily were similar to or more effective than three times a day. For example, in the early phase II study of a defensive-factor-enhancing agent A, three dose levels (400, 800, and 1600 mg) four times daily were to be used. However, the possibility of a twice daily regimen was also used in the study. The results are contained in Table 2, and overall safety in Table 3.

For this agent, twice daily was considered to be more appropriate for the phase III study. Since the healing rate of a defensive-factor-enhancing agent is not expected to

Table 2   Overall Reactions in the Early Phase II Study of Drug A

Adm. freq.	Daily dosage (mg)	Improvement			Unch.	Agg.	Total	Improvement rate (%)
		Marked	Moderate	Slight				
Four times a day	400	8	6	6	3	1	24	58.3
	800	10	9	3	3	1	26	73.1
	1600	13	10	1	1	1	26	88.5
Twice a day	800	14	13	1	1	0	29	93.1

Adm., administration; Unch., unchanged; Agg, aggravated.

Table 3 Overall Safety in the Early Phase II Study of Drug A

Adm. freq.	Daily dosage (mg)	No A.R.	Mild A.R.; adm. con.	Dosage reduced due to A.R.	Adm. disc.	Total
Four times a day	400	24	2	0	0	26
	800	28	0	0	1	29
	1600	27	1	0	0	28
Twice a day	800	31	1	0	0	32

A.R., adverse reaction(s); adm. con., administration could continue despite adverse reaction; adm. disc., administration discontinued.

be higher than that of a conventional anti-ulcer agent, it is reasonable to employ the more effective administration method if possible.

A similar tendency can also be observed for an aggressive factor depressant. For example, Asaki et al. [3,4] conducted a double-blind comparative study of 200 mg four times daily and 400 mg twice daily of cimetidine in the treatment of gastric ulcer. There was no significant difference in healing rate, improvement in subjective and objective symptoms, toxicity, or laboratory test values between 400 mg twice daily and 200 mg four times daily (see Fig. 1 and Table 4). Thus, it was concluded

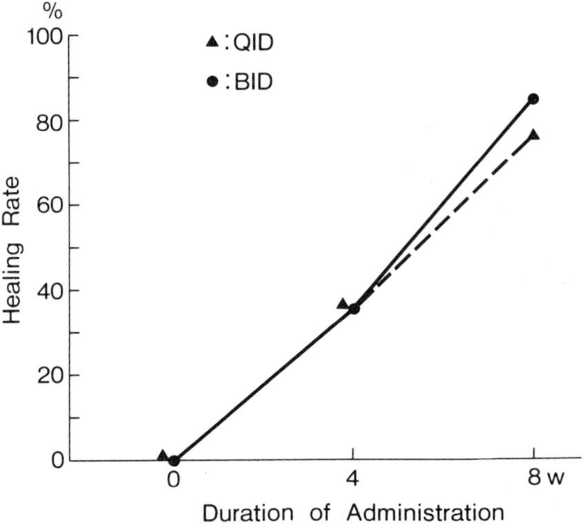

FIGURE 1 Changes in healing rate for gastric ulcer after the administration of cimetidine two (b.i.d.) and four (q.i.d.) times daily [3].

Table 4   Overall Safety of Cimetidine in the Treatment of Gastric Ulcer

Adm. freq.	No adverse reaction	Adverse reaction(s)			Total	Cannot assess	Tests
		Mild	Moderate	Severe			
Twice a day	65 (94.2)	3 (4.3)	1 (1.4)		69	1	N.S.
Four times a day	64 (92.8)	4 (5.8)		1 (1.4)	69		$(Z_0 = 0.343)$

Percent in parentheses. NS, not significant.
Source: Asaki et al. [3].

that a regimen of twice daily was easier for the patients to follow. Similar results were reported in the study of cimetidine in the treatment of duodenal ulcer (Fig. 2 and Table 5). Although these studies were conducted separately from the phase II dose-finding study, it is recommended to investigate the method of administration during phase II investigation.

More effective methods of administration have been investigated with various types of marketed drugs. At some time in the future, once-daily dosage is expected to be widely used.

Dosage and method of administration must be determined on the basis of results of pharmacology, pharmacokinetics, adverse reactions, and patient compliance. Al-

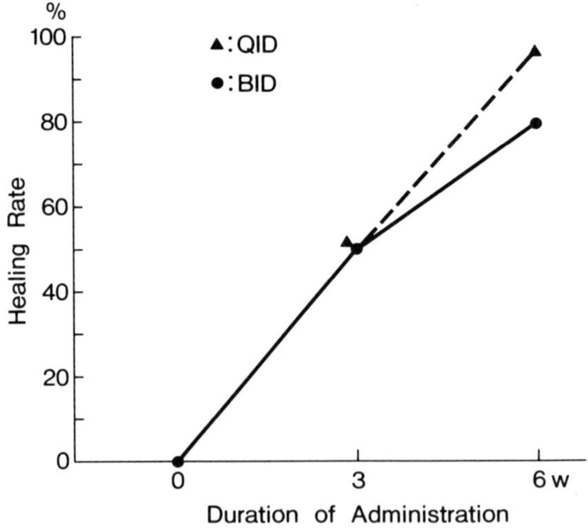

FIGURE 2   Changes in healing rate for duodenal ulcer after the administration of cimetidine two (b.i.d.) and four (q.i.d.) times daily [4].

Table 5   Overall Safety of Cimetidine in the Treatment of Duodenal Ulcer

Adm. freq.	No adverse reaction	Adverse reaction(s)			Total	Cannot assess	Tests
		Mild	Moderate	Severe			
Twice a day	50 (89.3)	5 (8.9)	1 (1.8)		56	1	N.S.
Four times a day	50 (92.6)	2 (3.7)	2 (3.7)		54		$(Z_0 = 0.552)$

Percent in parentheses. NS, not significant.
Source: Asaki et al. [4].

though adverse reactions can be estimated from the results of the preclinical investigations and phase I studies (including clinical pharmacology), patient compliance will be influenced by many factors. Thus, Figure 3 from the Japan Statistical Investigation K.K. is helpful.

B.   Patient Selection Criteria

Subjects with either gastric or duodenal ulcer will be included in this study. Subjects with serious concurrent diseases and pregnant or possibly pregnant women will be excluded from the study. In principle, subjects will be aged 15–79. Outpatients will be recruited primarily to the study of aggressive-factor depressants, and inpatients to the study of defensive-factor-enhancing agents. Washout of the premedication should be conducted as much as possible.

Experience has shown that 50–60 patients per dose group is satisfactory for aggressive-factor-inhibiting agents, while 100–120 per group are necessary for defensive-factor-enhancing agents.

In Japan, ulcers are classified into one of six stages: active stages A_1 and A_2, healing stages H_1 and H_2, and scarring stages S_1 and S_2, as defined below.

A_1.   A thick coating at the ulcer floor and marginal swelling are observed. No regenerative epithelium is seen. Hemorrhage and necrotic mass are sometimes observed.

A_2.   Marginal swelling is diminishing, and slight regenerative epithelium is appearing around ulcer margin. Mucosal rugae become visible and extend toward ulcer margin.

H_1.   White coating begins to thin. Regenerative epithelium protrudes into ulcer, but its area is not so wide as that of the white coating. Ulcer margin is distinctly outlined.

H_2.   Ulcer is almost covered with regenerative epithelium that is wider than white coating.

S_1.   Ulcer is covered by hyperemic epithelium and becomes reddish. This stage is called a *red scar*.

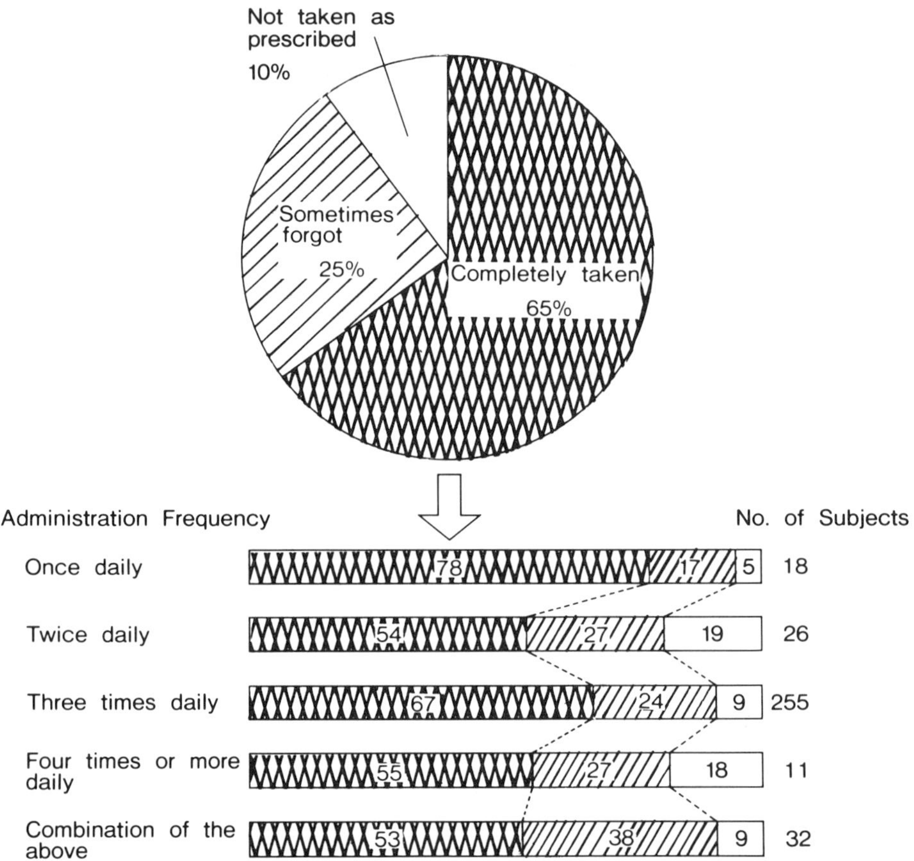

FIGURE 3 Patient compliance (342 people in Hanshin area were monitored). (Nihon Statistical Investigation K.K., 1983.)

S_2.   The covering epithelium turns normal, similar to the surrounding mucosa. This stage is called a *white scar*.

Ulcers at stage A_1 or A_2 will be investigated in the study of an aggressive-factor-depressant or a defensive-factor-enhancing agent, although the pharmacology of these agents is different.

Duration of administration and observation will be 8 weeks for gastric ulcer and 6 weeks for duodenal ulcer, in principle. In the case of a very potent anti-ulcer agent, it may be 6 weeks for gastric ulcer and 4 weeks for duodenal ulcer.

Regarding concurrent medication, in principle, anti-ulcer drugs other than the test article will be discouraged. However, as-needed use of them, if considered absolutely necessary, may be allowed for the treatment of severe subjective symptoms. Concurrent medication that cannot be discontinued for the treatment of other diseases will usually be continued, and stratified analysis will be performed.

C. Observations and Test Methods

The following observations and tests are made according to the schedule shown in Table 6.

1. Patient Background

Sex, age, body weight, date of patient's consent, diagnosis, in- or outpatient, ulcer site and description, present disease(s), premedication, concurrent disease(s), past history, hours of sleep, mealtimes, smoking habits, alcohol consumption, and so on will be recorded on the case card.

2. Subjective and Objective Findings

Examination will be made for the following at 1, 2, 4, and 8 weeks of treatment: pain, heartburn, eructation, nausea, vomiting, abdominal bloat, loss of appetite, diarrhea, constipation, epigastric tenderness, meteorism, clapotage, occult blood in stool, and body weight. The severity of the symptoms will be assessed according to four grades: severe $(+++)$, moderate $(++)$, mild $(+)$, and no symptom $(-)$.

Table 6 Examination Schedule for Gastric Ulcer

		Pretreatment	Week 1	2	4	8
1.	Patients background	x				
2.	Sub./obj. findings	x	x	x	x	x
3.	X-ray exam	x[a]				
4.	Endoscopy	x			x	x
5.	Gastric juice exam	x[a]				
6.	Clinical lab exam	x			x[b]	x
7.	Adverse reactions		x	x	x	x
8.	Patient compliance		x	x	x	x

In the case of duodenal ulcer, the above examinations will be conducted before treatment and at 1, 2, 3, and 6 weeks of treatment. For proton pump inhibitors, assessments will be conducted before treatment and at 2, 4, and 6 weeks of treatment for both gastric and duodenal ulcers.

Sub./obj., subjective/objective.

[a]If possible, conduct the examination.

[b]Ulcer was healed at 4 weeks after the treatment.

3. X-Ray Examination

If possible, x-ray examination will be conducted within 1 week before treatment begins, and the results [size, depth and location of ulcer(s), etc.] will be recorded on the case card. Although x-ray examination is not essential, it is considered to be one of the best methods for accurate measurement of ulcer size and depth.

4. Endoscopic Examination

Endoscopic examination will be conducted within 1 week before the treatment and at 4 and 8 weeks for gastric ulcer or 3 and 6 weeks for duodenal ulcer. The results will be recorded on the case card.

5. Measurement of Gastric Secretions

If possible, gastric secretions will be measured within 1 week before the treatment, and basal acid output (BAO) and maximal acid output (MAO) (tetragastrin 4 μg/kg) will be recorded on the case card. Gastric juice will be measured in accordance with the standard method recommended by the Japanese Society of Gastroenterology Committee for Secretory Function and Measurement of the Stomach.

6. Clinical Laboratory Tests and Vital Signs

A number of tests are conducted in the week prior to treatment and at the completion of the study. These include hematology (erythrocytes, hemoglobin, hematocrit, platelets, leukocytes, differentials), blood chemistry [serum cholesterol, total protein, A/G, GOT, GPT, ALP, TTT, r-GTP, LDH, total bilirubin (sometimes indirect bilirubin), uric acid, BUN, creatinine, Na, K, Cl], urinalysis (protein, glucose, urobilinogen, urinary sediment), and others (pulse, blood pressure, and if possible, ECG).

7. Adverse Reactions

When adverse reactions are observed, the symptoms, onset date, severity, course/ medical management, test article relatedness, etc., will be recorded on the case card.

8. Drug Compliance

The number of remaining test articles will be recorded on the case card by examining the compliance card kept by the subject.

D. Evaluation of Outcome

1. Subjective and Objective Findings

Improvement in symptoms and signs will be assessed according to five grades at 4 and 8 (or 3 and 6) weeks after the treatment:

1. Markedly improved
2. Moderately improved
3. Slightly improved

    4.   Unchanged
    5.   Aggravated
    6.   No symptom during the study

2. Endoscopic Findings and Healing Rate

Endoscopic findings will be assessed according to six grades at 4 and 8 (or 3 and 6) weeks after the treatment:

1. Healed (S_1 and S_2)
2. Markedly shrunk
3. Moderately shrunk
4. Slightly shrunk
5. Unchanged
6. Aggravated

The *healing rate,* defined as cumulative percent of patients with healed (S_1 and S_2) ulcers at specified times, is the most important measure of drug efficacy. Although S_1 is not totally healed, it is regarded as "healed" for purposes of drug evaluation because of the long time required for the ulcer scar to progress from S_1 to S_2.

3. Overall Improvement

Overall improvement will be assessed on the basis of changes in subjective and objective symptoms and endoscopic findings according to five grades at 4 and 8 (or 3 and 6) weeks after the treatment:

1. Markedly improved
2. Moderately improved
3. Slightly improved
4. Unchanged
5. Aggravated

4. Adverse Reactions

Adverse reactions will be assessed according to four grades:

1. No adverse reaction
2. Mild: administration continued without medical management of the adverse reaction
3. Moderate: administration continued with medical management of the adverse reaction
4. Severe: administration discontinued due to the adverse reaction

5. Usefulness

Usefulness of the test article will be assessed by taking into account the overall improvement and adverse reactions according to five grades:

1. Very useful
2. Useful
3. Slightly useful
4. Cannot specify
5. Not useful

6. Discontinuations

Patients who discontinue participation in the study are classified as follows:

1. Ulcer was healed.
2. Symptoms were aggravated, and the investigator in charge decided to discontinue administration of study drug.
3. Severe adverse reaction was observed, or patient requested the discontinuation of administration.

In such cases, the date of the discontinuation of administration, duration of administration, and reason for the discontinuation of administration will be recorded on the case card.

7. Dropouts and Withdrawals

Dropouts are patients who leave the study on their initiative for reasons other than those listed as discontinuations. Withdrawals are patients the investigator removes from the study for reasons other than those listed as discontinuations. The designation of these patients and the statistical handling of their data are determined by the key investigators, controllers, and the investigator in charge at the study site.

Since many ambiguities peculiar to ulcers exist in the present assessment methods, the following is expected to be conducted for evaluable patients:

1. Scoring the severity of subjective symptoms
2. Establishment of the standards of efficacy assessment

Item 1 is usually not controversial. Regarding item 2, the commonly used multiple standards of assessment (described previously) are often subjective and require clear definition and application by the clinical investigators.

V. PHASE III

A. Study Method

The appropriate dosage and method of administration as determined in the phase II study will be used in the phase III study. Because there are already drugs approved for the treatment of ulcers, ethical considerations require that the investigational drug be compared to a marketed drug as a control. It is recommended that the marketed drug have a mechanism of action similar to that of the test drug; however, it is not always possible to select an ideal control drug.

The objective of the phase III study is to compare the test article with the control in terms of efficacy and safety using a randomized double-blind clinical trial. Overall usefulness will be assessed based on the disappearance of subjective symptoms, ulcer healing, and incidence of adverse reactions.

The number of subjects depends on the efficacy of the test drugs, as evaluated by the results of the phase II study. Generally 50–100 patients per group will be recruited. A multicenter study is recommended, because enrollment of many participating institutions and investigators will reduce the bias in the assessment methods.

In general, the patient selection criteria, observations and test methods, and evaluation of outcome in the phase III study will be similar to those in the phase II study, as previously described.

B.   Determination of Evaluability (Data Fixing)

The evaluability of each patient will be determined by several key investigators at a joint meeting after completion of the clinical portion of the study. Inclusion of the subjects in the analysis will be determined by evaluating examination date lag, concurrent medication, patient compliance, concurrent diseases, adverse reactions, and so on. However, the method of fixing data varies slightly depending on the type of investigational drug and the method followed of the study.

In principle, a lag of an endoscopic examination up to 1 week is allowed. Although the use of concurrent medication is sometimes allowed for a few days, generally it is prohibited. Subjects with drug compliance lower than 75% will be excluded from the study. Subjects with concurrent diseases that affect ulcer healing will be excluded from the study or included in the stratified analysis.

After evaluability and outcome data are approved, the data are considered "fixed" or frozen and are not subject to revision. Then the treatment code is broken and the results are compiled for each treatment.

C.   Assessment of Outcome

The method of assessment in the phase II study will also be used in the phase III study. The most important factor is the healing rate at each endoscopic examination. In the clinical study of anti-ulcer drugs, ulcers at a stage of S_1 or S_2 are regarded as "healed," and the healing rate will be calculated.

It is expected that successful and desirable anti-ulcer drugs should meet two basic outcome criteria. First, the "healing rate" for gastric ulcer should be at least 60% and 70% at 8 weeks after the treatment with defensive-factor-enhancing and aggressive-factor-depressing agents, respectively. The "healing rate" for duodenal ulcer at 6 weeks after the treatment must be similar to that for gastric ulcer at 8 weeks after the treatment. Second, only mild adverse reactions are accepted, and the incidence must be lower than a certain percentage (usually less than 10%).

In Japan, there are many drugs that are considered to enhance protective factors, such as aldioxa, β-cyclodextrin, cetraxate, gefarnate, ornoprostil, plaunotol, proglumide, sofalcone, spizofurone, sucralfate, teprenone, and troxipide. These drugs have been investigated because it is thought that most ulcers are caused by reduction of protective factors. The efficacy of protective-factor-enhancing drugs is evaluated by comparison with a drug of similar pharmacological action that has clinically established effects and safety. This group of drugs does not produce as high an ulcer healing rate after 4 or 8 weeks as does treatment with antisecretory drugs. However, mucosal protectants can accelerate ulcer healing and inhibit relapse to some extent when used in combination therapy with antisecretory drugs.

VI. PHASE IV (POSTMARKETING SURVEILLANCE)

A. Efficacy and Adverse Reactions

The presence or absence of the efficacy established in the clinical study and reports of adverse reactions will be investigated by conducting postmarketing surveillance (PMS). Generally, the incidence of adverse reactions in the PMS tends to be lower than that in clinical investigations prior to marketing. However, surveying a large patient population provides an important opportunity to detect rate side effects of new drugs.

B. Expansion of Use

New methods of administration and new indications will also be investigated in specific clinical trials during the phase IV period. It is also important to investigate the effects of drugs used in combination for added benefit and also for drug–drug interactions.

Currently the dosage and administration methods for marketed anti-ulcer drugs to prevent ulcer recurrence are under clinical investigation. However, this work should be supported by much-needed preclinical investigations into the process of ulcer healing and recurrence, to provide a more fundamental understanding of ulcer recurrence and to better guide clinical investigations.

REFERENCES

1. Miyoshi A, Okabe H, eds. Problems in the healing assessment of peptic ulcers. Tokyo: Toyo Shoten, 1983.
2. Okabe S. Experimental ulcers and anti-ulcer agents. Drug activity symposium. Pharmaceutical Society of Japan and the Japanese Pharmacological Society. Kumamoto, Japan, 1979.
3. Asaki S, Goto Y, Tanaka T, Sakurada H, Miura K, Mochizuki F. Usefulness of cimetidine b.i.d. in the treatment of gastric ulcer; a double-blind comparison with cimetidine q.i.d. Med Consult New Rem 1982; 19(11):3026.
4. Asaki S, Goto Y, Tanaka T, Sakurada H, Miura K, Mochizuki F. Usefulness of cimetidine b.i.d. in the treatment of duodenal ulcer; a double-blind comparison with cimetidine q.i.d. Med Consult New Rem 1982; 19(11):3038.
5. Sakita T, Oguro Y, Takasu S, Ohmori K, Fukutomi H, Miwa T. Training in endoscopic examination of the alimentary tract. Tokyo: Chugai Igakusha, 1980.

24

Cost-Effectiveness in Treatment of Peptic Ulcer Disease

HARVEY E. ZIMMERMAN

Spectrum Research Services, Inc.,
Warwick, Rhode Island

KARL E. PEACE

Biopharmaceutical Research Consultants, Inc.,
Ann Arbor, Michigan

I. INTRODUCTION

It is estimated that roughly 10% of the population can expect to develop peptic ulcer disease during their lifetime. Data from the National Health Interview Survey indicate that the 1-year period prevalence of self-reported ulcer in the United States was between 1.7 and 1.9% between 1961 and 1981 [1]. Additional data through 1985 indicate that this prevalence rate has remained constant [2]. Thus about 4 million Americans suffer from peptic ulcers each year.

There are about four times as many duodenal ulcers as gastric ulcers. The incidence of duodenal ulcer increases continuously with age, whereas gastric ulcer occurs predominantly in people over 40 years of age [1]. Data from the 1960s showed that the male/female ratio for 1-year period prevalence was 2 : 1. Since the late 1970s the reported ratio has been about 1 : 1 [2].

Although self-reported prevalence rates for peptic ulcer disease has been relatively constant, the mortality rates and hospitalization rates for ulcer disease in the United States have been decreasing since the early 1960s. This may be due to improvements in therapy, changes in hospitalization criteria, changes in diagnostic practices, or coding changes [2].

This chapter reviews some basic principles of ulcer occurrence, recurrence, and treatment. Based on these principles, the cost-effective aspects of treatment of peptic ulcers over the period 1975–1989 are considered. Two major changes in treatment are considered in detail: First, the introduction of cimetidine was followed by significant reductions in ulcer surgery, and second, the acceptance of maintenance therapy, especially with newer agents, has reduced rates of symptomatic recurrences. Both of these changes improve the cost-effectiveness of treatment of peptic ulcer. Developments in the treatment of ulcer complications including endoscopic therapy for bleeding ulcers and nonoperative treatment of perforated ulcers are also considered, and the need for further analysis of the cost-effectiveness of these interventions is noted.

II. GENERAL PRINCIPLES

The etiology and pathogenesis of peptic ulcer disease are complex issues, and many of their aspects are still unknown. It is generally agreed that peptic ulcers occur as a result of an excess of "aggressive factors," notably gastric acid and pepsin, or a decrease in mucosal defense factors, or a combination of the two.

The validity of the dictum "no acid no ulcer" remains, and peptic ulcers occur only in areas of the gastrointestinal tract that are exposed to gastric acid. There is considerable overlap between ulcer patients and normal subjects in quantity of acid secretion, and ulcers frequently occur in the presence of normal acid secretion or hyposecretion.

The mechanisms responsible for mucosal defense have been the subject of intensive research. A number of defense factors have been identified, including mucosal secretion of mucus and bicarbonate, levels of mucosal endogenous prostaglandins, the status of mucosal blood flow, and the rate of mucosal cell renewal.

Both genetic and environmental factors play a role in the etiology of peptic ulcer disease through their influence on gastric acid secretion and mucosal defense. Prominent among environmental influences are smoking and ulcerogenic drugs, chiefly because of their adverse effects on mucosal defense. The potential role of *Helicobacter pylori* on the etiology and pathogenesis of peptic ulcer disease remains unsettled.

Ulcer therapy has traditionally been directed against gastric acid by neutralization or, more recently, suppression of its secretion. Increasingly more emphasis is being directed at the development of agents that enhance mucosal defense mechanisms.

Currently approved therapeutic modalities include intensive antacid regimens: sucralfate; misoprostol, the synthetic prostaglandin PGE_1 analogue; and the histamine H_2-receptor antagonists, four of which—cimetidine, ranitidine, famotidine, and nizatidine—have been approved for marketing by the regulatory authorities of various countries around the world. Other agents have demonstrated efficacy in ulcer healing. The substituted benzimidazoles, of which omeprazole is the prototype, are potent inhibitors of gastric acid secretion by virtue of their blocking action on the H^+/K^+-ATPase proton pump of the gastric parietal cell [3]. Other prostaglandin analogues have also been reported as effective in the healing of peptic ulcers. Of these, arbaprostil and enprostil have undergone the most extensive basic research and clinical studies [4]. Bismuth compounds have been shown to be effective, especially in ulcer and gastritis associated with *H. pylori* [5].

The goals of ulcer therapy are relief of symptoms, demonstration of healing, prevention of recurrence, prevention of complications, and minimization of side effects [6].

Guidelines for the management of duodenal ulcer may be modeled after suggestions given in the American Medical Association's *Drug Evaluations* [7]. These include:

1. Stop smoking and the use of ulcerogenic drugs.
2. Prescribe acute drug therapy for 4–6 weeks.
3. Since patients become asymptomatic long before healing occurs, discontinue drug therapy after 6 weeks only if symptoms have subsided.
4. Further therapy depends on whether the ulcer is asymptomatic, heals, or recurs. Maintenance therapy is usually not prescribed after an initial ulcer episode, but only in the event of at least one recurrence. If an acute ulcer recurs, a full course of therapy should be prescribed followed by maintenance therapy. In the event of therapeutic failure, evaluate patient compliance, adequacy of dosage, and the possibility of an erroneous diagnosis.
5. Bleeding due to ulcer stops spontaneously in about 90% of patients. Surgery may be required for intractable bleeding; however, interventional endoscopy is often able to avoid the need for surgery.
6. Diet and anticholinergics have little place in the therapy of peptic ulcer.

III. COMPARISON OF HOSPITALIZATION BEFORE AND AFTER THE INTRODUCTION OF CIMETIDINE

Before the introduction of cimetidine, the first approved H_2-receptor antagonist, the mainstays of treatment of peptic ulcer disease were antacids and ulcer surgery. Cimetidine was demonstrated to be safe and effective and was thought to increase patient compliance with doctor's dosage instructions. This treatment was more expensive than antacid therapy but much less expensive than ulcer surgery. The question of interest at that time was whether there were savings from reduced hospitalization or whether cimetidine costs were simply increasing the cost of ulcer medicines.

A number of studies undertaken soon after the introduction of cimetidine addressed this question. One such study is discussed here, and other corroborating studies are also noted.

From 1972 to 1980 all community short-term general hospitals in Rhode Island used the Professional Activity Study (PAS) of the Commission on Professional and Hospital Activities (CPHA). Copies of these data were maintained in a computerized database at Rhode Island Health Services Research, Inc. These medical records data include the patient's age, sex, census tract of residence, date of admission, date of discharge, primary and additional diagnoses, and major and minor surgical procedures.

These data were used to analyze the hospitalization of Rhode Islanders who had a principal diagnosis of a disease of the esophagus, stomach, or duodenum. Patients who had a diagnosis of cancer in any of the additional diagnosis fields of the medical abstract were identified and separated out. The exclusion of the cancers allowed concentration on the noncancerous peptic conditions, which were primarily ulcers and ulcer-related conditions.

The incidence of ulcer surgery was also investigated. The analysis of surgery stratified partial gastrectomy and vagotomy into groups based on the presence or absence of a diagnosis of cancer in any of the first three diagnosis fields. The stratification of these procedures into two groups is made because some of these surgeries (mainly partial gastrectomy) are used for cancer as well as for a variety of ulcers and ulcer-related conditions, such as duodenal, gastric, and gastrojejunal ulcers, duodenitis, gastritis, and reflux esophagitis.

Cimetidine was approved for sale in the United States in August 1977, and marketing began in September. Hence, data are grouped by years ending August 31. Hospitalization incidence was calculated for each year. If there was any significant trend prior to the introduction of cimetidine, the expected value from regression was compared to the observed post-cimetidine value, and a two-tailed t-test was used to measure significance. If no trend existed in the pre-cimetidine periods, a critical ratio was used.

From 1973 through 1980, Table 1 reports no significant changes in the incidence of hospitalizations for diseases of the esophagus, stomach, and duodenum. Table 2 shows that there were no significant changes in partial gastrectomy or vagotomy for cases with a diagnosis of cancer in the first three diagnosis fields. The stability of the

Table 1   Hospital Discharges and Discharge Rates for Disease of Esophagus, Stomach, and Duodenum—Rhode Island, 1973–1980

Year ending August 31	Number of hospitalizations	Discharge rate per 10,000 population[a]
1973	1999	21.1
1974	2215	23.2
1975	2271	25.0
1976	2035	22.3
1977	2019	22.0
1978	2006	22.0
1979	2039	22.4
1980	1965	21.5

[a]Rhode Island resident population.

Table 2 Hospital Discharges and Discharge Rates for Partial Gastrectomy and/or
Vagotomy—Rhode Island, 1973–1980

Year ending August 31	Partial gastrectomy and/or vagotomy without diagnosis of cancer		Partial gastrectomy and/or vagotomy with diagnosis of cancer	
	Number of hospitalizations	Discharge rate per 10,000 population	Number of hospitalizations	Discharge rate per 10,000 population
1973	412	9.4	47	0.5
1974	414	4.5	65	0.7
1975	373	4.1	67	0.7
1976	331	3.6	64	0.7
1977	324	3.6	69	0.8
1978	211	2.3	66	0.7
1979	192	2.1	63	0.7
1980	157	1.7	60	0.7

[a]Rhode Island resident population.

use of surgery here suggests no change in prevalence and choice of treatment by partial
gastrectomy for stomach cancer.

From 1973 through 1977, the use of partial gastrectomy and/or vagotomy to treat
ulcers and ulcer-related conditions declined ($p < .05$). Because a downward trend
exists in the pre-cimetidine periods, the expected post-cimetidine utilization for
1978, 1979, and 1980 was estimated using both linear and log-linear regression
equations, and actual utilization was compared with expected utilization. Actual
utilization was lower than predicted. Two-tailed t-tests indicate a significant decline
in the post-test periods using linear ($p < .05$) and log-linear ($p < .05$) regression
models. Figure 1 shows the data graphically.

The reduction in ulcer surgery following the introduction of cimetidine was
immediate, sustained, and statistically significant. However, caution is advisable in
attributing causality. Other factors that may have contributed to the accelerated
decline in ulcer surgery were investigated. First, a change in medical or surgical
personnel characteristics could affect the treatment choice. But there was no unusual
increase or decrease in the numbers of surgeons, internists, or gastroenterologists in
the state at the time cimetidine was introduced. Various types of ulcer surgery were
analyzed to see if there was any unusual shift from one type of ulcer surgery to
another—such as a move away from partial gastrectomy to selective or parietal cell
vagotomy—that might reflect a change in preference for certain procedures. No such
changes were found. Finally, a change in the prevalence of ulcer disease would be

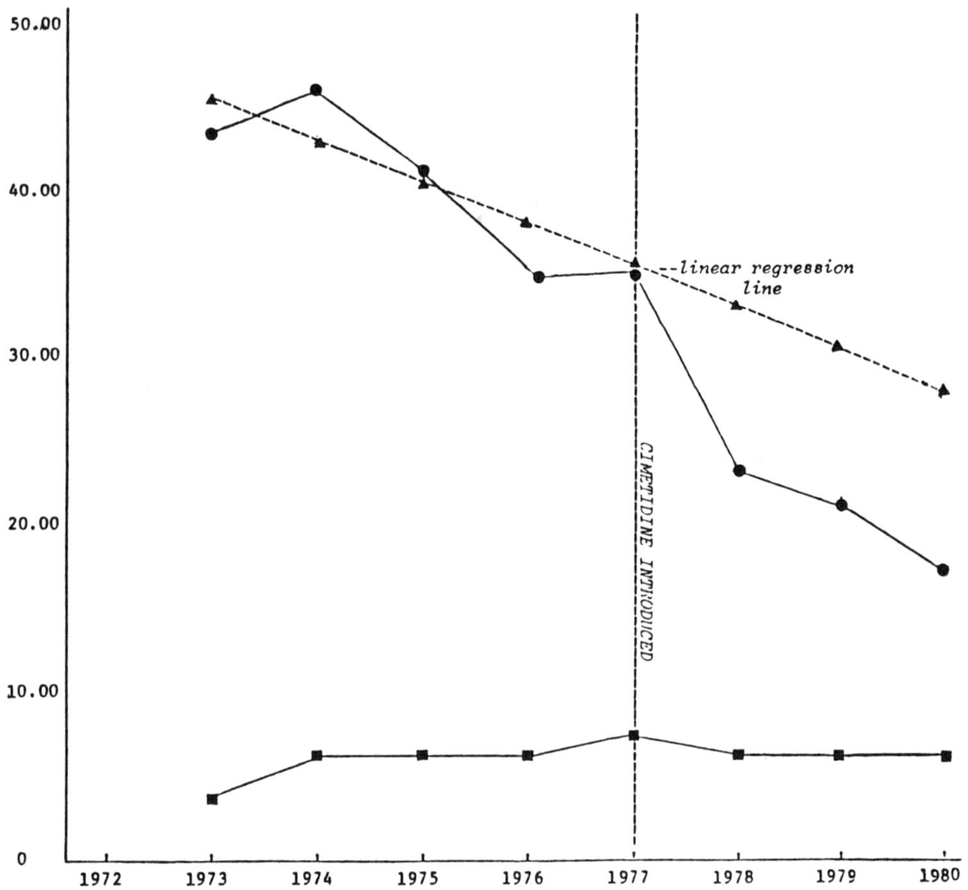

FIGURE 1 Rates of partial gastrectomy and/or vagotomy for Rhode Island residents per 100,000 for the period, August 31, 1973–1980. (●) Ulcer surgery; (▲) linear regression; (■) neoplasm. Reproduced from Paterson [10].

expected to affect the amount of ulcer surgery. Household interview surveys of the noninstitutionalized population of Rhode Island were done in 1975 and 1980 for the Rhode Island Department of Health. The 3-month period prevalence of ulcer disease in Rhode Island in 1975 was estimated to be 19.5 per 1000 population. This is similar to the 1-year period prevalence of 18.9 per 1000 population found in the 1975 National Health Interview Survey. The survey in 1980 found an estimated 3-month period prevalence of 25.5 per 1000 population. For the 1980 survey, respondents reporting that a household member had suffered from ulcer were asked for permission to recontact. Of these, 97% agreed to be recontacted. Of those who were reported to have ulcers, 18% were dropped on the basis of an ulcer-disease-specific questionnaire used on recontact. Of the remainder, 95% had physician-confirmed ulcers, and 91% reported confirmation with a gastrointestinal series or endoscopy. Allowing for overreporting, the self-reported prevalence of ulcer disease in Rhode Island still was higher, but the increase was not statistically significant.

Another means of investigating the face validity of the Rhode Island results is to compare this to utilization statistics in other areas. A similar study using data for the United States as a whole for partial gastrectomy and vagotomy surgeries found decreases in surgeries following the introduction of cimetidine [8]. Using data for 1966–1979 from the National Hospital Discharge survey, Fineberg and Pearlman [8] report that after the introduction of cimetidine, the numbers of partial gastrectomies and vagotomies were significantly below the long-term downward trend. They also found that the number of ulcer operations as a proportion of hospital admissions with ulcer disease declined from the range of 25–29% for 1966–1977 to 19% in 1978. The reduction in ulcer surgeries was estimated to be in the range between 21,000 and 31,000. These results were confirmed by Wylie [9], who also found reductions in hospital admissions and hospital days in the United States after the introduction of cimetidine. Other studies in the United States, England and Wales, France, and the Netherlands found similar results [10].

IV. COSTS OF ULCER SURGERY

All of the available evidence is consistent with the hypothesis that the use of cimetidine contributed to a decrease in ulcer surgeries. However, the evidence is mixed on whether there is also a decrease in hospital admissions for peptic ulcer disease. Thus, in calculating the reduction in surgical costs for treatment of ulcer disease following the introduction of cimetidine, separate estimates are made showing reduced and constant hospital admissions.

Data from Blue Cross and Blue Shield of Rhode Island for surgical and nonsurgical hospital stays and associated surgical fees for 1976 were adjusted for inflation between 1976 and 1978 and used as a basis for estimating charges. These data are reported in Table 3. The lower hospital charges for patients admitted without surgery reflect both the shorter average lengths of stay, which reduce routine costs, and the lesser ancillary costs due to not using the operating/recovery room services and so forth. Surgical charges include both surgeon and anesthesiologist fees. Overall a surgical case generates more than double the charges of a nonsurgical case. The savings that result from avoiding surgery on an ulcer patient who is admitted to the hospital is $2799. If the hospital admission can be avoided, the savings is $4875 in 1978 dollars for Rhode Island.

Per capita expenditures for hospital services in Rhode Island were 19% higher than national expenditures, and per capita expenditures for physician services were 20%

Table 3 Charges for Ulcer Surgery for Rhode Island Blue Cross/Blue Shield Patients, 1978 Dollars

Type of procedure	Hospital charges ($)		Surgical charges ($)	Total charges ($)
	Routine	Ancillary		
Partial gastrectomy	2228	1906	824	4958
Vagotomy	2289	1519	630	4438
Weighted average, vagotomy or partial gastrectomy	2238	1844	793	4875
Ulcer and ulcer-related without ulcer surgery	1492	584	—	2076
Savings from avoiding surgery during hospital stay	746	1260	793	2799

less [11]. Adjusting for these partially offsetting differences yields a projected national savings of $2680 per case for patients who are admitted to the hospital but not operated on and $4428 per case for patients who avoid a hospital admission at average U.S. expenditure levels.

The actual rate of ulcer surgery reported in Table 2 (and graphed in Figure 1) is 1 case per 10,000 population annually (or 10 cases per 100,000 population annually) less than was expected based on the trend from 1973 through 1977. Projected to a national population of 215 million, this results in an estimated 21,500 avoided ulcer surgeries. If hospitalization were avoided for all cases, the resultant savings would be $95,202,000. If patients were hospitalized but surgery were avoided, the savings would be $57,620,000. These are the upper and lower bounds of the estimated savings for the United States in 1978 dollars.

Ranitidine, famotidine, and nizatidine have action and safety profiles similar to those of cimetidine. Presumably, these agents, like cimetidine, would result in reductions in surgical costs. A choice among these agents depends on individual factors, including potential drug interactions and safety profiles, which may vary from patient to patient, as well as the costs of the medicines [12].

V. COMPARISON OF EFFECTIVENESS AND RELAPSE FREQUENCY BETWEEN MISOPROSTOL AND CIMETIDINE

Although the pharmacological agents have been reported to be effective in the treatment of peptic ulcer disease, none has had a significant beneficial influence on the natural course of the disease, which is characterized by frequent recurrences. "Once an ulcer, always an ulcer" appears to be a well-established dictum. For this reason, long-term maintenance therapy is frequently necessary.

Table 4 Proportion of Patients Healed at 4 Weeks

Treatment regimen[a]	Percent healed
Placebo	45.9
Misoprostol, 200 μg	65.4
Cimetidine, 300 mg	66.9

[a]All administered four times daily.

The usual ulcer therapy regimen consists of a full course of treatment for 4–8 weeks. Since some patients may experience only a single ulcer episode, maintenance therapy is usually not initiated after the first acute episode. If, as is usually the case, there are acute recurrences after the initial attack, maintenance therapy is usually initiated, generally in the form of a smaller daily dose administered at bedtime. Less often, full courses of short-term therapy are used for each exacerbation without intervening maintenance therapy. Most experts consider "demand" therapy, administered because of the presence of ulcer symptoms, as unacceptable.

Numerous studies have demonstrated that both misoprostol and cimetidine are significantly superior to placebo or no therapy in the healing of an acute peptic ulcer.

Table 4 reports the comparative duodenal ulcer healing rates for cimetidine, misoprostol, and placebo [13]. There is no statistical difference between the healing rates with misoprostol 200 μg four times daily or cimetidine 300 mg four times daily. Both are statistically superior to placebo.

Table 5 compares the relapse rates following acute ulcer therapy with the two therapeutic regimens and placebo and without the use of maintenance prophylactic treatment. The 6-months relapse incidence includes those patients who developed symptomatic (proven) recurrences (proved by endoscopy) during the 6-month period plus those asymptomatic recurrences demonstrated endoscopically at the end of the 6 months. These relapse statistics can be represented by a simple exponential decay

Table 5 Relapse Rates from Different Treatment Regimens

Acute treatment[a] regimen	% Relapse at 6 months	Median days to relapse	Implied relapse per month (%)
Placebo	31	247	8.2
Misoprostol, 200 μg	42	214	9.3
Cimetidine, 300 mg	46	188	10.5

[a]All administered four times daily.

Table 6 Percent of Patients Under Treatment by Alternative Therapies

Month	Placebo	Misoprostol, 200 µg	Cimetidine, 300 mg
0	100.00	100.00	100.00
1	54.10	34.60	33.10
2	33.03	18.05	17.98
3	23.36	13.87	14.56
4	18.92	12.81	13.79
5	16.89	12.54	13.61
6	15.96	12.47	13.57
7	15.52	12.45	13.57
8	15.33	12.45	13.57
9	15.23	12.45	13.57
10	15.19	12.45	13.57
11	15.17	12.45	13.57
12	15.17	12.45	13.57

[a]All administered four times daily.

Table 7 Percent of Patients Under Treatment Due to Relapse

Month	Placebo	Misoprostol, 200 µg	Cimetidine, 300 mg
1	—	—	—
2	3.76%	6.08%	7.02%
3	5.49	7.62	8.61
4	6.28	8.01	8.97
5	6.65	8.11	9.05
6	6.82	8.13	9.07
7	6.89	8.14	9.08
8	6.93	8.14	9.08
9	6.94	8.14	9.08
10	6.95	8.14	9.08
11	6.95	8.14	9.08
12	6.96	8.14	9.08

[a]All administered four times daily.

function with a constant percent relapse per month [14]. This derived monthly relapse rate is also depicted in Table 5.

From a 4-week healing rate and the monthly relapse rate, we can deduce the effects of each therapeutic regimen on an active ulcer population. Table 6 demonstrates the percent of patients per month who would be on drug therapy on average if we began a group of patients on each different therapy.

It may seem that the combinations of the healing rates and the relapse rates produce convergent series. The patients under treatment include two groups—those who have continued therapy because their ulcers did not heal and those who had relapses. Table 7 reports the patients under treatment due to relapse.

At first glance, Table 7 may seem to suggest that placebo patients are less likely to relapse. However, as shown in Table 6, more patients are under treatment with placebo than with either active therapy. The small numbers here reflect the fact that placebo-treated patients would have unhealed ulcers rather than recurring ulcers.

Further analysis of relapse rates considered the relationship between relapse rates and days to heal, ulcer history, smoking status, ulcer size, and gender. Of these variables, only history of previous ulcer was correlated with relapse rates [13]. Table 8 reports the rate of healing at 4 weeks for patients with a history of previous ulcers and for those without an ulcer history.

Table 9 depicts the relapse rates with and without a history of previous ulcers. Median days to relapse by treatment regimen are reported, as well as the implied rate of relapse per month.

These reported rates of healing and rates of relapse indicate that patients with a history of previous ulcers respond similarly to all treatment regimens. Patients without a history of previous ulcers show greater variance of healing, especially in rates of relapse.

In the remainder of this discussion we will consider all patients and patients

Table 8 Proportion of Patients Healed at 4 Weeks
With and Without a History of Previous Ulcer

	Percent healed	
Treatment[a]	Without previous ulcers	With previous ulcers
Placebo	55.1	39.7
Misoprostol, 200 μg	67.2	65.0
Cimetidine, 300 mg	73.0	63.4

[a]All administered four times daily.

Table 9 Relapse Rates from Different Treatment Regimens

	Without previous ulcers		With previous ulcers	
Treatment[a]	Median days to relapse	Implied relapse per month (%)	Median days to relapse	Implied relapse per month (%)
Placebo	288	7.0	198	10.2
Misoprostol, 200 μg	365	5.6	193	10.4
Cimetidine, 300 mg	169	11.7	191	10.5

[a]All administered four times daily.

Table 10 Percent of Patients Without Previous Ulcers Under Treatment by Alternative Therapies

		Treatment[a]	
Month	Placebo	Misoprostol, 200 μg	Cimetidine, 300 mg
0	100.00	100.00	100.00
1	44.90	32.80	27.00
2	24.02	14.52	15.83
3	16.10	9.55	14.12
4	13.10	8.20	13.86
5	11.96	7.83	13.82
6	11.53	7.73	13.81
7	11.37	7.71	13.81
8	11.31	7.70	13.81
9	11.29	7.70	13.81
10	11.28	7.70	13.81
11	11.27	7.70	13.81
12	11.27	7.70	13.81

[a]All administered four times daily.

Table 11 Comparative Costs of Misoprostol and Cimetidine

Country	Misoprostol, 200 μg	Cimetidine, 300 mg	Ratio
Canada	0.42 ($C)	0.57 ($C)	0.74
West Germany	0.56 (DM)	2.49 (DM)	0.63
Australia	0.38 ($A)	0.55 ($A)	0.69
Average			0.69

without a history of previous ulcers. Table 10 reports the percent of patients without a history of ulcers who are expected to be under treatment by alternative therapies.

VI. TREATMENT COSTS

Treatment patterns having been determined, it is now possible to estimate the costs involved for the regimens studied.

A standard treatment protocol is followed. Initial therapy is assumed to consist of a physician visit, an upper gastrointestinal endoscopy, and a prescription for an appropriate drug. The physician costs are based on Medicare rates prevailing in 1986 [15]. There is wide variability in charges for endoscopy. We use a charge of $400, which is in the range of costs allowed by private health insurance companies. Drug costs are based on prices reported in the *American Druggist Blue Book,* 1986–1987 edition, for cimetidine [16]. The retail markup is based on Pharmaceutical Manufacturers Association estimates [17]. Table 11 reports comparable costs for misoprostol and cimetidine in countries in which both drugs are sold. On average, the cost of misoprostol is 69% of that for cimetidine. In this analysis, placebos are free. Antacid use is assumed to be the same for each treatment and is not included here. At the end of the short-term treatment, the patient again sees a physician and either continues medication if not healed or discontinues medication if symptoms subside. Patients who relapse return to the physician for another full course of treatment.

At these rates, a full course of treatment for 1 month with added 2-week drug taper-off would cost $46.37 for physician services, $400 for endoscopy, and $86.10 for cimetidine at 1.2 g/day. The cost of the 200-μg regimen of misoprostol is estimated to be $59.41. As a first approximation, we will ignore cases in which more than one flare-up per year occurs, which would not have the endoscopy repeated. Table 12 reports the annual costs per 100 cohorts for all therapy and for relapse therapy both for the first year and for succeeding years.

Table 12 Costs ($) of Ulcer Therapy Under Alternative Regimens Considering Incidence and Relapse

	All therapy		Relapse therapy	
Treatment[a]	1st year	Later year	1st year	Later year
All patients				
Misoprostol, 200 μg	94,538	51,863	43,960	49,405
Cimetidine, 300 mg	106,115	61,729	46,921	58,018
Without previous ulcer				
Misoprostol, 200 μg	81,783	32,987	27,788	31,561
Cimetidine, 300 mg	116,304	67,491	58,082	64,408

[a]All administered four times daily.

Table 12 shows that per 100 patients initially diagnosed with duodenal ulcer and followed over time, cimetidine is the most expensive treatment. The cost per patient can be determined by moving the decimal point two places to the left.

VII. SIDE EFFECTS

Both misoprostol and cimetidine are considered to be safe medications. In a small percentage of cases cimetidine has been shown to cause a number of reversible adverse effects including granulocytopenia, gynecomastia, mental confusion, and adverse drug–drug interactions [6].

Adverse effects of short-term therapy serious enough to cause withdrawal of the drug have been reported in 1.5% of cimetidine patients (versus 1.2% of placebo patients), and untoward symptoms have been reported for 17% (versus 19% for placebo patients). Intermediate-term therapy (3–12 months) resulted in drug withdrawal due to side effects in 2.1% of cimetidine patients and 1.7% of placebo patients. Less serious side effects were reported for 22% of cimetidine patients and 15% of placebo patients in the intermediate term [18]. Most frequent side effects not causing withdrawal include diarrhea (1.8%), tiredness (1.7%), dizziness (1.3%), drowsiness (1.3%), and rash (1.2%). Even though these side effects are reported to be reversible upon dosage reduction or withdrawal, they would result in additional costs. A reaction severe enough to warrant withdrawal of medicine can be expected to result in a physician visit for examination and another follow-up visit to assess the return to normalcy. For mild to moderate symptoms, titration of drug dosages may be done by telephone with few, if any, additional office visits.

Diarrhea appears to be the most frequent adverse effect of misoprostol. Loose stools were reported in 8% of the patients receiving misoprostol, but only 0.4% had diarrhea serious enough to cause withdrawals from clinical trials [4].

Added treatment costs can be estimated on the basis of reported incidence of side effects serious enough to cause withdrawal. For cimetidine the expected withdrawals are 1.5% for short-term treatment and 2.1% for longer-term therapy. For misoprostol, 0.4% are expected to be withdrawn. Applying these rates to the patients under treatment reported in Table 6 would produce an estimated cost induced by side effects. The resultant frequency of side effects for the first and subsequent years as well as the corresponding costs are reported in Table 13.

VIII. WORK LOSS

It is estimated that 10% of the population can expect to develop a peptic ulcer during their lifetime. The 1-year period prevalence of self-reported peptic ulcer in the United States was 1.7–1.9% over the period 1961–1985. As noted previously, about 4 million Americans suffer active peptic ulcers in one year. In 1979, 21% of people with ulcers reported one or more "bed" days [19]. The next question is how long they could be expected to remain away from work. It is expected that most ulcers are

Table 13 Frequency and Treatment Costs of Serious Side Effects

	1st year		Later year	
Treatment[a]	Frequency	Cost/100 ($)	Frequency	Cost/100 ($)
All patients				
Misoprostol, 200 μg	1.06	41.34	0.60	23.40
Cimetidine, 300 mg	4.63	180.55	2.77	180.03
Without previous ulcer				
Misoprostol, 200 μg	0.88	34.32	0.37	14.43
Cimetidine, 300 mg	4.65	181.35	2.75	107.25

[a]All administered four times daily.

Table 14 Expected Days of Work Loss and Wages Lost Due to Duodenal Ulcer

	Work loss (days)		Wages lost ($)	
Treatment[a]	1st year	Later year	1st year	Later year
All patients				
Misoprostol, 200 μg	3.44	1.93	267.77	150.23
Cimetidine, 300 mg	3.54	2.10	275.55	163.46
Without previous ulcer				
Misoprostol, 200 μg	2.83	1.19	220.29	98.63
Cimetidine, 300 mg	3.45	2.14	268.55	166.58

[a]All administered four times daily.

reduced 50% in size in 14 days of medical management [20]. Thus, we use 10 days as an approximation for time lost from work per flare-up. Labor force participation of people above 17 years of age in the Health Interview Survey was 61.4%. Thus, the probability of having bed days × labor force participation × 10 days work loss per episode produces an estimated 1.29 days work loss per acute episode. This is reported in Table 14.

IX. COST SUMMARY

From the above analysis, we now summarize the costs of treating cohorts of duodenal ulcer patients by different strategies.

Table 15   Five-Year Costs of Duodenal Ulcer Treatment Under Alternative Regimens

| | Costs ($) | | | | Percent of cimetidine costs |
Treatment[a]	Therapy	Side effects	Work loss	Total	
All patients					
Misoprostol, 200 μg	3019.90	1.35	868.69	3889.94	70
Cimetidine, 300 mg	3530.31	6.13	929.39	4465.83	100
Without previous ulcer					
Misoprostol, 200 μg	2137.31	0.92	590.81	2729.04	57
Cimetidine, 300 mg	3862.68	6.10	934.87	4803.65	100

[a]All administered four times daily.

The costs reported in Table 15 are a simple 5-year sum undiscounted. The small costs associated with side effects point out the safety of both treatments.

Although misoprostol results in less total costs than cimetidine for all patients, it is for the subgroup of patients without a history of ulcer that this is the most dramatic. In the case of the 200 μg four times daily regimen of misoprostol, the treatment costs equal 55% of the treatment costs for cimetidine, and total costs equal 57% of total direct and indirect ulcer costs under treatment by cimetidine. In this particular instance, treatment with the less-expensive drug is clearly the most rational.

X.   COMPARISON OF SURGERY AND MEDICATIONS FOR MAINTENANCE THERAPY

An alternative to long-term medical maintenance therapy is surgical treatment. Recurrence rates of 2–3% per year have been reported for proximal vagotomy compared to 20–30% for medical therapy [21]. Sonnenberg [22] reported the results of a model of long-term treatment alternatives including no treatment, maintenance therapy, and intermittent intervention. In addition to these nonsurgical alternatives he also considers proximal gastric vagotomy an effective surgical intervention. This study shows that surgery is the least cost-effective treatment strategy in the United States even when cost streams for up to 15 years are considered and the surgical cost is amortized. However, at the lower surgical costs in the Federal Republic of Germany, surgical intervention is more cost-effective than medical maintenance when periods longer than 7 years are considered.

Maintenance therapy is estimated to result in the greatest amount of time (96%) free of acute duodenal ulcers over the 15-year horizon. With intermittent therapy, ulcer-free time drops to 89%. Over the 15-year period, it is estimated that the increased treatment costs under intermittent therapy offsets the cost of maintenance dosage of H_2-antagonist medication, so that there is no difference in costs [22].

XI. TREATMENT OF ULCER COMPLICATIONS

Two complications of peptic ulcer disease that have high mortality risks are hemorrhage and perforation of the ulcers. Emergency surgery has been the standard intervention for both complications.

Therapeutic endoscopy is an alternative to surgery for some bleeding ulcers. A 1989 NIH Consensus Development Conference [23] reviewed the current status of bleeding ulcers and endoscopic therapy. It was noted that more than 100,000 patients per year bleed from peptic ulcers in the United States and that the mortality rate of 6–10% has not changed in the past 30 years. Bleeding from peptic ulcers will stop spontaneously in 70–80% of patients. Endoscopic hemostatic therapy has an acceptable outcome profile but should be used only in patients with a high risk of persistent or recurrent bleeding. Bipolar electrocoagulation, heater probe, and neodymium: yttrium-aluminum-garnet (Nd:YAG) laser are the most promising techniques. Multicenter randomized clinical trials were recommended to further assess clinical efficacy and safety [23]. Cost-effectiveness analysis should also be included in the proposed trials.

Medical treatment has been reported as a nonoperative alternative to surgery for perforations of peptic ulcer. The overall mortality rate from perforated ulcers is about 5%. Equivalent results were demonstrated in a randomized clinical trial of surgical versus medical management of perforated ulcers [24]. Nonoperative treatment included nasogastric suction, intravenous antibiotic therapy, and intravenous ranitidine. Of the nonoperative patients, 73% responded to treatment and avoided surgery. However, the average hospital stay increased from 7.8 days for patients with immediate surgery to 12.0 days for patients treated nonoperatively. The combination of the nonoperative failure rate and the longer hospital stays suggest that surgical intervention may be more cost-effective than nonoperative management. This should be addressed in future studies. In addition, there was evidence from the study that elderly patients did not do as well with medical management.

ACKNOWLEDGMENTS

Part of this chapter was previously published in Lanza et al. [25]. We are grateful to Thomas W. Teal for permission to use this material.

REFERENCES

1. Kurata JH, Haile BH. Epidemiology of peptic ulcer disease. Clin Gastroenterol 1984; 13:289–307.

2. Kurata JH. Ulcer epidemiology: an overview and proposed research framework. Gastroenterology 1989; 96:569–80.

3. Friedman G. Omeprazole. Am J Gastroenterol 1987; 82:188–91.

4. Sontag SJ. Prostaglandins and acid peptic disease. Am J Gastroenterol 1986; 81:1021–28.

5. Blaser MJ. Gastric *Campylobacter*-like organisms, gastric and peptic ulcer disease. Gastroenterology 1987; 93:371–83.

6. Thomson ABR, Mahachai V. Medical management of uncomplicated peptic ulcer disease. In: Berk JE, ed. Gastroenterology. 4th ed. Vol. 2. Philadelphia: WB Saunders, 1985:1016–54.

7. American Medical Association. Agents used in disorders of the upper gastrointestinal tract. In: Lampke KF, ed. Drug evaluations, 6th ed. Chicago: AMA, 1986:937–57, Chap. 52.

8. Fineberg HV, Pearlman LA. Surgical treatment of peptic ulcer in the United States. Lancet, June 13, 1981; 1305–7.

9. Wylie CM. The complex wane of peptic ulcer. I. Recent national trends in deaths and hospital care in the United States. J Clin Gastroenterol 1981; 3:327–32.

10. Paterson ML. Cost-benefit evaluation of a new technology for treatment of peptic ulcer disease. Managerial Decision Econ 1983; 4:50–62.

11. Zimmerman H, Rinaldo D. Health expenditures in Rhode Island: 1977–78. SEARCH Reports No. 24. Providence: R.I. Health Services Research, Inc., May 1981.

12. Nostrant TT, Barnett JL. Peptic ulcer disease: new developments. Compr Ther 1989; 15:45–51.

13. Peace KE. An analysis of GD Searle in-house data on spontaneous ulcer recurrence. Data on file, Rep no. 581-87-07-001, February 9, 1987.

14. Pounder RE. Model treatment of duodenal ulcer. Lancet 1981; i:29–30.

15. Heath Care Financing Administration. Medicare directory of prevailing charges, 1984. Dept. of Health and Human Services. Washington, DC: U.S. Government Printing Office, 1985.

16. Lee FH, ed. American druggist blue book, 1986–87 ed. New York: Hearst Corp., 1986:467.

17. Trapnell G, Genuardi J, O'Brien J. Consumer expenditure for ethical drugs. PMA Report. Washington, DC: PMA, 1983.

18. McGuigan JE. A consideration of the adverse effects of cimetidine. Gastroenterology 1987; 80:181–92.

19. Jack SS. Current estimates from the National Health Interview Survey, U.S. 1979. Dept. of Health and Human Services, Ser. 10, No 136. DHHS Publication No (PHS) 81-1564. Washington, DC: U.S. Government Printing Office, 1981.

20. Roth JLA, Stein GN, Morrissey JF. Diagnosis of peptic ulcer. In: Berk JE, ed. Gastroenterology. 4th ed. Vol. 2. Philadelphia: WB Saunders, 1985:1060–115.

21. Lewis JH. Long-term management of peptic ulcer disease. Compr Ther 1989; 15:55–61.

22. Sonnenberg A. Costs of medical and surgical treatment of duodenal ulcer. Gastroenterology 1989; 96:1445–52.

23. NIH Consensus Development Conference. Therapeutic endoscopy and bleeding ulcers. J Am Med Assoc 1989; 262:1369–72.

24. Crofts TJ, Park KGM, Steele RJC, Chung SSC, Li AKC. A randomized trial of nonoperative treatment for perforated peptic ulcer. N Engl J Med 1989; 320:970–3.

25. Lanza F, Peace KE, Zimmerman H, Dickson B. Cost-effectiveness of cimetidine and misoprostol in peptic ulcer disease. Drug Inf J 1988; 22:449–57.

Index

About the Editors

Edward A. Swabb is Senior Director of Clinical Research at G. D. Searle & Co., Skokie, Illinois. He is the author of more than 80 articles, abstracts, and book chapters, including a chapter in *Beta-Lactam Antibiotics for Clinical Use* by Sherry F. Queener, J. Alan Webber, and Stephen W. Queener (Marcel Dekker, Inc.). A member of the American Society for Clinical Pharmacology and Therapeutics, American Society for Microbiology, Drug Information Association, and American Institute of Chemical Engineers, among others, Dr. Swabb received the B.E. (Ch.E.) (1969) degree from Vanderbilt University, Nashville, Tennessee, M.Ch.E. (1971) and Ph.D. (1973) degrees from the University of Delaware, Newark, and M.D. (1976) degree from the University of Pennsylvania School of Medicine, Philadelphia.

Sandor Szabo is Associate Professor of Pathology at the Harvard Medical School, Director of the Chemical Pathology Research Division, Department of Pathology, Brigham and Women's Hospital, and Lecturer on Occupational Medicine at the Harvard School of Public Health, all in Boston, Massachusetts. The author or editor of over 200 scientific publications, he is the Founding Editor of the *Boston Bulletin on Chemicals and Disease.* Dr. Szabo is Founding Chairman of the Chemical Pathology and Toxicology Subdivision, Division of Chemical Health and Safety, American Chemical Society; and a member of the Royal College of Pathologists, American Association of Pathologists, and American Society for Pharmacology and Experimental Therapeutics, among others. He received the M.Sc. (1971) and Ph.D. (1973) degrees from the University of Montreal, Canada, M.P.H. (1983) degree from the Harvard School of Public Health, Boston, Massachusetts, and M.D. (1968) degree from the University of Belgrade Medical School, Yugoslavia.